PEER ◗ IX

PHYSICIAN'S EVALUATION AND EDUCATIONAL REVIEW IN EMERGENCY MEDICINE

Volume 9

ANSWERS

Mary Jo Wagner, MD, FACEP
Editor-in-Chief

Chief Academic Officer/Designated Institutional Official
CMU Health
Saginaw, Michigan
Professor, Emergency Medicine
Central Michigan University College of Medicine
Mt. Pleasant, Michigan

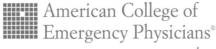

American College of
Emergency Physicians®

ADVANCING EMERGENCY CARE —⋀—

Table of Contents

Publisher's Notice

The American College of Emergency Physicians (ACEP) makes every effort to ensure that contributors to its publications are knowledgeable subject matter experts. Readers are nevertheless advised that the statements and opinions expressed in this publication are provided as the contributors' recommendations at the time of publication and should not be construed as official College policy. ACEP recognizes the complexity of emergency medicine and makes no representation that this publication serves as an authoritative resource for the prevention, diagnosis, treatment, or intervention for any medical condition, nor should it be the basis for the definition of, or standard of care that should be practiced by all health care providers at any particular time or place. To the fullest extent permitted by law, and without limitation, ACEP expressly disclaims all liability for errors or omissions contained within this publication, and for damages of any kind or nature, arising out of use, reference to, reliance on, or performance of such information.

To contact ACEP, call 800-798-1822 or 972-550-0911, or write to PO Box 619911, Dallas, TX 75261-9911, or email peer@acep.org. Your comments and suggestions are always welcome.

978-0-9889973-8-7

First printing, June 2017

About the Editor

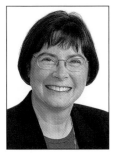

Mary Jo Wagner, MD, FACEP, has served as Editor-in-Chief of the PEER content review and self-assessment series since 2001.

Dr. Wagner is the Chief Academic Officer and Designated Institutional Official of Central Michigan University (CMU) Medical Education Partners in Saginaw, Michigan. She is Professor of Emergency Medicine at CMU College of Medicine and a clinical professor in the Department of Emergency Medicine at Michigan State University College of Human Medicine. She was the emergency medicine residency director in Saginaw from 2001 to 2014. Dr. Wagner also practices emergency medicine in two community hospitals. She earned her doctor of medicine degree from Boston University School of Medicine and completed her residency training at St. Vincent Medical Center/The Toledo Hospital Emergency Medicine Residency Program in Toledo, Ohio. She has been board certified by the American Board of Emergency Medicine since 1992.

In addition to the three previous editions of PEER, Dr. Wagner has edited *Last Minute Emergency Medicine, Emergency and Primary Care of the Hand, Emergency Medicine Clinics of North America—Endocrine and Metabolic Emergencies,* and ACEP's *Foresight.*

Dr. Wagner has chaired the national ACEP Education Committee, the Educational Meetings Subcommittee, and the Federal Government Affairs Committee and has also served on the Academic Affairs Committee, the Focused Meetings Task Force, and several other work groups both nationally and locally. In 2009, Dr. Wagner received one of the College's highest honors, the Outstanding Contribution in Education Award, in recognition of her work on behalf of excellence in emergency medicine clinical practice, teaching, and research. She is a past president of the Council of Emergency Medicine Residency Directors and was selected in 2012 as a Distinguished Educator by the CORD Academy for Scholarship in Education in Emergency Medicine.

PEER IX Editorial Board

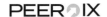
Rachel B. Liu, MD, FACEP
Director of Bedside Ultrasound Education
Associate Director, Emergency Ultrasound
  Section
Assistant Professor, Department of Emergency
  Medicine
Yale University School of Medicine
New Haven, Connecticut

Erik K. Nordquist, MD, FACEP
Assistant Professor of Emergency Medicine
Cook County Health and Hospitals System
Rush Medical College
Chicago, Illinois

Charles W. O'Connell, MD
Clinical Professor
Department of Emergency Medicine
Division of Medical Toxicology
University of California San Diego
Scripps Clinical Medical Group
San Diego, California

Joseph S. Palter, MD
Assistant Professor of Emergency Medicine
Cook County Health and Hospitals System
Rush Medical College
Chicago, Illinois

Aaron Schneir, MD, FACEP, FACMT, FAAEM
Professor of Clinical Medicine
Division of Medical Toxicology
Separtment of Emergency Medicine
University of California, San Diego Health
  System
San Diego, California

Semhar Z. Tewelde, MD, FACEP, FAAEM
Assistant Residency Program Director
Assistant Professor, Department of Emergency
  Medicine
University of Maryland School of Medicine
  Baltimore, Maryland

Adam Z. Tobias, MD, MPH, FACEP
Assistant Professor of Emergency Medicine
University of Pittsburgh School of Medicine
Assistant Program Director, University of
  Pittsburgh Emergency Medicine Residency
Pittsburgh, Pennsylvania

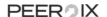

Contributors

Dr. Wagner and the PEER IX Editorial Board gratefully acknowledge the following individuals and organizations who contributed to PEER IX by donating images, participating in item testing, and providing and reviewing information.

Andrea Austin, MD
Aaron Bassett
Joshua S. Broder, MD, FACEP
Richard M. Cantor, MD, FAAP, FACEP
Ryan Coughlin, MD
Jill C. Crosby, MD
Jason Day, MD
Michael Harstaad, MD
Michael Heard, MD
Sharmin Kalam, MD
Timothy Kaufman, MD
Nicholas Kluesner, MD
Katrina Landa, MD
Jonathan Lau
Damali Nakitende, MD
Michael Paddock, MD
Joseph R. Pare, MD, MHS, RDMS
Brandi Sakai
Jeffrey Shih, MD
Brian Toupin
Robert J. Tubbs, MD

Residents from the Cook County Emergency Medicine Residency Program
Ari Edelheit, MD
Thomas W. Engel II, MD
Lindy Triebes, MD

Assistant Professor of Emergency Medicine at Cook County Health and Hospitals System—Rush Medical College and Clinical Educator of Emergency Medicine at NorthShore University Health Systems at the University of Chicago
Jessica Folk, MD

Director of Emergency Ultrasound in the Department of Emergency Medicine at Rush University Medical Center
Michael Gottlieb, MD

Attending Physician at the University of Pittsburgh Department of Emergency Medicine
Alanna C. Peterson, MD

Residents from the University of Pittsburgh Emergency Medicine Residency Program
Kimberly Fox, MD
Ashley A. Kilp, MD

Chief Resident from the University of Iowa
Brooks J. Obr, MD

Emergency Medicine Fellow and Clinical Instructor in the

Department of Emergency Medicine at Yale University School of Medicine
Anand Selvam, MD

Assistant/Associate Professors of Emergency Medicine at the University of Virginia
Nathan Charlton, MD
Thomas Hartka, MD
Heather Streich, MD
Amita Sudhir, MD
Christopher Thom, MD

Fellow in EMS and Instructor of Emergency Medicine at the University of Virginia
David Wilcocks, MD

Senior Residents of Emergency Medicine at the University of Virginia
Everett Austin, MD
Lee Cunningham, MD
Laura Grangeia, MD
Conwell Ottenritter, MD
Michael Wakim, MD

Fellow in Toxicology in the Department of Emergency Medicine at the University of Virginia
Jennifer L. Parker Cote, MD

Fellow at the University of Virginia Department of Emergency Medicine
Adam Nevel, MD

Assistant Professor at the University of Virginia Department of Emergency Medicine
Thomas Hartka, MD

Clinical Assistant Professor of Emergency Medicine/ Attending Physician at UT Southwestern Medical Center/ Parkland Memorial Hospital
Alex Koyfman, MD, FAAEM

Attending Emergency Physician and Assistant Professor of Military and Emergency Medicine/Associate Editor-in-Chief of Clinical Content at emDocs.net/SAUSHEC Emergency Medicine
Brit Long, MD

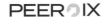

ACEP Educational Products

Marta Foster, Director
Jessica Hamilton, Educational Products Assistant
Nicole Tidwell, Sales and Marketing Manager
Robert Heard, MBA, CAE, Associate Executive Director, Membership and Education Division
Indexing: Sharon Hughes
Design: Susan McReynolds
Proofreading: Mary Anne Mitchell, Wendell Anderson
Printing: Modern Litho

Disclosures

In accordance with Accreditation Council on Continuing Medical Education (ACCME) Standards and ACEP policy, all persons who were in a position to control the content of this enduring material must disclose to participants the existence of significant financial interests in or relationships with manufacturers of commercial products that might have a direct interest in the subject matter. None of the individuals with control over the content of PEER IX reported significant financial interests or relationships.

ACEP expects all Editorial Board members and contributors to present information in an objective, unbiased manner without endorsement or criticism of specific products or services. ACEP also expects that the relationships they disclose will not influence their contributions.

In PEER IX, in most cases, drugs and devices are referred to by their generic names. In a few cases, however, brand names do appear for the sole purpose of clarification or easier recognition. In no instance is a drug or device listed by a brand name for a commercial purpose. No person who was in a position to control the content of PEER IX disclosed a relationship with a manufacturer of any drug or device referred to by its brand name.

PEER IX educational content includes links to other educational resources hosted on websites not owned, operated, or controlled in any way by ACEP. Some of these resources are videos that might be preceded by advertisements. ACEP has no control over the decision of a third-party website owner to include advertising and in no way endorses any product or service that appears on a third-party website. ACEP received no consideration for linking to any of these websites. ACEP assumes no responsibility for content on third-party websites.

PEER IX received no commercial support.

Not affiliated with the American Board of Emergency Medicine.

1. The correct answer is B, Flame-shaped hemorrhages, soft exudates, and papilledema.

Why is this the correct answer?

This patient is experiencing a hypertensive emergency — elevated blood pressure with evidence of ongoing, end-organ damage, which might be referred to as malignant hypertension. In this case, the microvasculature of the retina is overwhelmed by the elevated pressures, and the resulting endothelial injury results in an inflammatory reaction. The flame-shaped hemorrhages are a result of the intense pressure in vessels near the optic disc, and soft exudates result from ischemic infarction of nerve fibers. This condition can occur along with hypertensive encephalopathy, characterized by altered mental status, headache, vomiting, and papilledema. Other examples of ongoing end-organ damage in cases of hypertensive emergency include stroke, aortic dissection, congestive heart failure and pulmonary edema, and acute renal injury with hematuria. The condition should be managed with intravenous antihypertensive medications and hospital admission.

Why are the other choices wrong?

A cherry-red macula and ground-glass retina are the typical descriptions of a central retinal artery occlusion. This ischemic process usually results in sudden, painless vision loss.

A normal retina is the most common finding in patients with asymptomatic hypertension. Usually, hypertensive patients without symptoms do not require therapy in the emergency department but may be managed with close primary care follow-up. With the symptoms this patient is experiencing, it is likely that the patient has ophthalmologic findings.

Venous engorgement and an irregular, swollen optic disc occur with a retinal vein occlusion, also referred to as a blood and thunder appearance. This is often painful in later stages but can present with painless vision loss.

PEER POINT

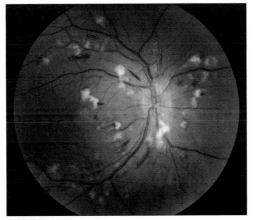

PEER Point 1

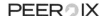

PEER REVIEW

- ✓ A hypertensive emergency is not defined by the absolute blood pressure but by the presence of end-organ injury.
- ✓ A hypertensive crisis can result in accelerated retinopathy, characterized by flame hemorrhages, soft exudates, and papilledema.
- ✓ Central retinal artery and vein occlusions can present with painless vision loss.

REFERENCES

Marx JA, Hockberger RS, Walls RM, eds. *Rosen's Emergency Medicine: Concepts and Clinical Practice.* 8th ed. St. Louis, MO: Elsevier; 2014;1113-1123.e3.

Tintinalli JE, Stapczynski JS, Ma OJ, et al, eds. *Tintinalli's Emergency Medicine: A Comprehensive Study Guide.* 8th ed. New York, NY: McGraw-Hill; 2012;1927-1936.

Wolfson AB, Hendey GW, Ling LJ, et al, eds. *Harwood-Nuss' Clinical Practice of Emergency Medicine.* 6th ed. Philadelphia, PA: Lippincott, Williams & Wilkins; 2014: 511-514.

2.   The correct answer is C, 0.75.

Why is this the correct answer?

There is no such thing as a perfect test. Each test has a set of intrinsic qualities that practitioners should take into consideration when incorporating their results into medical decision-making. The sensitivity of a test can be thought of as the true-positive rate. In other words, the sensitivity tells the provider what percentage of patients who have a given condition will have a positive test result. This can be calculated by dividing the number of true-positives by the total number of patients with the condition in question (TP/TP+FN). In this case, the calculation is 60 true-positives divided by the 80 patients with known pain for a sensitivity of 0.75, of 75%. Here is an illustration: Test Result Pain No pain Positive 60 true positive (TP) 10 false positive (FP) Negative 20 false negative (FN) 10 true negative (TN) 80 total with pain 20 total without pain 100 total Sensitivity = TP/(TP +FN) = 60/80 = .75 = 75% Specificity = TN/(FP + TN) = 10/20 = .50 Positive predictive value (PPV) = TP/(TP + FP) = 60/70 = .86 Negative predictive value (NPV) = TN/(TN+FN) = 10/30= .33

Why are the other choices wrong?

The first choice, 33%, is the negative predictive value. The formula is as follows: NPV = TN/(TN+FN). The calculation, then, is 10/30 = 0.33.

The specificity of the test is 50%. The formula is as follows: TN/(FP + TN), and the calculation in this case is 10/20 = 0.50.

The final choice, 86%, is the positive predictive value. The formula is as follows: PPV = TP/(TP + FP). The calculation is 60/70 = 0.86.

PEER POINT

Formulas for test sensitivity and specificity

- Sensitivity = TP/(TP + FN)
- Specificity = TN/(FP + TN)
- Positive predictive value = TP/(TP + FP)
- Negative predictive value = TN/(TN + FN)

PEER REVIEW

- ✓ The value of a medical test depends on its intrinsic sensitivity and specificity.
- ✓ Sensitivity can be thought of as the true-positive rate of a test.
- ✓ Specificity can be thought of as the true-negative rate of a test.

REFERENCES

Forthofer RN, Lee ES, Hernandez M. *Biostatistics: a guide to design, analysis and discovery*. 2nd ed. Philadelphia, PA: Academic Press; 2007.

3. The correct answer is A, Benign paroxysmal positional vertigo.

Why is this the correct answer?

Benign paroxysmal positional vertigo (BPPV) is suggested by the onset of vertigo with changes in head position and by the age of the patient. More important, the physical examination confirms that this patient has peripheral vertigo; the nystagmus has a long latency, transient duration, and is fatigable with provocative testing (the Dix-Hallpike maneuver). Furthermore, it is not associated with any other neurologic deficits. This is distinct from central vertigo such as that caused by strokes and tumors, which tends to have nystagmus with a short latency, a sustained duration, is not fatigable, and tends to be accompanied by other cranial and peripheral nerve deficits. Benign paroxysmal positional vertigo is the most common cause of vertigo overall, accounting for approximately 40% of vertigo diagnoses and affecting roughly 10% of all adults by age 80 years. The incidence of BPPV increases with age, with peak onset between 50 and 60 years old. Women are more commonly affected than men, with almost a 3-to-1 female-to-male ratio. Osteoporosis, vitamin D deficiency, and a history of prior head trauma have all been associated with the development of BPPV. Benign paroxysmal positional vertigo is believed to be caused by loose calcium carbonate otoliths moving aberrantly within the semicircular canals of the inner ear, ultimately resulting in the false sensation of rotation. The posterior semicircular canal is most commonly affected and accounts for approximately 60% to 90% of all cases of BPPV. Patients usually present with brief episodes of vertigo, typically lasting less than 1 minute, that are provoked by head position changes such as rolling over in bed, getting out of bed, tilting the head upward to reach objects on high shelves, or tilting the head downward to tie shoes. Diagnosis can be made with a series of bedside maneuvers known as the Dix-Hallpike maneuver, which provokes directional and torsional nystagmus depending on the involved semicircular canal. If a Dix-Hallpike

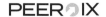

test is negative, a supine roll test may be performed to evaluate for lateral semicircular canal BPPV. The first-line treatment for BPPV is an attempt at repositioning the misplaced otolith with a procedure known as the Epley maneuver. This is effective in approximately 90% of cases. Pharmacologic treatments such as meclizine, ondansetron, and diazepam may be used to temper nausea and emesis in patients with BPPV but are not as effective as the Epley maneuver.

Why are the other choices wrong?

Meniere disease is not likely because the patient lacks the typical aural symptoms. The classic triad for Meniere disease is intermittent episodes of ear fullness, tinnitus, and vertigo.

A transient ischemic attack is an important consideration but is unlikely because of the lack of central signs on physical examination, including ataxia.

Vertebral basilar artery insufficiency is an important consideration in the differential diagnosis, but this condition is unlikely because of the lack of central signs on physical examination. This diagnosis should always be considered in patients with vertigo that occurs when they look up (when raising the head compresses the vertebral artery).

PEER REVIEW

- ✓ Peripheral vertigo is characterized by a lack of associated neurologic deficits and the demonstration of nystagmus with a long latency, transient duration, and fatigability.
- ✓ Benign paroxysmal positional vertigo is the most common cause of vertigo and has a peak onset in patients between 50 and 60 years old.
- ✓ The most widely accepted treatment is an otolith-repositioning procedure, most commonly the Epley maneuver.

REFERENCES

Marx JA, Hockberger RS, Walls RM, eds. *Rosen's Emergency Medicine: Concepts and Clinical Practice*. 8th ed. St. Louis, MO: Elsevier; 2014: 162-169.e1.

Tintinalli JE, Stapczynski JS, Ma OJ, et al, eds. *Tintinalli's Emergency Medicine: A Comprehensive Study Guide*. 8th ed. New York, NY: McGraw-Hill; 2012: 1164-1173, 1921-1927.

4. The correct answer is C, It is more likely in younger children than in older children.

Why is this the correct answer?

Spinal cord injury without radiographic abnormality, or SCIWORA, is thought to occur more commonly in children than in adults because of the relative laxity of the ligaments of the spine in children. In addition, the large size of the head and the increased mobility of the cervical spine in younger children are thought to contribute to this phenomenon. For the same reasons, SCIWORA is more common in younger children than in older children and adults. It is also thought to occur from mechanisms such as spinal traction or even spinal ischemia due to stretching, attributed to this relative mobility. That being said, elderly patients are also at risk due to spinal stenosis or kyphosis. Central cord syndrome is a manifestation of SCIWORA. The term SCIWORA was coined and recognized before the use of MRI became more commonplace in emergency departments. With the use of MRI, more of these injuries are being identified as spinal cord contusion or ischemia. At one time, high-dose steroids were thought to have benefit in patients with spinal cord injuries. But this therapy has fallen out of favor. It is now generally accepted that the benefits are somewhat controversial and are outweighed by the risks.

Why are the other choices wrong?

The most common mechanism of injury in SCIWORA is flexion and extension. This can happen in motor vehicle crashes. Axial loading injuries, usually from falls, less commonly cause SCIWORA.

The definition of SCIWORA is a neurologic deficit that does not demonstrate any bony radiographic abnormality on plain films or CT scans. With increased use of MRI, these injuries are being identified more often as spinal contusions or ischemia or ligament-related injuries.

Because of its relative mobility and laxity, the cervical spine is the most common location of SCIWORA. It is least commonly seen in the lumbar spine.

PEER REVIEW

- ✓ SCIWORA is more common in children than adults, although elderly persons can be affected.
- ✓ SCIWORA occurs most commonly in the cervical spine.
- ✓ Flexion and extension are the most common mechanisms of injury in SCIWORA.

REFERENCES

Marx JA, Hockberger RS, Walls RM, eds. *Rosen's Emergency Medicine: Concepts and Clinical Practice*. 8th ed. St. Louis, MO: Elsevier; 2014: 315, 326, 401-402.

Wolfson AB, Hendey GW, Ling LJ, et al, eds. *Harwood-Nuss' Clinical Practice of Emergency Medicine*. 6th ed. Philadelphia, PA: Lippincott, Williams & Wilkins; 2014: 1175, 1177, 1194-1195.

5. The correct answer is C, Pancreatitis.

Why is this the correct answer?

The image shows lipemic blood; this is a risk factor for acute pancreatitis. Although alcohol and gallstone obstruction are the most common causes, hypertriglyceridemia also results in pancreatitis. Hypertriglyceridemia and gallstone pancreatitis are associated with pregnancy and increase both maternal and fetal mortality rates. This form of pancreatitis correlates with triglyceride levels above 500 mg/dL, with more severe infections occurring at 1,000 mg/dL. Treatment for patients with hypertriglyceridemia-induced pancreatitis focuses on analgesia, antiemetics, intravenous fluid administration, insulin, and lipid-lowering agents.

More severe infections might require plasmapheresis or surgery if there is evidence for pancreatic necrosis. Antibiotic therapy is not indicated unless necrosis, abscess, or infected pseudocyst exists. Pancreatitis can be associated with pleural effusions and hypoxemia. The Ranson criteria are used after 48 hours to determine the severity of disease. Of interest, typical emergency department tests do not include the LDH value that is needed for calculating this formula. Although these criteria and other prediction rules are not helpful in the emergency department, in general, patients with increased inflammatory markers are at higher risk for death.

Why are the other choices wrong?

Cholecystitis should be considered in any patient presenting with upper abdominal pain and vomiting. In this case, however, the key is to recognize lipemic blood, as shown in the image.

Hyperemesis gravidarum presents with profuse vomiting and abdominal pain from gastric irritation. However, it typically is limited to the first trimester, and the patient in this case is in late second or early third trimester based on physical examination findings. It also does not produce lipemic blood.

Placental abruption is a complication of pregnancy that presents with vaginal bleeding and abdominal pain. Nausea and profuse vomiting are not usually features of this condition.

PEER POINT

Ranson criteria to determine severity of pancreatitis
Admission criteria

- Age >55 years old
- WBC count >16,000 mm^3
- Glucose level >200 mg/dL
- LDH level >350 IU/L
- AST level >250 IU/L

In the next 48 hours

- Decreasing hematocrit by >10%
- Fluid sequestration >6 L
- Calcium level <8 mg/dL
- Pa$_{O_2}$ <60 mm Hg
- Increased BUN >5 mg/dL after intravenous fluids
- Base deficit >4 mmol/L

PEER REVIEW

✓ Hypertriglyceridemia is a risk factor for pancreatitis and is associated with pregnancy.

✓ When you're treating pancreatitis, the focus should be on supportive care and intravenous fluids, lipid-lowering agents, and insulin if needed.

✓ In severe pancreatitis, plasmapheresis might be required to deal with the hypertriglyceridemia.

REFERENCES

Marx JA, Hockberger RS, Walls RM, eds. *Rosen's Emergency Medicine: Concepts and Clinical Practice*. 8th ed. St. Louis, MO: Elsevier; 2014: 1206-2012.

Tintinalli JE, Stapczynski JS, Ma OJ, et al, eds. *Tintinalli's Emergency Medicine: A Comprehensive Study Guide*. 8th ed. New York, NY: McGraw-Hill; 2012: 517-524.

6. The correct answer is D, Ventricular septal defect.

Why is this the correct answer?

In this case, the initial clinical clues to an underlying congenital cardiac disease include poor weight gain (weight loss in some infants), tiring while feeding (sweating in some cases), and signs of congestive heart failure (trouble breathing, as reported by the mother). Because she does not have signs of cyanosis or a ductal-dependent lesion, other types of congenital cardiac disease should be considered. Ventricular septal defect is the most common congenital cardiac lesion, and the degree of disease is dependent on the size of the defect. This can range from no issues to signs of congestive heart failure such as enlarged liver, which happens as the disease progresses.

Why are the other choices wrong?

Coarctation of the aorta would likely show a differential between the upper and lower extremity blood pressures.

Total anomalous pulmonary venous return is a cyanotic congenital cardiac disease and would likely present with some degree of cyanosis or alteration in pulse oximetry.

Transposition of the great arteries also is a cyanotic congenital cardiac disease and would likely present with some degree of cyanosis or alteration in pulse oximetry.

PEER REVIEW

✓ Ventricular septal defect is the most common congenital cardiac defect.

✓ A large ventricular septal defect can present as congestive heart failure with tachycardia, hepatomegaly, and poor weight gain.

REFERENCES

Marx JA, Hockberger RS, Walls RM, eds. *Rosen's Emergency Medicine: Concepts and Clinical Practice*. 8th ed. St. Louis, MO: Elsevier; 2014: 2139-2167.

Tintinalli JE, Stapczynski JS, Ma OJ, et al, eds. *Tintinalli's Emergency Medicine: A Comprehensive Study Guide*. 8th ed. New York, NY: McGraw-Hill; 2012: 822-835.

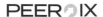

7. The correct answer is B, Start it with a target temperature of approximately 34°C (93.2°F).

Why is this the correct answer?

Therapeutic hypothermia, also referred to as induced hypothermia and more recently as targeted temperature management, can reduce the negative sequelae of cardiac arrest. Although the specific mechanism is unknown, therapeutic hypothermia likely involves the reduction in metabolic rate throughout the body as well as reduced electrical activity in the brain. This patient is a candidate because he had a shockable rhythm (either pulseless ventricular tachycardia or ventricular fibrillation) and was resuscitated in an out-of-hospital setting. The optimal timing of initiation of therapeutic hypothermia is broad, but initiation within the first 4 to 6 hours after resuscitation is best. Earlier applications are likely better. If clinically feasible, initiation as early as 15 to 30 minutes after resuscitation is appropriate. The target temperature for therapeutic hypothermia is 32°C (89.6°F) to 34°C (93.2°F), although temperatures as high as 36°C (96.8°F) have demonstrated benefit. Additional postresuscitation therapies, including advanced critical care and PCI, should be performed simultaneously with therapeutic hypothermia.

Why are the other choices wrong?

The presence of a STEMI by itself does not preclude the initiation of therapeutic hypothermia; in fact, STEMI and other ACS-related conditions are the most appropriate patient presentations for targeted temperature management.

Another indication for therapeutic hypothermia is unresponsiveness or other very significant mental status abnormality. Resuscitated patients who are alert or medically unstable are not candidates. Patients experiencing noncardiogenic cardiac arrest are likely not candidates either. Again, the ECG finding of STEMI is a reason to start targeted temperature management, not withhold it.

Therapeutic hypothermia may be started in the prehospital setting, emergency department, cardiac catheterization laboratory, or intensive care unit; the patient's clinical situation as well as the capabilities of the particular location dictate the most appropriate time of initiation.

PEER REVIEW

✓ Therapeutic hypothermia improves the chance of meaningful survival in patients resuscitated from cardiac arrest, particularly those resuscitated in the prehospital setting with shockable initial rhythms who are stable and remain unresponsive.

✓ Therapeutic hypothermia may be applied in a range of settings with minimal need for equipment.

REFERENCES

Adams JG, Barton ED, Collings J, et al, eds. *Emergency Medicine: Clinical Essentials.* 2nd ed. Philadelphia, PA: Saunders; 2013: 55-71.

Callaway CW, Donnino MW, Fink EL, et al. Part 8: Post-cardiac arrest care: 2015 American Heart Association Guidelines update for cardiopulmonary resuscitation and emergency cardiovascular care. *Circulation.* 2015;132(18 Suppl 2): S465-S482.

8. The correct answer is A, Erythema nodosum.

Why is this the correct answer?

Erythema nodosum (EN) is a form of panniculitis, inflammation of the subcutaneous fat tissue. Red or violet-hued nodules that are tender and mobile classically appear on the bilateral extensor surface of the legs, but they can occur anywhere there is fat under the skin, including on the extremities, trunk, face, and neck. Erythema nodosum has been associated with numerous systemic diseases such as inflammatory bowel disease, infections, and medications, and it can also be idiopathic. It typically occurs in conjunction with flulike symptoms and generalized arthralgia. The nodules progress in color from red to purple and eventually fade to a yellowish hue before self-resolution that occurs over several weeks to months. Management is supportive care with anti-inflammatories and treatment of the underlying condition (if one is present). Erythema nodosum has a strong association with the HLA-B27 histocompatibility antigen, which is present in about 65% of patients.

Why are the other choices wrong?

Henoch-Schonlein purpura (anaphylactoid purpura) is a systemic vasculitis most commonly seen in children. As a vasculitis, it has nonblanching, palpable lesions that are generally smaller than the lesions of EN. It involves the small vessels of the skin, the GI tract, and the kidneys. The hallmark of the disease is palpable purpura and petechiae located most commonly on the buttocks and lower extremities. The rash is seen in dependent areas, so the scrotum and hands might also be affected. Arthralgia is common and most often involves the large joints of the lower extremities, which can become edematous and tender with little movement. Abdominal pain occurs in about half or more of patients and is frequently colicky. In children there is a strong association with ileoileal intussusception. Renal involvement occurs in about half of patients and is usually seen as a microscopic hematuria and proteinuria.

Polyarteritis nodosa is a systemic vasculitis that causes necrotizing inflammatory lesions in the small and medium-sized blood vessels. This typically occurs where blood vessels bifurcate, resulting in microaneurysm formation, thrombosis, and ultimately organ ischemia or infarction. Multiple organ systems can be involved (joints, nerves, GI tract). Polyarteritis nodosa commonly affects the skin; the lesions range from subcutaneous nodules to purpura, ulcerations, and even gangrene, and distal ischemia can occur.

Pyoderma gangrenosum is an ulcerative cutaneous condition of uncertain etiology. It is associated with systemic diseases in about 50% of patients. It, like EN, is a common extraintestinal manifestation seen in inflammatory bowel diseases. The diagnosis is made by excluding other causes of similar-appearing cutaneous ulcerations, including infection, malignancy, vasculitis, collagen vascular diseases, diabetes, and trauma. Ulcers initially appear as small bites or papules and progress to larger ulcers. Ultimately the tissue becomes necrotic, resulting in deep ulcers that classically occur on the legs. Although the wounds rarely lead to death, they can

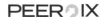

cause pain and scarring. One hallmark of pyoderma gangrenosum is pathergy, which is the appearance of new lesions at sites of trauma in those who already have the disease. Other organ systems can also be involved.

PEER REVIEW

✓ Erythema nodosum and pyoderma gangrenosum are two common rashes associated with inflammatory bowel disease.

✓ Here are the characteristics of erythema nodosum: painful reddish nodules, mobile lower legs below the knees, bilateral inflammation of the subcutaneous tissue.

✓ The flulike symptoms and generalized arthralgia that usually come with erythema nodosum can be treated with supportive care and NSAIDs.

REFERENCES

Adams JG, Barton ED, Collings J, et al, eds. *Emergency Medicine: Clinical Essentials.* 2nd ed. Philadelphia, PA: Saunders; 2013: 304-308, 949-967.

Marx JA, Hockberger RS, Walls RM, eds. *Rosen's Emergency Medicine: Concepts and Clinical Practice.* 8th ed. St. Louis, MO: Elsevier; 2014: 1558-1585, 2168-2187.

9. The correct answer is B, C3-C7.

Why is this the correct answer?

Unilateral facet dislocations most commonly occur at the level of C3-C7 due to the relatively flat articular processes in this region. These dislocations occur secondary to flexion-rotation forces causing anterior rotation of the inferior facet of one vertebra over the superior facet of the vertebra below. Typically, unilateral facet dislocations are stable injuries and might not present with any neurologic compromise. In the thoracic and lumbar spine, bilateral facet dislocations are much more common due to the relatively larger articular processes. Bilateral facet dislocations are unstable and typically present with neurologic deficits. Significant flexion-rotation forces at C1-C2 most commonly cause atlantoaxial dislocation, a highly unstable lesion.

Why are the other choices wrong?

Atlantoaxial dislocation, not unilateral facet dislocation, is the most common lesion that occurs at C1-C2 secondary to flexion-rotation forces. These lesions are extremely unstable and require emergent neurosurgical consultation.

Unilateral facet dislocations are even more rare in the lumbar spine than in the thoracic spine. Bilateral facet dislocations in the lumbar region are typically not associated with spinal cord deficits because the adult cord terminates at L1 into the cauda equina.

Flexion-rotation forces in the thoracic spine are more likely to cause bilateral facet dislocations, particularly at the thoracolumbar junction. A bilateral facet dislocation in the thoracic spine should raise significant concern for associated intrathoracic injuries.

PEER REVIEW

✓ Unilateral facet injuries are stable and most commonly occur at C3-C7.
✓ The prevalence of flexion-rotation injuries of the spine differs based on vertebral level.

REFERENCES

Marx JA, Hockberger RS, Walls RM, eds. *Rosen's Emergency Medicine: Concepts and Clinical Practice*. 8th ed. St. Louis, MO: Elsevier; 2014: 382-420.

Tintinalli JE, Stapczynski JS, Ma OJ, et al, eds. *Tintinalli's Emergency Medicine: A Comprehensive Study Guide*. 8th ed. New York, NY: McGraw-Hill; 2012: 1708-1724.

10. The correct answer is C, Pemphigus vulgaris.

Why is this the correct answer?

Pemphigus vulgaris (PV) is an autoimmune vesiculobullous disease seen in middle-aged to older-aged patients, with the majority having both skin and mucosal involvement. The primary lesion of PV is a flaccid, clear blister that becomes fragile and erupts, producing erosions. Pressure applied to these blisters/bullae results in sloughing, known as a positive Nikolsky sign. Before there is skin involvement, oral lesions occur in up to 60% of patients, often antedating the cutaneous lesions by several months. Triggers associated with PV include infections, medications, and emotional stress. Some patients require hospitalization to ensure optimal administration of fluids and electrolytes and control of pain and infection. The treatment options most commonly used are steroids and immunosuppressant therapy.

Why are the other choices wrong?

Bullous pemphigoid is also an autoimmune vesiculobullous disease. It is seen in slightly older patients (older than 65 years) than PV is. To distinguish it from PV, patients with bullous pemphigoid are much less likely to have mucosal involvement, and there is no positive Nikolsky sign. Pruritus is frequently present and can be the only manifestation of the disease. Generalized bullae can be seen anywhere, but there is a predilection for flexural areas. Treatment is similar to that for PV: mainly, supportive care with steroids and immunosuppressant therapy to decrease blister size and promote healing. Bullous pemphigoid is easier to treat than PV is.

Erythroderma (exfoliate dermatitis) is the term used to describe generalized erythema that affects more than 90% of the skin followed by scaling and sloughing. Typically, this condition causes the skin to be intensely tender and pruritic. Frequently, there is loss of both hair and nails. Patients should be treated as if they are burn victims because of the marked fluid loss and shifts and edema. Erythroderma is associated with skin and connective tissue disorders as well as cancer, medications, and heavy metals. These patients all require admission for optimal administration of fluids and electrolytes, for control of pain and infection, and for cancer workup and appropriate wound care. The recovery period is long, and there are frequent recurrences.

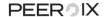

Toxic epidermal necrolysis (TEN, or Lyell disease) is a life-threatening dermatologic condition. It is characterized by a diffuse erythematous macular rash that coalesces, resulting in regions of skin with the epidermis separating from the dermis. There is both mucosal involvement and a positive Nikolsky sign. This rash is distinctive from PV in that PV starts with individual blisters without the typically large erythematous coalescing areas as seen with TEN. Symptoms of TEN first affect the eyes, then spread caudal to the thorax and upper extremities, and finally progress to the lower body, involving more than 30% of the body surface area. Toxic epidermal necrolysis is most commonly drug induced (sulfa, PCN, ASA, NSAIDs); however, it has also been associated with other potential etiologies (infection, malignancy, vaccines). Persons with AIDS who are on sulfa prophylaxis are 1,000 times more at risk of developing TEN. Treatment consists of hospitalization in the ICU or burn unit for optimization of fluids and electrolytes, control of pain and infection, and cessation of the offending agent. To date, no specific therapy has been proved effective. Despite hospitalization and aggressive resuscitation, the mortality rate of TEN remains high secondary to sepsis and multiorgan system failure.

PEER REVIEW

- ✓ Pemphigus vulgaris is an autoimmune vesiculobullous disease that frequently causes oral lesions then progresses to skin blisters.
- ✓ Patients with pemphigus vulgaris have a positive Nikolsky sign; those with bullous pemphigus do not.
- ✓ Treat pemphigus vulgaris with steroids and immunosuppressants.
- ✓ How can you distinguish pemphigus vulgaris from toxic epidermal necrolysis? Pemphigus vulgaris starts with individual blisters and doesn't have large erythematous coalescing areas.

REFERENCES

Adams JG, Barton ED, Collings J, et al, eds. *Emergency Medicine: Clinical Essentials*. 2nd ed. Philadelphia, PA: Saunders; 2013: 1598-1618.

Marx JA, Hockberger RS, Walls RM, eds. *Rosen's Emergency Medicine: Concepts and Clinical Practice*. 8th ed. St. Louis, MO: Elsevier; 2014: 1558-1585.

11. The correct answer is A, Flight of ideas.

Why is this the correct answer?

Flight of ideas is characterized by a nearly continuous flow of accelerated speech and is typically seen in patients with bipolar disorder. Patients shift rapidly between topics and, when the condition is severe, speech becomes disorganized or incoherent. Flight of ideas is not a feature of major depressive disorder.

Why are the other choices wrong?

Patients with major depressive disorder can exhibit either insomnia or hypersomnia. To meet a formal diagnosis of this disorder, at least five symptoms must be present continuously for a 2-week period; at least one must be depressed mood or loss of interest or pleasure.

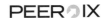

Patients with depression can exhibit either psychomotor agitation or retardation.

Patients with major depressive disorder can experience either decreased or increased appetite and might exhibit significant weight loss, that is, more than 5% of total body weight over 1 month.

PEER POINT

Diagnosing major depressive disorder

One of these symptoms:
- Depressed mood
- Loss of interest or pleasure

Plus four or more other symptoms:
- Change in appetite (weight gain or loss)
- Difficulty concentrating
- Fatigue or loss of energy
- Feeling worthless or inappropriate guilt
- Insomnia or hypersomnia
- Psychomotor agitation or retardation
- Suicidal ideation

For 2 weeks or longer

PEER REVIEW

✓ Major depressive disorder can be diagnosed when symptoms have been present continuously for 2 weeks.
✓ Patients with depression can have either insomnia or hypersomnia.
✓ Psychomotor agitation can be seen in patients with depression.

REFERENCES

American Psychiatric Association: Diagnostic and Statistical Manual of Mental Disorders. 5th ed. Washington, DC: American Psychiatric Association, 2013.

Tintinalli JE, Stapczynski JS, Ma OJ, et al, eds. *Tintinalli's Emergency Medicine: A Comprehensive Study Guide*. 8th ed. New York, NY: McGraw-Hill; 2012: 1963-1969.

12. The correct answer is B, Delay insulin administration if initial serum potassium is below 3.3 mEq/L.

Why is this the correct answer?

The management of diabetic ketoacidosis (DKA) involves administration of fluid, insulin, and potassium, in addition to searching for and treating any precipitant such as an infection. Initial hypokalemia is not common in DKA, and when present, represents extreme total body potassium depletion. In this situation, potassium administrations should be initiated before insulin. A reasonable guide is to delay insulin administration when the serum potassium level is below 3.3 mEq/L on presentation. Otherwise, as insulin and fluids are administered, hypokalemia worsens and predisposes patients to life-threatening respiratory paralysis and abnormal cardiac rhythms. Due to intracellular-to-extracellular shifting from acidosis and lack of insulin, most patients in DKA present with normal or slightly elevated serum potassium concentrations despite total-body depletion of potassium. In the absence of renal failure, it is appropriate to initiate potassium administration in DKA when the potassium is 5.3 mEq/L or lower.

Why are the other choices wrong?

Sodium bicarbonate administration in DKA can delay a decrease in ketonemia and worsen hypokalemia. If administered, it is reserved for when the pH is less than 6.90 (not 7.15).

Insulin boluses are not required in the management of DKA and have not demonstrated benefit over beginning with an insulin infusion. If used, a bolus dose of 0.10 to 0.14 units/kg (not 0.01 units/kg) is appropriate.

During DKA treatment, administration of dextrose might be needed when the serum glucose falls but significant ketoacidosis remains. Guidelines recommend dextrose administration when the serum glucose is less than 200 mg/dL (not 350 mg/dL).

PEER REVIEW

- ✓ Initial hypokalemia is not common in DKA. If you see it, the patient has extreme total body potassium depletion.
- ✓ When you're treating DKA and the patient's initial serum potassium is below 3.3 mEq/L, delay insulin administration.
- ✓ Start potassium if the patient's potassium level is 5.3 mEq/L or lower and if he or she isn't in renal failure.

REFERENCES

Van Ness-Otunnu R, Hack JB. Hyperglycemic crisis. *J Emerg Med.* 2013;45(5):797-805.

Wolfson AB, Hendey GW, Ling LJ, et al, eds. *Harwood-Nuss' Clinical Practice of Emergency Medicine.* 6th ed. Philadelphia, PA: Lippincott, Williams & Wilkins; 2014: 1011-1013.

13. The correct answer is D, The threshold for administering broad-spectrum antibiotics should be low.

Why is this the correct answer?

Thyroid storm is a life-threatening condition often precipitated by a significant physiologic stressor such as childbirth, an infection, surgery (particularly on the thyroid in a patient with thyrotoxicosis), and trauma. In addition to specific treatment of thyroid hormone excess, it is imperative to search for and treat the precipitating stressor. Since infections are a common precipitant and might not be clinically obvious, the clinician should have a low threshold for starting broad-spectrum antibiotics.

Specific treatment to address the thyroid hormone excess includes administration of these four agents: thionamide (propylthiouracil [PTU] or methimazole); iodine (an hour after the thionamide); corticosteroids; and beta blockers.

Why are the other choices wrong?

Corticosteroids (dexamethasone or hydrocortisone) decrease conversion of T4 to the more active T3 and decrease thyroid hormone release. They should be administrated routinely to patients in thyroid storm and not reserved just for those with coincident adrenal insufficiency.

The administration of a thionamide should precede that of iodine. Thionamides (propylthiouracil [PTU] or methimazole) inhibit thyroid peroxidase and decrease production of thyroid hormone. Iodine administration decreases the release and production of thyroid hormone by a feedback mechanism but must be given an hour or two following the thionamide to prevent the iodine from being used to produce even more thyroid hormone.

Plasmapheresis, a method of removing circulating thyroid hormone, can be considered for patients who are worsening despite maximal standard therapy and in those with contraindications to thionamide use. It is not a part of standard therapy and is not used routinely.

PEER REVIEW

✓ Infections commonly cause thyroid storm but might not be clinically obvious. So maintain a low threshold for starting broad-spectrum antibiotics.

✓ Here are the four agents used to treat thyroid hormone excess in thyroid storm, in order: a thionamide, iodine (an hour after the thionamide), corticosteroids, beta blockers.

REFERENCES

Tintinalli JE, Stapczynski JS, Ma OJ, et al, eds. *Tintinalli's Emergency Medicine: A Comprehensive Study Guide.* 8th ed. New York, NY: McGraw-Hill; 2012;1473, 1476-1478.

Wolfson AB, Hendey GW, Ling LJ, et al, eds. *Harwood-Nuss' Clinical Practice of Emergency Medicine.* 6th ed. Philadelphia, PA: Lippincott, Williams & Wilkins; 2014: 1025-1027.

14. The correct answer is C, Traditional ABC sequence is the recommended approach to CPR.

Why is this the correct answer?

The World Health Organization defines drowning as the process of experiencing respiratory impairment from submersion/immersion in liquid. The degree of hypoxic insult to the central nervous system is the main determinant of outcome. When cardiac arrest occurs from drowning, it is primarily due to hypoxia. This is why oxygenation and ventilation are paramount. The traditional ABC (airway-breathing-circulation) approach to CPR is recommended — not chest compression — only CPR. Resuscitation might be successful after initial rescue breathing alone.

Why are the other choices wrong?

The early radiographic appearance of water on chest xrays often leads to the misdiagnosis of pneumonia in the setting of drowning. Pneumonia develops in the minority of patients who have drowned, so prophylactic antibiotics should not be administered routinely. Prophylactic antibiotics can select resistant and aggressive organisms; administration should be reserved for the development of infectious systems.

Regurgitation of stomach contents is very common in resuscitation attempts of drowning victims.

Consistent with a systemic hypoxic etiology, cardiac arrest rhythms associated with drowning are typically asystole (most common) or pulseless electrical activity. Ventricular fibrillation is rare, and when it occurs, it suggests preexisting cardiac disease.

PEER REVIEW

✓ Use the ABC sequence when you perform CPR on drowning victims.
✓ Asystole is the predominant cardiac arrest rhythm in drowning.
✓ Don't use antibiotic prophylaxis routinely in patients who have survived a drowning episode.

REFERENCES

Lavonas EJ, Drennan IR, Gabrielli A, et al. Part 10: Special circumstances of resuscitation: 2015 American Heart Association Guidelines Update for Cardiopulmonary Resuscitation and Emergency Cardiovascular Care. *Circulation.* 2015;132(Suppl 2):S501–S518.

Szpilman D, Bierens JJ, Handley AJ, Orlowski JP. Drowning. *New Engl J Med.* 2012;366(22): 2102, 2104, 2106-2107.

15. The correct answer is A, Bark scorpion.

Why is this the correct answer?

The presentation of a child in severe pain associated with excessive oral secretions, muscular jerking, and wandering eye movements is classic for severe envenomation by a bark scorpion (Centruroides). The venom is primarily neurologically excitatory, leading to activation of the sympathetic and parasympathetic nervous systems. The most common presentation is localized pain and/or paresthesia. Systemic toxicity is rare but is most common in young children. Skeletal muscular dysfunction with jerking muscle movements, cranial nerve dysfunction, hypersalivation, and ataxia and opsoclonus (rapid multivectorial involuntary conjugate eye movements) are seen in severe envenomations. Without antivenom treatment, symptoms can last 24 to 48 hours. Management is supportive, with airway control as needed, pain control, and sedation. Antivenom is currently available in the United States and has proven efficacy, but it is very expensive and should be considered only in severe envenomations.

Why are the other choices wrong?

The main toxic component of the venom from a black widow spider (Latrodectus species) is alpha-latrotoxin. It causes the release of neurotransmitters, predominantly acetylcholine and norepinephrine. The release of acetylcholine can cause severe localized and occasional systemic myalgias. Localized diaphoresis might occasionally be seen near the bite site. Norepinephrine release can cause hypertension and tachycardia. Although patients might be very uncomfortable and restless due to the presence of pain, ataxia, excessive oral secretions, jerking muscular movements, and rapid, wandering eye movements are not expected manifestation of black widow spider envenomation.

The systemic toxicity described is not a manifestation of envenomation from the Loxosceles species, of which the brown recluse spider is the most notorious in the United States. Most bites do not cause any significant problem. The development of a necrotic skin wound is rare but possible. Children are at risk for hemolysis, the most feared but extremely rare systemic complication.

A significant portion of rattlesnake (Crotalus) bites are "dry," and no local or systemic effects occur. If signs of envenomation occur after a rattlesnake bite, manifestations are typically local tissue damage (swelling, muscle necrosis) and potentially hematologic abnormalities (thrombocytopenia and/or hypofibrinoginemia). Unlike scorpion stings and most spider bites, evidence of skin puncture (fang marks) is expected. Neuromuscular abnormalities such as myokymia (movement of individual muscle fibers) and fasciculations are occasionally seen after envenomation by rattlesnakes, and cranial nerve dysfunction, respiratory paralysis, and weakness can be seen with the Mojave rattlesnake.

PEER POINT

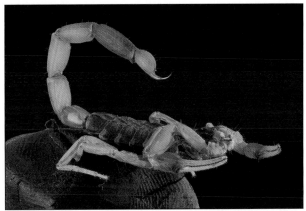

PEER Point 2

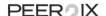

PEER REVIEW

- ✓ The most common symptom in bark scorpion envenomation is localized pain. But severe symptoms can develop in children: ataxia, cranial nerve dysfunction, hypersalivation, muscle jerking, and unusual eye movements.
- ✓ Black widow spider bite envenomation causes localized pain and diaphoresis that can spread systemically.
- ✓ North American rattlesnake envenomation causes pain and edema and can have severe hematotoxic effects.

REFERENCES

Hoffman RS, Howland MA, Lewin NA, et al. *Goldfrank's Toxicologic Emergencies*. 10th ed. New York, NY: McGraw-Hill; 2010: 1462-1470.

Tintinalli JE, Stapczynski JS, Ma OJ, et al, eds. *Tintinalli's Emergency Medicine: A Comprehensive Study Guide*. 8th ed. New York, NY: McGraw-Hill; 2012:1374, 1376, 1379.

16. The correct answer is D, Tobramycin 0.3% ophthalmic solution.

Why is this the correct answer?

As the image shows, this patient has a corneal abrasion, most likely as a result of wearing her contacts too long. The contact lens should be discarded, and an ophthalmic antibiotic solution should be instilled once all other foreign bodies have been ruled out. As a result of the contact lens use, pseudomonas should be covered by an antibiotic such as ciprofloxacin, ofloxacin, or tobramycin. Given that the abrasion is covering the central visual axis and the contact lens use, the patient needs to follow up with an ophthalmologist in 24 hours. Abrasions are important to differentiate from corneal ulcers, which have a more cavitary appearance and require very close ophthalmologic follow-up and management.

Why are the other choices wrong?

Cycloplegics like cyclopentolate 1% or homatropine 5% can help with the discomfort of a corneal abrasion theoretically by decreasing the associated ciliary spasm. However, atropine can last up to 2 weeks, which is too long for ongoing outpatient management of the corneal abrasion by an ophthalmologist.

Erythromycin ointment would have been an appropriate antibiotic selection if the patient did not wear contact lenses. However, it has inadequate pseudomonas coverage, so a fluoroquinolone or tobramycin should be used.

Proparacaine helps make examination of the eye possible and provides immediate pain relief but should not be used beyond the initial encounter. Prolonged use of topical anesthetics can blunt the normal protective mechanism of the cornea and delay healing.

PEER REVIEW

✓ Corneal abrasions in contact lens wearers require more aggressive antibiotic treatment and ophthalmologic follow-up.

✓ It is important to differentiate corneal abrasions from corneal ulcers.

✓ Other foreign bodies must be ruled out on eye examination.

REFERENCES

Tintinalli JE, Stapczynski JS, Ma OJ, et al, eds. *Tintinalli's Emergency Medicine: A Comprehensive Study Guide.* 8th ed. New York, NY: McGraw-Hill; 2012: 1211-1212. 1543-1579.

Wipperman JL, Dorsch JN. Evaluation and management of corneal abrasion. *Am Fam Physician.* 2013;87(2):114-120.

17. The correct answer is D, Indicated when the fetus is greater than 24 weeks of gestation.

Why is this the correct answer?

Before 24 weeks of gestation, survival of a fetus is unlikely even under ideal circumstances. Therefore, perimortem cesarean delivery (more recently termed resuscitative hysterotomy) should be performed only when the gestational age is greater than 24 weeks. If the age of the fetus is unknown, the procedure should be performed only when the uterine fundus can be palpated above the umbilicus. The procedure should also only be performed when there are fetal heart tones present, as survival of the fetus is unlikely once fetal heart tones have been lost. Cardiopulmonary resuscitation of the mother should continue during the procedure whenever possible. An emergency physician may perform this procedure under extreme circumstances. Nevertheless, the most experienced clinician should perform the procedure when possible, especially if an obstetrician or surgeon is available.

Why are the other choices wrong?

A standard horizontal incision does not provide enough exposure to deliver the fetus quickly. Although a horizontal incision might be ideal for cosmesis in an elective procedure, in this emergent situation, the initial incision should be vertical and is historically described as made from the maternal epigastric area extending to the pubic symphysis. This allows the greatest exposure of the uterus and fetus and ease of delivery. Some find that an incision from the umbilicus to the pubic symphysis is large enough to accomplish fetal delivery. The uterine incision should be vertical as well.

Perimortem cesarean delivery might actually improve maternal circulation and is better performed early rather than too late. There have been reports of maternal survival after perimortem cesarean delivery even when the mother has been in cardiac arrest. Theoretically, delivery of the fetus can help restore maternal circulation and remove pressure from the inferior vena cava.

The procedure is ideally performed within 4 to 5 minutes of the loss of maternal circulation. Survival of the mother and the fetus is unlikely if the procedure is performed too late and is virtually futile if performed after 20 minutes of maternal cardiac arrest.

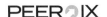
PEER REVIEW

✓ Don't perform a perimortem cesarean delivery unless fetal heart tones are present and the uterine fundus is above the umbilicus.

✓ Make vertical skin and uterine incisions when performing a perimortem cesarean delivery.

✓ Perimortem cesarean delivery is most successful when it's performed early, ideally within 4 to 5 minutes of maternal arrest.

REFERENCES

Marx JA, Hockberger RS, Walls RM, eds. *Rosen's Emergency Medicine: Concepts and Clinical Practice*. 8th ed. St. Louis, MO: Elsevier; 2014: 303-304.

Wolfson AB, Hendey GW, Ling LJ, et al, eds. *Harwood-Nuss' Clinical Practice of Emergency Medicine*. 6th ed. Philadelphia, PA: Lippincott, Williams & Wilkins; 2014: 324, 694.

18. The correct answer is B, Duration of symptoms.

Why is this the correct answer?

Panic attacks involve sudden-onset episodes of intense anxiety and fear. The episodes typically peak within 10 minutes and last up to 1 hour. The patient described in this question has been having symptoms for much longer than what is typical for a panic attack; this should prompt concern for another underlying medical problem. Further workup should be undertaken to rule out other serious pathology such as cardiac ischemia, aortic dissection, PE, or other life-threatening conditions. Various somatic and cognitive symptoms are associated with panic attacks. In addition to those listed above, they include paresthesias, shortness of breath, nausea, lightheadedness, inability to concentrate, and a fear of losing control or dying.

Why are the other choices wrong?

Chest pain is frequently a symptom of panic attacks. Naturally, other serious medical causes of chest pain should be considered and, where possible, ruled out before a diagnosis of panic attack is made in the emergency department. But chest pain is common enough that it does not raise the index of suspicion for an alternative diagnosis more than the duration of the patient's symptoms does.

Asthma is one of many medical conditions associated with panic disorder. Others include interstitial cystitis, hypertension, hyperthyroidism, COPD, and irritable bowel syndrome. The nature of these associations has not been elucidated. Like chest pain, it is not more compelling than the duration of symptoms.

Migraine headache also has been associated with panic disorder. There is also a high rate of comorbidity between panic disorder and other psychiatric illnesses, particularly other anxiety disorders such as major depression, bipolar disorder, and, most commonly, agoraphobia.

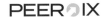

PEER REVIEW

✓ Panic attacks are usually acute in onset and peak within a few minutes.

✓ Chest pain is a frequent component of panic attacks.

✓ Various medical and psychiatric comorbidities have been associated with panic attacks and panic disorder.

REFERENCES
American Psychiatric Association: Diagnostic and Statistical Manual of Mental Disorders. 5th ed. Washington, DC: American Psychiatric Association, 2013: 608, 771, 772.
Tintinalli JE, Stapczynski JS, Ma OJ, et al, eds. *Tintinalli's Emergency Medicine: A Comprehensive Study Guide.* 8th ed. New York, NY: McGraw-Hill; 2012: 1963-1969.

19. The correct answer is C, Tension headache.

Why is this the correct answer?

A tension headache is the most common of the primary headache syndromes but also the least distinct. It is characterized by a gradual onset of pain, usually described as bandlike, and often associated with tightness in the muscles of the neck and shoulders. Because the pain from tension headaches usually does not interfere with the activities of daily living, patients can have symptoms for several days or weeks before seeking treatment. The pain in tension headaches does not increase with activity and is not affected by light and sound. Patients do not typically report nausea, vomiting, or neurologic symptoms. Tension headaches are, however, often associated with chronic conditions such as depression and anxiety. Besides screening for depression, clinicians evaluating patients with tension-type headaches should also consider other possible causes, including idiopathic intracranial hypertension, sinus disease, and intracranial mass. Nonsteroidal anti-inflammatory drugs or acetaminophen is usually sufficient to manage the pain of tension headaches, but most patients have tried this before seeking care in the emergency department and request a different approach. The antiemetic dopamine agonists used for migraine therapy can be helpful, and many clinicians favor muscle relaxants such as cyclobenzaprine. Another approach is to use trigger point injections into the tense muscles of the shoulder or neck. For patients with chronic symptoms, it is important to address the underlying stress and depression that are contributing to the headache syndrome. Nonpharmacologic approaches such as massage, meditation, and acupuncture can help some patients.

Why are the other choices wrong?

A cluster headache is a sharp, stabbing pain in one eye lasting 15 minutes to several hours and occurs in clusters throughout the week.

A migraine headache is abrupt-onset severe throbbing or pounding pain that is frequently associated with neurologic symptoms such as vision changes, photophobia, phonophobia, nausea, and even limb weakness or numbness.

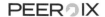

Trigeminal neuralgia is an episodic, shooting, electrical type of pain that occurs in one or more branches of the trigeminal nerve. These debilitating attacks can be brought on by stimulation of the nerve with talking, brushing teeth, or even a cold wind blowing on the face.

PEER REVIEW

✓ What are the primary headache syndromes? Cluster, migraine, and tension — and tension headaches are the most common.

✓ Tension headaches present with the gradual onset of bandlike, nondebilitating pain.

✓ Tension headaches can be managed with NSAIDs, acetaminophen, muscle relaxants, trigger point injections, or nonpharmacologic therapies.

REFERENCES

Marx JA, Hockberger RS, Walls RM, eds. *Rosen's Emergency Medicine: Concepts and Clinical Practice.* 8th ed. St. Louis, MO: Elsevier; 2014: 1386-1397.

Tintinalli JE, Stapczynski JS, Ma OJ, et al, eds. *Tintinalli's Emergency Medicine: A Comprehensive Study Guide.* 8th ed. New York, NY: McGraw-Hill; 2012: 1077-1085.

20. The correct answer is C, Factor VIII.

Why is this the correct answer?

von Willebrand disease is the most common inherited bleeding disorder. In patients with severe von Willebrand disease, factor VIII is the mainstay of therapy for bleeding. Typically, between 25 and 50 units/kg is the initial starting dose. The von Willebrand factor is a carrier protein for factor VIII and acts as a cofactor for platelet adhesion. An absence of von Willebrand factor causes a decrease in platelet adhesion and clinically appears similar to hemophilia A. Mucosal bleeding and cutaneous bleeding are common in von Willebrand disease and are typically milder than in hemophilia. Hemarthroses are not common, but GI bleeding and menorrhagia are typically seen.

Why are the other choices wrong?

Cryoprecipitate does contain von Willebrand factor, but its use is not recommended because of viral transmission risk.

Desmopressin is typically used to treat the milder and more common form of von Willebrand disease referred to as type I. In more severe von Willebrand disease, desmopressin may be used but usually along with factor VIII.

Factor IX is deficient in hemophilia B and is not associated with von Willebrand disease. Hemophilia B is clinically similar to hemophilia A but is much less common.

PEER REVIEW

- ✓ von Willebrand disease involves a dysfunction of factor VIII.
- ✓ Use desmopressin to treat bleeding patients in the milder and more common type 1 von Willebrand disease, but use factor VIII in severe cases.
- ✓ Mucosal and cutaneous bleeding are common in von Willebrand disease, typically GI bleeding and menorrhagia.

REFERENCES

Marx JA, Hockberger RS, Walls RM, eds. *Rosen's Emergency Medicine: Concepts and Clinical Practice.* 8th ed. St. Louis, MO: Elsevier; 2014:1606-1616.e1.

Tintinalli JE, Stapczynski JS, Ma OJ, et al, eds. *Tintinalli's Emergency Medicine: A Comprehensive Study Guide.* 8th ed. New York, NY: McGraw-Hill; 2012:1500-1504.

21. The correct answer is B, 50,000/mm³.

Why is this the correct answer?

Platelet transfusions are commonplace in patients with bone marrow disorders, but transfusion to prevent the risk of bleeding in other patients is less standard. Determining the patient's platelet level can help the clinician assess the risk of bleeding and guide transfusion practices. Patients with active bleeding require platelet transfusion when their platelet levels are below 50,000/mm³. When platelet levels fall below this number, the risk for further hemorrhage increases. Typically, patients who present with GI bleeding or trauma and those who are scheduled for surgery need more platelets when numbers are this low.

Why are the other choices wrong?

Platelet levels below 100,000/mm³ but greater than 50,000/mm³ very rarely cause bleeding. However, patients who are scheduled to have a more invasive surgery such as a cardiac or neurosurgical procedure should receive a platelet transfusion.

Levels below 20,000/mm³ require platelet transfusion in patients who have a coagulation disorder putting them at risk for other causes of bleeding.

Levels below 5,000/mm³ to 10,000/mm³ put patients at risk for spontaneous bleeding; these patients should be transfused prophylactically.

PEER REVIEW

- ✓ Platelet transfusion should occur for levels under 50,000 /mm³ in patients who present with trauma or active bleeding.
- ✓ Spontaneous bleeding is more likely at levels below 10,000/mm³, and prophylactic transfusion should occur for thrombocytopenia at this degree.
- ✓ Platelet transfusion in patients without primary bone marrow disorders should be guided by platelet levels to help predict hemostasis.

REFERENCES

Marx JA, Hockberger RS, Walls RM, eds. *Rosen's Emergency Medicine: Concepts and Clinical Practice.* 8th ed. St. Louis, MO: Elsevier; 2014: 1606-1616.e1.

Tintinalli JE, Stapczynski JS, Ma OJ, et al, eds. *Tintinalli's Emergency Medicine: A Comprehensive Study Guide.* 8th ed. New York, NY: McGraw-Hill; 2012: 1518-1524.

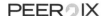

22.   The correct answer is C, Skin.

Why is this the correct answer?

The skin is a helpful indicator to distinguish between these two conditions. Dry skin is expected with anticholinergic toxicity, and damp or sweaty skin is expected with sympathomimetic toxicity. An anticholinergic (more accurately, antimuscarinic) toxidrome can result from exposure to a variety of agents, including drugs (atropine, benztropine, diphenhydramine, various antipsychotics, tricyclic antidepressants) and plants (angel's trumpet, jimsonweed). The antimuscarinic state results from antagonism at central and peripheral nervous system muscarinic receptors. Manifestations include coma, delirium, diminished bowel sounds, dry and at times flushed skin, hyperthermia, mydriasis, tachycardia, urinary retention, and picking behavior. The sympathomimetic toxidrome also includes hyperthermia, mydriasis, and tachycardia, but the presence of diaphoresis can help distinguish it from the anticholinergic toxidrome. Hypertension is expected with ingestion of sympathomimetic agents, although it can also occur with antimuscarinics. Agitation and psychosis rather than delirium are also more typical with sympathomimetic agents than with antimuscarinic agents. Exposure to cocaine and phencyclidine can result in a sympathomimetic toxidrome. So can various amphetamines, including ecstasy (methylenedioxymethamphetamine [MDMA]), methamphetamine, and cathinones, recently sold in the United States as bath salts.

Why are the other choices wrong?

Tachycardia is expected with both anticholinergic and sympathomimetic agents.

Mydriasis is expected with both anticholinergic and sympathomimetic agents.

Hyperthermia can occur with both anticholinergic and sympathomimetic agents.

PEER POINT

Is it anticholinergic (antimuscarinic) toxicity or sympathomimetic toxicity? Check the skin!

Anticholinergic (antimuscarinic) syndrome presents with dry skin:

- Other signs and symptoms include hyperthermia, mydriasis, tachycardia, delirium, coma, diminished bowel sounds, flushed skin (sometimes), urinary retention, picking
- Caused by exposure to drugs like atropine, benztropine, diphenhydramine, various antipsychotics, tricyclic antidepressants, and plants like angel's trumpet, jimson weed

Sympathomimetic syndrome presents with damp, sweaty skin:

- Other signs and symptoms include hyperthermia, mydriasis, tachycardia (sound familiar?), agitation, and psychosis (generally not delirium)
- Caused by exposure to cocaine, PCP, and amphetamines

PEER REVIEW

✓ It's typical for patients to present with elevated temperature, dilated pupils, and a rapid heart rate with both antimuscarinic and sympathomimetic toxidromes.

✓ But dry skin (antimuscarinic) and diaphoresis (sympathomimetic) can help you distinguish between the two.

REFERENCES

Hoffman RS, Howland MA, Lewin NA, et al. *Goldfrank's Toxicologic Emergencies.* 10th ed. New York, NY: McGraw-Hill; 2010: 26-29.

Wolfson AB, Hendey GW, Ling LJ, et al, eds. *Harwood-Nuss' Clinical Practice of Emergency Medicine.* 6th ed. Philadelphia, PA: Lippincott, Williams & Wilkins; 2014: 1316.

23. The correct answer is C, Indomethacin.

Why is this the correct answer?

The classic presentation of reactive arthritis (formerly referred to as Reiter syndrome) includes arthritis, urethritis, and uveitis; however, this triad is not necessary for making the diagnosis. This patient presents with an asymmetrical polyarthritis following a recent chlamydial infection, or urethritis, and that is enough to warrant a high level of suspicion for reactive arthritis. The treatment of choice for reactive arthritis is an NSAID, commonly indomethacin. Antibiotics have also been shown to have benefit in postchlamydial reactive arthritis. Long-term combination therapy of rifampicin with doxycycline or azithromycin may be used in addition to NSAIDs. In this syndrome, the Achilles tendon might be inflamed at the insertion point. The pain patients typically experience is in the weight-bearing joints of knees, ankles, and heels. In addition, the sacroiliac joints, ischial tuberosity, and ischial crest can be involved and cause pain with range of motion. Diarrhea caused by the invasive GI bacteria, *Campylobacter*, *Salmonella*, and *Shigella*, and *Yersinia* infection have also been known to cause a reactive arthritis picture. The NSAIDs are also the treatment of choice for postdysentery reactive arthritis, but antibiotics have been not shown to have benefit.

Why are the other choices wrong?

Antibiotics are not the first-line therapy for reactive arthritis. Chlamydial infections might respond to long-term antibiotic therapy, but ceftriaxone is not an antibiotic typically used in these cases.

Although not first-line therapy, the appropriate antibiotics have been shown to improve recovery time in cases caused by chlamydial infections. Typically, rifampicin is used in conjunction with either doxycycline or azithromycin, but NSAIDs are still the treatment of choice.

Methotrexate is not used for reactive arthritis but can be used in other forms of arthritis, most notably for rheumatoid arthritis.

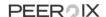

PEER REVIEW

✓ Reactive arthritis is an asymmetric polyarthralgia that typically affects weight-bearing joints.

✓ Reactive arthritis often develops following dysentery or a chlamydial infection.

✓ The treatment of choice for reactive arthritis is an NSAID, and if a chlamydial infection preceded the arthritis, adding an antibiotic might reduce recovery time.

REFERENCES

Marx JA, Hockberger RS, Walls RM, eds. *Rosen's Emergency Medicine: Concepts and Clinical Practice*. 8th ed. St. Louis, MO: Elsevier; 2014:1501-1517.e2.

Tintinalli JE, Stapczynski JS, Ma OJ, et al, eds. *Tintinalli's Emergency Medicine: A Comprehensive Study Guide*. 8th ed. New York, NY: McGraw-Hill; 2012:1927-1936.

24. The correct answer is B, Intravenous bolus.

Why is this the correct answer?

In this case, the patient exhibits signs of cardiovascular collapse — hypotension and tachycardia — along with his anaphylactic reaction. The initial intramuscular epinephrine injection was not effective, so intravenous administration is warranted. This dose is given first as a bolus — 0.1 mL epinephrine, using the 1:1,000 dilution in 10 mL of normal saline over 10 minutes. Any time intramuscular epinephrine is not working or a patient is showing signs of cardiovascular collapse, another dose must be given intravenously.

Why are the other choices wrong?

A repeat intramuscular dose of epinephrine would be warranted for a patient with continued anaphylactic symptoms except in cases where there is evidence of cardiovascular collapse. The intramuscular doses are not working, likely due to decreased perfusion and uptake of the medication in the musculature of the extremities.

An intravenous infusion of 1 mg epinephrine (1 to 4 mcg/min) is the next step in anaphylactic patients who do not respond adequately to the initial intravenous bolus administration. It is recommended that a bolus be given first over 5 to 10 minutes to assess for serious side effects such as serious arrhythmias or cardiac ischemia symptoms. If these occur during the bolus or drip, other vasopressors may be used.

Subcutaneous administration of epinephrine is not indicated in anaphylaxis and is certainly not indicated in anaphylaxis complicated by cardiovascular collapse.

PEER REVIEW

✓ In refractory anaphylaxis in the absence of cardiovascular collapse, use repeated intramuscular doses of epinephrine.

✓ An intravenous bolus of epinephrine is indicated in anaphylaxis with cardiovascular collapse.

✓ Treat refractory anaphylaxis with evidence of cardiovascular collapse first with intravenous bolus epinephrine, then an intravenous infusion of epinephrine.

REFERENCES

Marx JA, Hockberger RS, Walls RM, eds. *Rosen's Emergency Medicine: Concepts and Clinical Practice.* 8th ed. St. Louis, MO: Elsevier; 2014: 1543-1557.e2.

Tintinalli JE, Stapczynski JS, Ma OJ, et al, eds. *Tintinalli's Emergency Medicine: A Comprehensive Study Guide.* 8th ed. New York, NY: McGraw-Hill; 2012: 74-79.

25. The correct answer is A, Botulism immune globulin 0.5 mL/kg/hr.

Why is this the correct answer?

The classic presentation of infant botulism includes a history of constipation followed by an altered neuromuscular examination, with cranial nerve issues noted initially. Infant botulism is caused by ingestion of *Clostridium botulinum.* The mortality rate is 5% to 10% and can be attributed to ingestion of honey or corn syrup; it is more common in breastfed infants, as this can further affect the gastric acid or bile acids that would normally minimize the growth of Clostridium. *C. botulinum* can also be ingested on a fomite when local construction has caused it to be mobilized from the soil. The primary concern in infant botulism is paralysis of musculature related to breathing; deep tendon reflexes are spared and remain normal. Treatment includes supportive care, frequent evaluation of the respiratory status, and empiric treatment with botulism immune globulin intravenous. The time it takes to get results from stool sample testing is often too long given how difficult it is to obtain the sample in a constipated infant.

Why are the other choices wrong?

Dexamethasone is a steroid often used to treat croup, and there is evidence for its use in treating asthma in one or two doses (depending on the study). There is no role for steroids in the treatment of infant botulism.

Normal saline is best used as a volume expander and is dosed only at 10 mL/kg when the normal 20 mL/kg might be harmful (ie, increased intracranial pressure, congestive heart failure, renal dysfunction). The child has normal mentation and vital signs and does not warrant a fluid bolus at this time.

Vancomycin might be important in the treatment of wound botulism. although penicillin is still the preferred first-line agent. Vancomycin does not have any role in the treatment of infant botulism.

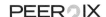

PEER REVIEW

✓ Botulism should be considered in an infant presenting with constipation followed by neuromuscular dysfunction.
✓ Monitoring the respiratory status is crucial in the care of infant botulism.
✓ Supportive care and botulism immune globulin are keys to treatment.

REFERENCES

Fleisher GR, Ludwig S, et al, eds. *Textbook of Pediatric Emergency Medicine.* 6th ed. Philadelphia, PA: Lippincott, Williams & Wilkins; 2010: 940-941, 1026-1027.

Wolfson AB, Hendey GW, Ling LJ, et al, eds. *Harwood-Nuss' Clinical Practice of Emergency Medicine.* 6th ed. Philadelphia, PA: Lippincott, Williams & Wilkins; 2014: 1493-1495.

26. The correct answer is C, NSAIDs.

Why is this the correct answer?

This patient has nonseptic olecranon bursitis, and the correct treatment for it is NSAIDs. It is often referred to as "carpetlayer's knee" or "student's elbow" because it most commonly occurs in the knee or elbow as a result of the prolonged pressure frequently exerted on these areas. This swollen area is typically nontender, and patients have full range of motion in their joint with no erythema or warmth noted. In contrast, septic bursitis typically presents more acutely with warmth, erythema, and tenderness of the areas. Patients with septic bursitis might also have a history of trauma or of a chronic disease such as diabetes or alcoholism.

Why are the other choices wrong?

Antibiotics are not indicated for the treatment of nonseptic bursitis. In patients with septic olecranon bursitis, the bursa should be aspirated, and the patient should be started on a 14-day course of antibiotics, typically first- or second-generation cephalosporins targeted at *Staphylococcus* and *Streptococcus*.

Incision and drainage is not indicated for nonseptic bursitis, but it is for septic bursitis. This procedure can be both diagnostic and therapeutic.

Surgical consultation is not necessary with the management of nonseptic bursitis. In a patient with a potentially septic joint, orthopedic consultation is necessary to determine the need for surgical washout.

PEER REVIEW

✓ Nonseptic bursitis is typically caused by repetitive pressure on the joint.
✓ You can generally tell the difference between septic and nonseptic bursitis by the presence of severe pain, redness, and warmth in septic bursitis.
✓ Treat nonseptic bursitis with NSAIDs and septic bursitis with incision and drainage, then antibiotics.

REFERENCES

Marx JA, Hockberger RS, Walls RM, eds. *Rosen's Emergency Medicine: Concepts and Clinical Practice.* 8th ed. St. Louis, MO: Elsevier; 2014: 1518-1526.e2.

Tintinalli JE, Stapczynski JS, Ma OJ, et al, eds. *Tintinalli's Emergency Medicine: A Comprehensive Study Guide.* 8th ed. New York, NY: McGraw-Hill; 2012: 1927-1936.

27. The correct answer is D, Raising the patient's straight right leg causes back pain and radiation of pain down the posterior left leg.

Why is this the correct answer?

Lumbar disc herniation is the most common cause of lumbar radiculopathy, or sciatica, a shooting or burning pain from the low back radiating down the posterior leg distal to the knee. Two tests used to evaluate these symptoms are the straight leg raise, which is performed by lifting the leg affected by the radiating pain, and the crossed straight leg raise, which is performed on the opposite leg. Of the two, the crossed straight leg raise test is highly specific for disc herniation that is causing the nerve root compression that manifests as sciatica. The straight leg raise test is highly sensitive but not very specific for disc herniation. The most common location of this herniation is at L5-S1. In the straight leg raise, the patient lies on his or her back with the knee extended. The examiner then raises the affected leg up to 70 degrees. Reproduction of low back pain that radiates down the posterior affected leg past the knee is considered a positive result. This test has been shown to be sensitive for a disc herniation but poorly specific. Conversely, performing the same test on the unaffected leg — the crossed straight leg raise test — and reproducing both the back pain and the radiation down the affected leg yield a low sensitivity but close to a 90% specificity for a sciatic disease.

Why are the other choices wrong?

The patient reported that his back pain radiated down his left leg. Reproducing the back pain only by raising his left leg is a negative result and therefore nondiagnostic.

Raising his left leg and reproducing both the back pain and the radiation represent a positive result that is very sensitive but not specific.

Again, regardless of which leg is raised, reproducing only the back pain is a negative test result.

PEER REVIEW

- ✓ The crossed straight leg raise test is more specific for a disc herniation and nerve root compression than is the straight leg test.
- ✓ Here's what constitutes a positive test result in a leg raise test: reproducing both the back pain and the radiation of pain down the posterior affected leg distal to the knee.
- ✓ Lumbar radiculopathies are most often caused by disc herniation, and the most common of those is an L5-S1 herniation that causes sciatica.

REFERENCES

Marx JA, Hockberger RS, Walls RM, eds. *Rosen's Emergency Medicine: Concepts and Clinical Practice*. 8th ed. St. Louis, MO: Elsevier; 2014: 643-655.e2.

Tintinalli JE, Stapczynski JS, Ma OJ, et al, eds. *Tintinalli's Emergency Medicine: A Comprehensive Study Guide*. 8th ed. New York, NY: McGraw-Hill; 2012: 1887-1894.

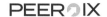
28. The correct answer is B, Pterygoid plate.

Why is this the correct answer?

The Le Fort classification system describes maxillary facial fractures and places them into four classes. Each of these classes of fractures involves the pterygoid plate, by definition. Le Fort I fractures involve the hard palate. Le Fort II fractures extend into the orbital floor. Le Fort III fractures also involve the zygoma and lead to craniofacial disruption. Le Fort IV fractures are Le Fort III fractures that also involve the frontal bone. In practice, with the routine use of CT scanning in these injuries, it is rare to have a pure Le Fort I, II, or III fracture; it is more common to see a mixed picture.

Why are the other choices wrong?

Le Fort I fractures do not involve the orbit. Only the higher classes do.

The vomer is a midline bone that helps to form the posterior aspect of the nasal septum. It might or might not be fractured as part of the Le Fort classification system but is not clearly defined in the classification system.

The zygoma is fractured only in Le Fort III and IV injuries.

PEER REVIEW

- ✓ Le Fort is a classification system of maxillary fractures defined by involvement of the pterygoid plate.
- ✓ Le Fort II fractures involve the orbit.
- ✓ Le Fort III fractures involve the zygoma.

REFERENCES

Marx JA, Hockberger RS, Walls RM, eds. *Rosen's Emergency Medicine: Concepts and Clinical Practice*. 8th ed. St. Louis, MO: Elsevier; 2014: 378-380.

Wolfson AB, Hendey GW, Ling LJ, et al, eds. *Harwood-Nuss' Clinical Practice of Emergency Medicine*. 6th ed. Philadelphia, PA: Lippincott, Williams & Wilkins; 2014: 162-163.

29. The correct answer is B, Evidence of head trauma.

Why is this the correct answer?

Patients with elevated intracranial pressure are at risk for herniation during performance of a lumbar puncture (LP). Noncontrast head CT can help evaluate for elevated intracranial pressure and should be performed in patients with evidence of head trauma, altered or deteriorating mental status, seizure, focal neurologic deficit, or papilledema. Interestingly, head trauma, even without obvious bony fracture, is a risk factor for meningitis. When a patient's signs and symptoms are concerning for meningitis, it is important to administer antibiotics early. Patients who meet the criteria for CT should receive empiric antibiotic treatment before neuroimaging: CSF cultures are not affected for 2 hours following administration of antibiotics.

Why are the other choices wrong?

There is some literature to support head CT prior to LP in patients older than 60 years.

Lumbar puncture is generally thought to be safe to perform in patients who have normal mental status before obtaining a head CT scan.

Patients who present with new seizure, not prior seizure disorder, fall into the group of patients who should undergo head CT before LP.

PEER REVIEW

- ✓ Lumbar puncture is a key test in diagnosing meningitis and can be safely performed without prior neuroimaging in most patients.
- ✓ Head CT should be obtained prior to LP for patients who present with altered mental status, seizure, focal neurologic deficit, evidence of head trauma, or papilledema. Immunocompromised patients are generally recommended for CT scan as well to evaluate for space-occupying lesion or abscess.
- ✓ Cerebral spinal fluid cultures are not affected until 2 hours after empiric antibiotic administration for meningitis.

REFERENCES

Marx JA, Hockberger RS, Walls RM, eds. *Rosen's Emergency Medicine: Concepts and Clinical Practice*. 8th ed. St. Louis, MO: Elsevier; 2014: 11417-1459.

Tintinalli JE, Stapczynski JS, Ma OJ, et al, eds. *Tintinalli's Emergency Medicine: A Comprehensive Study Guide*. 8th ed. New York, NY: McGraw-Hill; 2012: 1192-1199.

30. The correct answer is A, Crystallizing of fluid on microscopic examination.

Why is this the correct answer?

The approach to confirming rupture of membranes has three components: pooling of amniotic fluid in the vaginal vault, a positive Nitrazine test result, and ferning revealed on microscopic analysis of amniotic fluid. Of the three findings, ferning is the most specific. It occurs when amniotic fluid dries and sodium chloride crystals precipitate.

Why are the other choices wrong?

When exposed to a flame, vaginal secretions, not amniotic fluid, turn brown. Amniotic fluid turns white and displays the crystallized ferning pattern.

Nitrazine is a pH indicator that is more sensitive than litmus and is often used in the emergency department. Vaginal fluid is mildly acidic with a pH of approximately 4 to 5 and causes a Nitrazine strip to either remain yellow or turn slightly red (acidic). Amniotic fluid is basic with a pH of 7 to 7.5 and turns a Nitrazine strip blue. But

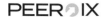

for several reasons, a Nitrazine test can have a false-positive result: lubricant use during speculum examination, the presence of semen, blood, or cervical mucus, or concurrent *Trichomonas vaginalis* infection.

When rupture of membranes is suspected, a speculum examination must be performed. Pooling fluid can have various sources: amniotic, vaginal, or urinary, so visualization of pooling is not specific.

PEER REVIEW

✓ The most specific finding for rupture of membranes is ferning — sodium chloride crystal precipitation.

✓ A Nitrazine test can yield a false-positive result for multiple reasons, so it shouldn't be the only test used to confirm rupture of membranes.

✓ Pooling of fluid in the vaginal vault is the least specific sign of rupture of membranes.

REFERENCES

Marx JA, Hockberger RS, Walls RM, eds. *Rosen's Emergency Medicine: Concepts and Clinical Practice*. 8th ed. St. Louis, MO: Elsevier; 2014: 2334, 2340-2341.

Tintinalli JE, Stapczynski JS, Ma OJ, et al, eds. *Tintinalli's Emergency Medicine: A Comprehensive Study Guide*. 8th ed. New York, NY: McGraw-Hill; 2012: 644-661.

31. The correct answer is C, Hyperflexing and abducting the mother's hips.

Why is this the correct answer?

Shoulder dystocia complicates about 1% of vaginal deliveries, typically when the anterior shoulder becomes trapped behind the pubic symphysis. One indication of shoulder dystocia is called the "turtle sign": the infant's head is delivered, then it retracts back against the mother's perineum. Several maneuvers can assist in successful delivery. The one that should be attempted first is the McRoberts maneuver. It is performed by hyperflexing and abducting the mother's hips, increasing sacroiliac joint mobility, which allows rotation of the pelvis and release of the fetal shoulder. In addition, delivery is often assisted when there is direct pressure applied for a minute or so to the suprapubic region to push the shoulder posterior from the pubic symphysis. Dystocia is most often seen in larger infants with macrosomia. Complications of delivery of these infants include fetal brachial plexus injury and fetal hypoxia from umbilical cord compression.

Why are the other choices wrong?

The Woods corkscrew maneuver should be attempted if the McRoberts maneuver fails to release the shoulder. It is performed by pushing the anterior shoulder toward the infant's chest, grasping the posterior scapula of the infant with two fingers, and rotating the shoulder girdle 180 degrees in the pelvic outlet in an attempt to rotate the posterior shoulder into the anterior position to deliver the shoulder.

Pushing the delivered head back into birth canal, a maneuver known as the Zavanelli maneuver, is a last resort in preparation for cesarean delivery.

The Leopold maneuver is intended to determine the position and size of a fetus by a series of systematic external palpations. This is generally done prior to delivery. It does not relieve shoulder dystocia; it is not diagnostic. Ultrasound examination is required to conclusively determine fetal position.

PEER POINT

The HELPERR mnemonic can help in emergency deliveries complicated by shoulder dystocia — this variation of it is adapted from the CALS program materials.

H — Call for help
E — Consider episiotomy
Legs — Perform the McRoberts maneuver
Pressure — Apply suprapubic pressure externally
Enter the vagina using internal pressure to reduce impacted shoulder; finally using a Woods corkscrew maneuver, bring the shoulders into oblique diameter and 180 degrees rotation, if necessary
Remove the posterior arm; finally, if all other maneuvers fail, cephalic replacement may be used in certain circumstances
Rotate the patient to her hands and knees

PEER REVIEW

✓ When an emergency delivery is complicated by shoulder dystocia, try the McRoberts maneuver first.
✓ The Woods corkscrew can be attempted if the McRoberts maneuver fails.
✓ Pushing the infant's head back into the birth canal is a last resort when other maneuvers don't work and cesarean delivery is required.

REFERENCES
Marx JA, Hockberger RS, Walls RM, eds. *Rosen's Emergency Medicine: Concepts and Clinical Practice*. 8th ed. St. Louis, MO: Elsevier; 2014: 2344-2345.
Tintinalli JE, Stapczynski JS, Ma OJ, et al, eds. *Tintinalli's Emergency Medicine: A Comprehensive Study Guide*. 8th ed. New York, NY: McGraw-Hill; 2012: 427-436.

32. The correct answer is B, Disorganized thinking.

Why is this the correct answer?

Disorganized thinking is one of the five clinical features of psychosis. It is typically inferred from a patient's speech and can include tangentiality, in which a patient's answers to questions are loosely related or unrelated; derailment, wherein the patient frequently switches from one topic to another; and word salad, in which the patient's speech becomes so disorganized that it is incomprehensible.

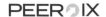

Why are the other choices wrong?

Delusions are one of the five clinical features of psychosis but are not exhibited by the patient in this case. Delusions are a fixed, incorrect belief held despite evidence to the contrary. They are classified by theme, including persecutory, grandiose, and erotomanic. Delusions are sometimes associated with hallucinations. Hallucinations are an apparent perception of a stimulus that does not exist. Hallucinations can be present in any sensory modality and are most commonly auditory in patients with schizophrenia.

Flight of ideas is often seen in patients with mania; they frequently shift from one topic to another with an almost continuous accelerated speech pattern. Features of mania can appear similar to psychosis but are not seen in schizophrenia. They are more likely to occur in bipolar patients. In mania, patients can present with pressured speech and accelerated thoughts, and they generally talk loudly and express grandiose ideas.

Negative symptoms, another feature of psychosis, include diminished emotional expression, avolition (decreased motivation), alogia (decreased speech), and anhedonia (decreased or absent ability to experience pleasure). Psychotic patients also can exhibit grossly disorganized or abnormal motor behavior ranging from unpredictable agitation to catatonia.

PEER POINT

Five clinical features of psychosis
- Delusions
- Disorganized thinking
- Hallucinations
- Negative symptoms
- Grossly disorganized or abnormal motor behavior

PEER REVIEW

- ✓ The five clinical features of psychosis are disorganized thinking, delusions, hallucinations, negative symptoms, and grossly disorganized or abnormal motor behavior.
- ✓ Patients with mania, not schizophrenia, have flight of ideas in which they frequently shift from one topic to another in an accelerated speech pattern.
- ✓ Grossly disorganized or abnormal motor behavior can range from unpredictable agitation to catatonia.

REFERENCES

Diagnostic and statistical manual of mental disorders: DSM-5. 5th ed. Washington, D.C.: American Psychiatric Association; 2013; Tintinalli JE, Stapczynski JS, Ma OJ, et al, eds. *Tintinalli's Emergency Medicine: A Comprehensive Study Guide.* 8th ed. New York, NY: McGraw-Hill; 2012: 1969-1972.

33. The correct answer is D, Synchronized cardioversion.

Why is this the correct answer?

This patient is presenting with unstable ventricular tachycardia with a pulse, which should be treated immediately with synchronized cardioversion. The ECG depicts a wide-complex tachycardia (QRS interval >120ms, rate greater than 100 bpm). The rhythm is likely ventricular tachycardia considering the patient's age, history of MI, and atrioventricular dissociation. As is typical of ventricular tachycardia, the rate is between 150 and 200 bpm. In a patient presenting with this rhythm and a pulse, it is important to differentiate whether the patient is stable or unstable. This patient is considered unstable due to the evidence of end-organ hypoperfusion, manifested by altered mental status, hypotension, and chest pain (likely ischemic). Other indicators of instability (not present in this patient) include evidence of respiratory compromise due to acute heart failure with pulmonary congestion. This patient should undergo synchronized electrical cardioversion. Sedation may be considered before cardioversion in an awake patient if time allows.

Why are the other choices wrong?

Adenosine is the treatment of choice for a stable supraventricular tachycardia (SVT). It can be difficult to determine the difference between ventricular tachycardia and SVT with aberrancy. However, in this case, the patient has risk factors for ventricular tachycardia. These include age older than 50 years and underlying heart disease. Moreover, the patient is unstable. Immediate treatment with synchronized cardioversion is the most appropriate treatment whether the rhythm is ventricular tachycardia or SVT with aberrant conduction.

Amiodarone is a first-line treatment for stable ventricular tachycardia. The dose is 150 mg IV over 10 minutes. This dose may be repeated for recurrent ventricular tachycardia up to a total dose of 300 mg. An infusion can be initiated at a rate of 1 mg/min for 6 hours. Procainamide is an alternative, 50 mg/min IV up to 17 mg/kg. Amiodarone is the preferred antiarrhythmic in the setting of acute MI, left ventricular dysfunction, or with unknown cardiac function.

Cardiac defibrillation is the appropriate treatment in a patient with ventricular fibrillation or ventricular tachycardia without a pulse. Defibrillation, as opposed to synchronized cardioversion, delivers the electrical shock at the moment the defibrillator button is pressed, which can be anytime during the cardiac cycle. Delivering the shock during the repolarization phase (QT interval), can induce ventricular fibrillation.

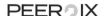

PEER REVIEW

✓ Treat unstable ventricular tachycardia immediately with synchronized cardioversion.

✓ Amiodarone is the first-line treatment for stable ventricular tachycardia.

✓ Evidence of end-organ hypoperfusion suggests the patient is unstable.

REFERENCES

Tintinalli JE, Stapczynski JS, Ma OJ, et al, eds. *Tintinalli's Emergency Medicine: A Comprehensive Study Guide.* 8th ed. New York, NY: McGraw-Hill; 2012: 112-134.

Winters ME, Bond MC, DeBlieux P, et al (eds). *Emergency Department Resuscitation of the Critically Ill.* Dallas, TX: American College of Emergency Physician Publishing; 2011: 51-68.

34.   The correct answer is B, Frontotemporal neurocognitive disorder.

Why is this the correct answer?

Major neurocognitive disorders, also referred to as dementia, are subtyped according to their presumed underlying etiologies. Each is associated with varying degrees and types of cognitive impairment and interference with everyday activities. Frontotemporal neurocognitive disorder is a common cause of dementia in patients younger than 65 years and is frequently associated with disruptive behavioral changes that are more prominent than the other cognitive impairments. These might include hyperorality, wandering, and generally disinhibited behavior. Based on this patient's relatively young age and behavioral changes, the most likely diagnosis of the choices listed is frontotemporal neurocognitive disorder. Median survival after diagnosis of frontotemporal neurocognitive disorder is 3 to 4 years, with a more rapid decline and shorter survival than with Alzheimer disease.

Why are the other choices wrong?

The biggest risk factor for development of Alzheimer disease is age. The age of onset is usually in the eighth or ninth decade of life, although it can be seen earlier in patients with a strong genetic predisposition. Patients typically present with memory loss and decline in executive functioning. Aphasia (language disturbance), apraxia (impaired motor ability), and agnosia (difficulty recognizing objects) are also sometimes seen.

Patients with neurocognitive disorder with Lewy bodies, in addition to developing problems with executive function and attention, also present with complex visual hallucinations and REM sleep behavior disorder. Their symptoms might wax and wane and appear similar to delirium, but no underlying cause is identified. Most patients develop symptoms in their mid-70s.

The neurocognitive disorders caused by prion disease typically manifest as, in addition to neurocognitive deficits, significant motor abnormalities such as ataxia, myoclonus, dystonia, or chorea. This category of neurocognitive disorders includes spongiform encephalopathies such as kuru, bovine spongiform encephalopathy ("mad cow" disease), and Creutzfeldt-Jakob disease. These diseases progress rapidly and can present at any age.

PEER REVIEW

✓ Neurocognitive disorders are classified by their presumed underlying cause.
✓ Frontotemporal neurocognitive disorder is typically associated with disinhibited behavior.
✓ Frontotemporal neurocognitive disorder is a common cause of dementia in patients younger than 65 years.

REFERENCES

Neurocognitive Disorders Diagnostic and Statistical Manual of Mental Disorders, 5th ed. American Psychiatric Association; 2013. Available at: http://dx.doi.org.foyer.swmed.edu/10.1176/appi.books.9780890425596.dsm17. Accessed May 19, 2017.
Zun L, Chepenik LG, Mallory MNS. *Behavioral Emergencies for the Emergency Physician*. Cambridge, NY: Cambridge; 2013: 117

35. The correct answer is A, Impotence.

Why is this the correct answer?

Priapism is a painful erection lasting longer than 2 hours. The most common sequela associated with priapism is impotence, occurring in up to 35% of cases and with increased rates when the erection lasts longer. Sickle cell disease is a common cause of priapism in children; a common cause in adults is injection of medications into the corpus cavernosum to treat erectile dysfunction. Other common causes are antihypertensive medications, anticoagulants, oral agents to treat erectile dysfunction, and some neuroleptic medications. Priapism is divided into the more common low-flow (ischemic) states characterized by slowed venous outflow and high-flow (nonischemic) conditions that result from a fistula between the cavernosal artery and corpus cavernosum. Urgent urologic consultation should be obtained for patients who present with priapism. Treatment consists of aspirating the blood from the corporal space then injecting an alpha-adrenergic agonist such as phenylephrine. This procedure is generally performed by a urologist but might need to be performed by the emergency physician, as time is of the essence. If the blood causing priapism is allowed to remain within the corpus cavernosum, penile fibrosis is a complication that can eventually lead to impotence. Patients who present with this condition with sickle cell disease might be eligible for exchange transfusion, so a hematology consultation should be obtained.

Why are the other choices wrong?

Penile stricture is a narrowing within the urethra. It is not caused by priapism.

Urethral transection may be considered in a patient who has a high-flow or nonischemic state who has experienced trauma. High-flow state can best be determined by looking at the color of the blood (should be bright red due to arterial involvement) and sending an arterial blood gas sample from material drained for analysis.

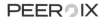

Urinary retention can develop while a patient is experiencing priapism, but this is not the most common complication.

PEER REVIEW

✓ Priapism is an erection lasting longer than 2 hours.

✓ Priapism is generally painless when it is related to trauma or some other high-flow state and painful when it is related to medications or sickle cell disease.

✓ The most common side effect of prolonged erection is impotence.

REFERENCES

Marx JA, Hockberger RS, Walls RM, eds. *Rosen's Emergency Medicine: Concepts and Clinical Practice.* 8th ed. St. Louis, MO: Elsevier; 2014: 1586-1605.

Tintinalli JE, Stapczynski JS, Ma OJ, et al, eds. *Tintinalli's Emergency Medicine: A Comprehensive Study Guide.* 8th ed. New York, NY: McGraw-Hill; 2012: 601-608.

36. The correct answer is A, Give a single dose of ciprofloxacin, 750 mg PO.

Why is this the correct answer?

Traveler's diarrhea is an exceedingly common ailment that affects up to half of all travelers returning from developing countries. It can usually be managed easily with a single dose of ciprofloxacin, 750 mg, along with symptomatic therapy, including loperamide. Multiple randomized controlled trials have proved the efficacy and safety of this approach. If the patient is having severe symptoms or if blood is visible in the stool (dysentery), treatment should be extended for 3 days, and the loperamide may be continued judiciously. In most areas of the world, enterotoxigenic *Escherichia coli* (ETEC) is the likely cause of the diarrhea. This is especially true in Mexico, Central America, and the Caribbean, where most travelers from North America are likely to visit. In southeast Asia, Campylobacter species are the most common. This is significant because Campylobacter has developed a high rate of quinolone resistance; azithromycin, 1,000 mg in a single dose, should be substituted for ciprofloxacin as first-line therapy for travelers returning from southeast Asia.

Why are the other choices wrong?

Metronidazole is first-line therapy for amoebiasis, which is characterized by the insidious onset of mucus and blood in the stools over a period of several weeks. This patient's symptoms are more acute and are more likely to have a bacterial or viral origin.

Traveler's diarrhea is self-limited and is unlikely to be harmful to an otherwise healthy patient. Reassurance and symptomatic therapy are a reasonable option. But extensive clinical evidence has demonstrated the safety and efficacy of antimicrobial therapy and a drastic reduction in the duration of symptoms. Since 75% of cases of traveler's diarrhea are caused by bacteria, antimicrobial treatment is warranted.

Traveler's diarrhea is a clinical diagnosis, and ordering laboratory stool studies, at least in this particular case, adds expense without adding value to the management of the patient. In the case of bloody stools or prolonged symptoms, laboratory testing can be useful.

PEER REVIEW

- ✓ If you're treating a patient who has just returned from a developing country with fever, cramps, nausea, and loose, nonbloody diarrhea, think traveler's diarrhea.
- ✓ Traveler's diarrhea is a self-limited disease usually caused by bacteria, and it is safely treated with a single-dose antimicrobial and an antimotility agent such as loperamide.
- ✓ Bloody diarrhea is dysentery, and the antimicrobial treatment should be extended for 3 days.

REFERENCES

Marx JA, Hockberger RS, Walls RM, eds. *Rosen's Emergency Medicine: Concepts and Clinical Practice*. 8th ed. St. Louis, MO: Elsevier; 2014: 254-260; 1233-1260.

Tintinalli JE, Stapczynski JS, Ma OJ, et al, eds. *Tintinalli's Emergency Medicine: A Comprehensive Study Guide*. 8th ed. New York, NY: McGraw-Hill; 2012: 1047-1057.

37. The correct answer is C, Thromboembolic event.

Why is this the correct answer?

From the history to the physical examination through the laboratory test results, this presentation is classic for nephrotic syndrome. One of the common risks associated with nephrotic syndrome is thromboembolic events. The cause of the hypercoagulable state in nephrotic syndrome is not well understood, but the condition creates an increased risk for thrombosis in the large vessels, including renal veins, deep veins, and the pulmonary vascular system. Another common complication is increased risk of severe infection, thought to be due to loss of complement, antibodies, and other immune-related proteins that are excreted via the urine. There is particular concern for *Streptococcus pneumoniae* spontaneous bacterial peritonitis among children who have developed ascites. Lower extremity edema, anasarca, periorbital edema, and ascites are common presenting complaints in nephrotic syndrome. They are the result of altered oncotic pressure from increased excretion of proteins due to alterations in the glomerular basement membrane. Nephrotic-range proteinuria is defined as more than 3.5 g of protein in 24 hours. There are many causes for nephrotic syndrome, ranging from primary renal disease to infection to medication side effects. Once this condition is recognized, it is important to obtain appropriate follow-up care and additional testing to confirm the diagnosis such as 24-hour urine collection and cholesterol levels (classically elevated to >200 mg/dL). Additional treatment might include diuretics with concomitant albumin administration and possible initiation of corticosteroids.

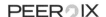

Why are the other choices wrong?

Diabetes mellitus might be a cause of nephrotic syndrome, but it does not occur as a result of the condition. Diabetic nephropathy would be suspected if there were glucose present on the urinalysis or hyperglycemia suggested by blood test results.

Patients with nephrotic syndrome have a hypercoagulable state, so a GI bleed is less likely to occur.

Urinary tract infection is generally not caused by nephrotic syndrome. Patients with nephrotic syndrome might be prone to more severe infections, but generally these are systemic, not focused on the urinary system.

PEER REVIEW

- ✓ Nephrotic syndrome clinically presents with edema — diffuse, periorbital, vulvar, scrotal, or in the extremities.
- ✓ Laboratory test results for patients with nephrotic syndrome include elevated protein levels on urinalysis and decreased albumin levels in the serum.
- ✓ The key risks for patients with nephrotic syndrome are thromboembolic events and severe infection.

REFERENCES

Marx JA, Hockberger RS, Walls RM, eds. *Rosen's Emergency Medicine: Concepts and Clinical Practice*. 8th ed. St. Louis, MO: Elsevier; 2014: 11291-1311.

Tintinalli JE, Stapczynski JS, Ma OJ, et al, eds. *Tintinalli's Emergency Medicine: A Comprehensive Study Guide*. 8th ed. New York, NY: McGraw-Hill; 2012: 881-888.

38. The correct answer is D, Woman with end-stage renal disease who goes to dialysis three times a week.

Why is this the correct answer?

Patients who regularly attend a dialysis clinic are considered at risk for health care-associated pneumonia (HCAP). Other risk factors include:

- Hospitalization within the past 3 months for 2 or more days
- Residence in a nursing home or long-term care facility
- Use of intravenous antibiotic therapy at home
- Chemotherapy
- Immunocompromise

Why are the other choices wrong?

Although the man with COPD has a chronic disease, his condition is stable, and he is not using immunocompromising medications, so he is not at risk to contract HCAP.

The nurse practitioner recently had surgery, but she was an outpatient. Because she did not stay in the hospital for 2 days or longer, she is not at risk either.

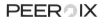

The paramedic most likely has been in and out of the emergency department and the hospital with sick patients multiple times, but because he has not been hospitalized, he does not meet the HCAP risk criteria.

PEER REVIEW

✓ Extended care facility patients are at risk for health care-associated pneumonia.

✓ Hospitalization for 2 days or longer within the previous 90 days is a risk factor for health care-associated pneumonia.

✓ Treatments and medications that increase the risk for health care-associated pneumonia: chemotherapy, prolonged intravenous antibiotic therapy, dialysis and wound care provided in specialty clinics, immunocompromising medications, including steroids, immunomodulators, and TNF-alpha inhibitors.

REFERENCES

Marx JA, Hockberger RS, Walls RM, eds. *Rosen's Emergency Medicine: Concepts and Clinical Practice*. 8th ed. St. Louis, MO: Elsevier; 2014: 978-987.

Tintinalli JE, Stapczynski JS, Ma OJ, et al, eds. *Tintinalli's Emergency Medicine: A Comprehensive Study Guide*. 8th ed. New York, NY: McGraw-Hill; 2012: 445-456.

39. The correct answer is B, Dyspnea.

Why is this the correct answer?

Although patients with PE can present in many ways, the most common uniting feature among them is dyspnea. It is present in more than 90% of patients with PE without infarction. Patients might present with dyspnea while at rest, but most have exertional dyspnea, both of which are due to irregular pulmonary blood flow from the occluded vessel. Pleuritic chest pain is a common presenting symptom as well but not as common as dyspnea. The Pulmonary Embolism Ruleout criteria (the PERC rule) are used to exclude the diagnosis of PE and avoid additional testing. These criteria rule out any patient with an oxygen saturation level above 94% on room air.

Why are the other choices wrong?

Chest pain is more likely with distal pulmonary emboli and is the second most common symptom, after dyspnea, for PE.

Hypotension is a physical examination finding, not a symptom. It is not likely to occur except in patients with very large hemodynamically compromising pulmonary emboli.

Hypoxia can occur, but it is not considered the most common finding. It is a sign, not a symptom.

PEER POINT

Pulmonary Embolism Ruleout Criteria (PERC Rule)

Can be applied to patients whom the treating physician believes are otherwise at low risk for PE based on clinical impression:

- Age younger than 50 years
- No exogenous hormone use
- No unilateral leg swelling
- Oxygen saturation above 94% on room air
- Pulse rate less than 100 beats per minute
- No prior history of PE or DVT
- No recent major surgery
- No hemoptysis

PEER REVIEW

✓ Symptoms are presenting complaints. Signs are found on physical examination.
✓ Hypoxia and hypotension can be present in large pulmonary emboli, but most pulmonary emboli are small and wouldn't cause these to occur.
✓ Dyspnea is the most common symptom found in patients presenting with PE.

REFERENCES

Marx JA, Hockberger RS, Walls RM, eds. *Rosen's Emergency Medicine: Concepts and Clinical Practice.* 8th ed. St. Louis, MO: Elsevier; 2014: 1157-1169.

Tintinalli JE, Stapczynski JS, Ma OJ, et al, eds. *Tintinalli's Emergency Medicine: A Comprehensive Study Guide.* 8th ed. New York, NY: McGraw-Hill; 2012: 388-399.

40. The correct answer is B, Lyme antibody.

Why is this the correct answer?

Syncope is a common presentation in emergency departments, up to almost 1% of visits. A good history and physical examination can often distinguish syncope from other confounding diagnoses (breath-holding spells, orthostatic hypotension). In children, syncope is most commonly vasovagal and least commonly cardiac (as opposed to adults). But in this case, the ECG shows a heart block that was causing episodes of syncope with such exaggerated myoclonic effects as to simulate a seizure. In endemic areas, rickettsial disease should be considered, especially when there is evidence of a heart block. Early disseminated disease can affect the heart and lead to the ECG changes as shown. Lyme carditis is found in up to 10% of untreated patients with Lyme disease and can present with nonspecific findings, including syncope or palpitations.

Why are the other choices wrong?

Antineutrophil antibody (ANA) is used in the evaluation of rheumatologic disease, which could lead to cardiac disease in time, but this is unlikely in an otherwise healthy child. Rheumatic cardiac disease is among the most common causes for acquired cardiac issues in children but is evaluated using testing for streptococcal infection and not an ANA titer.

Electrolyte abnormality is an important component of the evaluation of arrhythmia, and potassium levels can be inferred by the appearance of the T wave on the ECG. If there is a history of poor oral intake or increased losses due to vomiting or diarrhea, electrolyte evaluation would be needed, but in this otherwise well child and with no evidence of abnormal T waves on the ECG, this is not warranted.

Acute myocardial injury is rare in children except those with a history of Kawasaki disease, sickle cell anemia, or cardiac surgery. Although this child has a history of cardiac surgery, the ECG shows no evidence of ischemic injury.

PEER REVIEW

- ✓ Syncope has a broad differential diagnosis, but the most common type is vasovagal.
- ✓ The physical examination and history can narrow down the causes and guide additional testing.
- ✓ Does the patient live in a community where Lyme disease is endemic? If yes, consider that in the evaluation of syncope.

REFERENCES
Fleisher GR, Ludwig S, et al, eds. *Textbook of Pediatric Emergency Medicine*. 6th ed. Philadelphia, PA: Lippincott, Williams & Wilkins; 2010: 589-595, 1026-1027.
Wolfson AB, Hendey GW, Ling LJ, et al, eds. *Harwood-Nuss' Clinical Practice of Emergency Medicine*. 6th ed. Philadelphia, PA: Lippincott, Williams & Wilkins; 2014: 900-906, 1145-1149.

41. The correct answer is C, Provide supplemental oxygen.

Why is this the correct answer?

The mainstay of treatment for CO poisoning is removing the patient from the source of CO and delivering maximal oxygen as soon as possible. This patient has symptoms of acute CO poisoning with a corresponding elevated carboxyhemoglobin percentage. Providing the maximal amount of supplemental oxygen by nonrebreather facemask or endotracheal tube (if indicated for airway control) is the next best step in this scenario. The half-life of carboxyhemoglobin is drastically reduced from an average of 5 hours for patients breathing room air to roughly 1 hour when breathing 100% oxygen.

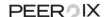

Why are the other choices wrong?

Exchange transfusion has no known role in the management of CO toxicity. It does have a role in the management of sickle cell disease, thrombotic thrombocytopenic purpura, and hemolytic disease of the newborn.

For inhalational CO exposures, serial measurements of carboxyhemoglobin are not necessary and do not change management. After the patient is removed from the CO source, the carboxyhemoglobin level predictably decreases, and oxygen therapy accelerates this.

Hyperbaric oxygen (HBO) therapy is a suitable treatment for this patient, but the most important first step is to supply maximal oxygen by nonrebreather mask or endotracheal tube. Providing HBO therapy for CO poisoning remains controversial. The primary goal of using it is to decrease the risk of persistent or delayed neurologic sequelae. The patient in this case does meet several suggested criteria for HBO treatment (syncope, coma, seizure, altered mental status or confusion, carboxyhemoglobin >25%, abnormal cerebellar function, age ≥36, prolonged CO exposure [≥24 hours], fetal distress in pregnancy). Transferring him to a facility for HBO treatment might certainly be considered — while he is already receiving supplemental oxygen.

PEER REVIEW

- ✓ Remember the mainstays of CO poisoning treatment: identify it, remove the victim from the source, and give oxygen.
- ✓ The primary goal of HBO therapy in CO poisoning is to decrease the risk of persistent or delayed neurologic sequelae.

REFERENCES

Hoffman RS, Howland MA, Lewin NA, et al. *Goldfrank's Toxicologic Emergencies*. 10th ed. New York, NY: McGraw-Hill; 2010: 1584-1588.

Tintinalli JE, Stapczynski JS, Ma OJ, et al, eds. *Tintinalli's Emergency Medicine: A Comprehensive Study Guide*. 8th ed. New York, NY: McGraw-Hill; 2012: 1439.

42. The correct answer is D, Upper sacral fractures can injure nerve roots and result in loss of perineal sensation and rectal tone.

Why is this the correct answer?

Upper sacral fractures can involve the neural foramina of the sacrum, thereby injuring the sacral nerve roots. Sacral nerve root injury can lead to difficulty voiding or sexual dysfunction. Patients might also present with decreased anal sphincter tone and changes in sensation or even loss of sensation in the perineum. There is a rich vascular supply to the pelvis, and sacral injury is commonly associated with pelvic vascular trauma and hemodynamic instability. Upper sacral fractures can be difficult to diagnose clinically and with plain films. Clues to possible injury of the sacrum include asymmetry of the sacral neural foramina and avulsion of the L5 transverse process or ischial spine.

Why are the other choices wrong?

Anteroposterior compression forces most commonly injure the pubic symphysis, leading to disruption or rupture. These forces can also injure the pubic rami, leading to vertical fractures of the rami. Severe AP compression such as that which occurs in a high-speed motor vehicle collision can also disrupt the posterior sacrospinous ligaments and lead to an "open book" fracture.

Anterior fractures with AP compression forces are more likely to injure the genitourinary tract than are fractures resulting from lateral compression or from sacral fractures, which are typically caused by a fall from a height in which there is vertical shear. Patients with anterior pelvic trauma might present with hematuria or an inability to void if the urethra is disrupted or obstructed by hematoma or clot.

Injury vectors that increase pelvic volume are much more likely to injure pelvic vessels due to stretching forces on the vessels. Compressive forces leading to decreased volume of the pelvis are less likely to cause significant bleeding, in general.

PEER POINT

The three main vectors leading to traumatic pelvic injuries can help you identify the injury pattern

- High-speed motor vehicle collision ⇒ AP compression ⇒ Bladder injury, hematuria, dislocation of pubic symphysis, fracture of pubic bones
- Fall from height ⇒ Vertical shear ⇒ Sacral fracture, sacral nerve root injury
- Fall from height or blow from the side ⇒ Lateral compression sacral fracture

PEER REVIEW

- ✓ Sacral fractures are the result of vertical shear or lateral compression forces and can lead to neurovascular injury.
- ✓ Injury to the sacral nerve roots can lead to decreased perineal sensation, decreased anal sphincter tone, and sexual dysfunction.
- ✓ Sacral fracture can be associated with significant vascular injury.

REFERENCES

Broder J. *Diagnostic Imaging for the Emergency Physician*. Philadelphia, PA: Saunders; 2011.

Marx JA, Hockberger RS, Walls RM, eds. *Rosen's Emergency Medicine: Concepts and Clinical Practice*. 8th ed. St. Louis, MO: Elsevier; 2014: 656-663.

Wolfson AB, Hendey GW, Ling LJ, et al, eds. *Harwood-Nuss' Clinical Practice of Emergency Medicine*. 6th ed. Philadelphia, PA: Lippincott, Williams & Wilkins; 2014: 277-284.

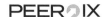

43. The correct answer is B, Enophthalmos.

Why is this the correct answer?

Enophthalmos occurs when the globe is posteriorly displaced within the orbit and a "sunken eye" can be seen on physical examination. This can occur as the result of an orbital blowout fracture of the affected eye or a loss of orbital contents. Another concerning physical examination finding in orbital blowout fracture is binocular diplopia, which can occur due to extraocular muscle entrapment in the fracture. An additional concerning examination finding is infraorbital numbness of the cheek or lip due to infraorbital nerve involvement. Subcutaneous emphysema can also occur and can indicate concomitant sinus fracture. Obvious displacement of the globe or a palpable step-off of the orbit is also indicative of fracture. A maxillofacial CT scan should be obtained if there is any concern for orbital or facial fracture on physical examination.

Why are the other choices wrong?

Ecchymosis can occur with or without fracture. The periorbital tissues are very susceptible to distention that can occur with blunt trauma, so swelling and ecchymosis are common even when a fracture is not present. Ecchymosis is not specific for orbital blowout fracture.

Exophthalmos occurs when the globe is displaced anteriorly. This can occur with retrobulbar hematoma, or it can occur insidiously due to nontraumatic causes such as orbital tumor or Graves disease. Exophthalmos is not specific for orbital blowout fracture.

Photophobia can occur for many reasons. The most common reason in trauma is traumatic iritis, resulting in ciliary spasm.

PEER REVIEW

- ✓ Orbital blowout fractures are highly suspected when the trauma results in enophthalmos.
- ✓ Diplopia, orbital step-off, and infraorbital numbness raise concern for orbital fracture.

REFERENCES

Marx JA, Hockberger RS, Walls RM, eds. *Rosen's Emergency Medicine: Concepts and Clinical Practice.* 8th ed. St. Louis, MO: Elsevier; 2014: 909-910.

Wolfson AB, Hendey GW, Ling LJ, et al, eds. *Harwood-Nuss' Clinical Practice of Emergency Medicine.* 6th ed. Philadelphia, PA: Lippincott, Williams & Wilkins; 2014: 160-161, 176-179.

44. The correct answer is C, Posterior fourchette.

Why is this the correct answer?

Approximately 1 in 6 women is sexually assaulted during her lifetime. Findings of the genital examination are frequently completely normal despite the sexual assault. However, when sexual assault-related vaginal injuries are present, the majority occur to the posterior fourchette, which is a tense band of mucous membrane connection formed at the posterior aspect by the labia minora. Although not routine, the use of colposcopy during the genital examination can increase the rate of detecting injury from 6% to 53%. Applying toluidine to the perineum can also enhance detection of genital injuries.

Why are the other choices wrong?

Novice examiners frequently concern themselves with detecting injuries to the hymen. However, hymenal injuries are rare in sexually active adult women and are more commonly observed in adolescents who had had minimal or no sexual intercourse before the assault. The hymen is a thin, membranous fold of tissue that is highly variable in appearance. It might not be clearly identifiable even in females who have not had sexual intercourse.

Labia are not the most commonly injured part of the female anatomy. Labial hematomas and lacerations are associated with straddle injuries. If such injuries are noted after a straddle injury, the patient should be evaluated for possible urethral injury or pelvic fractures.

Injuries to the vaginal wall are rare. However, injuries to the vaginal wall and cervix might be noted during speculum examination and should be carefully documented.

PEER POINT

Anatomical sites, female external genitalia

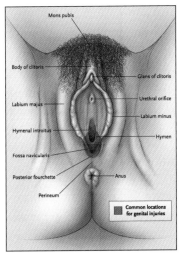

PEER Point 3

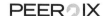

PEER REVIEW

✓ Genital examination findings are often normal following sexual assault.

✓ The genital area most commonly injured after sexual assault is the posterior fourchette.

✓ Colposcopy and toluidine application can increase the rate of detecting injury during the sexual assault examination.

REFERENCES

Marx JA, Hockberger RS, Walls RM, eds. *Rosen's Emergency Medicine: Concepts and Clinical Practice*. 8th ed. St. Louis, MO: Elsevier; 2014: 855-871.

Roberts JR, Hedges JR, eds. *Clinical Procedures in Emergency Medicine*. 6th ed. St. Louis, MO: WB Saunders; 2013: 1069-1074.

45. The correct answer is D, Left-sided weakness for the past 2 hours.

Why is this the correct answer?

Succinylcholine is a depolarizing neuromuscular blocking agent used in rapid sequence intubation. It has a more rapid onset and shorter duration of action than nondepolarizing neuromuscular blocking agents but carries the risks of bradycardia, hyperkalemia, masseter spasm, and malignant hyperthermia. Contraindications to succinylcholine include risk factors for hyperkalemia (burns over >10% BSA, crush injuries, neuromuscular diseases, spinal cord injuries, strokes, and intraabdominal sepsis), history of malignant hyperthermia, and recent amphetamine use. Of note, the risk for severe hyperkalemia is not significant until after the first 5 days for burns, crush injuries, spinal cord injuries, strokes, and intra-abdominal sepsis. The severe hyperkalemic response is due to acetylcholine receptor upregulation at the neuromuscular junction, which takes several days to develop. Therefore, a patient with an acute stroke may be given succinylcholine without increased risk for hyperkalemia. Bradycardia is more common in children and is typically self-limiting but may be treated with atropine. Masseter spasm may be treated with dantrolene or a nondepolarizing neuromuscular blocking agent.

Why are the other choices wrong?

Neuromuscular diseases (including amyotrophic lateral sclerosis and multiple sclerosis) result in upregulation of acetylcholine receptors at the neuromuscular junction, which can cause an exaggerated hyperkalemic response to succinylcholine. Succinylcholine is contraindicated in these patients regardless of time of diagnosis or severity of disease.

Succinylcholine is a known cause of malignant hyperthermia, and patients with a prior diagnosis of malignant hyperthermia should receive nondepolarizing neuromuscular blocking agents. Due to a pathophysiologic overlap between masseter spasm and malignant hyperthermia, all patients who develop masseter spasm should undergo future testing for susceptibility to malignant hyperthermia.

Patients who have recently used amphetamines (including cocaine) might have a prolonged duration of neuromuscular blockade because these agents competitively inhibit plasma cholinesterase, which reduces the amount of enzyme available for succinylcholine metabolism.

PEER POINT

Contraindications to succinylcholine use

- Burns covering more than 10% BSA (>5 days after injury until healed)
- Crush injuries (>5 days after injury until healed)
- Intra-abdominal sepsis (>5 days after onset until healed)
- Spinal cord injuries (>5 days after injury until healed)
- Strokes (>5 days onset until healed)
- History of malignant hyperthermia
- Neuromuscular diseases (amyotrophic lateral sclerosis, multiple sclerosis)
- Recent cocaine or amphetamine use

PEER REVIEW

✓ Don't use succinylcholine in patients with risk factors for hyperkalemia, history of malignant hyperthermia, and recent amphetamine use.

✓ Patients with burns, crush injuries, intra-abdominal sepsis, spinal cord injuries, and strokes are at high risk for severe hyperkalemia from succinylcholine use only starting 5 days after insult.

REFERENCES

Marx JA, Hockberger RS, Walls RM, eds. *Rosen's Emergency Medicine: Concepts and Clinical Practice*. 8th ed. St. Louis, MO: Elsevier; 2014: 855-871.

Tintinalli JE, Stapczynski JS, Ma OJ, et al, eds. *Tintinalli's Emergency Medicine: A Comprehensive Study Guide*. 8th ed. New York, NY: McGraw-Hill; 2012: 1620-1621.

46. The correct answer is B, 40-year-old woman with a respiratory rate of 20 and a strong radial pulse who is unable to follow simple commands.

Why is this the correct answer?

The purpose of any triage system is to sort patients by priority into categories for treatment and transport. Those categories typically are minor, delayed, immediate, expectant, and dead. In this situation, the 40-year-old woman is categorized as immediate (and thus the highest priority) because of her inability to follow simple commands. This categorization is based on one of the most commonly used systems in the United States: simple triage and rapid treatment, or START. Mass casualty triage becomes necessary whenever the available resources are insufficient to care for the number of patients at a given time. Triage is considered a dynamic process; as additional resources become available and as patients' conditions change,

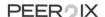
treatment priorities may be altered. However, it has been shown that there is a clear relationship between overtriage and poor patient outcomes during mass casualty incidents.

Why are the other choices wrong?

The 21-year-old man should be categorized as dead because he is apneic despite an airway-opening maneuver.

The 42-year-old man is ambulatory and can be considered minor.

The 85-year-old woman, because she has a normal respiratory rate and palpable radial pulse and is able to follow commands, should be categorized as delayed.

PEER POINT

START mass casualty triage card

M I N O R	D E C E A S E D	I M M E D I A T E		
				Move Walking Wounded
				No **Resp** after head tilt
				Breathing but **Unconscious**
				Resp -> 30
				Perfusion
				Cap refill > 2 sec or No radial Pulse *Control bleeding*
				Mental Status— Can't follow simple commands
		D E L A Y E D		Otherwise
				Remember R – 30 P – 2 M – Can do

PEER Point 4

PEER REVIEW

✓ When is it right to use a mass casualty triage approach? Anytime the number of patients exceeds available resources.

✓ Here are the five triage categories: minor, delayed, immediate, expectant, and dead.

✓ START stands for simple triage and rapid treatment. It's one of the most commonly used mass casualty triage tools.

REFERENCES

NAEMSP EMS Text, Prehospital Triage for Mass Casualties, Volume 4, Chapter 2

Tintinalli JE, Stapczynski JS, Ma OJ, et al, eds. *Tintinalli's Emergency Medicine: A Comprehensive Study Guide*. 8th ed. New York, NY: McGraw-Hill; 2012: 28.

47. The correct answer is B, Critical illness or injury with a high probability of deterioration.

Why is this the correct answer?

Critical care is a time-based billing designation that, if documented correctly, is an appropriately billable service for emergency departments and providers. To be eligible for critical care billing, the documentation of the encounter must show that the patient had a critical injury or illness. The American Medical Association defines critical illness or injury as one that acutely impairs one or more vital organ systems such that there is a high probability of imminent or life-threatening deterioration in the patient's condition. Some of the components of critical care time include direct patient care, time spent gathering history from old records and from family, interpretation of test results, time spent documenting the patient's record, and time spent discussing the case with consultants and other physicians.

Why are the other choices wrong?

Exclusive of separately billable procedures, emergency physicians must spend at least 30 minutes (not 45) on patient care to bill for critical care. The initial billing window is for 30 to 74 minutes; the next is for 75 to 104 minutes.

Previous definitions of critical care required that the patient have some level of hemodynamic instability or potential for instability, but this is no longer a requirement. Patients can be stable and still qualify for critical care time if they have critical illnesses or injuries and have the potential to deteriorate.

There is no specific requirement for vasopressors, invasive monitoring, airway management, or other specific interventions. These interventions, in most cases, qualify a patient for critical care, but they are not required to meet the definition.

PEER REVIEW

✓ To bill for critical care services, the physician must have cared for a patient with a critical illness or injury who had a high probability of deterioration.

✓ You must have spent at least 30 minutes on care to bill for critical care time.

✓ Billed critical care time may not include time spent on separately billable procedures.

REFERENCES

American Medical Association. *Current Procedural Terminology, 2016 Professional Edition*. Chicago, IL: AMA; 2017: 608, 771, 772.
Strauss RW, Mayer TA. *Emergency Department Management*. New York, NY: McGraw-Hill; 2014: 23.

48. The correct answer is A, Abdominal pain and vomiting are common.

Why is this the correct answer?

Alcoholic ketoacidosis typically occurs in undernourished alcoholics who have recently binged on alcohol and have had limited food intake. Abdominal pain and vomiting are common. These symptoms might be related to the condition, but a thorough evaluation for other etiologies such as pancreatitis is necessary. These patients characteristically have a normal mental status despite the presence of potentially severe acidosis, and this helps distinguish alcoholic ketoacidosis from poisoning with a toxic alcohol. The acidosis in alcoholic ketoacidosis predominantly results from the presence of beta-hydroxybutyrate (a ketoacid that is not typically detected as a ketone on urinalysis). As with most acidosis, tachypnea is expected. Treatment of alcoholic ketoacidosis involves hydration with glucose-containing solutions, thiamine, food intake, and treatment of any other underlying medical conditions.

Why are the other choices wrong?

As with other etiologies of metabolic acidosis such as diabetic ketoacidosis, tachypnea is expected as a normal compensatory mechanism, not bradypnea.

Preservation of mental status is characteristic of alcoholic ketoacidosis even when severe acidosis is present. This helps distinguish it from toxicity from toxic alcohols.

Although a not insignificant percentage of patients who present with alcoholic ketoacidosis have measurable ethanol levels, intoxication is not typical.

PEER REVIEW

- ✓ Abdominal pain and vomiting are common in alcoholic ketoacidosis, but look carefully for other causes such as pancreatitis.
- ✓ It's characteristic of alcoholic ketoacidosis for a patient to have a normal mental status despite significant acidosis.

REFERENCES

McGuire LC, Cruickshank AM, Munro PT. Alcoholic ketoacidosis. *Emerg Med J*. 2006;23(6):417-420.

Tintinalli JE, Stapczynski JS, Ma OJ, et al, eds. *Tintinalli's Emergency Medicine: A Comprehensive Study Guide*. 8th ed. New York, NY: McGraw-Hill; 2012: 1464-1465.

49. The correct answer is A, Aspirin.

Why is this the correct answer?

The decision to administer activated charcoal to prevent absorption requires multiple considerations: how dangerous an agent is in overdose, how effectively it is adsorbed by charcoal, the quantity ingested if known, how much time has passed since the ingestion, whether an effective antidote exists, the potential for unknown coingestants, and the presence of contraindications to administration. Of the agents listed, aspirin is the only one for which charcoal administration should be considered. Aspirin is adsorbed well by charcoal. Even non-enteric-coated aspirin can have very delayed absorption in overdose, making charcoal administration potentially effective even beyond 1 hour following ingestion.

Why are the other choices wrong?

Alcohols such as ethanol, ethylene glycol, and methanol are rapidly absorbed, so such patients are poor candidates for charcoal administration even if there is some adsorption.

Most metals such as iron and lithium demonstrate poor binding to charcoal.

Charcoal administration following the ingestion of a caustic agent such as sodium hydroxide is generally contraindicated. Toxicity from most caustic agents is predominantly from local tissue injury (not systemic absorption). Any vomiting precipitated by charcoal administration can be harmful. If endoscopy is performed, charcoal can obscure visibility.

PEER POINT

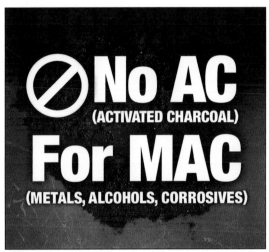

PEER Point 5

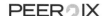

PEER REVIEW

✓ Aspirin, even the non-enteric-coated pills, is well adsorbed to activated charcoal. You can consider it even beyond an hour after ingestion.

✓ Don't use activated charcoal to treat a caustic agent ingestion.

REFERENCES
Hoffman RS, Howland MA, Lewin NA, et al. *Goldfrank's Toxicologic Emergencies*. 10th ed. New York, NY: McGraw-Hill; 2010:83-96.
Tintinalli JE, Stapczynski JS, Ma OJ, et al, eds. *Tintinalli's Emergency Medicine: A Comprehensive Study Guide*. 8th ed. New York, NY: McGraw-Hill; 2012: 1207-1213.

50. The correct answer is C, Severe hypertension.

Why is this the correct answer?

Noninvasive ventilation (NIV), which includes continuous positive-pressure ventilation (CPAP) and bilevel positive-pressure ventilation (BPAP), is an approach to providing positive-pressure airway support through the use of a face mask without the invasiveness of endotracheal intubation. In addition to assisting with work of breathing, NIV decreases both preload and afterload, which can augment cardiac output (which is one rationale for its benefit in acute heart failure). Thus while hypotension is a contraindication to NIV use, patients with hypertension might actually benefit from NIV. Noninvasive ventilation also has been shown to decrease hospital length of stay, frequency of endotracheal intubations, and mortality rates in specific patient groups when used appropriately. Contraindications include absent or agonal respiratory effort, altered level of consciousness, maxillofacial trauma, potential basilar skull fracture, life-threatening epistaxis, vomiting, and severe hypotension.

Why are the other choices wrong?

Altered level of consciousness is a contraindication to NIV because the patient might not be able to protect the airway and is at risk for aspiration. Any patient who presents concern for inadequate airway protection should undergo endotracheal intubation.

Maxillofacial trauma is a contraindication to NIV because of the potential for pneumocephalus, bacterial meningitis, and diffuse subcutaneous emphysema. Use of NIV in patients with any active nasopharyngeal or intraoral bleeding can increase the risk of aspiration as well. It is important to note that remote history of maxillofacial trauma is not a contraindication but might result in poor mask fit. Any patient with acute maxillofacial trauma should not receive NIV.

Vomiting is a contraindication to NIV because the positive pressure might force the vomit into the lungs, resulting in aspiration and possible chemical pneumonitis. Any patient with significant upper airway secretions, which includes both vomit and blood, should not receive NIV.

PEER POINT

Contraindications to NIV

- Absent or agonal respiratory effort
- Altered level of consciousness
- Life-threatening epistaxis
- Maxillofacial trauma
- Potential basilar skull fracture
- Severe hypotension
- Vomiting

PEER REVIEW

- ✓ Don't use noninvasive ventilation in patients with absent or agonal respiratory effort, altered level of consciousness, maxillofacial trauma, potential basilar skull fracture, life threatening epistaxis, vomiting, or severe hypotension.
- ✓ If you're worried about inadequate airway protection, use endotracheal intubation instead of noninvasive ventilation.

REFERENCES

Marx JA, Hockberger RS, Walls RM, eds. *Rosen's Emergency Medicine: Concepts and Clinical Practice*. 8th ed. St. Louis, MO: Elsevier; 2014: 25-26.

Tintinalli JE, Stapczynski JS, Ma OJ, et al, eds. *Tintinalli's Emergency Medicine: A Comprehensive Study Guide*. 8th ed. New York, NY: McGraw-Hill; 2012: 178-183.

51. The correct answer is A, Bidirectional ventricular tachycardia.

Why is this the correct answer?

Digoxin-induced ventricular tachycardia is life-threatening and should be managed by administration of digoxin-specific antibody fragments. Bidirectional ventricular tachycardia is an unusual rhythm caused by toxicity from very few agents, digoxin being one. Digoxin inhibits the Na+-K+-ATPase pump leading to increased intracellular calcium concentrations. In toxicity, this inhibition causes increased myocardial automaticity and excitability and/or vagally mediated bradycardic and conduction problems. Ventricular tachycardia, ventricular fibrillation, a wide variety of bradyarrhythmias, and various degrees of heart block can all be seen with digoxin toxicity. Digoxin toxicity can cause nearly every arrhythmia with the exception of rapidly conducted atrial tachyarrhythmias (such as atrial fibrillation with rapid ventricular response).

Why are the other choices wrong?

In the setting of chronic digoxin toxicity, the clinical status of the patient, predominantly the presence or absence of cardiac arrhythmias, not the digoxin concentration or hyperkalemia, should be the principal determinant of whether to administer digoxin-specific antibody fragments. In acute poisoning, the presence of

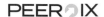
hyperkalemia and very elevated digoxin concentrations (>10 ng/mL) can guide the administration of digoxin-specific antibody fragments before arrhythmias develop.

The presence of hyperkalemia in chronic digoxin poisoning typically reflects underlying renal insufficiency and corresponding decreased potassium elimination. Renal insufficiency with the corresponding decreased clearance of digoxin is a common cause of chronic digoxin toxicity. In acute poisoning, hyperkalemia reflects poisoning of Na+-K+-ATPase, precedes the onset of arrhythmias, and is an indication for digoxin-specific antibody fragments, but hyperkalemia alone is not an indication to administer the antidote in chronic digoxin poisoning.

Vomiting is a symptom, albeit a very nonspecific one, of digoxin toxicity. Vomiting alone is not an indication to administer the antidote.

PEER REVIEW

✓ Digoxin-specific antibody fragments are indicated when a patient has life-threatening ventricular arrhythmias in the setting of digoxin toxicity.

✓ Digoxin and other cardiac glycoside toxicity can cause almost any arrhythmia except for rapidly conducted atrial arrhythmias.

REFERENCES

Hoffman RS, Howland MA, Lewin NA, et al. *Goldfrank's Toxicologic Emergencies*. 10th ed. New York, NY: McGraw-Hill; 2010: 898-899.

Tintinalli JE, Stapczynski JS, Ma OJ, et al, eds. *Tintinalli's Emergency Medicine: A Comprehensive Study Guide*. 8th ed. New York, NY: McGraw-Hill; 2012: 1284-1287.

52. The correct answer is B, Corrosive substance ingestion.

Why is this the correct answer?

Although there is no standard of care regarding gastric lavage in poisonings, some patients with potentially life-threatening ingestions can benefit if it is performed within 60 to 120 minutes of ingestion. The indication for lavage is simply that the benefits of gastric emptying outweigh the associated risks. Contraindications include the following: the patient has lost or will lose airway-protective reflexes; alkaline or acidic caustic ingestion; foreign body ingestion (body packers/drug pouch); ingestion of a substance with high aspiration potential in the absence of intubation; known esophageal strictures; and history of gastric bypass surgery. The ideal technique involves passing a lubricated gastric tube into the pharynx. The patient's chin should then be put to his or her chest to facilitate esophageal passage. Once the tube has been passed, correct placement in the stomach is confirmed by auscultation over the gastric area and aspiration with removal of gastric contents. Then small aliquots (200 to 300 mL in adults) of water are repeatedly delivered into the stomach with subsequent removal of the water while the patient is in the left lateral decubitus position. Of note, oral administration of charcoal alone is superior if the ingestion is adsorbed by charcoal. Corrosive substances cause rapid corrosive lesions in the GI tract, most often with alkali ingestions. The substance should be diluted with water or milk within 60 minutes, but lavage is contraindicated because it can worsen lesions and lead to other complications such as perforation or strictures.

Why are the other choices wrong?

Acetaminophen overdose is not a contraindication to lavage. However, acetaminophen is rapidly absorbed and has an antidote; thus gastric emptying is generally not recommended. Activated charcoal has been shown in the acute interval to minimize absorption and lower N-acetylcysteine requirements.

Intubation is not a contraindication to lavage. Rather, it is often ideal in patients at risk of losing airway patency or those who have ingested a substance with a high aspiration potential. Intubation reduces the risk of aspiration during lavage. Intubated patients may undergo lavage while supine for logistical reasons.

Gastric lavage is used to treat pesticide (organophosphate) ingestions given the elevated associated levels of toxicity. It is particularly common in Asia, where pesticides are the second most common toxic ingestion. However, given rapid symptom onset, it is unlikely to benefit patients except those who present within 60 to 120 minutes. Hydrocarbons are a relative contraindication given their elevated risk of aspiration unless the airway is protected.

PEER POINT

Contraindications to gastric lavage

- Unprotected airway
- Hydrocarbon ingestion (unless intubated)
- Corrosive ingestion
- Foreign body ingestion
- Bleeding diatheses
- Known esophageal strictures
- History of gastric bypass surgery
- Small children

PEER REVIEW

- ✓ In an acute presentation, gastric lavage can help decontaminate a toxic ingestion.
- ✓ With definitive airway protection, the risk of aspiration in gastric lavage significantly decreases.
- ✓ Outcomes for corrosive ingestions, particularly alkali ingestions, are worsened following lavage.

REFERENCES

Hoffman RS, Howland MA, Lewin NA, et al. *Goldfrank's Toxicologic Emergencies*. 10th ed. New York, NY: McGraw-Hill; 2010:83-85.

Roberts JR, Hedges JR, eds. *Clinical Procedures in Emergency Medicine*. 6th ed. St. Louis, Mo: WB Saunders; 2013: 838-843.

Tintinalli JE, Stapczynski JS, Ma OJ, et al, eds. *Tintinalli's Emergency Medicine: A Comprehensive Study Guide*. 8th ed. New York, NY: McGraw-Hill; 2012: 1211-1212.

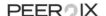

53. The correct answer is C, Normal mental status; serum sodium 104 mEq/L.

Why is this the correct answer?

The most feared complication in the treatment of hyponatremia is development of osmotic demyelination syndrome, which can manifest with permanent neurologic deficits and death. Patients at high risk for this, and in whom rapid serum sodium correction is contraindicated, primarily include those in whom hyponatremia has developed slowly. The patient in the case, who has an extremely low sodium level of 104 mEq/L and a normal mental status, must have a slow-developing hyponatremia. Hyponatremia manifests primarily with neurologic symptoms, the severity of which depends on the rate of hyponatremia development and its degree. When hyponatremia develops slowly, brain cells adjust intracellular solute concentration. This adaptation predisposes the cells to damage when serum sodium is corrected too rapidly. In acute-onset hyponatremia, water (but not sodium, due to the blood-brain barrier) from the hyposmolar serum can enter the hyperosmolar brain cells and cause cerebral edema. In these cases such as scenarios of acute large volume water ingestion and excessive water intake during a marathon, rapid correction with 3% hypertonic saline is considered safe.

Why are the other choices wrong?

A patient who rapidly ingests a large quantity of water and presents comatose with a serum sodium level of 117 mEq/L is manifesting a severe symptom (coma). Due to the rapidity of the onset of hyponatremia, such a patient is not at risk for complications from rapid serum sodium correction.

A patient who develops hyponatremia during a marathon has ingested too much free water over a relatively short period of time. Delirium is a severe symptom that might represent cerebral edema. Due to the rapidity of hyponatremia onset, the patient is not at risk for complications from rapid serum sodium correction.

A patient in status epilepticus with a serum sodium of 114 mEq/L is manifesting a life-threatening complication of hyponatremia, and so administration of 3% hypertonic saline is indicated.

PEER REVIEW

✓ Hypertonic saline administration for the treatment of hyponatremia should be reserved only for those patients with severe neurologic symptoms.

✓ Patients with severe hyponatremia but without severe neurological symptoms have had a gradual development of hyponatremia and are at high risk for osmotic demyelination syndrome with rapid serum sodium correction.

REFERENCES

Sterns RH. Disorders of plasma sodium—causes, consequences, and correction. *N Engl J Med.* 2015;372(1):55-64.

Tintinalli JE, Stapczynski JS, Ma OJ, et al, eds. *Tintinalli's Emergency Medicine: A Comprehensive Study Guide.* 8th ed. New York, NY: McGraw-Hill; 2012: 96-97.

54. The correct answer is A, Activate the cardiac catheterization laboratory.

Why is this the correct answer?

The patient described in this case is post-cardiac arrest with an ECG demonstrating an anteroseptal STEMI. Important early interventions in post-cardiac arrest patients with STEMI are blood pressure monitoring, activation of the cardiac catheterization laboratory for PCI, and consideration of therapeutic hypothermia. In patients who are appropriate candidates, therapeutic hypothermia may be initiated at the same time the catheterization lab is activated; some studies have shown improved outcomes without an increase in bleeding rates when these therapies are combined. Fibrinolytic therapy is a reasonable alternative in a non-PCI-capable facility.

Why are the other choices wrong?

This patient will be admitted to the ICU eventually, but he should be treated with PCI or fibrinolytic agents first. Activation of the cardiac catheterization laboratory should be considered in all post-cardiac arrest patients with evidence of STEMI on ECG.

Initiation of therapeutic hypothermia is recommended in all patients who remain comatose after resuscitation from cardiac arrest. However, this patient is awake, alert, and responding to commands and is thus not a candidate for therapeutic hypothermia.

Placement of a central venous catheter might be necessary in patients with fluid-refractory hypotension after cardiac arrest, but it does not need to be done emergently in most patients. It is also important to consider placement of an intra-aortic balloon pump (IABP) or percutaneous ventricular assist device in patients with refractory hypotension after STEMI or cardiac arrest.

PEER REVIEW

✓ Get an ECG in all post-cardiac arrest patients to assess for STEMI, which requires emergent coronary reperfusion.
✓ Consider therapeutic hypothermia in all comatose post-cardiac arrest patients.

REFERENCES

Marx JA, Hockberger RS, Walls RM, eds. *Rosen's Emergency Medicine: Concepts and Clinical Practice*. 8th ed. St. Louis, MO: Elsevier; 2014: 1022-1033.

Tintinalli JE, Stapczynski JS, Ma OJ, et al, eds. *Tintinalli's Emergency Medicine: A Comprehensive Study Guide*. 8th ed. New York, NY: McGraw-Hill; 2012: 175-176.

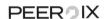

55. The correct answer is C, Pyridoxine.

Why is this the correct answer?

The primary manifestations of acute isoniazid poisoning are convulsions refractory to conventional therapy, coma, and metabolic acidosis. The principal treatment is the administration of pyridoxine (vitamin B6). Glutamate, the main excitatory neurotransmitter in the CNS is converted by a pyridoxine-dependent pathway to GABA, the main inhibitor neurotransmitter in the CNS. An overdose of isoniazid depletes pyridoxine by increasing excretion and causes inactivation of the active form of pyridoxine needed to convert glutamate to GABA. The combination of too much excitatory glutamate and not enough inhibitory GABA leads to convulsions that can be refractory to benzodiazepines (benzodiazepines require the presence of GABA to work). In this scenario, pyridoxine administration is required. Metabolic acidosis (lactic acidosis) predominantly occurs from the presence of convulsions.

Why are the other choices wrong?

Niacin (vitamin B3) is an essential dietary component. Deficiency causes pellagra characterized by the 3 Ds: dermatitis, diarrhea, and dementia. It does not have a role in the treatment of acute isoniazid poisoning.

Phytonadione (vitamin K1) is an essential fat-soluble vitamin. Its primary medical use is for the reversal of the effects of warfarin in the setting of bleeding or supratherapeutic effects. It does not have a role in the treatment of acute isoniazid poisoning.

Thiamine (vitamin B1) is water-soluble vitamin. Deficiency is responsible for wet beriberi, characterized by congestive heart failure, and dry beriberi, consisting of nervous system pathology such as Wernicke encephalopathy (triad of ataxia, altered mental status, and ophthalmoplegia) and Wernicke-Korsakoff syndrome. It does not have a role in the treatment of acute isoniazid poisoning.

PEER REVIEW

✓ The principal manifestation of acute isoniazid poisoning is convulsions.
✓ The antidote for isoniazid overdose is pyridoxine (vitamin B6).

REFERENCES

Hoffman RS, Howland MA, Lewin NA, et al. *Goldfrank's Toxicologic Emergencies*. 10th ed. New York, NY: McGraw-Hill; 2010:787-791.

Tintinalli JE, Stapczynski JS, Ma OJ, et al, eds. *Tintinalli's Emergency Medicine: A Comprehensive Study Guide*. 8th ed. New York, NY: McGraw-Hill; 2012: 1342-1343, 1347.

56. The correct answer is A, Exposed bone.

Why is this the correct answer?

Exposed bone in a fingertip amputation indicates that the injury can lead to significant complications and even death. The thumb and index finger are the most important digits in terms of hand function. Fingertip amputations are very common, and emergency physicians should understand what is within their scope of practice and when a hand surgery consultation is advised. An injury with enough tissue loss to reveal exposed bone can lead to osteomyelitis, poor sensation, cold intolerance, and even poor function. Significant tissue loss of the volar aspect of the digit is high risk. These patients often require surgical repair with a flap or skin graft performed by a hand surgeon, although outcomes are improved when patients undergo primary flap or closure.

Why are the other choices wrong?

Involvement of the fingernail is not necessarily a reason for hand surgeon consultation. If an avulsion is small and involves the distal tip of the nail, a good cosmetic outcome is usually achievable. These wounds can be cleansed and dressed with a nonadherent dressing in the emergency department and allowed to heal by secondary intention with close follow-up.

Pediatric patients do particularly well with fingertip avulsions and generally have better outcomes than adults, especially if only the tip of the digit is involved. Even when the wound approximates the bone, these patients have good regenerative capacity and can heal by secondary intention.

Injury to the volar aspect of the digit is more serious than a dorsal injury. However, these patients generally do well healing by secondary intention even if the volar fat pad is exposed as long as the injury is small (1 cm or less) and does not involve a large amount of soft tissue loss.

PEER REVIEW

✓ Get a hand surgery consultation if a fingertip amputation reveals exposed bone.

✓ Small fingertip avulsions can be managed by secondary intention.

REFERENCES

Marx JA, Hockberger RS, Walls RM, eds. *Rosen's Emergency Medicine: Concepts and Clinical Practice.* 8th ed. St. Louis, MO: Elsevier; 2014: 561-562.

Wolfson AB, Hendey GW, Ling LJ, et al, eds. *Harwood-Nuss' Clinical Practice of Emergency Medicine.* 6th ed. Philadelphia, PA: Lippincott, Williams & Wilkins; 2014: 274-275.

57. The correct answer is C, End-tidal capnography.

Why is this the correct answer?

There are multiple methods of assessing correct placement of the endotracheal tube after intubation. No technique is infallible, but the most reliable methods include direct visualization and end-tidal capnography. End-tidal capnography involves the use of a CO_2 monitor, which displays CO_2 concentration in real time. Capnometry is a similar though slightly less accurate method: it involves the use of a small adaptor with pH paper that changes colors in the presence of different concentrations of CO_2. Typically, the paper remains purple when exposed to low CO_2 concentrations (<4 mm Hg P_{CO_2}) and changes to yellow when exposed to higher CO_2 concentrations (15 to 38 mm Hg P_{CO_2}), indicating correct endotracheal location. It is important to note that no method is 100% accurate, and even end-tidal capnography can be rendered less accurate by cardiac arrest, hypopharyngeal placement, and recent ingestion of a carbonated beverage.

Why are the other choices wrong?

The 5-point auscultation involves listening with a stethoscope at four separate locations on the chest (typically, the bilateral axillae and bilateral anterolateral chest areas) and once near the epigastrium. Proper endotracheal placement is supported by bilateral breath sounds and the absence of gastric inflation. However, this has been shown to be much less reliable than capnography.

Chest radiography is used to identify mainstem bronchus intubation or a tube that is too high (not far enough into the trachea). A chest xray does not distinguish endotracheal versus esophageal placement.

Endotracheal tube condensation is an unreliable finding and can be seen with hypopharyngeal placement as well as with gastric distention. This finding should not be relied on as sole confirmation of correct endotracheal tube placement.

PEER POINT

Conditions associated with false colorimetric or capnographic readings

False-negative reading

- Low pulmonary perfusion: cardiac arrest, inadequate chest compressions during CPR, massive PE
- Massive obesity
- Severe pulmonary edema: secretions might obstruct the tube

False-positive reading

- Recent ingestion of carbonated beverage, but should not persist beyond six breaths
- Heated humidifier, nebulizer, or endotracheal epinephrine, but transient

Adapted with permission from *Tintinalli's Emergency Medicine: A Comprehensive Study Guide, 8th Ed.* Copyright McGraw-Hill Education.

PEER REVIEW

✓ End-tidal capnography is the most reliable way to confirm endotracheal intubation.

✓ No confirmation method is 100% accurate, so sometimes you'll have to use a combination of techniques.

✓ Don't use chest radiography to differentiate endotracheal from esophageal placement.

REFERENCES

Marx JA, Hockberger RS, Walls RM, eds. *Rosen's Emergency Medicine: Concepts and Clinical Practice.* 8th ed. St. Louis, MO: Elsevier; 2014: 7-8.

Tintinalli JE, Stapczynski JS, Ma OJ, et al, eds. *Tintinalli's Emergency Medicine: A Comprehensive Study Guide.* 8th ed. New York, NY: McGraw-Hill; 2012: 183-192.

58. The correct answer is D, O positive.

Why is this the correct answer?

Whenever possible, patients should receive typed and crossmatched blood for transfusion. However, blood typing and crossmatching can take time, and some patients require immediate transfusion of uncrossmatched blood. When giving uncrossmatched blood, it is important to use type O blood — no A or B antigens present on the cells. Men may receive either O-negative or O-positive blood, but most experts recommend transfusing O-positive blood in order to save the limited supply of O-negative blood for female transfusion patients. Women should receive O-negative (Rhesus antigen negative) blood to avoid Rh sensitivity, which can result in future childbearing complications. Transfusing incorrect or nontype O blood to a patient can result in an acute hemolytic reaction, which can be fatal. Rhesus antigen does not significantly increase the risk of acute hemolytic reaction in transfusion patients.

Why are the other choices wrong?

AB-negative blood has both A and B antigens on the red blood cells and carries the highest risk of causing an acute hemolytic reaction in an uncrossmatched blood transfusion.

Similar to AB-negative blood, AB-positive blood has both A and B antigens on the red blood cells and also carries a high risk of causing an acute hemolytic reaction in an uncrossmatched blood transfusion.

O-negative blood is the least reactive blood type and is recommended for empiric transfusion of all women who can bear children. Given the limited quantity of O-negative blood, men and postmenopausal women should receive O-positive blood in an emergent situation when feasible.

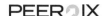
PEER REVIEW

✓ Any woman who can bear children should receive O-negative red blood cells if transfusion is needed.

✓ Men and postmenopausal women should receive O-positive red blood cells.

✓ Use typed and crossmatched blood for transfusions whenever it's feasible.

REFERENCES

Marx JA, Hockberger RS, Walls RM, eds. *Rosen's Emergency Medicine: Concepts and Clinical Practice*. 8th ed. St. Louis, MO: Elsevier; 2014: 75-78.

Tintinalli JE, Stapczynski JS, Ma OJ, et al, eds. *Tintinalli's Emergency Medicine: A Comprehensive Study Guide*. 8th ed. New York, NY: McGraw-Hill; 2012: 69-74.

59. The correct answer is D, Poorly controlled diabetes.

Why is this the correct answer?

Intraosseous (IO) access makes rapid vascular access possible and should be considered in hypovolemic patients when peripheral access is not obtainable. Contraindications to IO access include fracture of the same bone, previous IO attempt on the same bone, inferior vena cava injury, osteogenesis imperfecta, osteopetrosis, and overlying cellulitis. Poorly controlled diabetes is not a contraindication to IO line placement. The procedure typically involves cleansing the area with an iodine-based solution, anesthetizing the skin through the periosteum with a local anesthetic agent, and aiming the drill perpendicular to the bone while advancing in a slow and controlled manner. Bone marrow may be aspirated if specimens are needed for laboratory testing. After insertion, 40 mg (or 0.5 mg/kg in children) of 2% cardiac lidocaine should be injected into the bone marrow followed by a 10 mL bolus of normal saline. The currently approved sites for IO line insertion include the distal tibia, proximal tibia, and proximal humerus.

Why are the other choices wrong?

Concomitant fracture of the same bone is considered a contraindication to IO line insertion given the potential for fluid to exit the bone distally and cause a compartment syndrome.

Osteogenesis imperfecta is considered a contraindication because the fragile bones can easily break, resulting in loss of access and the potential for significant local tissue infiltration, which might lead to a compartment syndrome.

Sites with overlying cellulitis should be avoided because of the increased risk of associated osteomyelitis or systemic spread of the infection.

PEER POINT

Contraindications to IO line insertion

- Fracture of the same bone
- Previous IO attempt on the same bone
- Inferior vena cava injury
- Osteogenesis imperfecta
- Osteopetrosis
- Overlying cellulitis

PEER REVIEW

✓ Don' t attempt intraosseous infusion in patients who have a fracture of the same bone, a previous IO attempt on the same bone, inferior vena cava injury, osteogenesis imperfecta, osteopetrosis, or overlying cellulitis.

✓ These are the currently approved sites for IO line insertion: distal tibia, proximal tibia, and proximal humerus.

REFERENCES

Marx JA, Hockberger RS, Walls RM, eds. *Rosen's Emergency Medicine: Concepts and Clinical Practice*. 8th ed. St. Louis, MO: Elsevier; 2014: 307-308.

Roberts JR, Hedges JR, eds. *Clinical Procedures in Emergency Medicine*. 6th ed. St. Louis, Mo: WB Saunders; 2013: 457-458.

60. The correct answer is D, Glipizide 5 mg.

Why is this the correct answer?

Glipizide is a sulfonylurea used to treat noninsulin-dependent diabetes. Like other sulfonylureas that therapeutically act by inducing the release of preformed insulin, ingestion of a single pill can cause life-threatening hypoglycemia in children. Even potential accidental ingestions in children require a long observation period and typically admission to determine if hypoglycemia will develop. If hypoglycemia develops, it is treated with glucose and octreotide. Octreotide antagonizes the release of insulin and decreases the frequency of hypoglycemic episodes in the setting of sulfonylurea poisonings.

Why are the other choices wrong?

Ingestion of a single 500-mg acetaminophen pill in a 10-kg infant (50 mg/kg dose) will not cause liver injury and will not be life-threatening. Minimum doses that can potentially cause hepatotoxicity begin at approximately 200 mg/kg.

Ingestion of a single 325-mg aspirin pill in a 10-kg infant (32.5 mg/kg dose) will not cause significant toxicity and will not be life-threatening. Generally, toxicity begins to develop at 150 mg/kg, a dose that is easily reached with ingestions of even small volumes of oil of wintergreen, a highly concentrated formulation of methyl salicylate.

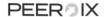

Ingestion of a single 325-mg pill of ferrous sulfate will not cause significant toxicity or be life-threatening in a 10-kg infant. The quantity of elemental iron is used as a guide for predicting toxicity. Ferrous sulfate is 20% elemental iron, meaning that a 325-mg pill will have 65 mg of elemental iron, a 6.5 mg/kg dose in this case. The toxic effects of iron begin to develop at approximately 10 mg/kg of elemental iron ingested, and potentially life-threatening ingestions are generally greater than 60 mg/kg.

PEER REVIEW

✓ Ingestion of one sulfonylurea pill can cause life-threatening hypoglycemia in an infant.

✓ The quantity of elemental iron in a pill is used as a guide for predicting toxicity.

REFERENCES

Hoffman RS, Howland MA, Lewin NA, et al. *Goldfrank's Toxicologic Emergencies*. 10th ed. New York, NY: McGraw-Hill; 2010:420, 450, 518, 617, 720.

Tintinalli JE, Stapczynski JS, Ma OJ, et al, eds. *Tintinalli's Emergency Medicine: A Comprehensive Study Guide*. 8th ed. New York, NY: McGraw-Hill; 2012: 1265-1276, 1307-1310.

61. The correct answer is B, Idiopathic facial paralysis.

Why is this the correct answer?

Idiopathic facial paralysis, better known as Bell palsy, is defined as paralysis of the peripheral portion of the seventh cranial nerve (facial nerve). The facial nerve provides motor innervation to the muscles of the face and scalp and taste sensation on the anterior two-thirds of the tongue. Patients with Bell palsy frequently present with pain adjacent to the ear as well as a facial droop on the affected side with inability to close the eye and effacement of facial folds. An important examination finding that helps distinguish Bell palsy from a central process is the inability to raise the eyebrow on the affected side. Patients with central lesions such as a stroke can raise the eyebrows and wrinkle the forehead symmetrically due to innervation of the upper face by both cerebral hemispheres. Treatment for Bell palsy consists of corticosteroids to decrease the inflammation and swelling of the facial nerve. The addition of antiviral medications for the treatment of Bell palsy is controversial. Many of the larger studies found no additional benefit to antiviral therapy; however, some smaller studies note higher rates of complete recovery with the addition of valacyclovir, with the most significant effects found in patients with severe facial paralysis. Patients who are unable to fully close the affected eye should be given a lubricating ophthalmic agent as well as instructions to patch the eye when sleeping to prevent corneal abrasions or other damage to the eye.

Why are the other choices wrong?

Herpes zoster oticus, also known as Ramsay Hunt syndrome, presents as unilateral facial paralysis with associated herpetic rash on the ear (including the tympanic membrane), face, mouth, or neck. The eighth cranial nerve might also be involved and cause hearing loss or dizziness (vertigo). There might be cases of Ramsay Hunt syndrome in which the paralysis precedes the development of a rash. Patients presenting with this condition should be treated with corticosteroids (prednisone) and an antiviral medication (valacyclovir or famcilovir).

It is important to perform a complete HEENT examination in patients presenting with symptoms of Bell palsy, especially those with pain around the ear. A diagnosis of mastoiditis would be supported if the patient has a fever or pain with palpation over the mastoid process. Mastoiditis can also cause paralysis of the seventh nerve, causing findings similar to Bell palsy. The diagnosis of mastoiditis can be further supported with CT; it should be promptly treated with intravenous antibiotics.

The most critical item in the differential diagnosis of patients presenting with unilateral facial paralysis is a middle cerebral artery stroke. Patients who are experiencing a stroke have sparing of the forehead muscles and can raise the eyebrow on the affected side. Additionally, they experience other neurologic symptoms, so it is imperative to perform and document a complete neurologic examination. If there is concern for possible stroke, neuroimaging should be obtained.

PEER POINT

The COWS mnemonic: elements of the examination for seventh cranial nerve palsy

<u>C</u>lose your eyes
<u>O</u>pen (the physician tries to open the patient's eyes)
<u>W</u>rinkle your forehead
<u>S</u>mile

PEER REVIEW

- ✓ Bell palsy presentation: paralysis of the facial nerve, facial droop of the affected side, can't raise the eyebrow on the affected side.
- ✓ Perform a thorough history and physical examination to distinguish Bell palsy from a stroke or ear/mastoid infection.
- ✓ Corticosteroids are the mainstay of therapy for Bell palsy.

REFERENCES

Marx JA, Hockberger RS, Walls RM, eds. *Rosen's Emergency Medicine: Concepts and Clinical Practice*. 8th ed. St. Louis, MO: Elsevier; 2014: 1409-1418.

Tintinalli JE, Stapczynski JS, Ma OJ, et al, eds. *Tintinalli's Emergency Medicine: A Comprehensive Study Guide*. 8th ed. New York, NY: McGraw-Hill; 2012:1178-1185.

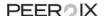

62. The correct answer is D, Patient with massive rectal bleeding.

Why is this the correct answer?

Nasogastric (NG) aspiration has recently become controversial in clinical settings in which it was previously recommended. Nasogastric tube placement is recommended in patients with hematemesis or massive rectal bleeding with hemodynamic instability. Severe persistent rectal bleeding with NG tube placement is useful if it identifies a potential upper GI bleed, which might be easier to control. However, some feel that NG aspiration lacks the sensitivity one would like to distinguish an upper from a lower GI source. Other indications include gastric decompression, persistent vomiting, administration of oral medications or contrast in those not able to take them orally, or to detect transdiaphragmatic stomach herniation, particularly in the setting of trauma. Nasogastric tube placement has been reported to be one of the most painful emergency department procedures, so at least 5 minutes prior to placement, topical anesthesia and oxymetazoline spray should be used. Complications include pain, epistaxis, vomiting, aspiration, perforation, intracranial placement, pulmonary placement, and pneumothorax.

Why are the other choices wrong?

Nasogastric aspiration and decompression are no longer routine for the treatment of adynamic ileus. Postoperative ileus has been shown to resolve quicker in patients without NG tube placement after abdominal surgery. While NG decompression may be useful in bowel obstruction, recent studies have shown safe medical management with octreotide or somatostatin.

Coagulopathy is a relative contraindication to NG tube placement, secondary to the risk of bleeding diatheses.

Gastric bypass and lap banding are other contraindications because the staples from the surgery can be torn and create an elevated risk of perforation. Additionally, it is not recommended to place an NG tube in the setting of midface injury, basilar skull fracture, esophageal stricture, or alkali injury.

PEER POINT

Indications for nasogastric aspiration

- Detect transdiaphragmatic stomach herniation
- Gastric decompression (obstruction/perforation)
- Give medication or contrast Intractable vomiting
- Monitor and evaluate upper GI bleeding

Contraindications to nasogastric aspiration

- Alkali injury/corrosive ingestion
- Basilar skull fracture or midface injury
- Coagulopathy
- Esophageal strictures
- History of gastric bypass or lap band surgery

PEER REVIEW

✓ Nasogastric tube intubation is controversial in minor bleeding but still recommended for GI bleeding associated with hemodynamic instability.

✓ Obstruction and perforation are indications for NG tube placement, but acute ileus should be managed medically.

REFERENCES

Roberts JR, Hedges JR, eds. *Clinical Procedures in Emergency Medicine*. 6th ed. St. Louis, Mo: WB Saunders; 2013: 809-816.

Tintinalli JE, Stapczynski JS, Ma OJ, et al, eds. *Tintinalli's Emergency Medicine: A Comprehensive Study Guide*. 8th ed. New York, NY: McGraw-Hill; 2012: 563-567.

63. The correct answer is D, Parent's kiss.

Why is this the correct answer?

Multiple techniques have been described to remove nasal foreign bodies in pediatric patients. The use of a "parent's kiss" or "mother's kiss" has been described as very successful (approximately 80% effective), and parents preferred the technique to others using instruments or patient restraint. The technique is performed by telling the patient that the parent is going "to give you a big kiss." The parent then occludes the nonaffected nostril and blows a short, quick breath into the patient's mouth. The technique can be repeated until successful removal of the foreign body. Before attempting any nasal foreign body removal technique, mucosal application of topical lidocaine and a vasoconstrictor such as phenylephrine reduces patient discomfort and helps make the attempt successful. If this and other techniques fail, otolaryngology consultation is warranted.

Why are the other choices wrong?

Back blows are used in infants and other young pediatric patients to remove suspected airway foreign bodies. This technique is not recommended for nasal foreign body removal.

The bag-valve-mask (BVM) positive pressure technique involves placing the BVM device sideways on the patient's face covering just the mouth. The provider occludes the nonaffected nostril and delivers positive pressure through the BVM. Although this technique is effective, it often requires restraint.

The forceps technique is also effective for nasal foreign body removal but requires physical restraint or procedural sedation to be successful.

PEER POINT

Nasal foreign body removal techniques and examples

- Direct instrumentation — forceps with or without using a nasoendoscope
- Positive pressure — "parent's kiss" technique, BVM positive pressure
- Balloon-catheter removal — small Foley catheter
- Glue — tissue adhesive
- Suction

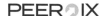
PEER REVIEW

✓ The "parent's kiss" technique is safe and effective for nasal foreign body removal.

✓ Using analgesia and a vasoconstrictor before nasal foreign body removal results in greater success and patient comfort.

✓ Other techniques — BVM positive pressure, catheter balloon extractors, forceps — work but often require physical restraint or procedural sedation.

REFERENCES

Botma M, Bader R, Kubba H. 'A parent's kiss': evaluating an unusual method for removing nasal foreign bodies in children. *J Laryngol Otol.* 2000;114(08):598-600.

Roberts JR, Hedges JR, eds. *Clinical Procedures in Emergency Medicine.* 6th ed. St. Louis, MO: WB Saunders; 2013: 1335-1337.

Tintinalli JE, Stapczynski JS, Ma OJ, et al, eds. *Tintinalli's Emergency Medicine: A Comprehensive Study Guide.* 8th ed. New York, NY: McGraw-Hill; 2012: 778-779.

64. The correct answer is C, Spine.

Why is this the correct answer?

Computed tomography is excellent at identifying bony injury in trauma patients, especially those with suspected spine injury. Trauma scans are typically performed without oral contrast: any delay in the time to scan is unacceptable, and patients in cervical spine precautions might be at risk for aspiration. Performing CT without contrast is especially beneficial in elderly patients who might have underlying renal dysfunction and for patients with limited intravenous access who are clinically stable. In these patients, even without contrast, CT can still identify bony trauma and significant solid organ injury. The use of intravenous contrast material helps reveal vascular injury and more subtle solid organ trauma, as well as identify active extravasation of contrast, and it does not inhibit identification of bony injury.

Why are the other choices wrong?

Computed tomography is excellent at identifying injuries to solid organs, with the exception of the pancreas. It often is not able to reveal pancreas injuries resulting from trauma.

Although CT is, again, excellent at identifying injuries to bone and solid organs, it is not as sensitive for mesenteric or hollow viscus injuries resulting from trauma to the small bowel area.

Retroperitoneal injuries and hemoperitoneum or retroperitoneal hematoma can be identified using CT. However, CT is not as sensitive when it comes to injuries to the stomach. If there is a high degree of suspicion for injury to any of these three organs, the patient should undergo further workup and management such as the addition of oral or rectal contrast material, serial abdominal examinations, or exploratory laparotomy if the patient has peritoneal signs or is ill.

PEER REVIEW

- ✓ Computed tomography is highly sensitive for solid organ trauma.
- ✓ Bony injuries can be detected on CT with or without contrast.
- ✓ Pancreas and hollow viscus injuries are often missed on CT.

REFERENCES

Marx JA, Hockberger RS, Walls RM, eds. *Rosen's Emergency Medicine: Concepts and Clinical Practice*. 8th ed. St. Louis, MO: Elsevier; 2014: 465-467.

Wolfson AB, Hendey GW, Ling LJ, et al, eds. *Harwood-Nuss' Clinical Practice of Emergency Medicine*. 6th ed. Philadelphia, PA: Lippincott, Williams & Wilkins; 2014: 221.

65. The correct answer is A, Abdominal and pelvic CT with contrast.

Why is this the correct answer?

The absence of gross and microscopic hematuria does not rule out upper urinary tract trauma or accurately correlate with degree of injury. To further evaluate for renal trauma, CT with intravenous contrast is the most appropriate radiographic study. This patient is hemodynamically stable with a negative FAST exam and does not require immediate surgical intervention, but the location of his wound is concerning for possible injury to the kidney. The use of CT with contrast allows for both identification and grading of renal injuries. Contusion, laceration, hematoma, perfusion abnormalities, and injuries to structures in the renal hilum can be noted. Obtaining additional delayed images after contrast is administered, once the material has been excreted into the urine, allows for identification of urinary extravasation as well. Renal injuries are graded on a scale of I to V, with most Grade I, II, and III injuries managed conservatively. Some Grade IV and most Grade V injuries require surgical intervention. Indications for operative management include active hemorrhage, expanding or noncontained retroperitoneal hematoma (thought to indicate renal avulsion), renal avulsion injury, and urinary extravasation from renal pelvis injury. Most penetrating traumatic injuries require surgical intervention. Urine dipstick and formal urinalysis are equally reliable studies to detect hematuria, but the presence or absence of hematuria (gross or microscopic) is not predictive of renal injury in the setting of penetrating trauma. In blunt trauma, both microscopic hematuria with hypotension as well as gross hematuria alone have been shown to have some predictive value for renal injury severity.

Why are the other choices wrong?

Cystography is used to identify bladder injuries, not renal parenchymal trauma. Delayed CT imaging or CT cystography (using intravenous contrast) can also be used to identify bladder injuries if there is concern.

Renal ultrasonography has been shown to have poor sensitivity for renal trauma, missing up to 78% of injuries. A FAST examination might reveal blood or extravasated urine, but most isolated renal injuries have no associated free intraperitoneal fluid. Again, CT is the radiographic modality of choice.

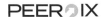

Retrograde urethrography is used to identify injury to the urethra, most commonly associated with pelvic fractures. It is not useful for identifying renal injury. Contrast-enhanced CT allows for evaluation of structures outside the urinary tract.

PEER REVIEW

- ✓ The presence or absence of hematuria is not predictive of penetrating trauma to the kidney.
- ✓ Contrast-enhanced CT is the imaging modality of choice for evaluation of traumatic renal injury.

REFERENCES

Marx JA, Hockberger RS, Walls RM, eds. *Rosen's Emergency Medicine: Concepts and Clinical Practice*. 8th ed. St. Louis, MO: Elsevier; 2014: 490-494.

Tintinalli JE, Stapczynski JS, Ma OJ, et al, eds. *Tintinalli's Emergency Medicine: A Comprehensive Study Guide*. 8th ed. New York, NY: McGraw-Hill; 2012: 1767-1768.

66. The correct answer is D, 90 degrees.

Why is this the correct answer?

Needle compartment pressure measurement is performed by inserting a needle perpendicular or at a 90-degree angle to the skin overlying the compartment. A pressure reading higher than 30 mm Hg is a positive finding for compartment syndrome. Extremity fractures, muscle injuries, prolonged compression, burns, bleeding from various etiologies (vascular injury, anticoagulation or antiplatelet therapy, underlying bleeding factor deficiencies), and certain medications and toxins (ergotamine, statins, snake venom) are all considered underlying etiologies for developing extremity compartment syndrome. Presence of risk factors and physical examination are critical to the evaluation, in addition to the direct measurement of compartments. The physical examination findings consist of compartment tension and pain with palpation, in addition to pain with passive extension, paresthesias, paresis/paralysis, pallor, and pulselessness (the "five Ps"). The presence of a distal arterial pulse does not exclude compartment syndrome, and there is often a lack of any of the other examination findings. The diagnosis should be carefully considered with pain out of proportion to the remainder of the examination.

Why are the other choices wrong?

Inserting the needle at 30 degrees to the skin overlying the compartment might result in inaccurately high or low compartment pressure measurements and can result in misdiagnosis.

Similarly, inserting the needle at 45 degrees to the skin can result in inaccurate compartment pressure measurements.

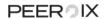

Ninety degrees, not 60, is the required angle for accurate measurement of a compartment pressure when evaluating a patient for compartment syndrome.

PEER POINT

Findings that should raise suspicion for compartment syndrome: the five Ps

- Pain with passive extension
- Paresthesias
- Paresis/paralysis
- Pallor
- Pulselessness

PEER REVIEW

- ✓ A patient doesn't have to show all five signs of compartment syndrome for the diagnosis to be correct, so keep a high degree of suspicion.
- ✓ You can't rule out compartment syndrome just because the patient has a distal arterial pulse.
- ✓ The needle should be inserted at a 90-degree angle to the skin when measuring compartment pressure. A pressure higher than 30 mm Hg is consistent with compartment syndrome.

REFERENCES
Roberts JR, Hedges JR, eds. *Clinical Procedures in Emergency Medicine.* 6th ed. St. Louis, MO: WB Saunders; 2013: 1099-111.
Sherman S. *Simon's Emergency Orthopedics.* 7th ed. New York, NY: McGraw-Hill; 2015: 77-78.

67. The correct answer is D, Wider tourniquets are more comfortable and less likely to cause nerve injury than narrow tourniquets.

Why is this the correct answer?

When one patient presents to the emergency department with bleeding, one clinician can manage the situation by applying direct pressure to the bleeding vessel. But in a multicasualty incident, managing several patients simultaneously with a limited number of clinicians is much more complex. In such a situation, application of a tourniquet allows for efficient control of life-threatening hemorrhage and frees up a clinician to tend to other critical needs and other patients. A wider tourniquet causes less soft tissue trauma than a narrow tourniquet because of its larger surface area. A wider tourniquet also causes less discomfort for the patient, as narrow tourniquets can be quite uncomfortable. Tourniquets may be left in place long enough to stabilize a patient for transport or control bleeding at the source surgically. Tourniquets are used in surgery for up to 2 hours at a time. However, the longer the tourniquet is in place, the greater the possibility of damage to tissue and nerves. The limb can also become acidotic at longer tourniquet application times.

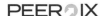

Why are the other choices wrong?

Tourniquets are less effective in controlling hemorrhage from the junctional areas such as the axilla, groin, and neck. Bleeding associated with injuries to these areas is much more difficult to control, and tourniquets are actually less useful in these areas of the body. Newer approaches are being developed and tested to control hemorrhage in these anatomic areas such as compression of the femoral vessels with a C-clamp and use of a compression device to the abdominal aortic bifurcation.

Strap-and-buckle tourniquets or simple gauze tourniquets are less effective in applying enough pressure to a bleeding vessel to be helpful. If a more secure device is available, it should be used.

A windlass mechanism uses an object to twist the tourniquet more tightly and provides a mechanical tightening advantage. This type of mechanism is actually very useful in tightening a tourniquet around a large vessel hemorrhage such as in the leg.

PEER REVIEW

✓ Wider tourniquets cause less trauma and are more comfortable.
✓ You can use tourniquets for brief periods of time in the situation of life-threatening hemorrhage.

REFERENCES:

Marx JA, Hockberger RS, Walls RM, eds. *Rosen's Emergency Medicine: Concepts and Clinical Practice*. 8th ed. St. Louis, MO: Elsevier; 2014: 2451.

Tintinalli JE, Stapczynski JS, Ma OJ, et al, eds. *Tintinalli's Emergency Medicine: A Comprehensive Study Guide*. 8th ed. New York, NY: McGraw-Hill; 2012: 2023-2024.

68. The correct answer is D, Retinal detachment.

Why is this the correct answer?

With floaters and visual field cuts, the patient must be evaluated by an ophthalmologist within 24 hours for concerns of a retinal detachment. Even with a direct ophthalmoscopic examination of the retina, most of the retinal tears seen in a detachment are in the periphery of the retina and might not be seen. Only large retinal detachments are seen on direct ophthalmoscopic examination as pale areas. To visualize smaller detachments, a dilated indirect and direct retinal examination must be done by an ophthalmologist. Emergency physicians are now also using ultrasonography of the eyeball to make this diagnosis. From the perspective of an emergency physician, the diagnosis is made primarily on symptoms and clinical history.

Why are the other choices wrong?

Acute angle-closure glaucoma is usually painful and sudden in onset with loss of visual acuity. Patients sometimes have a headache associated with the findings. The pupil is classically fixed and midpoint with a hazy cornea. The intraocular pressures must be quickly lowered using medications like timolol, and emergent ophthalmology consultation is required to avoid permanent vision loss.

A central retinal vein occlusion presents with a monocular vision loss that is typically painless. On ophthalmoscopic examination, the classic finding is a "blood-and-thunder" fundus. These patients require further evaluation by ophthalmology.

Giant cell arteritis, commonly called temporal arteritis, presents in patients in this age range but typically involves a headache. The patient frequently has other systemic symptoms as well, including fatigue, anorexia, fever, myalgias, and tenderness to palpation over the temporal artery. The diagnosis is made with an elevated ESR and temporal artery biopsy. The treatment is intravenous, then oral steroids.

PEER POINT

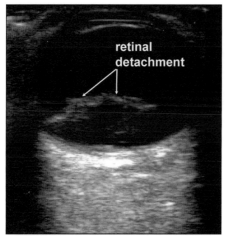

PEER Point 6

PEER REVIEW

✓ Retinal detachments are a diagnosis based on history and cannot be ruled out solely based on a normal direct ophthalmoscopic examination.

✓ Visual field cuts can be positionally dependent. Otherwise, patients still usually have baseline visual acuity.

✓ There is typically no pain in the eye or headache associated with a retinal detachment.

REFERENCES

Hollands H, Johnson D, Brox AC, Almeida D, Simel DL, Sharma S. Acute-onset floaters and flashes: is this patient at risk for retinal detachment? *JAMA*. 2009;302(20):2243-2249.

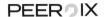

69. The correct answer is B, Pelvic fractures are associated with extremely high morbidity and mortality rates.

Why is this the correct answer?

Pelvic fractures are associated with extremely high morbidity and mortality rates in pregnant patients as well as in fetuses. Bony fragments can cause uterine perforation, rupture, hematoma, and contusion. These conditions can lead to uterine irritability, hemodynamic compromise of the fetus, fetal injury, and placental abruption. The pelvic veins are also relatively dilated during pregnancy, leading to an increased volume of bleeding with pelvic fractures. Any trauma during pregnancy is also associated with a high rate of fetal distress and demise.

Why are the other choices wrong?

Cardiotocographic monitoring is the most sensitive modality for identifying occult trauma to the uterus or to the fetus. A period of 4 to 6 hours of cardiotocographic monitoring is indicated after even the most minor trauma, either blunt or penetrating. Monitoring can identify subtle changes in fetal heart rate that might indicate fetal distress. In addition, monitoring can identify uterine irritability or early signs of placental abruption that can be missed with other diagnostic modalities.

Ultrasonography can be helpful in identifying uterine perforation, hematoma, or placental abruption but can miss more subtle injuries. A negative examination should prompt additional workup and monitoring.

Uterine perforation occurs most commonly during the third trimester when the uterus is relatively exposed. It can occur due to both blunt and penetrating trauma. During the first trimester, the uterus is small and relatively protected by the bony pelvis.

PEER REVIEW

- ✓ Pelvic fracture is associated with high morbidity and mortality rates in pregnancy.
- ✓ Cardiotocographic monitoring is the most sensitive modality for identifying occult injury.
- ✓ Ultrasonography can be useful but can miss many injuries.

REFERENCES

Marx JA, Hockberger RS, Walls RM, eds. *Rosen's Emergency Medicine: Concepts and Clinical Practice.* 8th ed. St. Louis, MO: Elsevier; 2014: 296-304.

Wolfson AB, Hendey GW, Ling LJ, et al, eds. *Harwood-Nuss' Clinical Practice of Emergency Medicine.* 6th ed. Philadelphia, PA: Lippincott, Williams & Wilkins; 2014: 321-325.

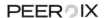

70. The correct answer is D, Torsades de pointes.

Why is this the correct answer?

Transcutaneous pacing has become a mainstay in the emergency department. Indications include AV block (Mobitz type II or complete heart block), sinus node dysfunction, and torsades de pointes. Although there are contraindications for transvenous pacing (such as poor vascular access, bleeding diathesis), there is no absolute contraindication to transcutaneous pacing. Transcutaneous pacing might not be effective in patients who have electrolyte abnormalities (hyperkalemia), obesity, air or fluid in the chest cavity, and past chest surgery with scarring. Transcutaneous pacing complications include chest wall burns and chest muscle pain; the most serious complication is the inability to identify a changing treatable rhythm.

Why are the other choices wrong?

Pacing is not recommended for asystole or a new right bundle-branch block (RBBB) with left axis deviation. Patients with asystole should be resuscitated with CPR and atropine if appropriate per ACLS guidelines.

Transcutaneous pacing is not recommended in severe hypothermia with bradycardia because it can induce ventricular fibrillation. These patients should be actively rewarmed and resuscitated.

First-degree and second-degree Mobitz type I (Wenckebach) blocks typically do not require pacing. In certain settings, both can progress to either second-degree Mobitz type II or complete heart block, conditions that would benefit from pacing.

PEER REVIEW

- ✓ Transcutaneous placing has largely replaced transvenous pacing in the emergency department.
- ✓ Here are the indications for pacing: certain types of AV block or sinus node dysfunction or other arrhythmias such as torsades de pointes that would benefit from overdrive pacing.
- ✓ Don't use pacing in patients with severe hypothermia; it can induce ventricular fibrillation.

REFERENCES

Roberts JR, Hedges JR, eds. *Clinical Procedures in Emergency Medicine.* 6th ed. St. Louis, MO: WB Saunders; 2013: 227-297.

Tintinalli JE, Stapczynski JS, Ma OJ, et al, eds. *Tintinalli's Emergency Medicine: A Comprehensive Study Guide.* 8th ed. New York, NY: McGraw-Hill; 2012: 218.

71. **The correct answer is B, Frozen shoulder complications decrease with immediate use of range of motion exercises.**

Why is this the correct answer?

Prolonged immobilization of the shoulder can lead to adhesive capsulitis. Therefore, patients who are treated with shoulder immobilization are often taught passive range of motion exercises to help prevent the frozen shoulder phenomenon. The treatment of closed clavicle fractures consists of ice, NSAIDs, and the use of an immobilization device such as a sling. Although a figure-of-eight bandage has been described in the literature, it is uncommonly used in treatment. A ready-made sling is usually easily available and comes in different sizes, both adult and pediatric. Traditionally, the patient is told to maintain immobilization until callus forms and is seen on xray in follow-up and, again, to perform passive range of motion exercises during the period of immobilization.

Why are the other choices wrong?

Clavicle fractures are divided into three groups based upon anatomy. They are classified as medial (proximal) third, middle third (midshaft), or distal third fractures, with middle third being the most common type.

Greenstick, or incomplete fractures of the clavicle, are common in children. They usually affect the middle third of the clavicle and generally heal uneventfully.

Nonunion of the clavicle is not uncommon. Comminuted fractures can lead to nonunion. Thirty percent of lateral clavicle fractures involving a torn coracoclavicular ligament result in nonunion and require surgical repair.

PEER REVIEW

- ✓ Most clavicle fractures involve the middle third of the bone.
- ✓ Treatment for a clavicle fracture includes a sling and orthopedic follow-up.
- ✓ Early range of motion exercises are encouraged to prevent adhesive capsulitis of the shoulder.

REFERENCES

Marx JA, Hockberger RS, Walls RM, eds. *Rosen's Emergency Medicine: Concepts and Clinical Practice.* 8th ed. St. Louis, MO: Elsevier; 2014: 621-624.

Wolfson AB, Hendey GW, Ling LJ, et al, eds. *Harwood-Nuss' Clinical Practice of Emergency Medicine.* 6th ed. Philadelphia, PA: Lippincott, Williams & Wilkins; 2014: 249.

72. The correct answer is A, Clear nasal discharge.

Why is this the correct answer?

Clear nasal discharge after blunt trauma to the face is a concerning finding. When the mechanism is a forceful blow to the bridge of the nose, the nasoethmoidal complex, or cribriform plate, can be injured, and a CSF leak is possible as a result. The physical finding of a CSF leak is clear rhinorrhea. The fluid may be sent to the laboratory for a beta-2 transferrin test to verify that it is truly CSF if the diagnosis is in question. Patients with this injury should have a maxillofacial CT scan to evaluate for other concomitant facial fractures. There might also be concern for intracranial injuries, pneumocephalus, or infection.

Why are the other choices wrong?

Epistaxis is common after blunt trauma to the nose and can occur with or without fracture. It is not indicative of cribriform plate injury. It is managed similarly to other etiologies of epistaxis.

Hemotympanum is seen in severe epistaxis when blood travels through the eustachian tube to the middle ear. It can also be seen with temporal bone fractures.

Septal hematoma is an important complication of nasal bone fracture. It appears as a grapelike mass in the naris after nasal trauma and is managed by incision and drainage followed by nasal packing. Failure to recognize and manage this complication can lead to nasal septal necrosis.

PEER REVIEW

- ✓ If you're treating a patient who got hit in the nose and has clear rhinorrhea, consider CSF leak and a cribriform plate injury.
- ✓ Hemotympanum can occur as a result of temporal bone fracture or epistaxis.
- ✓ Failing to drain a septal hematoma can lead to nasal septal necrosis.

REFERENCES

Marx JA, Hockberger RS, Walls RM, eds. *Rosen's Emergency Medicine: Concepts and Clinical Practice*. 8th ed. St. Louis, MO: Elsevier; 2014: 378-380.

Wolfson AB, Hendey GW, Ling LJ, et al, eds. *Harwood-Nuss' Clinical Practice of Emergency Medicine*. 6th ed. Philadelphia, PA: Lippincott, Williams & Wilkins; 2014: 161.

73. The correct answer is C, Lorazepam.

Why is this the correct answer?

For patients presenting with seizures lasting longer than 5 minutes or who experience multiple seizures within a short period of time without recovering from the postictal state (defined as status epilepticus), medications should be administered to stop the seizure activity. Benzodiazepines such as lorazepam, midazolam, and diazepam are first-line therapy to terminate the seizure until definitive treatment can be provided. On presentation to the emergency department, important initial interventions include

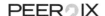

ensuring that the patient is in a safe environment and that he or she is able to maintain a patent airway. Patients who are experiencing a seizure should be placed on high-flow oxygen via nonrebreather mask. Many patients have seizures that self-terminate after a short period of time; however, patients who continue to have seizures as described above should be treated with benzodiazepines. Intravenous administration is common, given that access has already been established in many patients, but there are multiple dosing options available if needed, including intramuscular, buccal, and rectal. Patients who are treated with benzodiazepines should be closely monitored for respiratory depression and hypotension.

Why are the other choices wrong?

Fosphenytoin is a water-soluble prodrug preparation of phenytoin. It offers longer-acting antiepileptic therapy for patients with status epilepticus. But it is not first-line therapy; it is recognized as second-line drug therapy, following administration of a benzodiazepine. Advantages of fosphenytoin over phenytoin include a more rapid infusion rate and that it may be given intramuscularly, but it has similar cardiac side effects and a similar time of onset.

As with fosphenytoin, levetiracetam is a second-line, not first-line, agent for treatment of status epilepticus. It may be given in place of (or in addition to) a phenytoin preparation. This medication is favored in patients who take this drug as outpatients and have been noncompliant with therapy. Use of this medication to treat status epilepticus has been increasing due to its minimal side effect profile.

Phenobarbital (and other barbiturates) is regarded as "third-line therapy" for patients with seizures refractory to benzodiazepines and phenytoin. Patients who receive phenobarbital have a significant rate of respiratory depression, especially when it is administered along with benzodiazepines or other sedating medications. Careful observation of the patient's respiratory status is required, and intubation is often necessary if the patient's seizure has not been terminated by this time. It is important to remember that patients in status epilepticus can continue to have nonconvulsive seizures. Continuous EEG monitoring is recommended if the third-line treatment is required or if the patient has seizures for more than 30 minutes and does not wake up.

PEER REVIEW

- ✓ Status epilepticus: the seizure lasts longer than 5 minutes, and the patient doesn't regain consciousness. Treat it with medication to terminate the seizure activity.
- ✓ Benzodiazepines are first-line therapy for status epilepticus and refractory seizures.
- ✓ Second-line agents for refractory seizures: phenytoin or fosphenytoin, and levetiracetam.

REFERENCES

Marx JA, Hockberger RS, Walls RM, eds. *Rosen's Emergency Medicine: Concepts and Clinical Practice*. 8th ed. St. Louis, MO: Elsevier; 2014: 156-161.

Tintinalli JE, Stapczynski JS, Ma OJ, et al, eds. *Tintinalli's Emergency Medicine: A Comprehensive Study Guide*. 8th ed. New York, NY: McGraw-Hill; 2012: 1173-1178.

74. The correct answer is B, NSAIDs and topical aloe vera with primary care follow-up.

Why is this the correct answer?

This patient presents with small first-degree burn. The wound is painful, sensate, dry, and without blisters or necrosis. Management of a first-degree burn consists of providing NSAIDs, cooling the skin immediately using tap water or a cool compress (but not ice), and applying aloe vera topically. Antibiotics, either systemic or topical, are not indicated: there are no blisters or breaks in the skin with first-degree burns. Primary care follow-up is prudent, although these patients generally do quite well in the outpatient setting regardless of follow-up.

Why are the other choices wrong?

An occlusive dressing is not indicated for a first-degree burn. But for a partial-thickness burn, an occlusive dressing is indicated. If the wound has a moist surface or unroofed blisters or is insensate, an occlusive dressing can be considered.

Silver sulfadiazine is not indicated for first-degree burns. It can be used with a bulky dressing in the treatment of partial thickness burns. There is no indication for referral to a burn center in this case.

This patient does not require antibiotics or transfer to a burn center. Even with a partial-thickness burn, although topical antibiotics are indicated, systemic antibiotics are not indicated unless the patient develops a secondary infection.

PEER POINT

The Parkland formula for calculating fluid requirements for burn patients

Volume of lactated Ringer's solution

FOR THE FIRST 24 HOURS

4 mL x % of BSA burned x weight in kg

Give **HALF**

of the solution

FOR THE FIRST 8 HOURS

Give **THE OTHER HALF**

of the solution

FOR THE NEXT 16 HOURS

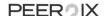

PEER REVIEW

✓ Patients with first-degree burns can be treated as outpatients with NSAIDs and aloe vera.

REFERENCES

Marx JA, Hockberger RS, Walls RM, eds. *Rosen's Emergency Medicine: Concepts and Clinical Practice*. 8th ed. St. Louis, MO: Elsevier; 2014: 808-817.

Wolfson AB, Hendey GW, Ling LJ, et al, eds. *Harwood-Nuss' Clinical Practice of Emergency Medicine*. 6th ed. Philadelphia, PA: Lippincott, Williams & Wilkins; 2014: 305-306.

75. **The correct answer is C, 63-year-old woman with a history of hypertension and diabetes presenting with chest pain and diaphoresis with an ECG demonstrating a wide-complex tachycardia.**

Why is this the correct answer?

The approach to arrhythmias begins with determining if the patient is stable or unstable. Unstable is defined as showing evidence of end-organ hypoperfusion (altered mental status, anginal chest pain, diaphoresis, presyncope, shortness of breath, or shock). If a patient is unstable, the condition may be further divided into bradyarrhythmias (treated with transcutaneous pacing) and tachyarrhythmias (treated with cardioversion or defibrillation). Of the patients presented, the 63-year-old woman and the 75-year-old woman both meet the criteria for cardioversion. But because multifocal atrial tachycardia (MAT) does not respond to cardioversion, only the 63-year-old woman with the wide-complex tachycardia is an appropriate candidate. Although almost all unstable tachyarrhythmias are treated with cardioversion, stable tachyarrhythmias are divided into narrow (supraventricular origin) and wide (ventricular origin or supraventricular origin with aberrancy) QRS complexes, followed by regular (typically single origin) versus irregular (multiple origins) frequency. Following this algorithm allows for rapid determination of likely etiologies and corresponding treatments.

Why are the other choices wrong?

Atrial fibrillation (a stable, irregular, narrow-complex tachycardia) is typically treated with rate control, but rhythm control or cardioversion may be considered if the patient presents within 72 hours. If the patient presents outside of 72 hours, the risk of embolic stroke after rhythm control is greater. Due to patient stability and the time of onset, this patient is not a candidate for cardioversion in the emergency department.

In patients presenting with an unstable bradyarrhythmia, treatment with transcutaneous pacing should be initiated, frequently followed by transvenous pacing. Atropine, epinephrine, and dopamine may be considered while preparing for cardiac pacing.

Although unstable tachyarrhythmias are typically treated with synchronized cardioversion, multifocal atrial tachycardia (MAT) is an exception, as cardioversion has been shown to have no effect due to the multiple sites of atrial ectopy. Treatment involves identifying and resolving the underlying disorder, which is frequently hypoxia.

PEER POINT

Adult cardiac arrest algorithm

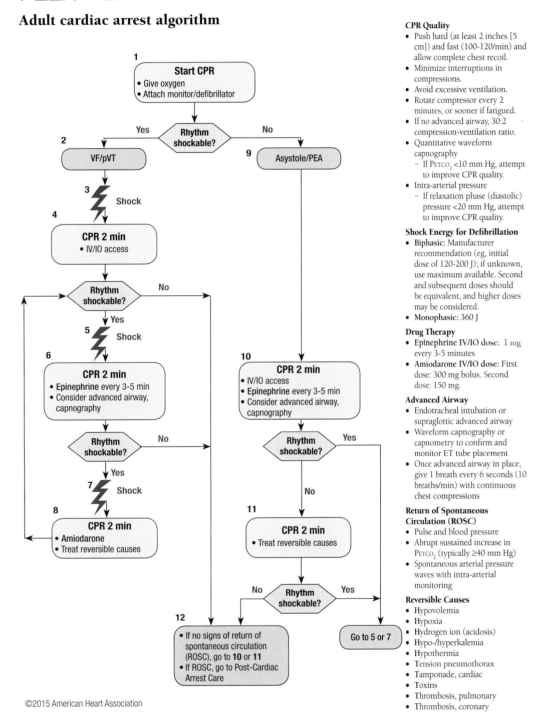

©2015 American Heart Association

CPR Quality
- Push hard (at least 2 inches [5 cm]) and fast (100-120/min) and allow complete chest recoil.
- Minimize interruptions in compressions.
- Avoid excessive ventilation.
- Rotate compressor every 2 minutes, or sooner if fatigued.
- If no advanced airway, 30:2 compression-ventilation ratio.
- Quantitative waveform capnography
  - If P_{ETCO_2} <10 mm Hg, attempt to improve CPR quality.
- Intra-arterial pressure
  - If relaxation phase (diastolic) pressure <20 mm Hg, attempt to improve CPR quality.

Shock Energy for Defibrillation
- Biphasic: Manufacturer recommendation (eg, initial dose of 120-200 J); if unknown, use maximum available. Second and subsequent doses should be equivalent, and higher doses may be considered.
- Monophasic: 360 J

Drug Therapy
- Epinephrine IV/IO dose: 1 mg every 3-5 minutes
- Amiodarone IV/IO dose: First dose: 300 mg bolus. Second dose: 150 mg.

Advanced Airway
- Endotracheal intubation or supraglottic advanced airway
- Waveform capnography or capnometry to confirm and monitor ET tube placement
- Once advanced airway in place, give 1 breath every 6 seconds (10 breaths/min) with continuous chest compressions

Return of Spontaneous Circulation (ROSC)
- Pulse and blood pressure
- Abrupt sustained increase in P_{ETCO_2} (typically ≥40 mm Hg)
- Spontaneous arterial pressure waves with intra-arterial monitoring

Reversible Causes
- Hypovolemia
- Hypoxia
- Hydrogen ion (acidosis)
- Hypo-/hyperkalemia
- Hypothermia
- Tension pneumothorax
- Tamponade, cardiac
- Toxins
- Thrombosis, pulmonary
- Thrombosis, coronary

PEER Point 7

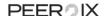

PEER REVIEW

✓ Unstable tachyarrhythmias, with the exception of multifocal atrial tachycardia, are typically treated with synchronized cardioversion.

✓ Unstable bradyarrhythmias are treated with transcutaneous and/or transvenous pacing.

REFERENCES

Link MS, Berkow LC, Kudenchuk PJ, et al. Part 7: Adult Advanced Cardiovascular Life Support: 2015 American Heart Association Guidelines Update for Cardiopulmonary Resuscitation and Emergency Cardiovascular Care. *Circulation.* 2015;132(18 Suppl 2):S444-S464.

Marx JA, Hockberger RS, Walls RM, eds. *Rosen's Emergency Medicine: Concepts and Clinical Practice.* 8th ed. St. Louis, MO: Elsevier; 2014: 1040-1063.

Tintinalli JE, Stapczynski JS, Ma OJ, et al, eds. *Tintinalli's Emergency Medicine: A Comprehensive Study Guide.* 8th ed. New York, NY: McGraw-Hill; 2012: 112-134.

76. The correct answer is B, Distended right atrium and ventricle on ultrasound.

Why is this the correct answer?

The risk of causing traumatic injuries while performing chest compressions is significant. These injuries include rib fracture and subsequent lung parenchymal damage and pneumothorax. When a patient is also given positive-pressure ventilation, intrapleural pressure increases, and tension pneumothorax can result as air continues to enter the pleural cavity but is unable to escape. This patient is beginning to show evidence of tension pneumothorax, specifically tachycardia, hypotension, hypoxia, increased central venous pressure, difficulty ventilating, and unilateral decreased or absent breath sounds. Other findings include jugular venous distention (from decreased right heart filling due to increased intrathoracic pressure), subcutaneous emphysema (from air being trapped beneath the skin), and tracheal deviation (from deviation of the mediastinum away from the involved side). If tension pneumothorax is clinically suspected, the patient should be immediately stabilized by performing a needle thoracostomy at the second intercostal space at the midclavicular line using a large-bore needle (at least 14 gauge). Alternatively, the needle may be placed laterally at the fourth or fifth intercostal space, which might allow for easier access to the intrapleural space, particularly in obese patients (when the needle is not long enough for an anterior approach). This intervention should not be delayed for radiographic confirmation.

Why are the other choices wrong?

Respiratory variation in the diameter of the inferior vena cava can be seen when central venous pressure is low, as is the case in hypovolemia or distributive shock. In this case, central venous pressure is likely elevated because the right heart cannot expand and fill properly due to the high intrathoracic pressure. Instead, the effect would be distention of the inferior vena cava and lack of variability throughout the respiratory cycle.

Sonographic evidence of right heart distention suggests right heart failure from a primary cardiac process or obstructive source such as PE. Although these conditions could be consistent with the patient's vital sign abnormalities and should be in the differential diagnosis, they do not explain the unilateral decrease in breath sounds or difficulty in ventilating.

Muffled heart sounds and enlarged globular cardiac silhouette in a patient with tachycardia and hypotension suggest pericardial effusion with cardiac tamponade. This can be caused by thoracic trauma but is more likely in penetrating trauma than blunt trauma. Although pericardial effusion can cause these vital sign abnormalities, it does not cause a unilateral decrease in breath sounds or difficulty in ventilating.

PEER REVIEW

✓ Chest compressions during CPR can cause rib fracture, pneumothorax, and other intrathoracic traumatic disorders.

✓ Patients with possible chest trauma who are receiving positive-pressure ventilation should be monitored closely for tension pneumothorax.

✓ Patients whose conditions are concerning for tension pneumothorax should be stabilized immediately by undergoing needle thoracostomy.

REFERENCES

Marx JA, Hockberger RS, Walls RM, eds. *Rosen's Emergency Medicine: Concepts and Clinical Practice*. 8th ed. St. Louis, MO: Elsevier; 2014: 437-440.

Tintinalli JE, Stapczynski JS, Ma OJ, et al, eds. *Tintinalli's Emergency Medicine: A Comprehensive Study Guide*. 8th ed. New York, NY: McGraw-Hill; 2012: 1750-1752.

## 77.	The correct answer is D, Perform trephination of the nail plate.

Why is this the correct answer?

A subungual hematoma develops when the nail bed vasculature is disrupted, as by trauma in this case, and blood accumulates under the nail plate. Hematomas occupying more than 50% of an intact nail plate can be adequately drained by trephination with either electrical cautery or an 18-gauge needle. This usually provides immediate pain relief for the patient. Even if the patient has an underlying fracture, trephination has not been shown to increase the risk of infection of the bone.

Why are the other choices wrong?

Discharge with instructions for analgesic pain relief is appropriate but only after drainage of the hematoma. The patient also should be instructed to soak the finger in water containing antibacterial soap for a few days. Oral antibiotics are usually not warranted.

Nail plate removal is performed to allow for exploration and repair of suspected nail bed lacerations. This patient presented with an intact nail plate, so in this case and others similar to it, trephination is adequate to drain the hematoma.

An emergent hand surgeon consultation is not necessary. Trephination can be performed by an emergency physician in the emergency department.

PEER POINT

Blood draining from a toenail hematoma following trephination

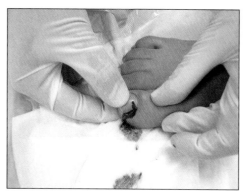

PEER Point 8

PEER REVIEW

✓ Subungual hematomas occupying more than 50% of the nail plate should be drained with trephination.

✓ Nail plate removal is indicated if there is nail avulsion or disruption of the nail fold.

REFERENCES

Marx JA, Hockberger RS, Walls RM, eds. *Rosen's Emergency Medicine: Concepts and Clinical Practice.* 8th ed. St. Louis, MO: Elsevier; 2014: 560-561.

Tintinalli JE, Stapczynski JS, Ma OJ, et al, eds. *Tintinalli's Emergency Medicine: A Comprehensive Study Guide.* 8th ed. New York, NY: McGraw-Hill; 2012: 294-295.

78. The correct answer is D, Hypoxia.

Why is this the correct answer?

Preventing hypoxia in patients with TBI is of the utmost importance because untreated hypoxia with associated hypercapnia correlates with significantly poorer outcomes and increased mortality rates. Hypotension is arguably the most important factor: it alone can increase mortality rates twofold to threefold through decreased cerebral perfusion. The patient in this case has a severe TBI, as evidenced by his GCS score and physical examination findings suggestive of basilar skull fracture. In patients with TBI, care must be taken to avoid hypoxia, hyperthermia, and hypotension because all of these factors increase morbidity and mortality rates. Hyperthermia is associated with poorer outcomes, although the mechanism remains unclear.

Why are the other choices wrong?

Heart rate alone does not seem to have an effect on morbidity and mortality rates in traumatic brain injury (TBI). However, tachycardia secondary to significant blood loss can increase the risk of death due to low-oxygen carrying capacity. Bradycardia can be a sign of Cushing reflex, a prequel to brain herniation.

Hypotension, not hypertension, is associated with increased morbidity and mortality rates in TBI. Maintaining cerebral perfusion is fundamental to improving outcomes, and actions to prevent hypotension should be taken.

Permissive hypothermia might actually improve outcomes in TBI, and some trauma centers recommend actively inducing hypothermia in patients with TBI. In all cases, hyperthermia should be avoided.

PEER REVIEW

- ✓ Hypotension, hypoxia, and hyperthermia all increase morbidity and mortality rates in patients with TBI.
- ✓ Early identification and treatment of hypotension, hypoxia, and hyperthermia will improve patient outcomes

REFERENCES:
Marx JA, Hockberger RS, Walls RM, eds. *Rosen's Emergency Medicine: Concepts and Clinical Practice.* 8th ed. St. Louis, MO: Elsevier; 2014: 339-367.
Wolfson AB, Hendey GW, Ling LJ, et al, eds. *Harwood-Nuss' Clinical Practice of Emergency Medicine.* 6th ed. Philadelphia, PA: Lippincott, Williams & Wilkins; 2014: 161-162.

79. The correct answer is B, Normal saline bolus.

Why is this the correct answer?

Approximately 30% to 50% of inferior STEMIs are associated with right ventricular infarction. This particular patient is experiencing an inferior STEMI with right ventricular infarction, and the hypotension, jugular venous distention, and clear lung sounds are signs of acute right-sided heart failure. Given that the patient is already hypotensive and preload dependent, the correct management is to administer a normal saline fluid bolus to increase preload and improve blood pressure. The patient's history and ECG findings match the diagnostic criteria for STEMI. These criteria include two contiguous leads with ST-segment elevation of more than 2 mm in leads V2 and V3 or more than 1 mm in all other leads. In this patient, the inferior STEMI is indicated by the ST-segment elevations in leads II, III, and aVF. Extension of the infarction into the right ventricle is indicated by the ST-segment elevation in lead V1. There is also evidence of respectively greater ST-segment elevation in lead III compared to lead II. These ECG changes require immediate evaluation by a cardiologist for potential PCI.

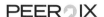

Why are the other choices wrong?

Morphine, oxygen, nitroglycerin, and aspirin (MONA) and STEMI protocols are appropriate for patients with STEMI who are not preload dependent. However, patients with right ventricular infarction are preload dependent with regard to maintaining adequate blood pressure. Medications such as nitroglycerin and opioids are contraindicated because they can lower preload and subsequently result in worsening hypotension and perfusion. Oxygen is not needed in this case because no respiratory distress is noted, and hypoxia is not present. Hyperoxia produced by supplemental oxygen therapy can be detrimental in a STEMI patient. Both can lower preload, resulting in worsening heart failure, hypotension, and coronary perfusion.

Oral beta blockers are indicated in STEMI within the first 24 hours of symptoms. However, beta blockers are not indicated for STEMI patients if they demonstrate signs of cardiogenic shock or heart failure. This patient is hypotensive and has signs of right-sided heart failure with distended neck veins.

Vasopressor therapy as the initial choice for resuscitation of a hypotensive event is rarely correct. In this particular situation, the patient is experiencing an inferior STEMI with right ventricular infarction. In such settings, the patient is preload dependent and requires initial intravenous fluid for initial resuscitation.

PEER POINT

Leads with ST-segment elevation and corresponding location of the MI

- V1-V4, anterior or anteroseptal
- I, aVL, V5-V6, lateral
- I, aVL, V1-V6, anterolateral
- V1-V2, septal
- II, III, aVF, inferior
- I, aVL, V5-V6, II, III, aVF, inferolateral
- V1-V4 / V8, V9, posterior indirect/posterior direct
- RV1-RV6 or RV4, right ventricular

PEER REVIEW

- ✓ Patients with right ventricular infarctions are preload dependent and susceptible to worsening hypotension via nitrates and opioids.
- ✓ Here are the diagnostic criteria for STEMI: two contiguous leads with ST-segment elevation of more than 2 mm in leads V2-V3 or more than 1 mm in all other leads.
- ✓ Beta blockers are contraindicated in STEMI patients with hypotension or heart failure.

REFERENCES

Mattu A, Brady WJ, et al (eds). *Cardiovascular Emergencies*. Dallas, TX: American College of Emergency Physicians Publishing; 2014: 11-35.

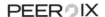
80. The correct answer is B, The patient can bite down on and break a tongue blade while the examiner twists it.

Why is this the correct answer?

The tongue blade test is performed by having a patient attempt to "clamp down on" a tongue blade between the teeth with enough force that the examiner is unable to pull it out from the teeth. When the examiner twists the blade, a patient should be able to generate enough force to break or crack the blade. The test is positive if the patient cannot clench the tongue blade between the teeth or if the examiner cannot break the blade while it is held in the patient's bite. This test is frequently used in the examination of a patient with blunt trauma to the face; if the result is positive, imaging is indicated. If the blade can be gripped by the patient and be broken by the examiner, fracture of the mandible is much less likely, and additional imaging is likely not needed. Patients with intraoral bleeding, tooth malocclusion, trismus, ecchymosis, and intraoral swelling are at higher risk for fracture.

Why are the other choices wrong?

Deviation of the chin toward the side of the face that is painful and swollen can indicate mandibular condyle fracture or unilateral dislocation. Dislocation is much more likely to occur as a result of yawning or extreme mouth opening, however, and is rare in trauma. Fracture is more likely in cases of trauma.

The presence of a sublingual hematoma is very rare, but when a patient has one, it is suggestive of mandibular fracture. The physician should be highly suspicious for fracture when sublingual hematoma is discovered.

When the interdental incisor distance at maximal mouth opening is less than 5 cm, there is a higher likelihood of mandibular trauma. Imaging would be more likely to reveal fracture in these cases.

PEER REVIEW

✓ Here are the signs of mandibular fracture: malocclusion, intraoral bleeding, trismus, and deviation of the chin.
✓ A positive tongue blade test in the right clinical setting should prompt imaging.
✓ A negative tongue blade test is reassuring in the evaluation of mandibular trauma.

REFERENCES
Marx JA, Hockberger RS, Walls RM, eds. *Rosen's Emergency Medicine: Concepts and Clinical Practice.* 8th ed. St. Louis, MO: Elsevier; 2014: 372-377.
Wolfson AB, Hendey GW, Ling LJ, et al, eds. *Harwood-Nuss' Clinical Practice of Emergency Medicine.* 6th ed. Philadelphia, PA: Lippincott, Williams & Wilkins; 2014: 163-165.

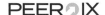

81. The correct answer is B, It is associated with fourth finger radial sensory dysfunction.

Why is this the correct answer?

Carpal tunnel syndrome is a median mononeuropathy and the most common mononeuropathy in the body. Classic symptoms include pain and paresthesias on the volar side of the first, second, and third fingers and radial half of the fourth finger with symptoms most notable at night. Fourth finger sensory dysfunction on the radial aspect of the finger only is very specific for the diagnosis of carpal tunnel syndrome. Extension and flexion at the wrist commonly exacerbate the condition and can aid in diagnosis. Using the Phalen test, by holding the wrists in maximum flexion for at least 1 minute, reproduction of the symptoms helps to point toward this diagnosis. A positive Tinel sign yields tingling after tapping on the wrist where the median nerve passes through the carpal tunnel between the carpal bones and the flexor retinaculum. Both of these tests have poor sensitivity, and if negative, do not effectively rule out the diagnosis. A more specific finding is divided sensation of the fourth finger, with dysfunction on the radial aspect only. Treatment for carpal tunnel syndrome includes a splint on the wrist and NSAIDs. Recurrent symptoms sometimes warrant steroid injections by a hand surgeon and possibly surgical decompression.

Why are the other choices wrong?

Some patients have weakness in the muscles of the hand, a condition known as Guyon canal syndrome or handlebar palsy. It is an ulnar mononeuropathy rather than a median neuropathy as with carpal tunnel syndrome. In this rare syndrome, there is compression of the ulnar nerve at the wrist that causes weakness of the intrinsic muscles of the hand. What often happens is that the sensory function of the ulnar nerve is spared or involves only the palmar aspect of the fifth finger and half of the fourth. Carpal tunnel can cause weakness in the thenar eminence, but not the traditional intrinsic muscles of the hand.

Carpal tunnel syndrome is caused by compression of the medial nerve in the inflamed carpal tunnel between the flexor retinaculum and carpal bones, not at the medial epicondyle. Compression here causes cubital tunnel syndrome, and patients have numbness and tingling in the fifth and lateral fourth digits.

Carpal tunnel syndrome is the most common mononeuropathy in the body and involves the median nerve, not the ulnar nerve. The most common ulnar nerve mononeuropathy is cubital tunnel syndrome. Patients typically have paresthesias of the fifth and lateral fourth fingers. Ultimately, weakness of the intrinsic muscles can ensue.

PEER REVIEW

- ✓ Symptoms of carpal tunnel syndrome: pain and paresthesias of the volar aspect of the first, second, and third fingers and radial side of the fourth.
- ✓ If you're treating a patient who has sensory dysfunction on the radial side of the fourth finger, suspect carpal tunnel syndrome.
- ✓ The Phalen test and the Tinel sign can help confirm the diagnosis of carpal tunnel syndrome but are not very sensitive or specific.

REFERENCES

Marx JA, Hockberger RS, Walls RM, eds. *Rosen's Emergency Medicine: Concepts and Clinical Practice*. 8th ed. St. Louis, MO: Elsevier; 2014: 1428-1440.

Tintinalli JE, Stapczynski JS, Ma OJ, et al, eds. *Tintinalli's Emergency Medicine: A Comprehensive Study Guide*. 8th ed. New York, NY: McGraw-Hill; 2012: 1179-1185.

82. The correct answer is C, Pelvic angiography followed by retrograde urethrography.

Why is this the correct answer?

Although this patient is at significant risk of having urethral injury, management of the hemodynamic instability and likely pelvic bleeding must take precedence. Urethral evaluation is not emergently necessary and can be performed later in the patient's course; resuscitation and control of his blood loss with angiography and embolization are more critical and time sensitive. If the patient is to undergo CT or angiography, retrograde urethrography should be delayed because the contrast material can interfere with the images obtained and jeopardize the chances for injury identification and treatment by vascular embolization. The proper order is angiography first, and once his condition is stabilized, retrograde urethrography. The first step in performing retrograde urethrography is to obtain a preinjection abdominal xray. Next is to inject contrast material into the urethral meatus, followed by a postinjection xray. A finding of contrast extravasation is consistent with urethral tear. Given the mechanism of injury in this case and the physical examination findings of perineal ecchymosis and blood at the urinary meatus, urethral injury is likely. Other findings might include penile, scrotal, or perineal hematoma, inability to void, high-riding prostate, and difficulty passing a Foley catheter. Urethral injuries are classified as anterior (distal to the prostate) and posterior (proximal to and including the prostatic urethra). Anterior urethral injuries are usually caused by direct perineal trauma; posterior urethral injuries are most often caused by pelvic fractures, particularly those involving the ischiopubic rami.

Why are the other choices wrong?

Although urethral injury can lead to significant morbidity if missed, it does not require emergent evaluation, particularly in a patient who is hemodynamically unstable and is in critical need of hemorrhage control. Retrograde urethrography should also be delayed in patients undergoing CT or angiography to avoid obscuring the images.

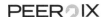

Retrograde cystography is used in the evaluation of bladder injury. It involves injecting contrast material into the bladder using a Foley catheter and assessing for extravasation on xray. Although bladder injury might also be of concern in this case, the patient is at higher risk for urethral injury, and a Foley catheter should not be placed until after retrograde urethrography is performed.

Placement of a Foley catheter should not be attempted in a patient with possible urethral injury (or high suspicion for urethral trauma) until retrograde urethrography is performed because it can worsen the injury. If close monitoring of urine output or bladder decompression is more urgently needed, a suprapubic catheter may be placed.

PEER POINT

Steps in performing retrograde urethrography

1. Obtain a preinjection abdominal xray.
2. Inject contrast material into the urethral meatus.
3. Obtain a postinjection xray.
4. Confirm the presence or absence of injury: contrast extravasation is consistent with urethral tear.

PEER REVIEW

✓ These signs and symptoms should raise concern for urethral injury: pelvic fracture, perineal hematoma or ecchymosis, blood at the urinary meatus, high-riding prostate, inability to void.

✓ If you suspect urethral injury, perform retrograde urethrography before placing a Foley catheter.

✓ Urethral evaluation should not be performed until the patient is stabilized and more critical injuries are assessed and managed.

REFERENCES

Marx JA, Hockberger RS, Walls RM, eds. *Rosen's Emergency Medicine: Concepts and Clinical Practice*. 8th ed. St. Louis, MO: Elsevier; 2014: 481-485.

Tintinalli JE, Stapczynski JS, Ma OJ, et al, eds. *Tintinalli's Emergency Medicine: A Comprehensive Study Guide*. 8th ed. New York, NY: McGraw-Hill; 2012: 1768-1769.

83. The correct answer is C, Nicardipine titrated to a MAP of 126.

Why is this the correct answer?

Severe headache, vomiting, and altered mental status in a patient with severe hypertension suggest hypertensive encephalopathy, a true hypertensive emergency. In this patient, the CT findings are consistent with the diagnosis as well. Goals for therapy include lowering the MAP back into a range where cerebral autoregulation can occur. Nicardipine, a peripherally acting calcium channel blocker given intravenously, has consistent effects on dilating vascular beds and is considered first-line therapy for hypertensive encephalopathy. Generally, the MAP should be lowered by 20% in the first hour but by no more than 25% in the first day. This formula can be used to estimate MAP: MAP = Diastolic BP + 1/3(Systolic – Diastolic pressure). Lowering the blood pressure too rapidly can provoke cerebral ischemia in a brain that is accustomed to higher blood pressures.

Why are the other choices wrong?

Hydralazine is not considered first-line therapy for hypertensive encephalopathy. It can unpredictably lower cerebral perfusion pressure, precipitating ischemia in the brain.

Metoprolol is a beta-1 selective adrenergic receptor blocker. It primarily affects the heart rate with no vasodilatory properties. Although metoprolol can lower blood pressure, direct-acting vasodilatory agents are considered better options. In addition, therapy for hypertensive encephalopathy does not normally focus on heart rate.

Nitroprusside, like hydralazine, can unpredictably lower cerebral perfusion pressure and paradoxically elevate intracranial pressure. It can be considered as second-line or third-line therapy but should not be used as a first-line agent.

PEER REVIEW

✓ What defines hypertensive encephalopathy? Central nervous system findings consistent with end-organ damage — not absolute blood pressure.

✓ Remember that lowering blood pressure too aggressively can result in ischemic symptoms in a chronically hypertensive patient.

REFERENCES

Manning L, Robinson TG, Anderson CS. Control of Blood Pressure in Hypertensive Neurological Emergencies. *Curr Hypertens Rep.* 2014;16:436.

Marx JA, Hockberger RS, Walls RM, eds. *Rosen's Emergency Medicine: Concepts and Clinical Practice.* 8th ed. St. Louis, MO: Elsevier; 2014: 1113-1123.

84. The correct answer is C, Retrograde cystography.

Why is this the correct answer?

This case presents a constellation of findings that should raise concern for bladder rupture: motor vehicle collision, pelvic fracture, and gross hematuria. To evaluate for bladder injury, the patient should undergo retrograde cystography. The first step is to get an xray or CT scan, after which the bladder is filled retrograde by syringe with contrast material until it is distended. Then imaging is performed again before and after the patient voids. Visualization of contrast material spilling into the peritoneal cavity or retroperitoneal area/pelvic outlet is diagnostic for bladder rupture. Bladder rupture can occur extraperitoneally and/or intraperitoneally. Extraperitoneal injuries are often secondary to shearing of fascial attachments from the anterolateral bladder wall or bladder laceration by bony pelvic fragments. Intraperitoneal injuries are usually the result of compressive forces causing increased intravesicular pressure and rupture into the peritoneal space through the thinnest part of the bladder,

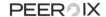

the dome. Gross hematuria is seen in more than 95% of cases and is the hallmark of bladder injury, warranting additional diagnostic workup. Once the patient is adequately stabilized, the urethra should first be evaluated for injury, as this can also cause hematuria in this setting, and then a Foley catheter should be placed. Extraperitoneal ruptures are generally managed conservatively with a Foley catheter, but intraperitoneal ruptures require surgical intervention to prevent subsequent infection and development of peritonitis and sepsis.

Why are the other choices wrong?

A CT scan of the pelvis with passive filling of the bladder with contrast is not adequate for evaluation of bladder injury. The muscular bladder wall might seal enough to prevent leakage of contrast material through the defect unless the bladder is sufficiently distended. Retrograde administration of contrast material is necessary to achieve this.

Pelvic ultrasonography can show free intraperitoneal fluid in the pelvis but has not been shown to be adequate for diagnosis of bladder rupture. Retrograde cystography is the gold standard study for this injury.

Retrograde urethrography is used to evaluate the urethra for injury. The urethra is also at high risk for injury in this scenario, and this should be ruled out before Foley catheter placement. Once this has been established, retrograde cystography is the appropriate study to evaluate for bladder rupture.

PEER REVIEW

- ✓ Your degree of suspicion for bladder rupture should go up if your patient has gross hematuria after blunt trauma, especially with a pelvic fracture.
- ✓ The gold standard study for diagnosing bladder rupture: retrograde cystography.

REFERENCES

Marx JA, Hockberger RS, Walls RM, eds. *Rosen's Emergency Medicine: Concepts and Clinical Practice*. 8th ed. St. Louis, MO: Elsevier; 2014: 485-490.

Tintinalli JE, Stapczynski JS, Ma OJ, et al, eds. *Tintinalli's Emergency Medicine: A Comprehensive Study Guide*. 8th ed. New York, NY: McGraw-Hill; 2012: 1769-1770.

85. The correct answer is C, Negatively birefringent crystals on aspirate.

Why is this the correct answer?

Gout and pseudogout are classified as inflammatory arthritides and are diagnosed by analyzing synovial fluid collected during arthrocentesis. These two can be identified by the level of the cell count along with the presence of crystals, which indicates a crystal-induced synovitis. If the underlying condition is gout, there are negatively birefringent uric acid crystals on aspirate. If it is pseudogout, there is positive birefringence. Patients with gout or pseudogout typically present with acute monoarthritis, seen most commonly seen in either the great toe or the knee, precipitated by factors such as alcohol, noncompliance of diet, infection, trauma, or other stressors. The treatment of choice for an acute attack starts with NSAIDs or colchicine only in the absence of renal dysfunction. If renal disturbance exists, recent guidelines recommend oral steroids, and a course of narcotic pain medications may be used if necessary.

Why are the other choices wrong?

Although the absence of bacteria on joint aspiration can help make the diagnosis of gout, it is not specific for gout itself and is not the gold standard test result. Only in conjunction with the presence of negative birefringent crystal can the absence of bacteria be used to confirm the diagnosis.

High levels of uric acid in the serum can be found in patients with gout, but the level can also be normal during an acute gout attack. Thus this finding should not be used to confirm the diagnosis of gout.

A WBC count less than 2,000 and PMNs less than 25% on arthrocentesis indicates the presence of a noninflammatory arthritis such as osteoarthritis. Gout is in the category of inflammatory arthritides, which have a WBC count between 2,000 and 100,000 and PMNs greater than 50% with a negative culture on arthrocentesis.

PEER REVIEW

- ✓ Gout and pseudogout are diagnosed by the presence of crystals on analysis of synovial joint fluid.
- ✓ Uric acid crystals with negative birefringence on aspirate confirm the diagnosis of gout.
- ✓ Gout and pseudogout are inflammatory arthritic conditions, and first-line treatment includes NSAIDs or colchicine in an acute attack as long as the patient's kidneys are functioning normally.

REFERENCES

Marx JA, Hockberger RS, Walls RM, eds. *Rosen's Emergency Medicine: Concepts and Clinical Practice.* 8th ed. St. Louis, MO: Elsevier; 2014: 1501-1517.

Tintinalli JE, Stapczynski JS, Ma OJ, et al, eds. *Tintinalli's Emergency Medicine: A Comprehensive Study Guide.* 8th ed. New York, NY: McGraw-Hill; 2012: 1927-1936.

86. The correct answer is B, Incision and drainage and suturing of cotton pledgets to the pinna.

Why is this the correct answer?

This patient has an auricular hematoma, and the timeframe indicates that the redness and swelling are likely caused by a hematoma and not profound infection or abscess. Incision and drainage of the hematoma, followed by the placement of sutured cotton pledgets, is indicated to prevent pressure necrosis of the underlying cartilage, which can result in a chronic deformity commonly known as cauliflower ear. If the skin is prepared with an antiseptic prior to incision and drainage, the

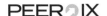

risk of infection is outweighed by the benefit of reduction in long-term deformity. Preparing the skin with alcohol, chlorhexidine, or Betadine reduces the risk of infection. Once proper bolsters have been placed, the ear is relatively protected from further trauma until the follow-up appointment.

Why are the other choices wrong?

The use of ice and NSAID pain medications is helpful if a hematoma is not present, but in the case of an auricular hematoma, it is not sufficient. An incision and drainage is performed to reduce the incidence of cartilaginous deformity later on.

Broad-spectrum antibiotics are not indicated unless the skin has been violated. In the case of an auricular hematoma, antibiotics may be prescribed after incision and drainage to protect the exposed cartilage from infection. But there is not an indication to prescribe them when there is no significant hematoma and when the skin has not been violated. Intravenous antibiotics should be reserved for treating significant infection.

The patient in this case is suffering from trauma and an auricular hematoma, not otitis externa. The reason to place a cotton wick is to facilitate drainage of the external auditory canal and to administer topical antibiotics in the case of otitis externa, an infectious process.

PEER POINT

Steps for draining an auricular hematoma

1. Cleanse with antiseptic.
2. Anesthetize with local anesthetic.
3. Use a scalpel to incise along skin folds to reduce scarring.
4. Drain the hematoma and irrigate with normal saline.
5. Suture dental rolls to the pinna to prevent reaccumulation of blood. Petrolatum or saline-soaked gauze may be applied as an alternative.
6. Apply gauze to either side of the ear and then elastic bandage to keep the gauze in place.
7. Prescribe an antistaphylococcal antibiotic to prevent infection.
8. Advise the patient to have the dressing removed in 1 week.

PEER REVIEW

- ✓ Perform incision and drainage on auricular hematomas.
- ✓ After draining an auricular hematoma, you'll need to apply a pressure dressing with cotton pledgets to prevent reaccumulation of blood.

REFERENCES

Marx JA, Hockberger RS, Walls RM, eds. *Rosen's Emergency Medicine: Concepts and Clinical Practice*. 8th ed. St. Louis, MO: Elsevier; 2014: 378.

Roberts JR, Hedges JR, eds. *Clinical Procedures in Emergency Medicine*. 6th ed. St. Louis, MO: WB Saunders; 2013: 1317-1320.

87. The correct answer is A, Alzheimer disease.

Why is this the correct answer?

One of the hallmarks of dementia is altered mental status that develops gradually and is insidious. Patients with dementia generally have a normal level of consciousness and normal attention. Alzheimer disease is a slowly progressing form of dementia that can be divided into early, middle, and late stages. In the late stage, disorientation can be more severe, and patients experience personality changes such as described in this case. It is also common for patients to have intact remote memory and difficulty with recent memories. Family members often bring loved ones in in the later stages because they are overwhelmed with their care at home. When patients present with symptoms consistent with dementia, it is important to evaluate for underlying medical causes and delirium, especially in the setting of a collateral historian reporting a change in behavior. Additionally, it is important to evaluate for reversible causes of dementia such as subdural hematoma, neurosyphilis, B12 or folate deficiency, or hydrocephalus.

Why are the other choices wrong?

Patients with delirium also present with altered mental status, but the onset is generally sudden in nature and fluctuating. Delirium is a medical emergency; it is important to look for an underlying cause, from medication reactions and drug overdoses to infections, just to name a few. Admission to the hospital is typically necessary, especially when the underlying cause is not found.

Depression is sometimes referred to as "pseudodementia," but the clinical distinctions between these two conditions can be a challenge for even an experienced clinician. It is important to remember that patients in early stages of dementia can have depression symptoms. Patients with depression are more likely to have a psychiatric history, are generally completely oriented, and present shortly after symptom onset.

Normal pressure hydrocephalus presents with the classic triad of dementia, ataxia, and urinary incontinence. Head CT reveals enlarged ventricles. Patients are generally younger; about half are younger than 60 years.

PEER REVIEW

✓ Dementia: gradual onset, difficulty with memories, personality changes.
✓ Look for reversible causes of dementia with basic laboratory testing and noncontrast head CT and tools guided by history and physical examination.
✓ Remember, in elderly patients, depression can look a lot like early dementia; this patient is oriented and likely to have a history of depression.

REFERENCES
Marx JA, Hockberger RS, Walls RM, eds. *Rosen's Emergency Medicine: Concepts and Clinical Practice.* 8th ed. St. Louis, MO: Elsevier; 2014: 1398-1408.
Tintinalli JE, Stapczynski JS, Ma OJ, et al, eds. *Tintinalli's Emergency Medicine: A Comprehensive Study Guide.* 8th ed. New York, NY: McGraw-Hill; 2012: 1156-1161.

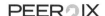

88. The correct answer is C, Place a three-sided occlusive dressing over the wound.

Why is this the correct answer?

In this case, the patient's penetrating traumatic injury resulted in an open pneumothorax. When an open pneumothorax is identified, the appropriate next step in stabilization is to place an occlusive dressing of petrolatum gauze over the wound and secure it to the patient on three sides. This occlusion converts the open pneumothorax to a closed one. The fourth side is left open to allow for escape of any air building up in the pleural space from associated pulmonary tree injuries (particularly if the patient is receiving positive-pressure ventilation) and to prevent a tension pneumothorax. Open pneumothoraces are seen most often in military injuries. Among civilian injuries, they are most commonly caused by shotgun wounds. The defect in the chest wall caused by the penetrating trauma is large enough that air is able to move freely between the chest cavity and the outside atmosphere. If the resistance of air moving through the wound is less than that of the tracheobronchial tree, air preferentially flows in through the wound instead of into the airway when intrathoracic pressure decreases during inspiration. The lung itself paradoxically collapses on inspiration and expands during expiration. Ventilation and gas exchange are subsequently significantly impaired. These wounds are also called "sucking" chest wounds because air can sometimes be heard moving through the wound during respiration. Simultaneously or soon after an occlusive dressing is applied, a large-bore thoracostomy tube should be placed in a separate site in the chest wall to manage the pneumothorax. Again, the occlusive dressing should be secured on three sides rather than four. Securing it on all four sides can convert the open pneumothorax to a tension pneumothorax. Allowing air to escape prevents tension physiology while continuing to prevent air from flowing in through the wound during inspiration.

Why are the other choices wrong?

While placement of a thoracostomy tube is indicated in this patient for management of the pneumothorax, this should not be placed through the site of the chest wound, as the tube is likely to track along the course of the object causing the trauma. This prevents the tube from being placed properly for appropriate functioning and has high risk of further injury to the lung, diaphragm, or other intrathoracic structures. A separate site in the affected hemithorax should be chosen.

In this patient with audible air movement through a large chest wound, it is clinically evident that an open pneumothorax is already present. Needle thoracostomy is indicated for stabilizing a suspected tension pneumothorax and does so by creating an opening to the outside atmosphere, essentially converting it to an open pneumothorax and allowing release of building intrathoracic pressure. In this patient, the problem is the paradoxical physiology caused by the large open pneumothorax, and a needle thoracostomy would not improve this.

Most patients do not need emergent surgical treatment for an open pneumothorax. In this case, before the patient is transported from the emergency department, the sucking chest should be immediately stabilized as described above. Other injuries can be identified and reviewed, and if thoracotomy is needed later, the patient may be taken to the OR in a more controlled, elective manner.

PEER REVIEW

✓ How to perform initial stabilization of an open pneumothorax: place a three-sided occlusive dressing over the wound.

✓ Don't seal the occlusive dressing on an open pneumothorax on all four sides — that will convert it to a tension pneumothorax.

REFERENCES

Marx JA, Hockberger RS, Walls RM, eds. *Rosen's Emergency Medicine: Concepts and Clinical Practice*. 8th ed. St. Louis, MO: Elsevier; 2014: 437-440.

Tintinalli JE, Stapczynski JS, Ma OJ, et al, eds. *Tintinalli's Emergency Medicine: A Comprehensive Study Guide*. 8th ed. New York, NY: McGraw-Hill; 2012: 1750-1752.

89. The correct answer is B, Burst fracture.

Why is this the correct answer?

In this case, the patient presents after a motor vehicle collision with a wedge-shaped compression fracture noted on xray. This clinical presentation and fracture pattern should raise concern for a burst fracture, which can be missed on plain films and is best visualized using spinal CT. Burst fractures are associated with motor vehicle crashes, especially with seatbelt use, as well as falls from height. Compression fractures involve only the anterior column and are stable unless loss of vertebral height is greater than 50%. However, burst fractures are inherently unstable due to the potential for the retropulsion of bone fragments into the spinal canal secondary to disruption of the posterior column. For this reason, additional imaging should be performed if there is clinical suspicion for a burst fracture, and neurosurgery consultation is required.

Why are the other choices wrong?

On plain radiographs, bilateral facet dislocations appear as vertebral subluxations and should be obvious. They are inherently unstable and typically associated with neurologic deficits.

A Chance fracture is a complete disruption through the vertebral body and associated structures in a horizontal plane. These fractures also commonly occur in motor vehicle crashes due to seatbelt injuries. However, these fractures are actually best visualized on lateral plain radiographs or on sagittal reconstructions of spinal CT.

Transverse process fractures are stable. They are considered minor spinal injuries and do not require neurosurgery evaluation. They might, however, indicate serious intrathoracic or intraabdominal trauma due to the force required to fracture the bones.

PEER REVIEW

✓ Burst fractures can be misdiagnosed as compression fractures.

✓ Compression fractures, burst fractures, and Chance fractures are common in motor vehicle collisions, especially with seatbelt use.

✓ Transverse process fractures are stable.

REFERENCES

Marx JA, Hockberger RS, Walls RM, eds. *Rosen's Emergency Medicine: Concepts and Clinical Practice*. 8th ed. St. Louis, MO: Elsevier; 2014: 382-420.

Wolfson AB, Hendey GW, Ling LJ, et al, eds. *Harwood-Nuss' Clinical Practice of Emergency Medicine*. 6th ed. Philadelphia, PA: Lippincott, Williams & Wilkins; 2014: 193-199.

90. The correct answer is C, Make a unilateral longitudinal incision lateral to the infection to drain the wound.

Why is this the correct answer?

This patient has a felon. A felon is an infection of the pulp space of the distal finger or thumb. An incision and drainage is necessary to treat the infection and prevent more serious complications. The procedure is usually accomplished by making a unilateral longitudinal incision lateral to the infection and distal to the distal interphalangeal joint to prevent damaging the nerves and vessels in the finger pad. Usually, the thumb and fifth finger are incised radially, and the second, third, and fourth fingers are incised on the ulnar side to avoid the sensate finger pad and areas most vulnerable to contact. An infection in this area usually starts off as a superficial cellulitis that ultimately progresses into a deeper infection. This infection spreads through the septae present in the pulp space to form multiple abscesses. Left untreated, the infection can progress to flexor tenosynovitis, a joint infection, or even osteomyelitis. In the evaluation and treatment of finger infections, it is very important to be able to distinguish a felon from herpetic whitlow because the treatments are very different. Herpetic whitlow is a viral infection. It can be caused by herpes simplex I or II. Health care workers are at risk of getting infected given their increased exposure to oral secretions and should wear gloves during the evaluation. Herpetic whitlow appears as small vesicles on an erythematous base, usually on the volar surface of the finger, much like a felon, but it can also be on the dorsal surface and be mistaken for a paronychia. A patient might describe itching and burning. Again, it is extremely important that herpetic whitlow not be mistaken for a felon. With herpetic whitlow, no incision or drainage should be performed: it can result in a secondary bacterial infection or even poor healing.

Why are the other choices wrong?

Applying a clean dressing and prescribing an NSAID are appropriate in the treatment of herpetic whitlow, not felon. Immobilizing and elevating the finger can be helpful, and antiviral medications might help in infections with a long course. The patient should be educated that herpetic whitlow is highly contagious, and that keeping the area covered with a clean dressing is very important.

Elevating the eponychial fold for a wound to drain is a procedure used for a paronychia, not a felon. Paronychia is a nail infection that develops on the paronychium, ie, lateral nail fold. There is usually an accompanying history of a hangnail or a minor trauma such as nail biting. Any fluctuance or pus noted requires an incision and drainage that involves lifting the paronychium or the eponychium with a blade and allowing the infected fluid to drain. Occasionally, the lateral one fourth of the nail plate must be removed to allow for drainage.

A felon is not a surgical emergency and does not require consultation with a hand surgeon or parenteral antibiotic administration; that would be the correct disposition and treatment for flexor tenosynovitis. Felons do typically have an overlying cellulitis and are treated with oral antibiotics, but rarely are intravenous antibiotics indicated. Patients may be referred to hand surgeons for follow-up and long-term treatment, but rarely is an emergency department consultation required for treatment of a felon.

PEER POINT

Characteristics of fingertip infections

- Felon — Located on the finger tuft, treated with lateral fingertip incision and drainage
- Paronychia — Located on the nail bed edge, treated with elevation of the paronychium for drainage
- Whitlow — Located anywhere on the finger, a small ulcerative lesion, don't cut it! Treated with a clean dressing, NSAIDs, elevation, possibly antiviral medication

PEER REVIEW

- ✓ A felon is a bacterial pulp space infection of the distal finger or thumb requiring incision and drainage.
- ✓ The incision made to treat a felon should be longitudinal unilateral to spare the sensate finger pad.
- ✓ You need to be able to tell the difference between a felon and herpetic whitlow to prevent serious consequences. Whitlow should not be treated with incision and drainage.

REFERENCES

Marx JA, Hockberger RS, Walls RM, eds. *Rosen's Emergency Medicine: Concepts and Clinical Practice*. 8th ed. St. Louis, MO: Elsevier; 2014: 148-183.

Tintinalli JE, Stapczynski JS, Ma OJ, et al, eds. *Tintinalli's Emergency Medicine: A Comprehensive Study Guide*. 8th ed. New York, NY: McGraw-Hill; 2012: 1921-1927.

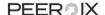

91. The correct answer is D, Stain extruding from the laceration.

Why is this the correct answer?

Eyelid lacerations within 5 to 7 mm of the medial canthus can result in lacrimal duct injury. The risk of this injury is high, and the degree of suspicion should be as well when a patient presents with a laceration near the medial canthus. If the duct is involved, fluorescein dye will enter the lacrimal system and then flow from the laceration itself. Lacrimal duct injuries should never be repaired by an emergency physician. These injuries require oculoplastic consultation.

Why are the other choices wrong?

Flow of aqueous fluid through the fluorescein stain, or a positive Seidel test, is diagnostic of an open globe injury. Open globe injuries are associated with pupillary defects, eye pain or irritation, and decreased visual acuity.

Localized corneal uptake of fluorescein stain is consistent with a corneal abrasion. Corneal abrasions are typically very painful, but some patients describe only a sensation of foreign body or irritation. Excessive tearing and photophobia are also signs of a corneal abrasion.

Pooling of the stain in a localized area suggests conjunctival laceration. This injury is associated with foreign body sensation or eye irritation as well as mild tearing. The Seidel test should be performed to evaluate for a globe rupture.

PEER REVIEW

- ✓ Eyelid lacerations close to the medial canthus are at high risk for lacrimal duct injury.
- ✓ Complex eyelid lacerations require ophthalmology or oculoplastic consultation.
- ✓ Fluorescein staining is crucial to the evaluation of injuries secondary to eye trauma.

REFERENCES

Tintinalli JE, Stapczynski JS, Ma OJ, et al, eds. *Tintinalli's Emergency Medicine: A Comprehensive Study Guide.* 8th ed. New York, NY: McGraw-Hill; 2012: 1543-1579.

Wolfson AB, Hendey GW, Ling LJ, et al, eds. *Harwood-Nuss' Clinical Practice of Emergency Medicine.* 6th ed. Philadelphia, PA: Lippincott, Williams & Wilkins; 2014: 181-182.

92. The correct answer is C, Intubation.

Why is this the correct answer?

Angioedema from ACE inhibitors is caused by decreased metabolism of bradykinin; it does not respond to the typical anaphylactic treatment medications. This patient presents with symptoms concerning for airway compromise. Admitting him to the hospital for close observation is the correct disposition, but the first best step in the emergency department is to perform emergent intubation to protect his airway. It is often prudent to request an anesthesia or ENT consultation due to the high risk to the airway. There are no approved medications for treatment of angioedema; supportive care and close observation are indicated. There are some reports that administration of fresh frozen plasma is beneficial for patients with hereditary angioedema.

Why are the other choices wrong?

C1 inhibitor replacement protein is very useful for hereditary angioedema but is not indicated in patients with angioedema caused by medications, as is implied in this case. Treatment for ACE-inhibitor-induced angioedema is supportive, and airway protection is indicated.

Although epinephrine is often used in the treatment of patients who present with angioedema, there is no proven benefit of using it in the treatment of kinin-mediated angioedema. Antihistamines such as diphenhydramine are similarly unhelpful. This patient's use of an ACE inhibitor provides a strong clue to the cause of his symptoms, but when a patient presents with these symptoms and the cause is not clear, considering an anaphylactic reaction is reasonable. In these cases, epinephrine administration may be considered.

Methylprednisolone is often used in anaphylaxis to help reduce inflammation, but there is no indication that it produces benefit in angioedema.

PEER REVIEW

✓ Evaluate patients with angioedema with airway compromise immediately for intubation.
✓ Traditional medicines for allergic and anaphylactic reactions like diphenhydramine, steroids, and epinephrine have no proven benefit or indication in angioedema.
✓ Treatment for angioedema is largely supportive and includes close observation for airway protection.

REFERENCES

Marx JA, Hockberger RS, Walls RM, eds. *Rosen's Emergency Medicine: Concepts and Clinical Practice*. 8th ed. St. Louis, MO: Elsevier; 2014: 1543-1557.

Tintinalli JE, Stapczynski JS, Ma OJ, et al, eds. *Tintinalli's Emergency Medicine: A Comprehensive Study Guide*. 8th ed. New York, NY: McGraw-Hill; 2012: 74-79.

93. The correct answer is C, Start infusion of 50 units/kg of factor VIII then obtain a head CT scan.

Why is this the correct answer?

Hemophilia A is a bleeding disorder: the patient's blood contains a variant form of factor VIII and lacks clot-forming properties. In patients with hemophilia A who are bleeding, the decision to start factor replacement therapy should be made based on the type of injury. In the case of head trauma, factor should be given prophylactically and not delayed for a head CT due to the potential for life-threatening consequences. The guideline for severe, life-threatening CNS bleeding always requires 50 units/kg of factor VIII. In the general management of hemophilia A with factor replacement therapy, 1 unit/kg of factor VIII increases the amount of circulating factor by 2%. This is the method for determining the dosage: desired factor VIII level (%) × 0.5 × patient weight (kg). It is important to remember that when treating a hemophiliac patient in an emergency, the patient's factor level should be assumed to be zero. In this case, the patient has the potential for major intracranial bleeding, and factor should be replaced to 100%.

Why are the other choices wrong?

In the setting of severe head trauma, factor VIII replacement should not be deferred for a head CT and should instead be performed prophylactically. Of the other answer choices, 12.5 units/kg is a dose within the range typically given to patients with a minor risk of bleeding. Head trauma should always be considered a major risk for bleeding.

The 25 units/kg dose is within the range typically given to patients with a moderate risk of bleeding. Events that would be included in the moderate risk injuries might include known bleeding into a joint, large muscle bleeding, or traumatic oral or nasal bleeding.

Finally, 100 units/kg is not a dose that is calculated for factor replacement; 50 units/kg is typically the highest dose. Instead, factor VIII should be replaced to 100% in patients who have a major risk of bleeding.

PEER POINT

How to calculate dosing for factor replacement therapy in hemophilia A

Desired factor VIII level (%) × 0.5 × patient weight (kg)

PEER REVIEW

✓ If you're treating head trauma in a patient with hemophilia A, do the factor VIII replacement immediately — don't delay it for a head CT.
✓ Here's the dosing formula for factor VIII replacement in a bleeding hemophiliac patient: desired factor VIII level (%) × 0.5 × patient weight (kg).
✓ The desired factor VIII replacement in a hemophiliac patient with a head injury (ie, severe risk of bleeding) is 100%, and the appropriate dose is 50 units/kg.

REFERENCES

Marx JA, Hockberger RS, Walls RM, eds. *Rosen's Emergency Medicine: Concepts and Clinical Practice.* 8th ed. St. Louis, MO: Elsevier; 2014: 1606-1616.

Tintinalli JE, Stapczynski JS, Ma OJ, et al, eds. *Tintinalli's Emergency Medicine: A Comprehensive Study Guide.* 8th ed. New York, NY: McGraw-Hill; 2012: 1500-1504.

94. The correct answer is D, Symptoms are related to the degree of herniation of abdominal contents.

Why is this the correct answer?

This patient has a diaphragmatic rupture with herniation of the abdominal contents into the thoracic cavity, thus leading to severe respiratory distress and decreased breath sounds. The degree of his respiratory distress is related to both the size of the diaphragmatic tear as well as the amount of abdominal viscera that is herniated into the hemithorax. Large injuries can be identified on chest xray, but smaller injuries are harder to detect when they do not involve herniation of visceral contents into the thoracic cavity. A CT scan can help identify these injuries when they are not visible on chest xray, but smaller injuries can be missed on CT scan as well and can be notoriously difficult to identify. Patients occasionally present months to years later with symptoms from a previously undiagnosed injury. Patients with smaller tears typically have fewer symptoms. These injuries occur most commonly with blunt trauma due to violent compression of the abdominal cavity and the pressure gradient between the thoracic and abdominal cavities. It is important to proceed cautiously if considering chest tube placement in these patients to avoid iatrogenic visceral injury.

Why are the other choices wrong?

Blunt trauma typically causes larger tears in the diaphragm than penetrating trauma due to the forces involved in the injury. Blunt trauma can cause tears as large as 5 to 15 cm typically, and at the posterolateral portion of the diaphragm, due to the inherent weakness of the diaphragm in this area.

Diaphragmatic tears were previously thought to be much more common on the left side of the body because the right hemidiaphragm is relatively protected by the liver. Right-sided injuries do occur, but typically these injuries cause more hemodynamic compromise due to the greater force required to cause injury, and because the mortality rate is higher in the field with right-sided injuries. In addition, right-sided injuries can be underdiagnosed due to the protective effect of the liver. It is now thought that left-sided and right-sided injuries occur at about the same frequency.

The mortality rate for diaphragmatic rupture is higher with blunt trauma than penetrating trauma because penetrating trauma typically causes smaller defects, and larger forces are required to tear the diaphragm with blunt trauma. Blunt traumatic diaphragm rupture can cause immediate or delayed herniation of abdominal contents into the thoracic cavity that results in complications such as tension gastrothorax, visceral ischemia, or perforated viscus.

PEER REVIEW

✓ Blunt trauma causes larger defects in the diaphragm than penetrating trauma does.

✓ Herniation of abdominal contents can be immediate or delayed even months to years after the initial injury.

✓ The degree of complications and symptoms is related to the degree of herniation of abdominal contents.

REFERENCES

Broder J. *Diagnostic Imaging for the Emergency Physician*. Philadelphia, PA: Saunders; 2011:323.

Tintinalli JE, Stapczynski JS, Ma OJ, et al, eds. *Tintinalli's Emergency Medicine: A Comprehensive Study Guide*. 8th ed. New York, NY: McGraw-Hill; 2012: 1762.

Wolfson AB, Hendey GW, Ling LJ, et al, eds. *Harwood-Nuss' Clinical Practice of Emergency Medicine*. 6th ed. Philadelphia, PA: Lippincott, Williams & Wilkins; 2014: 209-211.

95. The correct answer is B, Cultures of the pharynx and vagina.

Why is this the correct answer?

Gonococcal septic arthritis is the most common form of septic arthritis in adolescents and young adults, and it has a greater female:male predominance. Because cultures of synovial fluid are positive less than 50% of the time, the clinician should obtain specimens for culture from other parts of the body where Neisseria gonorrhoeae might be found — the posterior pharynx, urethra/cervix, or rectum. The patient in this case has the typical symptoms — the classic triad of a migratory arthritis in multiple joints, papular or pustular rash, and inflammation of the tendon sheaths. Confirming the diagnosis is important because the treatment of gonococcal septic arthritis is different from that for the nongonococcal type. Gonococcal septic arthritis often may be treated with intravenous antibiotics only, thus avoiding surgical joint irrigation, because it rarely results in the joint destruction that is more typical of nongonococcal septic arthritis. The most effective antibiotic for treating gonococcal septic arthritis is a third-generation cephalosporin such as the classic ceftriaxone, and this approach should continue until all culture results are in. When the diagnosis is unknown initially, many practitioners add vancomycin. Vesiculopustular lesions should be looked for on a skin examination, including the classic rash on the palms and soles. This rash is seen in nearly half of patients with this disease, so it can help make the diagnosis. The rash can range from hemorrhagic papules to pustules.

Why are the other choices wrong?

Taking a patient to surgery for joint irrigation is usually required in the treatment of nongonococcal septic arthritis because it is highly associated with joint destruction. Joint aspiration is essential to diagnose septic arthritis, but the sensitivities of the results are not great. Septic arthritis is usually considered with the accepted cutoff of 50,000 cells/mm^3. Measuring ESR and C-reactive protein can also help make the diagnosis but are nonspecific indictors. Nongonococcal

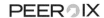

septic arthritis is usually just monoarticular; polyarticular involvement is present in fewer than 20% of adult cases.

Lyme arthritis also starts with a migratory polyarthritis but then typically evolves into a monoarticular process. In contrast to patients with gonococcal arthritis, those with Lyme arthritis typically have recurrent, brief attacks from weeks to months after infection that cause joint swelling and pain and progresses to a chronic arthritis. These patients live in or have traveled to areas known to be associated with Lyme disease. They might or might not have a history of tick bite or rash.

Measuring a patient's serum uric acid level would be reasonable if the suspected diagnosis were gout. However, patients with gout are usually older than 40 years and typically present with symptoms in the great toe or the knee. Gout usually is a monoarthritis that is often preceded by trauma, surgery, a change in medication, or illness. When diagnosing gout, a serum uric acid level is not very helpful: up to 30% of patients have a normal level during an acute attack.

PEER REVIEW

✓ In gonococcal septic arthritis, joint fluid cultures are positive for *N. gonorrhoeae* infection less than half the time, so be sure to get samples from other areas such as the posterior pharynx, urethra/cervix, and rectum for culture.

✓ What are the clues? Gonococcal arthritis is typically associated with a migratory arthritis. Gout is usually monoarticular. Lyme can be either, or it can start as polyarthritis and evolve into monoarthritis.

✓ Gonococcal arthritis may be treated with intravenous antibiotics — usually a third-generation cephalosporin — and avoid surgical joint irrigation, but nongonococcal septic arthritis typically requires surgical management.

REFERENCES

Marx JA, Hockberger RS, Walls RM, eds. *Rosen's Emergency Medicine: Concepts and Clinical Practice.* 8th ed. St. Louis, MO: Elsevier; 2014: 1831-1850.

Tintinalli JE, Stapczynski JS, Ma OJ, et al, eds. *Tintinalli's Emergency Medicine: A Comprehensive Study Guide.* 8th ed. New York, NY: McGraw-Hill; 2012: 1927-1936.

96. The correct answer is D, Urinary retention.

Why is this the correct answer?

Cauda equina syndrome is a type of epidural compression syndrome similar to spinal cord compression and conus medullaris syndrome. The presentation of each of these syndromes is similar except for the level of neurologic deficit. In a patient with cauda equina syndrome, the most common presenting symptom is urinary retention with or without resultant overflow urinary incontinence. The symptom of urinary retention has a sensitivity of approximately 90% and specificity of 95%. The etiology in cauda equina is usually an intervertebral disc rupture, commonly at level L4–L5. Conus medullaris is distinct from cauda equina syndrome, as the former

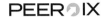

can have upper motor neuron findings (increased muscle tone) with lower motor neuron findings and is generally bilateral. In contrast, cauda equina syndrome is more likely to occur gradually, often unilaterally, with only lower motor neuron symptoms (incontinence or retention, numbness, or weakness).

Why are the other choices wrong?

Sciatica can be a presenting complaint in patients with cauda equina, but it can present either bilaterally or unilaterally. A better predictor for cauda compression is a presentation of bilateral sciatica along with urinary retention. A more common sensory complaint is saddle anesthesia.

Lower extremity weakness is another common complaint among patients with cauda equine syndrome, but it is not the most common or consistent finding. It is often described as either a weakness or stiffness.

Stool incontinence is another common presentation in cauda equina and is associated with decreased anal sphincter tone. Anal tone is usually decreased in 60% to 80% of cases.

PEER REVIEW

- ✓ The most common and sensitive symptom for cauda equina syndrome is urinary retention.
- ✓ What causes it? Cauda equina syndrome is usually caused by an intervertebral disc herniation at level L4-L5.
- ✓ Cauda equina syndrome, spinal cord compression, and conus medullaris syndrome have similar presentations and fall under the general diagnosis of epidural compression syndrome.

REFERENCES

Marx JA, Hockberger RS, Walls RM, eds. *Rosen's Emergency Medicine: Concepts and Clinical Practice*. 8th ed. St. Louis, MO: Elsevier; 2014: 1419-1427.

Tintinalli JE, Stapczynski JS, Ma OJ, et al, eds. *Tintinalli's Emergency Medicine: A Comprehensive Study Guide*. 8th ed. New York, NY: McGraw-Hill; 2012: 1887-1894.

97. The correct answer is D, Perform endotracheal intubation.

Why is this the correct answer?

This patient has sustained a Zone II neck injury. He is demonstrating signs of impending airway obstruction with an expanding anterior neck hematoma, dysphagia, and dysphonia. The primary focus in the care of this patient and any other patient presenting following a traumatic injury should be the ABCs. This particular patient should be intubated right away: he is at risk for rapid deterioration and respiratory failure. Indications for establishing a definitive airway in the setting of penetrating neck trauma include respiratory distress, altered mental status, bloody secretions in the oropharynx, subcutaneous emphysema, expanding hematoma, and tracheal shift. Other signs of potential airway compromise include

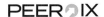

dysphagia and dysphonia. Orotracheal intubation is preferred in penetrating neck injury, but backup airway techniques should be available. If quickly available, awake fiberoptic intubation may be considered.

Why are the other choices wrong?

The patient's presentation is critical. As soon as the airway is established, he should be transported immediately to the OR. Performing angiography would inappropriately delay management. All symptomatic patients with penetrating injuries to Zone II require surgical exploration.

Again, sending the patient for a CT scan would delay appropriate management. Additionally, CT is more appropriate in the evaluation of blunt trauma.

Cricothyrotomy should be avoided when an anterior neck hematoma is present. If the patient were more stable on arrival, intubation could be delayed until the patient reached the OR.

PEER REVIEW

- ✓ Zone II neck injuries require surgical exploration in the OR.
- ✓ Airway stabilization is of primary importance in patients with penetrating neck trauma and respiratory distress or an expanding hematoma.

REFERENCES
Tintinalli JE, Stapczynski JS, Ma OJ, et al, eds. *Tintinalli's Emergency Medicine: A Comprehensive Study Guide.* 8th ed. New York, NY: McGraw-Hill; 2012: 1733-1740.
Wolfson AB, Hendey GW, Ling LJ, et al, eds. *Harwood-Nuss' Clinical Practice of Emergency Medicine.* 6th ed. Philadelphia, PA: Lippincott, Williams & Wilkins; 2014: 183-188.

98. The correct answer is D, Recommend light daily activities.

Why is this the correct answer?

Although back pain can be a symptom of a serious illness or injury, the patient in this case has a benign condition known as lumbago or idiopathic back pain. This is a clinical diagnosis and one that is not associated with any risk factors or neurologic deficits. Imaging is rarely needed, and the cost and radiation exposure can be avoided by conservative management. Symptoms of lumbago typically resolve on their own. Patients who resume light daily activities as they can tolerate them improve faster than those who go on bed rest. High-intensity exercise is not recommended. Because lumbago is a diagnosis of exclusion, the clinician should be on the lookout for signs of other diagnoses and ask all patients presenting with back pain questions to find out if the symptoms indicate more serious conditions. Some of those more concerning symptoms that warrant further workup and are cannot-miss diagnoses include midline back tenderness and trauma concerning for fracture; history of weight loss, fever, or night sweats concerning for cancer or infection; and bowel or bladder changes, weakness, or neurologic deficit concerning for cord compression.

Why are the other choices wrong?

Computed tomography is not indicated in acute lumbago because this disease process usually resolves on its own. It is mainly used to evaluate for trauma such as fractures involving the spine and does not visualize the spinal cord or canal as well as MRI.

Magnetic resonance imaging is not indicated in acute lumbago, again, because the condition is usually self-limiting and does not yield radiographic findings. But MRI is the diagnostic imaging modality of choice to diagnose the major back-related emergencies like neoplasms, infections, and cord compression.

Bed rest is not recommended as treatment for lumbago. Patients who go on bed rest have been shown to have a longer recovery times than those who resume light daily activities. Physical therapy has no proven benefit for acute lumbago.

PEER REVIEW

✓ Your aftercare instructions for patients with lumbago should recommend light daily activities, not bed rest.

✓ Lumbago resolves on its own; imaging isn't needed in patients with nonspecific back pain.

✓ Here are some "red flag" symptoms of a back pain presentation: fever, weight loss, night sweats, bowel or bladder changes, trauma, weakness, history of cancer. These warrant imaging to help make a diagnosis.

REFERENCES

Marx JA, Hockberger RS, Walls RM, eds. *Rosen's Emergency Medicine: Concepts and Clinical Practice*. 8th ed. St. Louis, MO: Elsevier; 2014: 643-655.

Tintinalli JE, Stapczynski JS, Ma OJ, et al, eds. *Tintinalli's Emergency Medicine: A Comprehensive Study Guide*. 8th ed. New York, NY: McGraw-Hill; 2012: 1887-1894.

99. The correct answer is B, Hyperuricemia.

Why is this the correct answer?

Because this patient has non-Hodgkin lymphoma and recently started chemotherapy, he is at risk for the development of tumor lysis syndrome (TLS). Rapid tumor breakdown produces various metabolic derangements and causes the associated clinical picture in this syndrome. In particular, the ions of potassium, calcium, and phosphorus are affected, as well as nucleic acids that metabolize to uric acid. Hyperuricemia is a clinical feature of TLS due to the DNA breakdown. Depending on the degree of hyperuricemia, a urate nephropathy can result and is commonly the cause of the resultant renal failure. Hyperuricemia causes a buildup of uric acid in renal tubules, which leads to the renal failure and subsequent hyperkalemia. This hyperkalemia can cause cardiac arrhythmias and thus makes TLS an emergency. Patients are at higher risk for TLS hours to days after starting chemotherapy or radiation for hematologic cancers like non-Hodgkin lymphoma, leukemia, and some solid tumors.

Why are the other choices wrong?

Hypocalcemia, not hypercalcemia, is a hallmark of tumor lysis syndrome (TLS). Malignant cells have a large amount of phosphorous that is suddenly released into the circulation causing the drop in serum calcium. Hypocalcemia has been known to cause seizures, muscle cramps, tetany, and possibly arrhythmias in TLS patients.

Hyponatremia is not a hallmark of TLS, and sodium has not been shown to be an ion of particular concern in this syndrome. Hyponatremia is more commonly associated with malignancy in syndrome of inappropriate diuretic hormone (SIADH) secretion. Clinicians should have a high degree of suspicion for SIADH when caring for patients with normovolemic hyponatremia and cancer.

Hyperphosphatemia, not hypophosphatemia, has been shown in TLS. Malignant cells carry an excessive amount of phosphorous, and as these cells are lysed, a large amount of phosphorous is released into the circulation, causing this metabolic derangement. Hyperphosphatemia has also been shown to cause renal failure in TLS, possibly as a result of a precipitation of phosphorous with calcium in the renal tubules.

PEER REVIEW

✓ Hallmarks of tumor lysis syndrome: hyperuricemia, hyperkalemia, hyperphosphatemia, and hypocalcemia.
✓ Renal failure contributes to morbidity in tumor lysis syndrome and is usually the result of a urate nephropathy.
✓ Hyperkalemia puts patients at risk for ventricular arrhythmias, which makes tumor lysis syndrome an emergency.

REFERENCES

Marx JA, Hockberger RS, Walls RM, eds. *Rosen's Emergency Medicine: Concepts and Clinical Practice*. 8th ed. St. Louis, MO: Elsevier; 2014: 1617-1628.
Tintinalli JE, Stapczynski JS, Ma OJ, et al, eds. *Tintinalli's Emergency Medicine: A Comprehensive Study Guide*. 8th ed. New York, NY: McGraw-Hill; 2012: 1535-1539.

100. The correct answer is B, Disseminated intravascular coagulation is a late complication.

Why is this the correct answer?

Rhabdomyolysis is diagnosed by laboratory analysis: a CK level at least five times the level of normal in addition to the presence of myoglobin in the urine. If rhabdomyolysis is left undiagnosed or progresses to advanced stages, disseminated intravascular coagulation (DIC) and myoglobin-induced kidney injury can ensue. Early in the course of rhabdomyolysis. complications such as compartment syndrome, hypovolemia, and hepatic dysfunction are known to occur. Electrolyte disturbances and acidosis pose the greatest threat; hyperkalemia and hypocalcemia are the most common electrolyte abnormalities and pose the greatest risk for

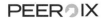

arrhythmias. Later in the course is when kidney failure begins, the result of myoglobin being deposited in renal tubules and obstructing them in the presence of aciduria. This, combined with hypovolemia, further reduces the glomerular filtration rate and worsens renal failure. The worse the renal failure, the worse the hyperkalemia can be. In severe forms of this condition, prothrombotic substances are released and cause DIC and hemorrhagic complications.

Why are the other choices wrong?

There is no evidence to suggest that urine alkalinization is a necessary goal in the treatment of rhabdomyolysis. What is known is that aggressive intravenous hydration is necessary and that urine output should be targeted to 2 to 3 mL/kg per hour. Avoiding acidosis is important, and some continue to use sodium bicarbonate in conjunction with intravenous fluids to avoid this complication.

Mannitol and other diuretics have not been shown to provide any benefit in the treatment of rhabdomyolysis. Mannitol might actually cause an osmotic diuresis that can worsen a patient's hypovolemic state.

The urine dipstick cannot differentiate among hemoglobin, myoglobin, and RBCs. Thus the presence of any of these on the dipstick yields a positive test result. Myoglobin should be suspected if there is blood detected in the urine but no RBCs on microscopy.

PEER POINT

Tea-colored urine from *The Atlas of Emergency Medicine*

The color change is caused by a high level of myoglobin in a patient's urine, a sign of rhabdomyolysis. ©MHEducation

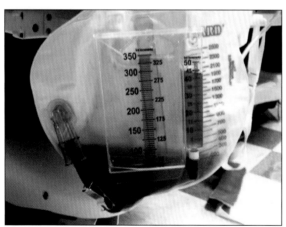

PEER Point 9

PEER REVIEW

✓ There's no evidence to suggest that urine alkalinization or mannitol is necessary in the treatment of rhabdomyolysis.

✓ If the urine dipstick is positive for blood but microscopy is negative for RBCs, suspect myoglobin.

✓ These are the severe complications of rhabdomyolysis: renal failure, hyperkalemia, hypocalcemia, and DIC.

REFERENCES

Marx JA, Hockberger RS, Walls RM, eds. *Rosen's Emergency Medicine: Concepts and Clinical Practice*. 8th ed. St. Louis, MO: Elsevier; 2014: 1667-1675.

Tintinalli JE, Stapczynski JS, Ma OJ, et al, eds. *Tintinalli's Emergency Medicine: A Comprehensive Study Guide*. 8th ed. New York, NY: McGraw-Hill; 2012: 581-584.

101. The correct answer is D, Posterior inferior cerebellar artery.

Why is this the correct answer?

In this case, the patient has suffered a stroke from occlusion of the blood supply to the cerebellum. The vessel most commonly associated with a cerebellar infarct is the posterior inferior cerebellar artery, a branch of the vertebral artery that feeds the brain from the posterior side. Cerebellar infarcts present with ataxia, vertigo, nystagmus, and difficulty with coordination. The nystagmus in cerebellar infarcts is often "direction-changing" and has a fast beat component in the same direction as the patient's gaze. Patients can also have difficulty with finger-to-nose or heel-to-shin tests. One of the most significant clinical findings in patients with cerebellar infarcts is the severe ataxia: patients are unable to balance and walk normally. This is a very useful clue to distinguish a patient with benign positional vertigo from one who has had a cerebellar stroke. Other clues to a stroke in this case include the patient's age and comorbidities, all of which are strongly associated with stroke risk.

Why are the other choices wrong?

A stroke from occlusion of the anterior cerebral artery results in gait impairment due to weakness and sensory loss in the contralateral foot and can result in mental slowing for frontal cortex release signs. This patient has normal mentation and no weakness or sensory loss.

A thrombosis of the cerebral venous sinus results in headache, motor weakness, difficulty speaking, and seizures, but the neurologic deficits do not clearly follow the path of arterial blood supply. This patient's predominant symptoms are vertigo and ataxia.

A stroke from occlusion of the middle cerebral artery results in contralateral paralysis of the arms and legs and, if it occurs on the left side of the head, aphasia. This patient denies motor complaints and is speaking normally.

PEER REVIEW

✓ A stroke of the cerebellar artery should be considered in any patient presenting with vertigo and ataxia. Two clues that favor a cerebellar stroke over peripheral vertigo are the presence of stroke risk factors and the finding of severe, unrelenting ataxia.

✓ The posterior inferior cerebellar artery is the vessel most often associated with cerebellar infarcts and arises from the vertebral artery.

✓ Infarcts of the middle cerebral artery cause contralateral limb paralysis. If the stroke occurs on the left side of the brain, it may affect the Wernicke or Broca area and result in aphasia.

REFERENCES

Adams JG, Barton ED, Collings J, et al, eds. *Emergency Medicine*. Philadelphia, PA: Saunders; 2008: 870-880.

Marx JA, Hockberger RS, Walls RM, eds. *Rosen's Emergency Medicine: Concepts and Clinical Practice*. 8th ed. St. Louis, MO: Elsevier; 2014: 1363-1374.

102. The correct answer is A, Admit her to the hospital for intravenous antibiotic therapy and ENT consultation.

Why is this the correct answer?

In this case, the patient has symptoms concerning for mastoiditis. Mastoiditis is most common in children between 1 and 3 years old. It is a complication of acute otitis media with extension of the infection into the mastoid bone. Patients typically present with ear proptosis, fever, an injected tympanic membrane on the infected side, and postauricular erythema. Organisms involved in this infection are similar to those in otitis media, including *Streptococcus pyogenes*, *Staphylococcus aureus*, and *Pseudomonas aeruginosa*. Diagnosis is confirmed by CT, and consultation with ENT is indicated. If the patient has not taken antibiotics before, the initial treatment is with oral antibiotics if the disease is mild and close follow-up can be ensured. If a patient develops mastoiditis after an appropriate course of oral antibiotics, then admission, ENT consultation, and intravenous antibiotic therapy are warranted. Antibiotics with good gram-positive coverage like ampicillin-sulbactam or third-generation cephalosporins are the first-line choice.

Why are the other choices wrong?

This patient has already completed one course of antibiotic therapy, so starting her on a different oral antibiotic is not appropriate. Admission is warranted for more aggressive management.

Discharging the patient with instructions for supportive care is not the right course of action, again, because initial antimicrobial treatment failed. Admission and additional antibiotics are needed to treat the acute infection process.

At this point in the patient's care, intravenous antibiotic therapy is the next step. Mastoidectomy should be considered only if intravenous antibiotic therapy fails and the infection spreads beyond the mastoid.

PEER REVIEW

✓ If you're treating a patient with mild mastoiditis who hasn't taken antibiotics for it yet, start a course of oral antibiotics with close follow-up.

✓ But if oral antibiotics have failed to resolve the mastoiditis, admit the patient for intravenous antibiotic therapy and ENT consultation.

✓ Surgical intervention is indicated for mastoiditis only after parenteral antibiotic therapy fails.

REFERENCES
Pai S, Parikh SR. Current Diagnosis & Treatment in Otolaryngology- Head & Neck Surgery. 3rd ed. Chapter 49: Otitis Media.
Tintinalli JE, Stapczynski JS, Ma OJ, et al, eds. *Tintinalli's Emergency Medicine: A Comprehensive Study Guide*. 8th ed. New York, NY: McGraw-Hill; 2012: 757-764.

103. The correct answer is C, Discharge home with oral analgesics and close follow-up instructions.

Why is this the correct answer?

Sternal fractures occur most commonly as a result of head-on motor vehicle collisions and in persons who were restrained: the seatbelt overlies the sternum and transmits to it a significant amount of force during sudden deceleration. Sternal fractures are generally managed conservatively with pain control and usually require no further intervention. Most patients with an isolated nondisplaced sternal fracture such as the patient in this case can be safely discharged home if they have normal vital signs, a normal initial ECG, adequate pain control with oral analgesics, and normal findings on an ECG repeated several hours later. Older patients are more likely to have sternal fractures because younger patients have more compliant chest walls. Traditionally, sternal fractures were thought to indicate a high risk for severe intrathoracic trauma; the belief was that the force required to break the sternum was likely to cause other significant injury in the chest. However, evidence has shown more recently that patients with isolated sternal fractures have a low rate of other significant traumatic thoracic injuries. This is thought to be due to the sternum's dissipating the force of impact and subsequently lessening the kinetic force received by underlying structures. The injuries most commonly associated with sternal fracture are pulmonary contusion and rib fractures. Sternal fractures are often difficult to see on PA or AP chest xray but can be diagnosed using a lateral view; ultrasonography has been shown to be an even more effective test than xray. Patients for whom there is a significant concern for sternal fracture should undergo CT of the chest, as this is the best study for diagnosis and can also evaluate for other thoracic and mediastinal injury. An ECG should also be obtained to evaluate for cardiac injuries such as myocardial contusion, which can occur in a small subset of patients.

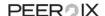

Why are the other choices wrong?

Although sternal fractures were traditionally thought to create significant risk for myocardial injury, cardiac complications are seen in only a small number of patients. This patient has normal vital signs, two normal ECGs, and an otherwise negative workup. She can be safely discharged home and does not require additional cardiac evaluation or monitoring.

If this patient had a displaced fracture or overlying bone fragments, she might need to undergo surgical fixation to manage or prevent respiratory compromise, severe pain, nonunion, or physical deformity. But her injury is a nondisplaced fracture. She has no respiratory compromise or obvious deformity and is unlikely to require operative management. The vast majority (95%) of sternal fractures are managed conservatively with pain control.

Sternal fractures were originally thought to be indicators of other severe chest trauma, particularly cardiovascular injury. They have since been shown to have low incidence of cardiac injury and a mortality rate of less than 1%. There is no association with aortic injury. Rib fracture and pulmonary contusion are the most common associated injuries, but there is no evidence of these injuries in this case. This patient underwent CT and has no other injuries. Her vital signs are normal, and her respiratory status is reassuring, so observation overnight is not necessary.

PEER REVIEW

✓ Sternal fractures: low rate of associated major intrathoracic trauma, low mortality rate.

✓ Most sternal fractures are managed conservatively with pain control.

REFERENCES

Marx JA, Hockberger RS, Walls RM, eds. *Rosen's Emergency Medicine: Concepts and Clinical Practice*. 8th ed. St. Louis, MO: Elsevier; 2014: 432-433.

Tintinalli JE, Stapczynski JS, Ma OJ, et al, eds. *Tintinalli's Emergency Medicine: A Comprehensive Study Guide*. 8th ed. New York, NY: McGraw-Hill; 2012: 1750-1752.

104. The correct answer is B, Nodes in the proximal interphalangeal and distal interphalangeal joints of the hand.

Why is this the correct answer?

Osteoarthritis (OA) is a polyarticular condition that is worse with activity and better with rest, although it can present with acute monoarticular pain. Bouchard and Heberden nodes can be found in the PIP and DIP joints of the hands in these patients. Osteoarthritis most commonly affects the knees. In contrast to rheumatoid arthritis, patient with OA do not complain of any systemic symptoms. The clinician can also expect to see joint space narrowing on radiographs.

Why are the other choices wrong?

"Bamboo spine" is a radiographic finding in ankylosing spondylitis, a seronegative spondyloarthropathy that causes symptoms mostly in the spine and pelvis. Patients complain of morning stiffness, similar to rheumatoid arthritis (RA), but the rheumatoid factor is negative. Uveitis is known to be a common extra-articular sign, but patients might also experience plantar fasciitis or Achilles tendinitis or aortic root disease more rarely. This affects male patients about three times more often than female patients and is usually diagnosed in patients before the age of 40 years. Radiographic findings of sacroiliitis and squaring of the vertebral bodies help confirm this diagnosis. This vertebral body squaring is where the term "bamboo spine" comes from.

Swan neck deformities, which are the result of increased extension of the PIP joint, are characteristic of RA, not OA. Patients with RA can also have boutonnière deformities, an extension of the DIP joint caused by retraction of the extensor hood.

Swelling in the MP and PIP joints of the hand is commonly seen in RA, a progressive polyarticular symmetric arthritis that is often accompanied by fever, weakness, and fatigue. Patients typically complain of morning stiffness lasting more than an hour. The absence of DIP involvement in the hands helps distinguish RA from OA.

PEER POINT

Swan neck deformity

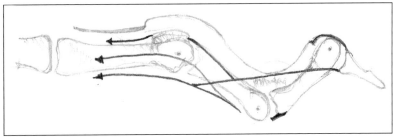

PEER Point 10

Boutonnière deformity

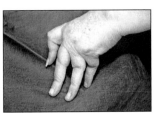

PEER Point 11

PEER REVIEW

✓ How can you distinguish osteoarthritis from rheumatoid arthritis? If there's DIP joint involvement, it's osteoarthritis. If there are systemic symptoms, it's rheumatoid arthritis.

✓ Characteristic of osteoarthritis: joint pain that gets worse with activity and better with rest.

✓ Swan neck and boutonnière deformities are found in rheumatoid arthritis, not osteoarthritis.

REFERENCES

Marx JA, Hockberger RS, Walls RM, eds. *Rosen's Emergency Medicine: Concepts and Clinical Practice.* 8th ed. St. Louis, MO: Elsevier; 2014: 1501-1517.

Tintinalli JE, Stapczynski JS, Ma OJ, et al, eds. *Tintinalli's Emergency Medicine: A Comprehensive Study Guide.* 8th ed. New York, NY: McGraw-Hill; 2012: 1927-1936.

105. The correct answer is D, Foreign body aspiration.

Why is this the correct answer?

In this case, a child presents with acute onset of respiratory distress. The mother's description of the event and his symptoms is consistent with a history of choking, which is the most reliable predictor of foreign body aspiration. Signs and symptoms are related to the location of the obstructing foreign body. If the obstruction is in the upper airway, stridor and respiratory or cardiopulmonary arrest can be expected. If it is in the lower airway, coughing, wheezing, retractions, decreased breath sounds, and cyanosis are likely. More than half of cases of foreign body aspiration are in children 1 to 2 years old, and the vast majority are in children younger than 5 years. The foreign bodies are usually food such as candy or nuts or wieners, or coins, marbles, or batteries. Foreign body aspirations are fatal most often in infants younger than 1 year. A balloon is the most commonly fatal foreign body aspirated. In patients who present with suspected partial obstruction, imaging includes AP and lateral xrays of the upper airway; extending the view from the nasopharynx to the abdomen covers the diaphragm as well. Additional studies, including inspiratory and expiratory chest xrays and bilateral decubitus views, might be needed.

Why are the other choices wrong?

Asthma exacerbation is a common cause of respiratory distress. But the signs of respiratory distress described in this case are more associated with upper airway illness (stridor, retractions noted at suprasternal and supraclavicular areas) than lower airway. There are no findings of wheeze on examination to further indicate lower airway disease, and although cough is the most common presenting symptom, this child presented with a history of cough and choking, which makes the presence of a foreign body more likely than asthma in a child with no history of asthma or reactive airway disease.

Again, in this case, the patient's respiratory distress had an acute onset. Although there is a history of an upper respiratory infection, his temperature is normal, making croup and epiglottitis less likely. Croup, otherwise known as laryngotracheobronchitis, is associated with a barking or seal-like cough. It can have associated laryngitis, respiratory distress, and even stridor due to upper airway edema. Physical signs and symptoms of fever, malaise, and other influenza-like illnesses can be present. The most common infectious agent is parainfluenza virus, although there are many other infectious agents that can cause croup. Croup is more commonly seen in fall and winter.

Epiglottitis is a life-threatening infectious process that was most commonly caused by *Haemophilus influenzae* type b. But, due to increasing use of the Hib vaccine, the incidence of epiglottitis has declined dramatically. There is a rapid deterioration of the upper airway due to the edema of the aryepiglottic folds, potentially leading to respiratory arrest. There is no seasonal aspect to epiglottitis as there is to croup.

PEER REVIEW

- ✓ Upper airway obstruction: stridor, respiratory or cardiopulmonary arrest.
- ✓ Lower airway obstruction: coughing, wheezing, retractions, decreased breath sounds, and cyanosis.
- ✓ A history of choking is the most reliable predictor of foreign body aspiration.
- ✓ The most common presenting symptom for asthma or reactive airway disease is cough.

REFERENCES

Fleisher GR, Ludwig S, et al, eds. *Textbook of Pediatric Emergency Medicine*. 6th ed. Philadelphia, PA: Lippincott, Williams & Wilkins; 2010: 277-278; 281-282.

Schafermeyer RW, Tenenbein M, Macias CG, et al, eds. *Strange and Schafermeyer's Pediatric Emergency Medicine*. 4th ed. New York, NY: McGraw-Hill; 2015: 213.

Wolfson AB, Hendey GW, Ling LJ, et al, eds. *Harwood-Nuss' Clinical Practice of Emergency Medicine*. 6th ed. Philadelphia, PA: Lippincott, Williams & Wilkins; 2014: 1218-1219.

106. The correct answer is C, Obstruction of the drainage of CSF.

Why is this the correct answer?

The CT scan shows enlargement of the lateral ventricles with compression of the otherwise normal surrounding brain. This patient is suffering from hydrocephalus and has evidence of increased intracranial pressure. Since she was previously healthy at age 44, this is likely an acquired rather than congenital cause of hydrocephalus. The CSF is generated in the choroid plexus, then flows to lateral ventricles, through the foramen of Monro into the third ventricle, then through the aqueduct of Sylvius into the fourth ventricle and finally out the foramen of Magendie and foramina of Luschka into the subarachnoid space. A space-occupying lesion developing anywhere along this tract can lead to obstructive or noncommunicating hydrocephalus. In adults, hydrocephalus most commonly results from obstruction due to a subarachnoid hemorrhage. Patients with hydrocephalus can present with

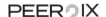

headache, declining mental function, nausea, vomiting, ataxia, and incontinence. Headaches are typically worse on rising in the morning. The classic triad of normal pressure hydrocephalus, a chronic form of communicating hydrocephalus, is altered mental status, ataxia, and incontinence.

Why are the other choices wrong?

Cerebral ischemia from a stroke initially appears normal on a head CT scan and then later develops into a wedge-shaped area of hypodensity.

The glioblastoma multiforme is the most common malignant tumor of the CNS and develops from glial cells. It usually appears as an irregular mass with surrounding edema.

A rupture of a cerebral aneurysm causes bright hyperdense bleeding throughout the subarachnoid space, usually in the base of the brain. Head CT scanning misses up to 5% of subarachnoid hemorrhages, especially if the patient presents more than 6 hours after the onset of headache.

PEER REVIEW

- ✓ What's the most common cause of obstruction in the CSF production and drainage pathway? Blood from a subarachnoid hemorrhage.
- ✓ If that pathway gets blocked, a noncommunicating hydrocephalus and increased intracranial pressure develop.
- ✓ The classic triad for normal-pressure hydrocephalus is altered mental status, ataxia, and incontinence.
- ✓ Head CT is 95% sensitive in detecting subarachnoid hemorrhages and almost 100% for patients who undergo imaging within 6 hours of headache onset.

REFERENCES
Marx JA, Hockberger RS, Walls RM, eds. *Rosen's Emergency Medicine: Concepts and Clinical Practice*. 8th ed. St. Louis, MO: Elsevier; 2014: 142-150.

107. The correct answer is B, *Staphylococcus aureus*.

Why is this the correct answer?

S. aureus is the most common organism causing spinal epidural abscesses, with a large portion of those being methicillin-resistant *S. aureus*. Antibiotic coverage started in the emergency department must include vancomycin. Gram-negative bacilli coverage is also recommended until culture results have returned, as these bacteria are often present in intravenous drug users. The incidence of spinal epidural abscess has increased due to growing numbers of intravenous drug users and immunocompromised patients.

Why are the other choices wrong?

Pseudomonas is seen commonly in intravenous drug users with spinal epidural abscesses, but it is not the most common organism among all patients.

S. epidermidis is found in spinal epidural abscesses but is not the most common cause.

Again, *S. pneumoniae* infection does occur in spinal epidural abscess but is not the most common.

PEER REVIEW

- ✓ *S. aureus* is the most common pathogen in spinal epidural abscesses.
- ✓ Use vancomycin for spinal epidural abscess to cover methicillin-resistant infection.
- ✓ A growing number of cases of spinal epidural abscess are associated with immunocompromise, so until culture results are in, cover gram-negative bacilli, too.

REFERENCES

Marx JA, Hockberger RS, Walls RM, eds. *Rosen's Emergency Medicine: Concepts and Clinical Practice*. 8th ed. St. Louis, MO: Elsevier; 2014: 643-655.

Tintinalli JE, Stapczynski JS, Ma OJ, et al, eds. *Tintinalli's Emergency Medicine: A Comprehensive Study Guide*. 8th ed. New York, NY: McGraw-Hill; 2012: 1192-1199.

108. The correct answer is A, Fluctuance of the mass when palpated.

Why is this the correct answer?

Overall, this patient presentation is concerning for a malignancy, most likely of the thyroid. The only sign that makes a malignancy less likely is the fluctuant nature of the mass, which is more consistent with a cyst. There are five features to consider in the evaluation of a mass concerning for malignancy. Without all five of them, there is a 99.7% accuracy that the mass is not malignant in 80% of the cases. The five features are associated skin ulcer, onset when the patient is a neonate, fixation of the mass to skin or fascia, progressive enlargement, and size greater than 3 cm with a hard consistency. Other significant clinical features in this case are fever and possible weight loss reported by the mother. Further examination is likely to reveal diffuse lymphadenopathy. Given these findings, and since the patient has no source of regular care, the emergency physician should get a consultation. If the patient's airway is intact, the best course of treatment is consultation and close follow-up with a pediatric oncologist for definitive diagnosis with fine needle aspiration, biopsy, or imaging.

Why are the other choices wrong?

The size of the mass is suggestive of a malignant lesion. An ultrasound examination of the mass might help delineate its size and consistency.

The mother says that the mass has grown over the past month, which means that it was likely present before the baby was 4 weeks old. Onset as a neonate is one of the indicators for a malignancy.

Ulceration of the skin is another of the five features consistent with malignancy in neck masses.

PEER POINT

Five features associated with malignancy in neck masses

- Skin ulcer
- Onset of the mass when the patient is a neonate
- Nonmobile, fixed to skin or fascia
- Progressive enlargement
- Size greater than 3 cm and hard

PEER REVIEW

✓ If a neck mass can be moved around and compressed, it's less likely to be malignant. Those features are more consistent with a cyst.

REFERENCES

Lal G, Clark OH .Thyroid, Parathyroid, and Adrenal. In: Brunicardi F, Andersen DK, Billiar TR, et al, eds. *Schwartz's Principles of Surgery*. 10th ed. New York, NY: McGraw-Hill; 2015. http://accessmedicine.mhmedical.com/content.aspx?bookid=980&sectionid=59610880. Accessed May 18, 2017.

Tintinalli JE, Stapczynski JS, Ma OJ, et al, eds. *Tintinalli's Emergency Medicine: A Comprehensive Study Guide*. 8th ed. New York, NY: McGraw-Hill; 2012: 786-793.

109. The correct answer is A, Delirium.

Why is this the correct answer?

Making the diagnosis of delirium is challenging. Patient presentations vary widely: rapid onset or somewhat rapid onset, hypoactivity or hyperactivity, confusion, trouble with memory and language, hallucinations, disorientation. Sometimes it is difficult to distinguish delirium from dementia and psychosis clinically. In this case, however, the patient's family describes one of the characteristic features, a rapid fluctuation of symptoms, and that helps narrow down the diagnostic process. Delirium is a syndrome, a collection of symptoms of cognitive dysfunction that has an underlying organic condition. Hallmarks include development of cognitive disturbance within hours or days of presentation that change throughout the course of the day, along with an identifiable underlying medical cause. The medical causes of delirium are many and varied and include infectious, metabolic, and substance-related conditions. It is important to obtain an accurate history from either the patient or family members to help determine the underlying cause. Patients who present with delirium should be admitted to the hospital unless a clear reversible cause can be found (such as adverse medication reaction, substance abuse, or hypoglycemia) due to a high associated mortality rate.

Why are the other choices wrong?

Dementia, in contrast to delirium, is characterized by a gradual progressive decline in memory or cognitive function. It can be reversible, but most cases are irreversible. Alzheimer-type dementia is one of the more common causes in the United States. Patients presenting with dementia generally have normal vital signs and no fluctuations in level of consciousness. It is important to consider that patients with a known history of dementia might experience an episode of delirium and demonstrate the characteristics noted above.

Patients who present with confusion related to psychosis often have a history of underlying psychiatric illness or similar prior behavior. Additionally, fluctuation of the confusional state is absent. An acute confusional state related to psychosis may be treated with medication, but recurrences are common.

Seizure can cause confusion during the postictal state. The diagnosis of seizure would be supported by evidence of trauma or oral injury, witnessed seizure activity, or incontinence of urine or stool. The length of time of a postictal state varies but can last anywhere from a few minutes to a few days.

PEER POINT

Is it delirium, dementia, or psychosis?

	Delirium	Dementia	Psychosis
Acuteness	Very rapid	Gradual	Rapid
Systemic findings	Common, including fever, other vital sign changes	None	None
Prior mental health problems	Rare	Unlikely	Likely
Psychomotor activity	Seen in some patients	None	Variable
Involuntary activity	Trembling, shaking (seizure)	None from dementia	Might have some from medications
Hallucinations	Possible auditory or visual	None	Auditory most common
Disease course	Rapidly changing	Steady progression	Constant
Outcome	With treatment of underlying problem, most resolve	Progressively worse	Responds with therapy but can recur

Why is this patient altered?
Remember AEIOU TIPS

A Alcohol (drugs), acidosis

E Electrolytes, epilepsy, endocrine, encephalopathy, environment

I Insulin, intussusception

O Overdose, opiates

U Uremia

T Trauma, temperature, tumor

I Infection

P Psychogenic, poisoning, psychiatric

S Shock, seizure, stroke, shunt, syncope

PEER REVIEW

✓ Hallmark features of delirium: fluctuating mental status over short time course, development over prior hours to days, altered level of consciousness.

✓ There is always an underlying organic cause for delirium.

✓ Dementia is a gradually progressive disease process.

REFERENCES

Marx JA, Hockberger RS, Walls RM, eds. *Rosen's Emergency Medicine: Concepts and Clinical Practice.* 8th ed. St. Louis, MO: Elsevier; 2014: 1398-1408.

Tintinalli JE, Stapczynski JS, Ma OJ, et al, eds. *Tintinalli's Emergency Medicine: A Comprehensive Study Guide.* 8th ed. New York, NY: McGraw-Hill; 2012: 1156-1161;1958-1963.

110. The correct answer is B, Perform lumbar puncture.

Why is this the correct answer?

This patient's presentation of severe sudden-onset headache during exertion is classic for the diagnosis of subarachnoid hemorrhage (SAH). Patients who present to the emergency department with "thunderclap" headache have been found to have an 11% to 25% incidence of SAH. Noncontrast head CT is the most appropriate initial imaging study for a patient in whom there is concern for SAH. Some of the most recent studies have shown a sensitivity of 98% to 100% for noncontrast CT obtained within the first 6 hours. It is important to note that as time from symptom onset increases, the sensitivity of noncontrast head CT decreases: recent studies show sensitivity above 90% at 24 to 48 hours, but then old studies seem to indicate a further decrease to 50% at 1 week. The gold standard test to diagnose SAH remains a lumbar puncture with laboratory evaluation for xanthochromia and RBC count. There is a growing body of literature that discusses other options, including CT angiography following a negative CT scan, but no definitive change in practice has been standardized. Family history in these patients is important; it has been found that with a first-degree relative with history of aneurysm, there is a four times higher risk for ruptured intracranial aneurysm.

Why are the other choices wrong?

Administration of antibiotics is the best next step for meningitis, which should be considered as a serious cause of a secondary headache. If this patient had had, in addition to the headache, fever, meningismus, rash, or other concerns, meningitis would be suspected. In such a case, antibiotics should not be withheld for any reason and may be given before head CT and lumbar puncture without decreasing the sensitivity of CSF culture.

Repeat head CT is sometimes indicated following traumatic SAH to assess whether the amount of bleeding has changed. Repeat head CT does not have a role in diagnosing a spontaneously ruptured intracranial aneurysm. There is an increasing role for CT angiography or MRI/MRA imaging following a negative head CT. In a mathematical probability model study, it was calculated that a negative CT combined with CT angiography might have sensitivity as high as 99.4%.

Patients with primary headache may be treated symptomatically and discharged from the emergency department. In this patient's history, there are red flags for the diagnosis of SAH, making symptomatic treatment and discharge inappropriate.

PEER REVIEW

✓ Noncontrast head CT is the most appropriate initial test when evaluating suspected SAH.

✓ Lumbar puncture is still the gold standard for diagnosing spontaneously ruptured intracranial aneurysm.

REFERENCES

Edlow JA, Caplan LR. Avoiding pitfalls in the diagnosis of subarachnoid hemorrhage. *N Engl J Med.* 2000;342:29.

Edlow JA, Panagos PD, Godwin SA, et al. Clinical policy: Critical issues in the evaluation and management of adult patients presenting to the emergency department with acute headache. *Ann Emerg Med.* 2008;52(4):407-436.

Marx JA, Hockberger RS, Walls RM, eds. *Rosen's Emergency Medicine: Concepts and Clinical Practice.* 8th ed. St. Louis, MO: Elsevier; 2014: 170-175.

McCormack RF, Hutson A. Can computed tomography angiography of the brain replace lumbar puncture in the evaluation of acute-onset headache after a negative noncontrast cranial computed tomography scan? *Acad Emerg Med.* 2010;17(4):444-451.

111. The correct answer is D, Oxygen 12 L via nonrebreather mask.

Why is this the correct answer?

Cluster headaches present with recurrent episodes of severe unilateral headache lasting a few hours or less at a time. Initial treatment consists of high-flow oxygen, 7 to 12 L via nonrebreather mask. One study found this treatment to be effective within the first 15 minutes in 78% of patients. Oxygen via nasal cannula has not been shown to be effective. Other treatments that have been shown to provide relief are the use of selective serotonin agonists such as sumatriptan. Associated symptoms of cluster headaches include ipsilateral lacrimation, rhinorrhea, nasal congestion, and conjunctival injection. On physical examination, ipsilateral miosis and ptosis might also be noted. Cluster headaches are the only primary headache syndrome that is more common in men and generally diagnosed after patients are 20 years old.

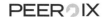

Why are the other choices wrong?

Ketorolac is an NSAID, and NSAID therapy using drugs such as ketorolac intravenously or ibuprofen orally is first-line treatment for both tension-type and migraine headaches. The NSAIDs are not indicated in the treatment of cluster headaches, and many cluster headaches resolve before these medications become therapeutic.

The antiemetic metoclopramide and dopamine antagonists such as prochlorperazine and chlorpromazine are often regarded as first-line treatment for migraine headache. They are generally well tolerated with a minimal side effect profile. These medications have an unclear mechanism of action, but it is thought that dopamine pathways have a role in migraine headache pathogenesis. They are not typically used to treat cluster headaches.

Morphine and other narcotic medications are not advised for the treatment of headaches. Patients who take opioid medications for headache treatment have been found to develop rebound headaches that are at times more severe than the initial headache.

PEER REVIEW

- ✓ Cluster headaches are the only primary headache disorder that is more common in men.
- ✓ Classic presentation of cluster headache: unilateral sharp and stabbing eye pain, headache with recurrent episodes lasting minutes to a few hours over a period of a few weeks.
- ✓ Treat cluster headache initially with high-flow oxygen by nonrebreather mask.

REFERENCES

Gooriah R, Buture A, Ahmed F. Evidence-based treatments for cluster headache. *Ther Clin Risk Manag.* 2015;11:1687-1696. PMC. Web. 22 May 2016.

Marx JA, Hockberger RS, Walls RM, eds. *Rosen's Emergency Medicine: Concepts and Clinical Practice.* 8th ed. St. Louis, MO: Elsevier; 2014: 1386-1397.

Petersen AS, Barloese MC, Jensen RH. Oxygen treatment of cluster headache: a review. *Cephalalgia.* 2014;34(13):1079-1087.

Tintinalli JE, Stapczynski JS, Ma OJ, et al, eds. *Tintinalli's Emergency Medicine: A Comprehensive Study Guide.* 8th ed. New York, NY: McGraw-Hill; 2012: 1131-1137.

112. The correct answer is A, Idiopathic endolymphatic hydrops.

Why is this the correct answer?

Idiopathic endolymphatic hydrops, commonly known as Meniere disease, is a type of peripheral vertigo. Associated tinnitus and hearing loss are hallmarks of the presentation. The exact cause is unknown but is thought to be related to increased endolymph within the inner ear. Patients experience intermittent episodes of vertigo lasting from minutes to much of a day, associated with the typical symptoms of dizziness, nausea, and vomiting. The attacks often come in clusters. If Meniere disease is suspected, the patient should be referred to otolaryngology for follow-up. Episodes of vertigo can generally be managed symptomatically with antihistamines or betahistine, but the hearing loss and tinnitus are often refractory to treatment. Patients who present with the chief complaint of dizziness can pose a diagnostic challenge. Having the patient describe the sensation he or she is experiencing can help distinguish between vertigo — the illusion of movement — and a near-syncopal sensation or feeling as if he or she might pass out. If the patient reports a vertiginous sensation, the next step is to determine if the cause is peripheral or central. According to classic teaching, peripheral vertigo has a sudden and severe onset with episodes lasting from seconds to minutes or hours. The symptoms are often related to position, and nystagmus is unidirectional and horizontorotary. Central vertigo has a more gradual and insidious nature. It is not affected by position changes; nystagmus is often vertical and downbeating, and there can be associated neurologic symptoms. This distinction is crucial since a missed diagnosis of a central process causing vertigo can be catastrophic.

Why are the other choices wrong?

Labyrinthitis is caused by an infection of the labyrinth in the inner ear. Patients present with typical acute otitis media and the addition of vertigo and possibly hearing loss. It can be caused by measles or mumps viral infection or can be due to an extension of acute bacterial otitis media, which causes suppurative labyrinthitis. Suppurative labyrinthitis should be treated with intravenous antibiotics and ENT referral.

Lateral medullary infarction of the brainstem, also known as Wallenberg syndrome, is caused by occlusion of the posterior inferior cerebellar artery. It presents with ipsilateral findings of facial numbness and decreased pain and temperature sensation, paralysis of the soft palate or pharynx, Horner syndrome, and loss of corneal reflex. Contralateral findings include loss of pain and temperature sensation in the limbs and trunk. Dizziness is not a normal manifestation of this syndrome.

The etiology of vestibular neuritis is a viral infection. Patients often experience severe intermittent vertigo for a few days, often associated with a viral syndrome. Vestibular neuritis is seen often in the emergency department. Patients are very symptomatic initially, but the symptoms seem to resolve completely after it runs its course.

PEER POINT

Is it central or peripheral vertigo?

	Central	Peripheral
Onset	Gradual, subtle	Sudden, severe
Nystagmus	Multidirectional and vertical/downbeating	Unidirectional, horizontorotary
Affected by position?	No	Yes

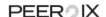

PEER REVIEW

✓ Characteristics of peripheral vertigo: sudden, severe onset lasting seconds to hours, positional.

✓ Meniere disease presents with recurrent bouts of vertigo lasting minutes to hours with associated hearing loss and tinnitus.

REFERENCES

Marx JA, Hockberger RS, Walls RM, eds. *Rosen's Emergency Medicine: Concepts and Clinical Practice*. 8th ed. St. Louis, MO: Elsevier; 2014: 162-169.

Tintinalli JE, Stapczynski JS, Ma OJ, et al, eds. *Tintinalli's Emergency Medicine: A Comprehensive Study Guide*. 8th ed. New York, NY: McGraw-Hill; 2012: 1164-1173.

113. The correct answer is A, Benztropine.

Why is this the correct answer?

The patient in this case is experiencing an acute dystonic reaction to haloperidol, an antipsychotic medication that is commonly used to sedate agitated patients. Haloperidol is associated with extrapyramidal side effects and dystonia. Typical or first-generation antipsychotics and metoclopramide commonly cause dystonic reactions in the emergency department that can be quite alarming for both patient and provider. Acute dystonia can present with involuntary movements of the neck, eyes, mouth, or trunk. Physical examination findings can be mistakenly identified as acute stroke. Treatment for dystonic reaction is either diphenhydramine 25 to 50 mg or benztropine 1 to 2 mg IV or IM. Treatment should be continued for 3 days to prevent recurrence. Coadministration of diphenhydramine or benztropine with possible causative agents is common preventive practice for acute dystonia in many emergency departments.

Why are the other choices wrong?

Dantrolene, along with aggressive supportive care, is used to treat neuroleptic malignant syndrome, a rare but serious adverse reaction to typical antipsychotic medications. Patients with neuroleptic malignant syndrome have hyperthermia, autonomic instability, muscle rigidity, and altered mental status.

Flumazenil is the antidote to benzodiazepine overdose. If the patient had been overly sedated or exhibited a depressed respiratory rate, flumazenil administration might be considered. Flumazenil should not be used in patients who take benzodiazepines regularly because it can precipitate seizures refractory to treatment.

Risperidone is an atypical or second-generation antipsychotic medication that may be used to manage agitation in the emergency department. Other atypical antipsychotics include ziprasidone, olanzapine, and quetiapine. These agents have fewer extrapyramidal side effects and are less likely to cause dystonia and tardive dyskinesia in long-term use than typical antipsychotic medications are.

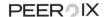

PEER REVIEW

- ✓ Agitation in emergency department patients is commonly managed with typical antipsychotic medications plus benzodiazepines.
- ✓ Treat acute dystonia with benztropine or diphenhydramine.
- ✓ Don't use flumazenil to reverse benzodiazepine overdose or toxicity in a patient who regularly takes benzodiazepines.

REFERENCES

Marx JA, Hockberger RS, Walls RM, eds. *Rosen's Emergency Medicine: Concepts and Clinical Practice.* 8th ed. St. Louis, MO: Elsevier; 2014: 2414-2428.

Tintinalli JE, Stapczynski JS, Ma OJ, et al, eds. *Tintinalli's Emergency Medicine: A Comprehensive Study Guide.* 8th ed. New York, NY: McGraw-Hill; 2012: 1952-1958.

114. The correct answer is A, Nonsteroidal anti-inflammatory agents.

Why is this the correct answer?

Pericarditis is, of course, inflammation within the pericardial space involving the pericardial surfaces. The clinical presentation is generally that of sharp pleuritic chest pain that improves with sitting up. The diagnosis in this case is supported by the ECG findings: normal sinus rhythm, diffuse ST-segment elevation along with diffuse PR segment depression. Leads I and aVR can show reciprocal ST-segment depression in acute pericarditis. Management involves NSAIDs of typical doses provided in the outpatient setting for uncomplicated cases. Adding colchicine has been shown in several studies to decrease the incidence of recurrent pericarditis. Pericarditis is often idiopathic or related to a viral infection, but it can be caused by various underlying disease states. There is often a prodromal period of low-grade fever, malaise, or flu-like symptoms. On examination, a pericardial friction rub can sometimes be appreciated. A bedside echocardiogram can be obtained to evaluate for an associated pericardial effusion. Patients with large effusions or pericardial tamponade benefit from inpatient evaluation and management.

Why are the other choices wrong?

Heparin is indicated in suspected PE or in certain ACS presentations. Although pulmonary embolus could cause ECG changes, most commonly tachycardia and classically S1Q3T3, it is not expected to cause diffuse ST-segment elevation as seen on this patient's ECG.

Cardiac catheterization with PCI is indicated for STEMI. The clinical presentation and ECG in this case are not consistent with STEMI: it is uncommon for an MI to produce diffuse ST-segment elevation. The PR segment depression seen on this ECG is also much more consistent with acute pericarditis.

The presentation is most consistent with acute pericarditis due to the diffuse

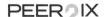

changes seen in essentially all leads. This is not a typical pattern indicating cardiac ischemia which might have ST changes in contiguous leads consistent with specific cardiac vessels (inferior ischemia seen in leads II, III, aVF) Thus nitrates are of no benefit to this patient.

PEER REVIEW

✓ Characteristic ECG findings of acute pericarditis: diffuse ST-segment elevation and diffuse PR interval depression.

✓ The clinical presentation of acute pericarditis is sharp pleuritic chest pain that gets worse when the patient lies down — and sometimes you can hear a pericardial friction rub.

✓ Treatment for uncomplicated pericarditis includes NSAIDs and colchicine.

REFERENCES

Marx JA, Hockberger RS, Walls RM, eds. *Rosen's Emergency Medicine: Concepts and Clinical Practice*. 8th ed. St. Louis, MO: Elsevier; 2014: 1091-1105.

Tintinalli JE, Stapczynski JS, Ma OJ, et al, eds. *Tintinalli's Emergency Medicine: A Comprehensive Study Guide*. 8th ed. New York, NY: McGraw-Hill; 2012: 380-387.

115. The correct answer is C, Idiopathic intracranial hypertension.

Why is this the correct answer?

Idiopathic intracranial hypertension (IIH), also known as pseudotumor cerebri and benign intracranial hypertension, is a rare condition that presents with gradual onset and chronic headache, vision changes, nausea, vomiting, and tinnitus. The image shows papilledema, or swelling of the optic disc. It is noted by the edema around the edge of the disc that can obscure the insertion of the blood vessels when the pressure gets severe. The classic presentation of IIH is a young obese female. An association has been found with this diagnosis and the use of oral contraceptive medications, tetracycline, anabolic steroids, and vitamin A. The pathophysiology is not well understood, but IIH is thought to be caused by an imbalance in CSF production and reabsorption. Diagnostic criteria include an alert patient with either a normal neurologic examination or findings consistent with papilledema, visual field defect, or an enlarged blind spot. Lumbar puncture done in a recumbent position reveals an elevated CSF opening pressure of more than 200 mm Hg in an obese patient (normal being up to 25 mm Hg). Results of CSF analysis are normal. Other possible causes of intracranial hypertension should be ruled out, including venous sinus thrombosis. Treatment consists of regular outpatient lumbar puncture for drainage of CSF to a normal pressure and acetazolamide. Possible offending agents such as oral contraceptive medications should be discontinued. It is important to note that permanent loss of vision can occur in up to 10% of patients.

Why are the other choices wrong?

Acute glaucoma also presents with severe headache with associated vision change, but this usually presents acutely. On examination, the disc is normal, but the affected eye has a fixed mid-dilated pupil and a shallow anterior chamber. Intraocular pressure is markedly elevated, in the 60 to 90 mm Hg range (normal is approximately 21 mm Hg). The opening pressure of a lumbar puncture is normal in this disease entity. Emergent vision-saving treatment consists of topical beta blockers and miotics, acetazolamide, possible mannitol diuresis, and ophthalmologic evaluation.

Giant cell arteritis (temporal arteritis) is a vasculitis of small and medium-sized arteries, primarily affecting branches of the aortic arch and ophthalmologic arteries. Like IIH, temporal arteritis presents with gradual-onset headache with associated vision changes and usually some vague systemic symptoms such as fever, anorexia, and weight loss. Physical examination can show a swollen pale disc due to ischemia, possibly an afferent pupillary defect, and classically tenderness over the temporal artery. Diagnosis is confirmed by temporal artery biopsy and supported by a markedly elevated erythrocyte sedimentation rate. This condition occurs most commonly in elderly women. Treatment consists of prompt initiation of high-dose systemic steroids.

Cerebral venous sinus thrombosis is a rare diagnosis that is often associated with thrombophilic states (hypercoagulable, pregnancy, or vasculitis). It generally affects younger patients and can potentially lead to stroke. Patients often complain of a persistent headache with symptoms progressing to include neurologic deficits. Similar to IIH, an elevated opening pressure on a lumbar puncture is found, and both diagnoses must be considered in these cases. Diagnosis is confirmed by MRI/MRA imaging. Noncontrast CT is insensitive for this diagnosis.

PEER REVIEW

✓ Features of idiopathic intracranial hypertension: headache and vision changes, papilledema, visual field defect, or an enlarged blind spot.

✓ Diagnosis of idiopathic intracranial hypertension is confirmed with elevated CSF opening pressures (>20 mm Hg) with a normal CSF analysis.

✓ Treatment of idiopathic intracranial hypertension consists of intermittent CSF drainage and acetazolamide.

REFERENCES

Marx JA, Hockberger RS, Walls RM, eds. *Rosen's Emergency Medicine: Concepts and Clinical Practice*. 8th ed. St. Louis, MO: Elsevier; 2014: 1386-1397.

Tintinalli JE, Stapczynski JS, Ma OJ, et al, eds. *Tintinalli's Emergency Medicine: A Comprehensive Study Guide*. 8th ed. New York, NY: McGraw-Hill; 2012: 1131-1137.

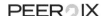

116. The correct answer is D, Urinary excretion of protein leading to decreased oncotic pressure in the plasma.

Why is this the correct answer?

The boy in this case is presenting with a nephrotic syndrome, which could be induced by a number of different pathological changes in the glomerulus. Any of these processes leads to increased permeability of the glomerulus to proteins and the loss of these in the urine, hence the large amount of protein detected on urinalysis. This leads to decreased serum albumin and hypoproteinemia with a loss of oncotic pressure in the plasma and resulting generalized edema. The kidney also retains salt and water in response to increased aldosterone secretion, and the edema worsens. The liver attempts to counter the loss of albumin by increasing protein production of all kinds, including lipoproteins, leading to hyperlipidemia and hypercoagulability. In this patient, the most likely renal pathology is minimal change disease. It is the most common primary glomerulonephritis in children and one of the few that is unlikely to have concomitant hematuria. A similar complaint with a recent upper respiratory tract infection is a typical presentation for post streptococcus glomerulonephritis. Other causes of glomerulonephritis include Henoch-Schönlein purpura, focal segmental glomerulonephritis, and membranous glomerulonephritis (as seen in systemic lupus erythematosus).

Why are the other choices wrong?

When faced with decreased blood flow to the glomerulus, the kidney responds appropriately by decreasing filtration and retaining sodium and free water as much as possible. This decreased filtration leads to the uremia seen in acute kidney injury from shock or severe dehydration. This patient has increased filtration, which has become less selective, and he is losing proteins from the plasma.

In the nephrotic syndrome, the liver increases production of albumin and other proteins to compensate for the loss in the urine. This results in hyperlipidemia and hypercoagulability.

Anaphylaxis is the result of sudden degranulation of mast cells in response to an antigen. These granules contain preformed vasoactive substances, including histamine and nitric oxide that lead to increased vascular permeability and edema. This patient is suffering from the gradual onset of nephrotic syndrome rather than the sudden and immediate effects of anaphylaxis.

PEER REVIEW

✓ Minimal change disease is the most common cause of the nephrotic syndrome in children.

✓ Characteristics of nephrotic syndrome: loss of protein in the urine leading to generalized edema, increased risk of infections, hyperlipidemia, and increased risk of thromboembolic disease.

✓ The presence of protein and blood in the urine is consistent with nephritis.

REFERENCES
Marx JA, Hockberger RS, Walls RM, eds. *Rosen's Emergency Medicine: Concepts and Clinical Practice*. 8th ed. St. Louis, MO: Elsevier; 2014: 1291-1311.
Tintinalli JE, Stapczynski JS, Ma OJ, et al, eds. *Tintinalli's Emergency Medicine: A Comprehensive Study Guide*. 8th ed. New York, NY: McGraw-Hill; 2012: 843-852.

117. The correct answer is D, *Streptococcus pneumoniae*.

Why is this the correct answer?

Although patients with HIV, because they are immunocompromised, are prone to contracting pneumonia caused by uncommon pathogens, they are also more likely to get the common types and have severe disease as a result. *S. pneumoniae* is the most common cause of community-acquired pneumonia among both immunocompetent and HIV-positive patients. Pulmonary infections are the most common cause of serious illness and death among patients with HIV, and while upper tract infections are most common, the incidence of lower tract infection increases as the CD4 count decreases.

Why are the other choices wrong?

Pneumocystis pneumonia (PCP) is caused by infection with *P. jirovecii* and is a serious cause of pneumonia for HIV-infected patients. But it is still less common than infection with *S. pneumoniae* and is usually present only when the CD4 count drops below 200. It is considered an AIDS-defining illness.

Pseudomonas infection is a concern among immunocompromised patients and recently hospitalized patients, particularly those who are in a hospital setting for more than 48 to 72 hours. But *P. aeruginosa* is decidedly less common than *S. pneumoniae* as a cause of community-acquired pneumonia.

S. aureus can be a common cause of pneumonia; the illness can follow another infection, and it can be severe, but it is a less common cause of community-acquired pneumonia than *S. pneumoniae*.

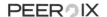

PEER REVIEW

✓ Pulmonary infections are the leading cause of morbidity and mortality among HIV-positive patients, and the incidence of lower tract disease increases as the CD4 count decreases.

✓ What's the most common source of pneumonia among persons who are HIV positive? *S. pneumoniae*, and opportunistic infections increase particularly when the CD4 count falls below 200.

REFERENCES

Marx JA, Hockberger RS, Walls RM, eds. *Rosen's Emergency Medicine: Concepts and Clinical Practice.* 8th ed. St. Louis, MO: Elsevier; 2014: 978-987; 1751-1767.

Tintinalli JE, Stapczynski JS, Ma OJ, et al, eds. *Tintinalli's Emergency Medicine: A Comprehensive Study Guide.* 8th ed. New York, NY: McGraw-Hill; 2012: 445-456; 1047-1057.

118. The correct answer is B, It is caused by abnormal absorption of cerebrospinal fluid.

Why is this the correct answer?

This case describes a classic presentation of normal-pressure hydrocephalus (NPH), a form of dementia with urinary incontinence and ataxia. The enlarged ventricles revealed by head CT are thought to be caused by abnormal absorption of CSF by the arachnoid villa. This diagnosis should be considered in patients who are experiencing dementia at a young age, as the symptoms of NPH can develop in individuals younger than 60 years. The enlarged ventricles revealed by head CT are thought to be caused by abnormal absorption of CSF by the arachnoid villa. Normal-pressure hydrocephalus can be reversible. Treatment is placement of a ventriculoperitoneal shunt.

Why are the other choices wrong?

Gait disturbance (ataxia) and urinary symptoms generally develop early in the disease course rather than late.

The dementia associated with NPH is characterized as reversible. With shunt placement, some patients experience resolution or significant improvement of their symptoms. Between 3% and 10% of all dementia cases are reversible. Other causes of reversible dementia include subdural hematoma, depression, and drug and alcohol dependence syndromes.

Donepezil is a medication used to treat Alzheimer disease, the most common form of dementia. It provides no benefit in NPH.

PEER REVIEW

✓ Normal-pressure hydrocephalus classically presents with memory loss, ataxia, and urinary incontinence, which develop early in the illness course. Head CT will reveal enlarged ventricles.

✓ Half of patients with normal-pressure hydrocephalus are younger than 60 years on initial presentation.

✓ Normal-pressure hydrocephalus can be reversed. It's treated with a ventriculoperitoneal shunt.

REFERENCES

Marx JA, Hockberger RS, Walls RM, eds. *Rosen's Emergency Medicine: Concepts and Clinical Practice*. 8th ed. St. Louis, MO: Elsevier; 2014: 1398-1408.

Tintinalli JE, Stapczynski JS, Ma OJ, et al, eds. *Tintinalli's Emergency Medicine: A Comprehensive Study Guide*. 8th ed. New York, NY: McGraw-Hill; 2012: 1156-1161.

119. The correct answer is A, CT angiography of the neck with contrast.

Why is this the correct answer?

Dissection of the carotid or vertebral arteries is a common cause of stroke among young and middle-aged persons. Diagnosis is made first and foremost by considering this disorder in the differential and then by obtaining CT angiography of the neck. Although it might take longer to obtain, MRA is also an acceptable diagnostic test. Carotid or vertebral artery dissection is often caused by minor trauma in the setting of neck manipulation or a minor sports injury. There are some case reports of these injuries occurring from riding roller coasters. Carotid and vertebral dissections are also seen more commonly in patients with connective tissue disorders. Classic presentations include neck pain and headache that might precede development of neurologic symptoms by hours or up to 14 days. Symptoms associated with vertebral artery dissection include unilateral facial numbness, dizziness, ataxia, vision disturbances (diplopia), and nausea or vomiting or both. Treatment for carotid or vertebral artery dissection is anticoagulation with heparin intravenously followed by warfarin.

Why are the other choices wrong?

Although CT without contrast can help identify acute fractures and bony injuries, it cannot provide additional information about vessel patency.

Duplex scans of the carotid arteries are not adequate to diagnose dissections. A CT scan with contrast or MR imaging with contrast is indicated.

As with duplex scans of the carotid arteries, duplex scans of vertebral arteries are not the right choice in this case. Duplex ultrasonography is a good test to diagnose chronic vessel atherosclerosis and assess patients for stroke risk.

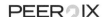

✓ Carotid and vertebral artery dissections present with headache and neck pain, usually first, and neurologic symptoms.

✓ What causes carotid and vertebral artery dissections? Usually minor trauma such as neck manipulation, roller coaster riding, or sports injuries.

✓ Carotid and vertebral dissections are diagnosed using CT angiography or MR angiography and treated with heparin followed by warfarin.

REFERENCES

Marx JA, Hockberger RS, Walls RM, eds. *Rosen's Emergency Medicine: Concepts and Clinical Practice*. 8th ed. St. Louis, MO: Elsevier; 2014: 1363-1374.

Tintinalli JE, Stapczynski JS, Ma OJ, et al, eds. *Tintinalli's Emergency Medicine: A Comprehensive Study Guide*. 8th ed. New York, NY: McGraw-Hill; 2012: 1142-1155.

120. The correct answer is C, Ciprofloxacin orally for 30 days.

Why is this the correct answer?

The patient is presenting with signs and symptoms consistent with prostatitis: fever and chills, urinary symptoms, and low back pain. Patients with prostatitis who do not have systemic signs of infection may be treated as outpatients. First-line treatment consists of a fluoroquinolone such as ciprofloxacin for a period of 4 to 6 weeks. Fluoroquinolones have the greatest concentration into the prostate of the urologic antibiotics, but the length of treatment must be extended due to limited antibiotic penetration of the prostate. As with most urologic infections, *Escherichia coli* is by far the most common bacteria. Other infectious agents include Klebsiella, Enterobacter, Proteus, and Pseudomonas. In patients with prostatitis, rectal examination reveals a tender and boggy prostate. Urinalysis might be positive for leukocyte esterase, and the patient might have an elevated WBC count. The culture should be sent, but this diagnosis is a clinical one; treatment should not be withheld if laboratory test results are normal.

Why are the other choices wrong?

If the patient appears systemically ill (fever, vital sign abnormalities) or is immunosuppressed or diabetic, then hospitalization and parenteral antibiotic therapy might be indicated. Appropriate intravenous antibiotics for prostatitis include ceftriaxone with the possible addition of gentamycin or a fluoroquinolone.

Oral cephalexin might be appropriate for a patient with uncomplicated cystitis, depending on local resistance patterns, but it is not first-line therapy for prostatitis because of its lack of concentration in the prostate. Length of treatment for cystitis is generally shorter, ranging from 3 to 10 days.

Trimethoprim-sulfamethoxazole is an alternative to ciprofloxacin, but the patient should take it for 30 days, not just 10. It is important to note that treatment failure rates might be higher in patients treated with trimethoprim-sulfamethoxazole, likely due to local resistance patterns.

PEER REVIEW

✓ What's the most common pathogen in prostatitis? *E. coli.*

✓ Outpatient treatment for prostatitis should include a prolonged course of oral antibiotics.

REFERENCES

Marx JA, Hockberger RS, Walls RM, eds. *Rosen's Emergency Medicine: Concepts and Clinical Practice.* 8th ed. St. Louis, MO: Elsevier; 2014: 1326-1354.

Tintinalli JE, Stapczynski JS, Ma OJ, et al, eds. *Tintinalli's Emergency Medicine: A Comprehensive Study Guide.* 8th ed. New York, NY: McGraw-Hill; 2012: 601-609.

121. The correct answer is D, Right middle cerebral artery.

Why is this the correct answer?

The middle cerebral artery is a common location for clot formation in ischemic stroke, making the pattern associated with blockage important to recognize early. Motor and sensory alterations are contralateral to the affected vessel, with the arm and face generally affected more commonly than the leg. So in this patient's situation, with left-sided weakness and sensory deficit, the lesion is most likely in the right middle cerebral artery. Other findings associated with a middle cerebral artery stroke include hemianopsia and gaze deviation toward the lesion. Aphasia, expressive, receptive, or both, is commonly associated with middle cerebral artery stroke of the dominant hemisphere (generally the left).

Why are the other choices wrong?

The anterior cerebral arteries are associated with loss of frontal lobe function. Patients with anterior cerebral artery occlusion might present with lack of judgment or insight into their conditions. Primitive reflexes such as suck and grasp can reappear, and some patients experience incontinence. Weakness and sensory findings are contralateral to the lesion and more pronounced in the lower extremity.

Patients with a left middle cerebral artery stroke experience weakness and sensory deficit on the right side. Most people are left-hemisphere dominant, making aphasia more common in strokes involving the left middle cerebral artery.

The anterior cerebral arteries are associated with loss of frontal lobe function. Patients with anterior cerebral artery occlusion might present with lack of judgment or insight into their conditions. Primitive reflexes such as suck and grasp can reappear, and some patients experience incontinence. Weakness and sensory findings are contralateral to the lesion and more pronounced in the lower extremity.

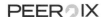

PEER REVIEW

✓ Strokes of the middle cerebral artery: weakness contralateral to the lesion, gaze deviation and hemianopsia ipsilateral to the lesion, upper extremities and face affected more commonly than lower extremities.

✓ Strokes of the anterior cerebral artery: loss of frontal lobe function, weakness, sensory findings contralateral to the lesion, lower extremities affected more commonly than upper extremities and face.

✓ Aphasia is a common and prominent presenting symptom in ischemic stroke, especially when the dominant hemisphere is involved.

REFERENCES

Marx JA, Hockberger RS, Walls RM, eds. *Rosen's Emergency Medicine: Concepts and Clinical Practice*. 8th ed. St. Louis, MO: Elsevier; 2014: 1363-1374.

Tintinalli JE, Stapczynski JS, Ma OJ, et al, eds. *Tintinalli's Emergency Medicine: A Comprehensive Study Guide*. 8th ed. New York, NY: McGraw-Hill; 2012: 1142-1155.

122. The correct answer is D, Traumatic aortic dissection.

Why is this the correct answer?

This patient presentation — upper extremity hypertension, decreased pulses in the lower extremities, systolic murmur, deceleration mechanism with steering column damage — is consistent with a diagnosis of traumatic aortic dissection. The upper extremity hypertension and decreased pedal pulses can result as a syndrome of pseudocoarctation thought to be due to a periaortic hematoma causing compression of the thoracic aorta. In addition, systemic reflex hypertension can result from stretching of the aortic isthmus. Turbulent flow across an area of aortic transection can lead to a systolic murmur, as is present in this patient. A high-speed deceleration mechanism places this patient at risk for this injury in particular. Findings on chest xray can include a wide mediastinum, although a normal chest xray does not rule out this diagnosis. The mediastinal widening, when present, is usually wider than 8 cm in a supine trauma patient. Most patients with complete disruption die in the field or en route to the hospital; therefore, these uncommon injuries, while less severe than complete disruption, are life-threatening and must remain on the differential diagnosis.

Why are the other choices wrong?

A patient with cardiac tamponade presents with tachycardia and hypotension. Performing a FAST examination reveals a pericardial effusion and helps the emergency physician make the diagnosis.

A patient with severe pulmonary contusion presents with dyspnea, tachypnea, and hypoxia. This patient's oxygen saturation is 98%. The hypoxia with severe pulmonary contusion is usually refractory to supplemental oxygen by nasal cannula.

A patient with a tension pneumothorax presents with hypotension and might also have decreased breath sounds on one side and tracheal deviation.

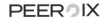
PEER REVIEW

✓ Maintain a high degree of suspicion for traumatic aortic disruption in patients with a high-speed deceleration mechanism in blunt trauma.

✓ Pseudocoarctation syndrome caused by periaortic hematoma can present with upper extremity hypertension and decreased pedal pulses.

REFERENCES

Marx JA, Hockberger RS, Walls RM, eds. *Rosen's Emergency Medicine: Concepts and Clinical Practice*. 8th ed. St. Louis, MO: Elsevier; 2014: 451-455.

Wolfson AB, Hendey GW, Ling LJ, et al, eds. *Harwood-Nuss' Clinical Practice of Emergency Medicine*. 6th ed. Philadelphia, PA: Lippincott, Williams & Wilkins; 2014: 208-212.

123. The correct answer is C, Paraphimosis.

Why is this the correct answer?

Paraphimosis is a condition that affects uncircumcised males. It develops when the foreskin is retracted and cannot be pulled back over the head of the penis. Paraphimosis is an acute urologic emergency because the distal glans penis can develop ischemia and eventually gangrene. Predisposing factors include masturbation, infection, and trauma. Treatment consists of reducing the foreskin; this can be done by reducing the swelling through the application of ice or with mild, prolonged compression and manual reduction. If no other measures are successful, dorsal band traction or a dorsal slit procedure should be performed. Patients can generally be safely discharged home following a voiding trial with close urologic follow-up. If there is any evidence of infection, admission to the hospital for treatment with intravenous antibiotics is indicated.

Why are the other choices wrong?

Balanoposthitis is inflammation of the glans penis and foreskin. It is mainly caused by infection with either gram-negative or gram-positive organisms. Treatment emphasis should be placed on proper hygiene. Antibiotics are needed in patients with evidence of infection.

Fournier gangrene is a necrotizing infection of the perineal tissues, including the penis, scrotum, or perianal area. It is polymicrobial. Immunocompromised patients, especially diabetic patients and alcoholics, are predisposed to development of Fournier gangrene. Treatment consists of emergent surgical or urologic consultation, surgical debridement, and broad-spectrum antibiotics.

Phimosis is the inability to retract the foreskin from an uncircumcised penis. It is important to note that, in most newborns, the foreskin cannot be retracted, and this resolves as the babies get older. Treatment for phimosis is generally circumcision, although recently topical steroid treatment has been shown to have good effect.

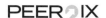
PEER REVIEW

✓ Phimosis: inability to retract the foreskin back from covering the penis.

✓ Paraphimosis: inability to return the retracted foreskin to its natural anatomic position.

✓ Paraphimosis is an acute surgical emergency, so it's important to know how to recognize it quickly and reduce it to prevent ischemia and gangrene.

REFERENCES

Marx JA, Hockberger RS, Walls RM, eds. *Rosen's Emergency Medicine: Concepts and Clinical Practice*. 8th ed. St. Louis, MO: Elsevier; 2014: 2205-2223.

Tintinalli JE, Stapczynski JS, Ma OJ, et al, eds. *Tintinalli's Emergency Medicine: A Comprehensive Study Guide*. 8th ed. New York, NY: McGraw-Hill; 2012: 601-609.

124. The correct answer is C, Penicillin G benzathine intramuscularly.

Why is this the correct answer?

Syphilis, also known as "the great imitator," can present in many different forms throughout the natural course of the disease. In the primary and secondary phases of the disease, the appropriate treatment is penicillin G benzathine 2.4 million units IM. It is important to treat with the long-acting form of penicillin, as shorter-acting preparations can result in treatment failure. Patients with penicillin allergy should be desensitized when treating the late phases of syphilis. Syphilis is a sexually transmitted infection caused by the spirochete *Treponema pallidum*. A chancre, as shown in the question, is the main manifestation of primary syphilis. The chancre is a painless lesion classically with well-defined edges that develops 2 to 4 weeks following exposure. Because it does not cause pain, it can go unnoticed, and as a result, the disease is left to progress to its secondary form. Secondary syphilis is often associated with a classic macular rash that involves the palms and soles, condyloma lata, lymphadenopathy, and the typical systemic symptoms of fever, weakness, and body aches. If untreated in this phase, latent and then tertiary syphilis develop. Tertiary syphilis has mainly cardiac and neurologic sequelae.

Why are the other choices wrong?

Azithromycin 1 g PO is appropriate treatment of both *Neisseria gonorrhoeae* infection and *Chlamydia trachomatis* urethritis. These conditions present with dysuria and vaginal or penile discharge. Azithromycin is recommended as the second antibiotic for just *N. gonorrhoeae* infection for combination therapy with ceftriaxone to help decrease resistance from the use of a single antibiotic, according to the CDC. This treatment regimen is also appropriate for *Haemophilus ducreyi* infection, which presents with chancroid, painful genital ulcers, and inguinal lymphadenopathy.

Ceftriaxone 250 mg IM, like azithromycin, is appropriate treatment for *N. gonorrhoeae* but not syphilis.

Genital herpes is the most common sexually transmitted disease in the United States. Patients with primary herpes infection present with vesicles progressing to multiple grouped ulcers that are painful — an important distinction from the painless lesions seen in syphilis — along with systemic symptoms such as fever and malaise. Treatment regimens include acyclovir, famciclovir, or valacyclovir. The advantage of valacyclovir is that it is dosed only twice daily, compared with acyclovir that must be taken five times a day. It is important to note that herpes is incurable; treatment reduces symptoms, but most patients experience recurrent outbreaks.

PEER REVIEW

✓ Patients can easily overlook the primary manifestation of primary syphilis — it's a painless genital lesion.

✓ Treat primary and secondary syphilis with penicillin G benzathine, the long-acting preparation if necessary.

✓ Chancroid caused by *H. ducreyi* and HSV infection presents with painful genital ulcers.

REFERENCES

Marx JA, Hockberger RS, Walls RM, eds. *Rosen's Emergency Medicine: Concepts and Clinical Practice*. 8th ed. St. Louis, MO: Elsevier; 2014: 1312-1325.

Tintinalli JE, Stapczynski JS, Ma OJ, et al, eds. *Tintinalli's Emergency Medicine: A Comprehensive Study Guide*. 8th ed. New York, NY: McGraw-Hill; 2012: 1007-1017.

125. The correct answer is B, She was conscious but confused during the primary survey.

Why is this the correct answer?

Distinguishing a seizure from a syncopal episode in the emergency department can be quite challenging. Important first steps are to obtain a good history and perform a thorough physical examination and to try to get information from persons who witnessed the event. Of the four pieces of information provided by the paramedics, the one about the patient being confused is what distinguishes this incident from a syncopal episode. It is also important to find out if the patient has a history of seizure or of substance abuse. A period of postictal confusion ranging from 10 minutes to hours (sometimes days) follows all generalized tonic-clonic seizures. Patients who experience syncope generally are not confused following the event. Other historical clues that support a diagnosis of seizure include abrupt onset, brief duration (90 to 120 seconds), loss of consciousness, purposeless behaviors, and that the event was unprovoked (ie, no association with emotional stimuli). Laboratory tests performed shortly after a generalized tonic-clonic seizure reveal a significant lactic acidosis. Other possible diagnoses when making this distinction include pseudoseizure, hyperventilation syndrome, migraine, and movement disorders.

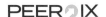

Why are the other choices wrong?

An HEENT examination is an important part of the physical examination when considering the differential diagnosis of seizure versus syncope. Oral trauma supports the diagnosis of seizure, but its absence does not rule it out. A bump on the head is not a helpful finding for making the distinction.

Many patients who experience a syncopal episode are observed to have some shaking behavior or myoclonus associated with the event. Observed shaking activity alone is not enough to make a distinction. However, shaking activity related to a generalized tonic-clonic seizure is generally more forceful than that associated with a syncopal episode.

Some patients who experience seizures also experience urinary or fecal incontinence. This information can support the diagnosis of seizure and should be noted in the history, but the absence of this finding does not rule it out.

PEER REVIEW

- ✓ It's hard to distinguish seizure from syncope, so a good history and physical examination are necessary.
- ✓ Pretty much every person who has a seizure has postictal confusion.
- ✓ Evidence of incontinence of urine or stool and oral trauma can be associated with seizure.

REFERENCES

Marx JA, Hockberger RS, Walls RM, eds. *Rosen's Emergency Medicine: Concepts and Clinical Practice*. 8th ed. St. Louis, MO: Elsevier; 2014: 158-161.

Tintinalli JE, Stapczynski JS, Ma OJ, et al, eds. *Tintinalli's Emergency Medicine: A Comprehensive Study Guide*. 8th ed. New York, NY: McGraw-Hill; 2012: 1173-1178.

126. The correct answer is B, Cephalexin 500 mg PO four times daily for 10 days.

Why is this the correct answer?

The causative agents of UTI are similar in pregnant and nonpregnant patients, and *Escherichia coli* is the culprit in approximately 75% of infections. Appropriate antibiotic choices for pregnant patients with UTI include nitrofurantoin, cephalexin, or amoxicillin for 10 to 14 days. The increased rate of UTI in pregnancy is thought to be related to physiologic changes to the renal system, which include decreased peristalsis through the collecting system and a dilated ureter and renal pelvis. It is important to note that pregnant patients with asymptomatic bacteriuria, as well as those with symptoms consistent with cystitis, should be treated with antibiotics to minimize the risk of development of pyelonephritis and prevent preterm labor. Urine cultures should be ordered on all pregnant patients with concerning urinalysis results to ensure correct antibiotic selection.

Why are the other choices wrong?

Most pregnant patients who present with urinary tract infection (UTI) may be treated as outpatients. Consideration for hospital admission and intravenous administration of antibiotics such as ceftriaxone, should be given to patients with intractable nausea and vomiting, concern for pyelonephritis, and third trimester presentations.

Ciprofloxacin is a pregnancy category C drug and should not be administered to pregnant patients. In nonpregnant patients, ciprofloxacin might be an appropriate choice for UTI treatment, depending on local resistance patterns.

Metronidazole is the treatment of choice for bacterial vaginosis, a common cause of vaginal infection predominantly caused by *Gardnerella*. It can present in a similar manner to cystitis and can be distinguished based on pelvic examination, sexual history, and testing for the causative organisms. It is important to treat bacterial vaginosis if suspected in a pregnant patient because it is also associated with preterm labor, spontaneous abortion, and other complications of pregnancy.

PEER REVIEW

✓ Treat asymptomatic bacteriuria and cystitis in all pregnant patients.

✓ Choose nitrofurantoin, cephalexin, or amoxicillin (10 to 14 days) to treat UTI in pregnant patients.

✓ Should you admit a pregnant patient who has a UTI? Indications include intractable nausea and vomiting, pyelonephritis, and third trimester infection.

REFERENCES

Marx JA, Hockberger RS, Walls RM, eds. *Rosen's Emergency Medicine: Concepts and Clinical Practice*. 8th ed. St. Louis, MO: Elsevier; 2014: 1326-1354.

Tintinalli JE, Stapczynski JS, Ma OJ, et al, eds. *Tintinalli's Emergency Medicine: A Comprehensive Study Guide*. 8th ed. New York, NY: McGraw-Hill; 2012: 590;636-643;661-668.

127. The correct answer is A, Extract it with a glue-covered cotton applicator.

Why is this the correct answer?

The use of cyanoacrylate, a glue, should be considered only in special cases. In this case, the foreign body is round and large enough to fill the entire external auditory canal, and the strategies for removal are limited. Use of a fast-acting glue to attach to the foreign body and pull it out has been described for years and might be the only option in this scenario when the object is not amenable to alternative removal methods. The downside to the use of glue is that it might get stuck to surrounding tissue and not the object. The use of suction to remove foreign bodies is useful only if the object is small or light; otherwise, it rarely helps. The use of a small Foley balloon that is inflated posterior to the foreign body is extremely effective but is dependent on the ability to pass the deflated catheter past the object.

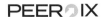

Why are the other choices wrong?

Irrigation is not likely to work because there is no room for the liquid to go around the obstruction and build up against the tympanic membrane to move the bead. Additionally, the water should be body temperature, not room temperature; otherwise it could trigger a vestibuloocular reflex and lead to nausea, disorientation, or even nystagmus. Irrigation should be used only if the tympanic membrane is intact. This can be inferred from noting no difference in hearing acuity between the affected and the unaffected ear. The tympanic membrane provides about 30 decibels of hearing due to the vibration of the membrane. An effusion or perforation of the tympanic membrane affects this and leads to asymmetric hearing; this should be a determining factor in any decision to use irrigation. If the tympanic membrane is perforated, some liquids can affect natural healing. Irrigation should be strongly considered when the object is adjacent to the tympanic membrane because direct manipulation of the object can cause significant discomfort.

Forceps, alligator or otherwise, generally cannot grasp spherical objects well enough to allow for removal. As the object also encompasses the whole external auditory canal, there is no room for the object to be grasped.

This is also the case with the ear hook method: there is not enough room around the bead to insert the hook.

PEER REVIEW

- ✓ Removal of a foreign body from the ear requires planning based on the object and clinical examination.
- ✓ If the patient is cooperative, you can do a gross examination of hearing and decide if the tympanic membrane is intact.
- ✓ Irrigation should be performed using body-temperature fluid.

REFERENCES

Fleisher GR, Ludwig S, et al, eds. *Textbook of Pediatric Emergency Medicine*. 6th ed. Philadelphia, PA: Lippincott, Williams & Wilkins; 2010: 1298; 1770-1771.

Wolfson AB, Hendey GW, Ling LJ, et al, eds. *Harwood-Nuss' Clinical Practice of Emergency Medicine*. 6th ed. Philadelphia, PA: Lippincott, Williams & Wilkins; 2014: 1247.

128. The correct answer is B, Hematuria is present in 85% of stone presentations.

Why is this the correct answer?

Renal colic and nephrolithiasis are common diagnoses in the emergency department. The classic presentation of a patient with an acute kidney stone consists of colicky flank pain that radiates to the groin with associated nausea and vomiting. Hematuria is present in most patients presenting with a kidney stone (15% have no microscopic hematuria), with only a minority (30%) experiencing gross hematuria.

It is important to note that the absence of hematuria does not rule out the possibility of kidney stone. The pain associated with kidney stone is caused by hydronephrosis associated with ureteral obstruction or the stone passing through the ureter. There are three common locations where kidney stones get stuck: the ureteropelvic junction, the pelvic rim, and the ureterovesicular junction. In patients who have obstructing stones, the creatinine level is frequently normal because the unaffected kidney can increase its workload. The differential diagnosis for flank pain should always include abdominal aortic aneurysm, especially in a middle-aged or elderly patient. Stones larger than 5 to 6 mm and stones lodged more proximally are less likely to pass spontaneously.

Why are the other choices wrong?

Of the four types of kidney stones, calcium stones (either oxalate or phosphate) predominate, making up between 75% and 80%. The cause of calcium stones is hyperexcretion of calcium within the renal collecting system. Uric acid calculi account for 10% of stones among patients in the United States and are associated with gout and increased uric acid excretion.

Nephrolithiasis is more common in men in the United States, with a male:female ratio of 2:1. Men generally experience the first stone at around 30 years old; it is rare for a man to have a first kidney stone over the age of 60 years. Women present with kidney stones in a bimodal distribution around age 35 and then 55.

Struvite (magnesium-ammonium-phosphate) stones are large stones "staghorn calculi") that form in the renal pelvis. They make up 15% of renal stones and are caused by urea-splitting bacteria such as *Proteus, Klebsiella, Corynebacterium, Staphylococcus* species, and *Providencia*. These urea-splitting bacteria increase urinary pH levels to more than 7.2, which might be noted in urinalysis. Struvite stones frequently require surgical removal. Of note, nitrate-reducing bacteria such as *Escherichia coli* are associated with nitrite-positive urinalysis results and UTIs.

PEER REVIEW

- ✓ About 85% of patients with kidney stones present with blood in the urine.
- ✓ The differential diagnosis of new-onset flank pain in men older than 60 years must include aortic aneurysm because first-time kidney stone is unlikely.
- ✓ Struvite stones are caused by urea-splitting bacteria. Urinalysis will reveal an elevated urinary pH.

REFERENCES

Marx JA, Hockberger RS, Walls RM, eds. *Rosen's Emergency Medicine: Concepts and Clinical Practice*. 8th ed. St. Louis, MO: Elsevier; 2014: 1326-1354.

Tintinalli JE, Stapczynski JS, Ma OJ, et al, eds. *Tintinalli's Emergency Medicine: A Comprehensive Study Guide*. 8th ed. New York, NY: McGraw-Hill; 2012: 609-613.

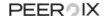

129. The correct answer is D, Surgical exploration.

Why is this the correct answer?

Given the physical findings, the patient's complaints of pain, and her description of how rapidly the redness is progressing, the most likely diagnosis is necrotizing fasciitis. Necrotizing infections can spread very rapidly, and some of these polymicrobial infections are more insidious. The result is soft tissue destruction and a mortality rate as high as about 25%. The gold standard for diagnosing this condition is also its treatment: surgical exploration — a process of direct visualization and subsequent fasciotomies. The diagnosis of necrotizing fasciitis is frequently missed because it can appear benign on examination early in its course. The early symptoms can appear similar to cellulitis, and as the disease progresses, examination might reveal crepitus or brawny edema. Patients typically have pain out of proportion to examination findings, which is one of the most important diagnostic features. But as the disease progresses, the affected area can become insensate and obscure this important sign. Later in the course, drainage or bullae can also manifest. The disease can progress to systemic manifestations such as fevers and tachycardia; late in necrotizing infections, patients develop severe sepsis and die. Causative factors include events that result in skin penetrations — trauma, bites, rashes, surgery. But some patients present with no preceding event. Persons with immunocompromising diseases and those who take immunosuppressant medications are at risk for necrotizing soft tissue infections. Antibiotics are an extremely important component of treatment, but they are rarely curative. If clinical suspicion is high based on examination findings, early surgical consultation is of paramount importance and should be pursued before obtaining any radiographic images.

Why are the other choices wrong?

Computed tomography has a higher sensitivity than plain film radiography, about 80%, and can reveal edema and gas formation, but the lack of findings cannot rule out the disease. Direct visualization is ultimately the best method of diagnosing this potentially fatal condition.

Magnetic resonance imaging has the highest radiographic sensitivity, as high as 90% to 100%, but again its negative predictive value has not been well determined. Furthermore, the time it takes to obtain MRI results in a delay to the ultimate treatment of surgical intervention in this time-sensitive condition.

Plain film radiographs might show gas that could indicate a necrotizing soft tissue infection, but the absence of this finding does not rule out this condition.

PEER REVIEW

✓ The gold standard for diagnosing and treating necrotizing soft tissue infections is surgical exploration.

✓ One of the key clinical signs of necrotizing soft issue infection is pain out of proportion to examination findings.

✓ Radiographic testing might help make the diagnosis of necrotizing fasciitis but takes time and does not rule it out.

REFERENCES

Marx JA, Hockberger RS, Walls RM, eds. *Rosen's Emergency Medicine: Concepts and Clinical Practice*. 8th ed. St. Louis, MO: Elsevier; 2014: 1851-1863.

Tintinalli JE, Stapczynski JS, Ma OJ, et al, eds. *Tintinalli's Emergency Medicine: A Comprehensive Study Guide*. 8th ed. New York, NY: McGraw-Hill; 2012: 1029-1039.

130. The correct answer is D, If he complies, he is three times less likely to return for more care or hospitalization.

Why is this the correct answer?

Multiple randomized controlled trials have demonstrated a strong benefit from a short burst of oral corticosteroid therapy for the prevention of relapse in asthma. Based on a 2007 Cochrane Database meta-analysis, the relative risk for relapse (return emergency department visit or hospitalization) in patients receiving therapy was 0.35 to 0.38. The same analysis showed that the number needed to treat for steroid therapy was only 9 to 11 to prevent one return visit or hospitalization. Corticosteroids are a mainstay of therapy in asthma. They work to reduce the inflammation and reactivity of the airways that is otherwise the hallmark of the disease. The onset of benefit is within 1 to 2 hours of the initial dose, whether given orally or intravenously. The peak benefit comes at about 24 hours after initiation. The risks of therapy are the usual side effects of corticosteroids, including elevated plasma glucose, hyperactivity and difficulty sleeping, hypertension, weight gain, osteoporosis, and accelerated cataract formation. Most of these side effects are significant only for those taking steroids long term. An asthma patient with diabetes should be warned about elevated blood sugars, but the benefit of the short course of steroids very likely outweighs the risk.

Why are the other choices wrong?

The onset of action of intravenous corticosteroids is the same as it is for the oral route, which is 1 to 2 hours. In the emergency department, steroids should be given to a patient with asthma intravenously if the patient cannot tolerate oral pills.

For patients with asthma that is mildly persistent or more severe, inhaled corticosteroids are recommended for maintenance therapy. They reduce the frequency of exacerbations and the need for rescue therapy with beta-agonists.

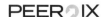

Oral corticosteroids stimulate cortisol secretion and act on the liver to release glycogen stores. They commonly increase plasma glucose and might be challenging to tolerate for a patient with diabetes.

PEER REVIEW

✓ A short course of oral corticosteroids following an emergency department visit for an asthma exacerbation significantly reduces the risk (by about one-third) of a return visit or hospitalization.

✓ The onset of action of intravenous corticosteroids is the same as for the oral route, which is 1 to 2 hours.

✓ Steroid therapy has a number of unfortunate side effects, including elevated plasma glucose, hyperactivity and difficulty sleeping, hypertension, weight gain, osteoporosis, and accelerated cataract formation.

REFERENCES

Marx JA, Hockberger RS, Walls RM, eds. *Rosen's Emergency Medicine: Concepts and Clinical Practice*. 8th ed. St. Louis, MO: Elsevier; 2014: 941-955.

Rowe BH, Spooner CH, Ducharme FM, et al. Corticosteroids for preventing relapse following acute exacerbations of asthma. *Cochrane Database Syst Rev.* 2007; (3): CD000195.

Tintinalli JE, Stapczynski JS, Ma OJ, et al, eds. *Tintinalli's Emergency Medicine: A Comprehensive Study Guide*. 8th ed. New York, NY: McGraw-Hill; 2012: 489-492.

131. The correct answer is A, CT scanning of the abdomen and pelvis followed by urgent urology follow-up.

Why is this the correct answer?

The presentation of an older patient with painless intermittent hematuria should prompt suspicion for a urinary tract carcinoma, most often bladder or renal cell cancer. Patients with this complaint should undergo CT imaging of the abdomen and pelvis, which is likely to reveal a complex mass in the kidneys if the patient has renal cell cancer. Bladder cancer, however, might not be detectable on CT in its early stages. Therefore, regardless of the imaging results, the patient should be urgently referred to a urologist for appropriate screening by cystoscopy and, if necessary, biopsy. Risk factors for bladder cancer include tobacco use, excessive analgesic use, radiation to the pelvis, exposure to cyclophosphamide, and occupational exposure to aromatic amines or benzenes. For patients in tropical areas, especially Africa, infection with *Schistosoma haematobium* is associated with an increased rate of bladder cancer. The strongest risk factors for renal cell cancer are tobacco use, obesity, and hypertension.

Why are the other choices wrong?

Patients with large amounts of gross hematuria with visible clots are prone to develop urinary obstruction from a blood clot in the urethra. Typically, a patient with a urinary tract structural abnormality or surgery who is taking anticoagulants can develop this complication. The intermittent, mild (only 30 RBCs/hpf) bleeding of the patient in this case is unlikely to cause acute obstruction.

Painless intermittent hematuria with blood appearing at the conclusion of the stream can be caused by benign prostate hypertrophy. Although initiating therapy for prostate enlargement might be reasonable, patients with this complaint and multiple risk factors for neoplastic disease should undergo imaging then be referred. Reassurance only is not the ideal management.

Older men with prostate enlargement and incomplete bladder emptying can develop UTIs, which present with hematuria and dysuria. They do not typically complain of painless, intermittent bleeding. Initiating antibiotic therapy and sending a urine culture might be reasonable for the patient in the case, but he should undergo advanced imaging first because of the high risk of cancer.

PEER POINT

Risk factors for urinary tract neoplasms

Bladder cancer

- Age >40 years
- Analgesic abuse
- Cigarette smoking
- Cyclophosphamide
- Occupational exposures
- Pelvic irradiation
- Schistosoma haematobium infection

Renal cell cancer

- Alcohol consumption
- Cigarette smoking
- Genetic factors
- Hypertension
- Obesity
- von Hippel-Lindau disease

PEER REVIEW

- ✓ If you're treating an older man who has painless intermittent hematuria, consider urinary tract cancer.
- ✓ Risk factors for bladder cancer: tobacco use, analgesic abuse, pelvic radiation, and exposure to certain chemicals.
- ✓ Excessive hematuria with clots can cause urinary obstruction and requires bladder irrigation.

REFERENCES

Marx JA, Hockberger RS, Walls RM, eds. *Rosen's Emergency Medicine: Concepts and Clinical Practice*. 8th ed. St. Louis, MO: Elsevier; 2014: 1326-1354.

Tintinalli JE, Stapczynski JS, Ma OJ, et al, eds. *Tintinalli's Emergency Medicine: A Comprehensive Study Guide*. 8th ed. New York, NY: McGraw-Hill; 2012: 609-613.

132. The correct answer is B, Intubate with a large endotracheal tube into the right mainstem bronchus.

Why is this the correct answer?

The acute management of life-threatening pulmonary hemorrhage follows the same principle as any other resuscitation: airway, breathing, and circulation. This patient needs a definitive airway, and it should be established in a way that protects the remaining functional lung; the right lung can still ventilate and should be protected from blood pooling from the left lung hemorrhage. In this case, the best approach is a standard intubation, but the endotracheal (ET) tube should be pushed in deeply until it meets resistance. A single-lung intubation of the right lung (the unaffected side in this case) is fairly easy to achieve without special equipment. Selectively intubating the left lung requires finesse and experience and is made easier with the use of bronchoscopy. Without a bronchoscope, it is possible to maneuver the ET tube into the left mainstem bronchus by turning the tube 90 degrees to the left after passing the cords. Regardless, a large ET tube should be used in a patient with pulmonary hemorrhage so that a bronchoscope can be passed through it later for closer examination of the lung injury and possible sclerotic therapy of the bleeding vessel. Based on the history, the patient is most likely taking rivaroxaban, one of the novel anticoagulants. These medications do not require the frequent monitoring and adjustment necessary with warfarin use. But their function is not easily reversed; vitamin K has no role in their reversal. In addition to recently approved specific fab-fragment antidotes, there are some general therapies that can help the severely bleeding patient. Dabigatran has low protein binding and can be removed via dialysis, or an activated prothrombin complex concentrate (factor VIII inhibitor bypass activity [FEIBA]) might help. The anticoagulation effect of rivaroxaban and apixaban can be lessened by the use of a prothrombin complex concentrate.

Why are the other choices wrong?

An immediate, emergent open thoracotomy is an extreme measure with a high risk of death. Localized treatment of the bleeding vessel with a bronchoscope is a preferred approach. Regardless, the patient's airway must be secured and the anticoagulation reversed before a thoracotomy is possible.

In theory, a patient with pulmonary hemorrhage should be placed with the bleeding side down (left in this case, not right) so that the blood pools in the "bad" lung and the "good" lung can continue to ventilate. This practice has not been validated by scientific study and might increase ventilation-perfusion mismatching.

Continuous positive airway pressure is very effective in patients with ventilator failure such as those with COPD and congestive heart failure. But it would be disastrous to attempt in a patient who is struggling to clear the blood from his airway.

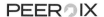

Emergency stabilization of severe, life-threatening pulmonary hemorrhage: position the patient on his or her side with the bleeding lung down, and attempt to intubate the nonbleeding lung.

PEER REVIEW

✓ If you're intubating a patient who has hemoptysis, use a large ET tube so a bronchoscope can be passed later.

✓ Novel anticoagulant agents cannot be reversed with vitamin K; various prothrombin complex concentrates can help, and specific antidotes are preferred.

REFERENCES

Marx JA, Hockberger RS, Walls RM, eds. *Rosen's Emergency Medicine: Concepts and Clinical Practice*. 8th ed. St. Louis, MO: Elsevier; 2014: 203-205.

Tintinalli JE, Stapczynski JS, Ma OJ, et al, eds. *Tintinalli's Emergency Medicine: A Comprehensive Study Guide*. 8th ed. New York, NY: McGraw-Hill; 2012: 436-440.

133. The correct answer is D, *Streptococcus pneumoniae*.

Why is this the correct answer?

Streptococcus pneumoniae, a gram-positive diplococci, is the most common pathogen causing bacterial meningitis in adult patients, causing 50% of the disease in the United States. *S. pneumoniae* and *N. meningitidis* are encapsulated organisms that generally invade the host via the upper airway: they work their way into the subarachnoid space and in turn cause infection of the CSF. There is some evidence to support an association between *S. pneumoniae* meningitis and recent head trauma. It is important to note that there are increasing vaccination rates for *S. pneumoniae*, *N. meningitidis*, and *Haemophilus influenzae* type b leading to decreased prevalence of infection overall. Empiric administration of dexamethasone with the initial antibiotic dose (and continued for 4 to 6 days) has been shown to reduce morbidity and mortality rates among adult patients with *S. pneumoniae* meningitis. It is believed this might be due to decreasing the inflammatory cascade caused by these encapsulated organisms.

Why are the other choices wrong?

Listeria monocytogenes infection represents only about 2% of cases of meningitis but carries a mortality rate as high as 40%. It is generally thought to affect very young patients (<1 month) or older patients (>50 years) or immunocompromised patients. In addition to standard empiric antibiotic therapy, high-dose ampicillin should be added if the patient is in one of the high-risk age groups for Listeria meningitis.

The most common cause of pneumonia in school-aged children is infection with *M. pneumoniae*, but it is a rare cause of CNS infection.

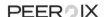

Risk factors for *N. meningitidis* infection include close living quarters such as dormitories or military barracks, and for that reason it is the most common pathogen in patients younger than 45 years. *N. meningitidis* can be associated with a petechial or purpuric rash on the extremities and trunk. The incidence of meningococcal meningitis has decreased dramatically with increased use of vaccines.

PEER REVIEW

✓ Most cases of bacterial meningitis among adults in the United States are caused by infection with *Streptococcus pneumoniae*.
✓ The incidence of meningitis caused by common pathogens has decreased because more people are getting vaccinations.

REFERENCES

Centers for Disease Control and Prevention. Pneumococcal disease. CDC website. Available at: https://www.cdc.gov/pneumococcal/clinicians/clinical-features.html. Accessed May 23, 2017.

Marx JA, Hockberger RS, Walls RM, eds. *Rosen's Emergency Medicine: Concepts and Clinical Practice*. 8th ed. St. Louis, MO: Elsevier; 2014: 1447-1459.

Tintinalli JE, Stapczynski JS, Ma OJ, et al, eds. *Tintinalli's Emergency Medicine: A Comprehensive Study Guide*. 8th ed. New York, NY: McGraw-Hill; 2012: 1192-1199.

134. The correct answer is A, Esophagogastroduodenoscopy.

Why is this the correct answer?

This patient is suffering from a food impaction, which most often occurs in the distal esophagus. The best management is esophagogastroduodenoscopy (EGD) and manual retrieval or advancement of the food bolus. Medical approaches to encourage esophageal relaxation are unlikely to be successful, and feeding agents to dissolve the food can be harmful. Esophageal food impaction develops for multiple reasons, aside from simply trying to swallow a mouthful that is too large. Patients might have structural abnormalities such as strictures, a Schatzki ring, esophageal webs, or a Zenker diverticulum. The narrowest point in the esophagus is the cricopharyngeus muscle or upper esophageal sphincter. Children account for 80% of presentations of swallowed foreign bodies, and they tend to get objects trapped in the upper esophagus. Adults, especially prisoners and psychiatry patients, who ingest foreign bodies most often get theirs stuck at the lower esophageal sphincter. Anything that passes through the pylorus is likely to complete transit of the GI tract. Although expectant management is reasonable for a patient who is tolerating the obstruction, food impactions should not be allowed to persist for more than 24 hours; they can lead to esophageal perforation. Dangerous objects such as sharp objects or button batteries need to be removed immediately.

Why are the other choices wrong?

Glucagon has been widely advocated for use in food bolus impaction to relax the esophageal smooth muscle and allow passage of the material. But in the few times it has been studied against a control, it was demonstrated to be ineffective. It also can be associated with vomiting. It is likely not harmful and could be offered while awaiting the availability of an EGD, but it is not the best approach.

The theory of using effervescent beverages (sodium bicarbonate along with a mild acid such as lemon juice or simply a brand-name cola) to dislodge a food impaction is to generate carbon dioxide in the esophagus to push the food bolus along. There are case reports of this approach occasionally being effective. The disadvantages are that the beverages are difficult to administer and prone to induce aspiration in patient like the one in this case who has a complete obstruction.

Papain, a trypsin-like enzyme, is used as a meat tenderizer. It has been suggested in the past as an option for dissolving food boluses, but in practice it can dissolve the esophagus itself, leading to perforation. It has been associated with fatal outcomes and should never be considered as a potential therapy.

PEER REVIEW

✓ Eighty percent of esophageal foreign body ingestions occur in children, and they most often get lodged in the upper esophagus.

✓ Some adult patients have a congenital ring or web that impairs normal transition of the esophagus, and food can get stuck just above the lower esophageal sphincter.

✓ If you're treating a patient with an impacted food bolus and you're waiting for definitive treatment with EGD, it's OK to try relaxing the esophageal smooth muscle with glucagon just to see if it works.

REFERENCES

Marx JA, Hockberger RS, Walls RM, eds. *Rosen's Emergency Medicine: Concepts and Clinical Practice*. 8th ed. St. Louis, MO: Elsevier; 2014: 1170-1185.

Tintinalli JE, Stapczynski JS, Ma OJ, et al, eds. *Tintinalli's Emergency Medicine: A Comprehensive Study Guide*. 8th ed. New York, NY: McGraw-Hill; 2012: 525-532.

135. The correct answer is B, Apply warm compresses.

Why is this the correct answer?

Of the conditions that present with a red eye, two that can be clinically indistinguishable are chalazion and hordeolum. This particular patient has a chalazion, which is a lump in the eyelid caused by blockage of a meibomian gland. To help promote resolution, the patient should be instructed to apply warm compresses. A chalazion is usually painless, but some patients experience mild tenderness. The chalazion is preceded by the hordeolum, either external (stye) or internal. Both types of hordeolum are more painful than a chalazion and are associated with mild conjunctival hyperemia, but all three conditions are treated in the same way, with warm compresses and no antibiotics. Nonurgent referral (within 30 days) is recommended for both chalazia and hordeola if they continue to grow and do not resolve or if they begin to affect vision. If that happens, the ophthalmologist might perform biopsy or excision.

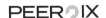

Why are the other choices wrong?

An over-the-counter topical vasoconstrictor-antihistamine medication might be effective as a second-line treatment for allergic conjunctivitis if systemic antihistamines fail. The patient in this case, however, does not report itching, which is characteristic of allergic conjunctivitis. Other symptoms include binocular tearing, conjunctival hyperemia, swelling, and watery discharge.

The patient's vision is still intact, so excision of the chalazion in the emergency department is not indicated. The patient should be instructed to follow up with an ophthalmologist if the lump grows or starts to affect his vision.

Oral antibiotics are not indicated because the inflammation is localized and is not caused by a bacterial infection. If the patient had pain with extraocular movement, cellulitis would be a concern. In that case, intravenous antibiotic therapy and an emergent ophthalmologic consultation are indicated.

PEER REVIEW

✓ First comes hordeolum, then comes chalazion. Treatment is the same for both — warm compresses.

✓ A patient with a chalazion should see an ophthalmologist if he or she has vision changes or if it gets bigger or doesn't go away.

✓ Antibiotics are not indicated for either chalazion or hordeolum.

REFERENCES

Tintinalli JE, Stapczynski JS, Ma OJ, et al, eds. *Tintinalli's Emergency Medicine: A Comprehensive Study Guide*. 8th ed. New York, NY: McGraw-Hill; 2012: 757-764.

Trobe JD. *The Physician's Guide to Eye Care*. 4th ed. San Francisco, CA: American Academy of Ophthalmology; 2012: 60-62; 78-79.

Valeri MR, Sullivan JH, Correa ZM, et al. *Vaughn & Asbury's General Ophthalmology*. 18th ed. New York, NY: McGraw-Hill; 2011. http://accessmedicine.mhmedical.com/content.aspx?bookid=387&sectionid=40229321. Accessed May 16, 2017.

136. The correct answer is B, Benztropine.

Why is this the correct answer?

Benztropine is an anticholinergic medication used to treat Parkinson disease and well known for causing constipation. Constipation has a wide range of causes, roughly divided into primary and secondary. Primary causes are intrinsic to the intestines and have no apparent cause such as irritable bowel or functional bowel disease. Secondary causes are local anatomic causes or systemic medical causes, including iatrogenic from medication therapy. Almost every medication has been documented to be associated with constipation, but some drugs are more prone to inhibiting bowel motility. Chief among them are opioids, iron supplements, and anticholinergics (such as benztropine, diphenhydramine, and tricyclic antidepressants). Calcium channel blockers, antiepileptics, and most psychiatric medications are also often associated with constipation. Constipation should be a diagnosis of exclusion in the emergency department. Before assigning a patient's abdominal pain to "just constipation," the clinician should thoroughly consider other more life-threatening conditions. This is especially true for elderly patients in whom the chief complaint of abdominal pain carries a high mortality rate (up to 10%).

Why are the other choices wrong?

Amoxicillin-clavulanate is more often associated with diarrhea. Mild diarrhea is expected with amoxicillin-clavulanate, but severe diarrhea developing several days after starting therapy should prompt investigation for *Clostridium difficile* infection.

Bisacodyl, a laxative, is used as a therapy for constipation. But long-term use of laxatives can result in atonic colon, the so-called lazy bowel syndrome, a condition in which the colon no longer responds to normal stimuli to evacuate.

Colchicine, a therapy for gout, is more commonly associated with diarrhea. Patients are advised to titrate their use of the medication, depending on the degree of diarrhea they develop.

PEER POINT

Most common medications associated with constipation

- Anticholinergics
- Antidepressants
- Antiepileptics
- Antipsychotics
- Antiparkinson drugs
- Calcium
- Calcium channel blockers
- Diuretics
- Iron
- Opiates

PEER REVIEW

✓ Many medications are associated with constipation, but most commonly? Opioids, iron supplements, and anticholinergics.

✓ Undiagnosed abdominal pain in the elderly is associated with a 10% mortality rate.

✓ Antibiotic-associated diarrhea begins very soon after starting therapy.

✓ Diarrhea accompanying *Clostridium difficile* infection can be very severe and typically begins several days after starting therapy.

REFERENCES

Adams JG, Barton ED, Collings J, et al, eds. *Emergency Medicine*. Philadelphia, PA: Saunders; 2008: 309-314.

Hoffman RS, Howland MA, Lewin NA, et al, eds. *Goldfrank's Toxicologic Emergencies*. 10th ed. New York, NY: McGraw-Hill; 2015: 564-574.

Marx JA, Hockberger RS, Walls RM, eds. *Rosen's Emergency Medicine: Concepts and Clinical Practice*. 8th ed. St. Louis, MO: Elsevier; 2014: 261-265.

137. The correct answer is B, Chest CT with contrast.

Why is this the correct answer?

Superior vena cava (SVC) syndrome is caused by occlusion of the SVC by a thrombus or mediastinal mass, and it should be easily identified with a CT scan of the chest with contrast. The symptoms usually develop over weeks to months as a tumor grows and compresses venous return from the head and neck. The tumor is most commonly a non-small-cell cancer of the lung but can also be small-cell lung cancer or lymphoma. The syndrome can develop more quickly in the case of a thrombus, which is the most common nonmalignant cause of the condition. Other nonmalignant causes include restrictive pericarditis, mediastinal fibrosis, and goiter. Patients with SVC syndrome present with gradual onset of periorbital edema and facial swelling that is most prominent in the early morning after spending a night lying flat. This can progress to plethora of the face, edema of the upper extremities and neck, and headaches from cerebral venous backflow. Patients typically have a cough, either from the lack of venous drainage or primarily from irritation of the tumor itself. Some develop dyspnea and hypoxia, leading to cyanosis.

Why are the other choices wrong?

An SVC compression from a tumor could cause cerebral sinus congestion and cerebral edema that can be identified using MRI, but CT of the chest to evaluate the vena cava is a more reasonable approach.

Pulmonary embolism should always be considered in a patient with dyspnea and chest discomfort, and identifying a deep venous thrombosis in the leg is sufficient to make the diagnosis by inference. But this patient has a more gradual onset of symptoms, and facial swelling is not a recognized symptom of PE.

Lumbar puncture is indicated to rule out meningitis or subarachnoid hemorrhage, but facial swelling and cough are not usually symptoms of these conditions. Idiopathic intracranial hypertension is diagnosed and relieved with a lumbar puncture, but imaging should be done first to ensure the patient is not at risk of herniation.

PEER REVIEW

- ✓ Superior vena cava syndrome is caused by compression and occlusion, usually by lung cancer or thrombus.
- ✓ Signs and symptoms of superior vena cava syndrome: gradual-onset facial swelling, periorbital edema, cough, dyspnea, headaches, and plethora of the face.
- ✓ Pulmonary embolism can be presumptively diagnosed using CT of the chest with contrast or by finding a DVT using lower-extremity Doppler ultrasonography.

REFERENCES

Marx JA, Hockberger RS, Walls RM, eds. *Rosen's Emergency Medicine: Concepts and Clinical Practice*. 8th ed. St. Louis, MO: Elsevier; 2014: 129-134.

Tintinalli JE, Stapczynski JS, Ma OJ, et al, eds. *Tintinalli's Emergency Medicine: A Comprehensive Study Guide*. 8th ed. New York, NY: McGraw-Hill; 2012: 1500-1504.

138. The correct answer is B, de Quervain tenosynovitis.

Why is this the correct answer?

In this case, the patient has de Quervain tenosynovitis, an overuse syndrome that affects the extensor pollicis brevis and abductor longus tendons at the radial styloid. de Quervain syndrome is diagnosed clinically by performing the Finkelstein test, as follows: tell the patient to place the affected thumb in the palm of his or her affected hand ("bend it across"), then tell the patient to deviate the wrist in the ulnar direction ("toward the little finger"). The test result is positive if this motion reproduces the patient's presenting pain, usually at the base of the thumb or radial styloid, and has been shown to be pathognomonic for de Quervain tenosynovitis. On physical examination, swelling at the radial styloid is sometimes present. This condition is treated with a thumb spica splint and NSAIDs; recurrence might necessitate steroid injections or surgical decompression.

Why are the other choices wrong?

The question describes the steps of the Finkelstein test, which is used to diagnose de Quervain syndrome, not carpal tunnel syndrome. In contrast, carpal tunnel syndrome is entrapment of the median nerve that leads to paresthesias along the volar thumb, second and third fingers, and radial aspect of the fourth finger. Traditionally, the tests used to diagnose carpal tunnel syndrome have focused on eliciting the Phalen sign and the Tinel sign.

Dupuytren contracture is a fibrosis causing a flexing of the fingers; it is not diagnosed with the Finkelstein test. The finding of this contracture, and possibly the palpation of a fibrotic nodule in the palm, helps make this diagnosis.

Lateral epicondylitis, known as "tennis elbow," is pain at the lateral epicondyle of the humerus; it does not involve the wrist. The Cozen test, holding a clenched hand in extension against resistance while the arm is fully extended, can reproduce the symptoms.

PEER POINT

The Finkelstein Test

Cup the thumb, close the fist, and ulnar deviate the wrist to reproduce pain along the extensor pollicis and abductor pollicis.

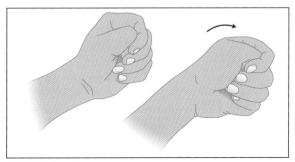

PEER Point 12

✓ de Quervain tenosynovitis is an overuse syndrome that causes pain at the radial styloid.

✓ The diagnosis of de Quervain tenosynovitis is supported by a positive Finkelstein test.

✓ de Quervain tenosynovitis is treated with NSAIDs and a thumb spica splint.

REFERENCES

Marx JA, Hockberger RS, Walls RM, eds. *Rosen's Emergency Medicine: Concepts and Clinical Practice*. 8th ed. St. Louis, MO: Elsevier; 2014: 1518-1526.

Tintinalli JE, Stapczynski JS, Ma OJ, et al, eds. *Tintinalli's Emergency Medicine: A Comprehensive Study Guide*. 8th ed. New York, NY: McGraw-Hill; 2012: 1921-1927.

139. The correct answer is C, Replacement of hepatic tissue with fibrosis causing portal vein hypertension.

Why is this the correct answer?

This patient likely has cirrhosis following long-standing alcoholic liver disease. Excessive, chronic ingestion of alcohol destroys hepatocytes by a variety of mechanisms, especially by the metabolization of alcohol into toxic degradation products. If the liver injury exceeds the rate of regeneration, fibrotic tissue replaces normal liver architecture and liver function deteriorates. The most significant impact is on the portal venous system, where obstructed flow leads to portal hypertension and increased hydrostatic pressure in the veins draining the intestines. This induces collateral flow from the vessels. In the stomach and esophagus, varices can form. Midgut collaterals are manifested as caput medusa, engorgement of the periumbilical veins radiating out from the umbilicus. Vessels in the hindgut can form hemorrhoids as collaterals. The increased hydrostatic pressure pushes transudate out into the peritoneal space, leading to ascites. Portal hypertension from cirrhosis develops slowly, leaving time for collateral flow to form. Portal hypertension from a portal vein thrombosis can develop very quickly and is manifested by primarily ascites without significant variceal vein development. Ascites from portal hypertension is best managed by relieving the obstructed flow directly, either through liver transplantation or a transjugular intrahepatic portal shunt. But before these procedures can be done, a patient is managed on a low-sodium, fluid-restricted diet and diuretics to minimize the fluid retention.

Why are the other choices wrong?

A low-sodium, fluid-restricted diet minimizes fluid retention and reduce the progression of ascites.

Intraperitoneal carcinomas such as ovarian cancer can seed the omentum and develop omental "caking." This can lead to an exudative leaking of plasma and the development of ascites. It is not the mechanism seen in cirrhosis.

Thrombosis of the inferior vena cava leads to bilateral lower extremity edema, but likely not ascites. Portal vein thrombosis is associated with portal hypertension and ascites.

PEER REVIEW

✓ Cirrhosis is replacement of hepatic tissue with fibrosis. It leads to portal hypertension.

✓ Portal hypertension is manifested by ascites, esophageal and gastric varices, caput medusae, hemorrhoids, and hepatic encephalopathy.

✓ Metastatic ovarian cancer can seed the omentum, developing omental "caking," and can present with ascites.

REFERENCES

Adams JG, Barton ED, Collings J, et al, eds. *Emergency Medicine.* Philadelphia, PA: Saunders; 2008: 347-355.

Marx JA, Hockberger RS, Walls RM, eds. *Rosen's Emergency Medicine: Concepts and Clinical Practice.* 8th ed. St. Louis, MO: Elsevier; 2014: 1186-1204.

140. The correct answer is B, Chest xray and an infectious disease workup.

Why is this the correct answer?

In second-degree heart block, atrioventricular (AV) conduction is intermittent; some atrial impulses do reach the ventricles, but others are blocked. In this case, the ECG demonstrates a second-degree type I (Mobitz) heart block (Wenckebach). It typically is transient. Even though this patient recently underwent cardiac surgery, he does not have any specific cardiac symptoms such as shortness of breath, syncope, or dyspnea on exertion. His symptoms — chest pain with a productive cough and fever — more likely have an infectious etiology such as pneumonia, so a chest xray and infectious disease workup are indicated. Second-degree type I (Mobitz) block occurs when successive depolarizations produce a prolongation of the refractory period at the AV node. Subsequent depolarizations arrive at the AV node during a refractory period, and conduction is thus slower through the AV node. Eventually, an atrial impulse attempts to conduct during an absolute refractory period; conduction is blocked completely, and a nonconducted, or "dropped," beat occurs. The PR interval prolongs until a dropped QRS complex, the dropped beat, occurs. Generally, the P wave-P wave interval is constant and the R wave-R wave interval shortens. Second-degree type I block can be seen after an acute inferior MI, digoxin toxicity, myocarditis, or cardiac surgery. It can also occur after the AV node is subject to rapid atrial rates.

Why are the other choices wrong?

Cardiology consultation is likely needed if the patient is admitted. However, the rhythm strip and symptoms do not indicate any signs of ischemia that require cardiac catheterization. Again, the patient has a likely pulmonary infection and a stable rhythm that is a normal variant.

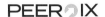

Extensive laboratory evaluation is not warranted in a patient who is stable from a cardiovascular perspective. This form of AV block is rarely compromising and is frequently a normal variant.

Typically, second-degree type I (Mobitz) blocks do not require intervention if the patient is asymptomatic. Hemodynamic instability is usually not encountered, and permanent pacing is rarely required. This patient is hemodynamically stable and does not need transcutaneous pacing. If he were to become symptomatic (syncope, shortness of breath, hypotensive, and so on) then transcutaneous pacing would be indicated.

PEER REVIEW

✓ Classic findings of second-degree type I (Mobitz) heart block (Wenckebach): a rhythm in which the PR interval prolongs until a dropped QRS complex, the dropped beat, occurs.

✓ Second-degree type I (Mobitz) heart block (Wenckebach) is generally a transient rhythm that does not need extensive workup.

REFERENCES

Tintinalli JE, Stapczynski JS, Ma OJ, et al, eds. *Tintinalli's Emergency Medicine: A Comprehensive Study Guide.* 8th ed. New York, NY: McGraw-Hill; 2012: 112-134.

Winters ME, Bond MC, DeBlieux P, et al (eds). *Emergency Department Resuscitation of the Critically Ill.* Dallas, TX: American College of Emergency Physician Publishing; 2011: 51-68.

141. The correct answer is D, Place a Foley catheter into the bladder to relieve the obstruction.

Why is this the correct answer?

This patient is suffering from acute kidney injury (AKI) from postrenal obstruction of the bladder outflow from a large prostate mass. The next step should be to relieve the obstruction with a urinary catheter, which might be sufficient to reverse the AKI. One of the first steps in evaluating AKI is to determine if the problem is prerenal, renal, or postrenal. Prerenal AKI is the appropriate compensatory renal response to low circulating plasma volume. If a patient is severely dehydrated or has relative hypovolemia from sepsis, the kidneys respond by restricting urinary output, leading to rising BUN and creatinine levels (azotemia). Intrinsic kidney insults such as exogenous toxins, nephrotoxic medications leading to acute tubular necrosis, or glomerulonephritis result in decreased renal function. Prerenal AKI should be treated primarily by adequate intravenous volume replacement. Postrenal obstruction restricting the output of urine flow also leads to decreased renal function and azotemia. Theoretically, this should happen only when there is bilateral obstruction: one normally functioning kidney should be able to compensate for the decreased function of the other obstructed kidney. In practice, however, patients with chronic conditions such as diabetes and hypertension might have a baseline subclinical renal dysfunction and demonstrate significant azotemia and renal failure from a single obstructed kidney. Large kidney stones and surgical misadventures severing a ureter are two examples of unilateral postrenal obstruction. Bladder, cervical, and prostate cancers are well recognized causes of bilateral postrenal obstruction. A quick bedside ultrasound examination can easily identify urinary obstruction; examiners might see hydronephrosis of one or both kidneys or enlargement of the bladder. Any urinary obstruction identified should be promptly relieved by placing a urinary catheter or arranging for urgent nephrostomy stenting.

Why are the other choices wrong?

The patient's medication list should be thoroughly examined for any nephrotoxic medications or drugs that require adjustment for renal dysfunction. But it takes time to reverse acute tubular necrosis, and other more expedient solutions should be examined first (such as relieving bladder obstruction).

Radiographic exploration for the extent of the tumor might be indicated after the initial obstruction is relieved, but the use of contrast is contraindicated in the setting of AKI.

The use of urinary electrolytes to calculate the fractional excretion of sodium, or FENa, is very helpful in separating prerenal from renal causes of AKI, but the process of obtaining the urine sample in this patient treats the underlying problem. The formula for calculating FENa is (plasma Cr × urinary Na) / (plasma Na × urinary Cr) × 100.

PEER POINT

Clinical features that are rapid bedside clues to the cause of AKI

Prerenal
- Clinically dehydrated; FENa <1%

Renal
- Euvolemic or hypervolemic, FENa >2%

Postrenal
- Bedside ultrasonography to examine for hydronephrosis of the kidneys, bladder size

PEER REVIEW

- ✓ Acute kidney injury can be classified as prerenal, renal, or postrenal.
- ✓ A quick bedside ultrasound examination of the kidneys and bladder can rule in or rule out urinary obstruction; any obstruction should be promptly relieved.
- ✓ Treat prerenal AKI with intravenous volume replacement.

REFERENCES

Marx JA, Hockberger RS, Walls RM, eds. *Rosen's Emergency Medicine: Concepts and Clinical Practice.* 8th ed. St. Louis, MO: Elsevier; 2014: 1291-1311.

Tintinalli JE, Stapczynski JS, Ma OJ, et al, eds. *Tintinalli's Emergency Medicine: A Comprehensive Study Guide.* 8th ed. New York, NY: McGraw-Hill; 2012: 575-581.

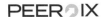

142. The correct answer is C, Indomethacin.

Why is this the correct answer?

The classic presentation of reactive arthritis (formerly referred to as Reiter's syndrome) includes arthritis, urethritis, and uveitis; however, this triad is not necessary for making the diagnosis. This patient presents with an asymmetrical polyarthritis following a recent STD (most commonly a chlamydial infection), or urethritis, and that is enough to warrant a high level of suspicion for reactive arthritis. The treatment of choice for reactive arthritis is an NSAID, commonly indomethacin. Antibiotics have also been shown to have benefit in postchlamydial reactive arthritis. Long-term combination therapy of rifampicin with doxycycline or azithromycin may be used in addition to NSAIDs. In this syndrome, the Achilles tendon might be inflamed at the insertion point. The pain patients typically experience is in the weight-bearing joints of knees, ankles, and heels. In addition, the sacroiliac joints, ischial tuberosity, and ischial crest can be involved and cause pain with range of motion. Diarrhea caused by infection with the invasive GI bacteria — *Campylobacter*, *Salmonella*, *Shigella*, and *Yersinia* — has also been known to cause a reactive arthritis picture. The NSAIDs are also the treatment of choice for postdysentery reactive arthritis, but antibiotics have not been shown to have benefit.

Why are the other choices wrong?

Antibiotics are not the first-line therapy for reactive arthritis. Chlamydial infections might respond to long-term antibiotic therapy, but ceftriaxone is not an antibiotic typically used in these cases.

Although not first-line therapy, the appropriate antibiotics have been shown to improve recovery time in patients with reactive arthritis caused by chlamydial infections. Typically, rifampicin is used in conjunction with either doxycycline or azithromycin, but NSAIDs are still the treatment of choice.

Methotrexate is not used for reactive arthritis but may be used in other forms of arthritis, most notably rheumatoid arthritis.

PEER REVIEW

- ✓ Reactive arthritis is an asymmetric polyarthralgia that typically affects weight-bearing joints.
- ✓ Reactive arthritis often develops following dysentery or a chlamydial infection.
- ✓ The treatment of choice for reactive arthritis is an NSAID, and if a chlamydial infection preceded the arthritis, adding an antibiotic might reduce recovery time.

REFERENCES

Marx JA, Hockberger RS, Walls RM, eds. *Rosen's Emergency Medicine: Concepts and Clinical Practice*. 8th ed. St. Louis, MO: Elsevier; 2014: 1501-1517.

Tintinalli JE, Stapczynski JS, Ma OJ, et al, eds. *Tintinalli's Emergency Medicine: A Comprehensive Study Guide*. 8th ed. New York, NY: McGraw-Hill; 2012: 1927-1936.

143. The correct answer is B, Retained foreign body.

Why is this the correct answer?

Vaginal foreign bodies are a rare cause of pediatric vulvovaginitis but are largely believed to be under-reported in the pediatric and adolescent literature. Obtaining an accurate history from pediatric patients can be very challenging, and a subjective history is most commonly obtained from parents. Importantly, a high level of suspicion must be maintained for possible sexual abuse in all pediatric patients presenting with vulvovaginitis. Blood-stained vaginal discharge is the most common presenting symptom, occurring in approximately 80% to 90% of all cases. Wads of tissue paper are the most common retained vaginal foreign body and comprise approximately 80% of all cases. Very young pediatric patients are generally unaware of the vagina; later in childhood, in the process of self-exploration, they sometimes insert larger objects or toys. However, sexual abuse must always be strongly considered in this cohort as well. Placing the patient in the supine position, knees to chest, often allows for optimal physical examination of the vaginal vault. If a vaginal foreign body can be directly visualized, attempted removal using either forceps or irrigation with warmed saline is a reasonable first approach. Vaginal foreign bodies that cannot be directly visualized or are not amenable to simple removal in the emergency department as described require further workup, including vaginal ultrasonography, xrays, vaginoscopy, examination under general anesthesia, or consultation with a pediatric gynecologist, depending on resources immediately available.

Why are the other choices wrong?

A normal examination is certainly possible, but if the parents are bringing the child in because of discharge, it is likely she has some discharge. Although examining the genitals of a young child is difficult, care must be taken to look for foreign bodies, lacerations, and other trauma as well as to localize the source of the blood.

Urethral prolapse presents with spotting on the underwear and is identified as a red-purple mass at the opening of the urethra. It is far less common than retained foreign bodies.

Vaginal neoplasms are relatively rare in children. When they occur, they are usually rhabdomyosarcomas, but they can occasionally present as germ cell tumors or clear cell adenocarcinoma.

PEER REVIEW

✓ Always consider sexual abuse in all cases of pediatric vulvovaginitis and retained vaginal foreign body.

✓ What's the most common symptom of retained vaginal foreign body? Blood-stained vaginal discharge, occurring in 80% to 90% of cases.

✓ Pieces of tissue paper are the foreign body most commonly retained, occurring in roughly 80% of cases.

REFERENCES

Marx JA, Hockberger RS, Walls RM, eds. *Rosen's Emergency Medicine: Concepts and Clinical Practice*. 8th ed. St. Louis, MO: Elsevier; 2014: 835-842.

Tintinalli JE, Stapczynski JS, Ma OJ, et al, eds. *Tintinalli's Emergency Medicine: A Comprehensive Study Guide*. 8th ed. New York, NY: McGraw-Hill; 2012: 1500-1504.

144. The correct answer is B, Prepare for intubation and administer intravenous antibiotics.

Why is this the correct answer?

Bacterial tracheitis is a rare condition that can cause severe upper airway obstruction in children. In a presentation such as the one described in the case, with signs of near-total airway obstruction, airway control takes priority over diagnostic evaluation. This patient requires intubation followed by intravenous administration of antibiotics — vancomycin and a third-generation cephalosporin such as ceftriaxone. Bacterial tracheitis generally occurs in the first 8 years of life. It is characterized by purulent secretions of the tracheal mucosa below the vocal cords caused by bacterial infection. *Staphylococcus aureus* is the most common cause, but *Streptococcus pneumoniae*, *Streptococcus pyogenes*, *Moraxella catarrhalis*, and *Haemophilus influenzae* are other known causes. It often occurs following damage to the airway mucosa or inflammation that accompanies viral upper respiratory infections. Clinical features of bacterial tracheitis include signs of airway obstruction: stridor, cough, and respiratory distress. Fever is common, and drooling is uncommon. Patients appear toxic with high fever and a rapidly progressing croup-like syndrome. Nebulized epinephrine and steroids are ineffective. Patients often prefer to lie flat. Overall, bacterial tracheitis can appear very similar to croup. Imaging classically shows the steeple sign — a narrowing of the subglottic trachea that is indistinguishable from croup on plain films. Neck radiographs are not needed to make the diagnosis. Laboratory analysis is not helpful; WBC count and C-reactive protein results vary widely in bacterial tracheitis and are not prognostic.

Why are the other choices wrong?

Giving dexamethasone and repeated doses of nebulized racemic epinephrine is usually sufficient to improve the condition of a patient with severe croup. But this patient's clinical picture — toxic appearance, high fever — suggests a disease more severe than croup. Bacterial tracheitis or epiglottitis should be considered, and airway control is essential.

Guidelines from the American Academy of Pediatrics indicate that bronchodilators, steroids, and antibiotics are ineffective in bronchiolitis and that only supportive care is recommended. If this patient had bronchiolitis, suctioning and supplemental oxygen would be correct management. But this patient is older and has a more severe presentation than is expected for bronchiolitis. Intervention with airway management and antibiotics is indicated.

The development of bacterial pneumonia is common following influenza. Intravenous antibiotic therapy and a chest xray are indicated, but control of his impending respiratory failure is more urgent.

PEER REVIEW

✓ Bacterial tracheitis should be suspected in children who present with acute onset of airway obstruction in the setting of viral upper respiratory infection and in children who are febrile, toxic appearing, and have a poor response to treatment with nebulized epinephrine or corticosteroids.

✓ Empiric antimicrobial therapy for bacterial tracheitis should include a third-generation cephalosporin and an anti-MRSA medication such as vancomycin.

✓ Croup usually responds to corticosteroids and bronchodilator therapy.

REFERENCES

Ralston SL, Lieberthal AS, Meissner HC, et al. Clinical Practice Guideline: The Diagnosis, Management, and Prevention of Bronchiolitis. *Pediatrics*. 2014;134:e1474–e1502.

Stephan M, Carter C, Ashfaq S, et al. Pediatric Emergencies. In: Stone C, Humphries RL, eds. *CURRENT Diagnosis & Treatment Emergency Medicine*. 7th ed. New York, NY: McGraw-Hill; 2011. http://accessmedicine.mhmedical.com/content.aspx?bookid=385&sectionid=40357266. Accessed May 18, 2017.

Tintinalli JE, Stapczynski JS, Ma OJ, et al, eds. *Tintinalli's Emergency Medicine: A Comprehensive Study Guide*. 8th ed. New York, NY: McGraw-Hill; 2012: 764-775.

145. The correct answer is D, Procainamide and synchronized cardioversion.

Why is this the correct answer?

The patient is presenting with atrial fibrillation in Wolff-Parkinson-White (WPW) syndrome. The ECG findings in WPW include a rapid, irregularly irregular rhythm with widened QRS complexes; the QRS complexes vary in morphology from beat to beat. Conduction occurs via both the atrioventricular node and the accessory pathway, producing a fusion of the two impulses and varying QRS complexes from one beat to the next. Medical management options include antiarrhythmic therapy; procainamide is the most appropriate antiarrhythmic agent in this setting. It is administered at a dose of 17 mg/kg over approximately 30 to 45 minutes. In unstable patients or those who do not respond to procainamide, electrical cardioversion is indicated. After conversion to sinus rhythm, the patient should be admitted to the hospital for further monitoring and electrophysiologic testing.

Why are the other choices wrong?

Atrioventricular node blocking agents, including adenosine (despite its short half-life), must be avoided in patients with WPW and atrial fibrillation. They inhibit conduction via the atrioventricular node with increased impulse conduction via the accessory pathway. Ultimately, these patients could experience cardiovascular collapse, potentially with ventricular fibrillation.

Amiodarone is not appropriate because of its beta-blocking and calcium channel-blocking effects. Using it in conjunction with procainamide can increase the likelihood of cardiovascular collapse. The most recent guidelines by the AHA in 2014 indicates that amiodarone and other antiarrhythmics can slow the AV conduction, but not alter the accessory path which can increase the ventricular rate. Those patients with one or more accessory paths are at greater likelihood for this treatment to lead to ventricular fibrillation. Procainamide both slows the AV rate and prolongs the refractory period of the accessory path, making this safer to use in these patients.

Calcium channel blockers such as diltiazem and beta-adrenergic blocking agents are contraindicated in these patients, as explained above.

PEER POINT

Atrial fibrillation and WPW syndrome

This ECG shows an irregular wide complex rhythm with extremely rapid rates (>200 to 250 bpm) in some areas. The QRS complexes do not have a typical bundle-branch block morphology, and they vary beat to beat. These characteristics are indicative of the presence of a bypass tract. Reproduced from Mattu et al, *Cardiovascular Emergencies*, ©2015 American College of Emergency Physicians

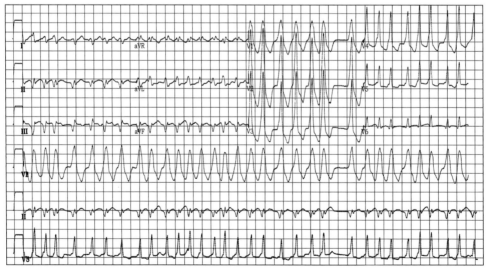

PEER Point 13

PEER REVIEW

✓ A rapid, irregularly irregular rhythm with widened QRS complexes and beat-to-beat variation in the QRS complex morphology suggests WPW-related atrial fibrillation.

✓ Don't use atrioventricular node blocking agents in patients with this WPW rhythm presentation.

REFERENCES
January CT, Wann LS, Alpert JS, et al. 2014 AHA/ACC/HRS guideline for the management of patients with atrial fibrillation: a report of the American College of Cardiology/American Heart Association Task Force on Practice Guidelines and the Heart Rhythm Society. J Am Coll Cardiol. 2014;64(21):2305-2307.
Link MS, Berkow LC, Kudenchuk PJ, et al. Part 7: adult advanced cardiovascular life support: 2015 American Heart Association Guidelines Update for Cardiopulmonary Resuscitation and Emergency Cardiovascular Care. *Circulation.* 2015; 132(Suppl 2):S444–S464.
Tintinalli JE, Stapczynski JS, Ma OJ, et al, eds. *Tintinalli's Emergency Medicine: A Comprehensive Study Guide.* 8th ed. New York, NY: McGraw-Hill; 2012: 112-134.

146. The correct answer is C, Herpes simplex virus.

Why is this the correct answer?

This case describes the presentation of a less common form of herpes simplex virus (HSV) keratitis, HSV disciform keratitis. Although the most common form of HSV keratitis is epithelial keratitis manifesting with the classic dendrites, other forms, including disciform, stromal, and keratouveitis, are all manifestations of HSV keratitis. Disciform keratitis is a deeper, disc-shaped, localized area of corneal edema. Patients might have pain and decreased vision. In most patients, there is a history of orolabial or genital herpes infections. The slit lamp examination is useful for separately examining the layers of the eye to determine the source of the vision defect. Treatment usually consists of antiviral eye drops and topical steroids.

Why are the other choices wrong?

The consistently elevated blood sugar levels in diabetes lead to accelerated cataract formation, but this patient has signs of corneal disease, not lens disease.

Exposure to bright sunlight, especially when reflected off sand or snow, can result in ultraviolet keratitis, which is diffuse and bilateral, not one spot in one eye.

Several systemic autoimmune diseases present with eye findings, for example, anterior uveitis in reactive arthritis. This patient has no evidence of anterior chamber disease; there is no cell or flare and no irritation with iris constriction (no photophobia).

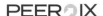

PEER POINT

Examination findings in HSV keratitis

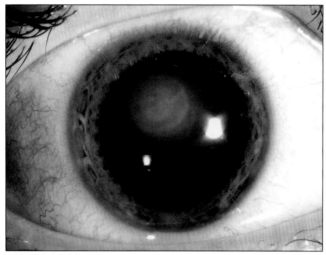

PEER Point 14

PEER REVIEW

✓ The classic description of HSV keratitis is dendritic lesions, but it can manifest in a number of other forms, including ulcerative and disciform.

✓ The treatment for HSV keratitis is topical steroids and oral antiviral therapy.

✓ The slit lamp examination is useful for separately examining the layers of the eye to determine the source of the vision defect.

REFERENCES

Marx JA, Hockberger RS, Walls RM, eds. *Rosen's Emergency Medicine: Concepts and Clinical Practice.* 8th ed. St. Louis, MO: Elsevier; 2014: 909-930.

Tintinalli JE, Stapczynski JS, Ma OJ, et al, eds. *Tintinalli's Emergency Medicine: A Comprehensive Study Guide.* 8th ed. New York, NY: McGraw-Hill; 2012: 1504-1512.

147. The correct answer is B, Obtain a cardiology consultation for cardiac catheterization.

Why is this the correct answer?

Wellens syndrome is a high-grade stenosis of the proximal left anterior descending coronary artery and a high-risk emergency department presentation. The natural history of Wellens syndrome is anterior wall STEMI within 30 to 90 days of initial presentation, so the correct disposition is to obtain a cardiology consultation. The patient in this case is most appropriately admitted to the hospital with involvement of a cardiologist. The most appropriate diagnostic and therapeutic approach is cardiac catheterization and PCI. Provocative testing should be avoided. Wellens syndrome is characterized by ECG findings (deeply inverted or biphasic T waves in leads V1 to V4), ongoing or recent chest pain, the absence of acute MI (no ECG or cardiac marker evidence of MI), and proximal left anterior descending artery occlusion. Importantly, the patient demonstrates the characteristic ECG findings during periods of pain as well as when pain free; these findings resolve only with definitive management of the coronary obstruction.

Why are the other choices wrong?

Admitting the patient for immediate PCI is not necessary. The ECG and presentation are highly characteristic of Wellens syndrome, but not an acute myocardial infarction.

A workup that is negative for acute cardiac injury (serial troponin and ECG determinations) with discharge and cardiology follow-up is not appropriate, primarily from the perspective of the disposition: the discharge is not appropriate. Given the natural history of STEMI within 30 days, the patient should be admitted to the hospital for further evaluation and management.

Exercise stress testing after a negative rule-out MI is not appropriate. With a high likelihood of proximal left anterior descending coronary artery obstruction, provocative testing could produce a negative outcome, either STEMI or cardiac arrest.

PEER REVIEW

- ✓ A patient with Wellens syndrome can present without chest pain and continue to demonstrate the characteristic ECG abnormalities.
- ✓ The natural history of Wellens syndrome presentation is anterior wall STEMI 30 to 90 days after initial presentation.
- ✓ Cardiac catheterization with subsequent PCI is the most appropriate diagnostic-treatment approach to Wellens syndrome.
- ✓ A patient with Wellens syndrome should not undergo provocative testing in the evaluation of the chest pain and ECG abnormalities.

REFERENCES

Marx JA, Hockberger RS, Walls RM, eds. *Rosen's Emergency Medicine: Concepts and Clinical Practice.* 8th ed. St. Louis, MO: Elsevier; 2014: 997-1033.

Mattu A, Brady WJ, et al (eds). *Cardiovascular Emergencies.* Dallas, TX: American College of Emergency Physicians Publishing; 2014: 16-17.

148. The correct answer is D, Rating pain greater than 10 on a 10-point scale.

Why is this the correct answer?

Drug-seeking behavior, a form of malingering, is a common concern for emergency physicians. According to one source, prescription drug abuse increased 400% from 1999 to 2010. Certain behaviors tend to be associated with patients who are misusing or abusing prescription opioid medications. In a case-control study of 152 patients enrolled in a case-management program due to prescription abuse, the factor most associated with abuse was reporting pain levels at more than 10 out of 10. Requesting parenteral medications, claiming to be out of medications, and having at least three visits in 7 days were also associated with prescription abuse. In a different retrospective analysis, patients requesting a specific medication by name, making multiple visits for the same complaint, and having a "suspicious history" were indicators of drug-seeking behavior. Although estimates of prevalence vary widely, patients demonstrating this behavior represent a small minority of emergency department visits. It is important to recognize that patients with chronic pain who are undertreated might demonstrate some of these behaviors. This can be labeled "pseudoaddiction" and tends to resolve once the pain is adequately treated.

Why are the other choices wrong?

Patients in pain should be expected to ask for pain relief, and it is the duty of emergency physicians to provide prompt, effective pain relief for patients with acutely painful conditions. Asking for a specific medication might be suspicious behavior, but seeking pain control in general is why these patients chose the emergency department for their care.

Patients with sickle-cell disease often struggle with frequent episodes of severe pain, and inadequately treated pain can lead to pseudoaddiction and the demonstration of drug-seeking behaviors. An appropriate case management plan for these high-utilizing patients can help to provide more consistency and continuity in care.

Many emergency department patients lack access to primary care follow-up, but that problem in and of itself has not been identified as a high-risk factor for patients inappropriately seeking narcotic medications. Socioeconomic challenges are not a reason to deny appropriate use of opioid analgesia for acutely painful conditions.

PEER POINT

Most common behaviors associated with prescription abuse, ranked by odds ratio (Grover et al)

- Specifically asking for the parenteral route
- Reporting pain worse than 10 out of 10
- Making three visits in 7 days

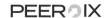

- Having more than three different pain complaints
- Claiming to have run out of medication
- Requesting a certain drug by name
- Noting a chief complaint of needing a medication refill
- Reporting a lost or stolen medication

PEER REVIEW

✓ Here are three behaviors commonly associated with prescription drug abuse: asking for a parenteral route, reporting pain that is greater than 10 out of 10, and asking for a specific drug.

✓ Inadequately treated chronic pain can lead to pseudoaddiction.

REFERENCES

Grover CA, Close RJH, Wiele ED, Villarreal K, Goldman LM. Quantifying drug-seeking behavior: a case control study. *J Emerg Med.* 2012;42(1):15-21.

Marx JA, Hockberger RS, Walls RM, eds. *Rosen's Emergency Medicine: Concepts and Clinical Practice.* 8th ed. St. Louis, MO: Elsevier; 2014: 31-49.

Tintinalli JE, Stapczynski JS, Ma OJ, et al, eds. *Tintinalli's Emergency Medicine: A Comprehensive Study Guide.* 8th ed. New York, NY: McGraw-Hill; 2012: 256-261.

149. The correct answer is B, Obtain surgical consultation while considering imaging and intravenous antibiotics.

Why is this the correct answer?

Most gastrostomy tube (G-tube) tracts mature after 2 to 3 weeks, so dislodgement of the G-tube puts the patient at risk for intestinal content leakage and peritonitis. Imaging, antibiotics, and surgical consultation are typically recommended. Attempting to replace a G-tube or Foley catheter into the tract before the tract matures can create a false lumen or even worsen intraperitoneal leakage. On the other hand, if the G-tube had been in place long enough for the tract to mature (2 to 3 weeks), emergent replacement with another G-tube is indicated (within hours) to maintain tract patency. Maintaining temporary patency with a Foley catheter (16F or 18F, typically) is an acceptable alternative. To confirm that the tube has been replaced correctly, about 25 mL of a water-soluble contrast material (eg, Gastrografin) should be injected through the tube then checked with a supine abdominal radiograph.

Why are the other choices wrong?

Conservative wound management — applying an occlusive dressing — might be the right thing to do after surgical consultation, but the patient likely requires observation and potentially alternative parenteral access.

Again, inserting a replacement G-tube or temporary Foley catheter to maintain tract patency is the appropriate intervention only after the tract has matured, which takes about 2 to 3 weeks.

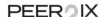

Using a wire to insert a similarly sized G-tube carries the risk of creating a false lumen, but this procedure may be performed by a consultant with sufficient experience.

PEER REVIEW

✓ Don't try to replace a G-tube in the first 2 to 3 weeks after it was placed — get a consult instead.

REFERENCES:

Marx JA, Hockberger RS, Walls RM, eds. *Rosen's Emergency Medicine: Concepts and Clinical Practice*. 8th ed. St. Louis, MO: Elsevier; 2014: 581-584.

Tintinalli JE, Stapczynski JS, Ma OJ, et al, eds. *Tintinalli's Emergency Medicine: A Comprehensive Study Guide*. 8th ed. New York, NY: McGraw-Hill; 2012: 256-261.

150. The correct answer is A, Cool compresses to the eyes and diligent handwashing.

Why is this the correct answer?

This patient has viral conjunctivitis, the most common cause of acute red eye. The image shows the characteristic diffuse hyperemia and mild discharge. Adenovirus is the most likely cause; it is highly contagious, and antibiotic treatment is of no use. Viral conjunctivitis is self-limited; it typically lasts 1 to 3 weeks and requires supportive therapy only such as cool compresses and diligent hand hygiene to minimize the risk of spread. It is most contagious when discharge is present; patients should stay away from work, school, and daycare during that time. Many infections start in one eye then quickly spread to the other. The clinical presentation of viral conjunctivitis includes fullness, tightness, warmth, or a scratchy sensation, but not pain, in the affected eye; diffuse hyperemia on the conjunctiva; watery or mucoid discharge; and a tender, swollen preauricular node. Symptoms commonly develop after (or while) the patient has had an upper respiratory infection. One or both eyes can be affected. Some patients also have keratitis, characterized by slight vision defect, light sensitivity, and a foreign body sensation. If keratitis is suspected, follow-up with an ophthalmologist within 48 hours is recommended. The same is true if the condition worsens after 3 days or does not improve after 7 days.

Why are the other choices wrong?

If there are concerns for a more aggressive infection like endophthalmitis, then intravenous antibiotic medications and immediate ophthalmology involvement are warranted. However, since the patient has no vision deficits and an otherwise normal eye examination, this more aggressive type of infection is likely not present.

The patient has no signs of dendritic lesions on fluorescein exam, so it is unlikely that a herpes simplex keratoconjunctivitis is present. Therefore, oral acyclovir is not the right pharmacotherapy.

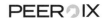

Antibiotic drops are indicated when treating bacterial conjunctivitis. Since this patient's symptoms are bilateral and the discharge is watery rather than mucopurulent, a bacterial infection is unlikely, and antibiotics are not warranted.

PEER REVIEW

✓ Viral conjunctivitis is the most common form of conjunctivitis.

✓ Is it viral or bacterial? Viral conjunctivitis is most likely monocular (at least early on) with a watery discharge, and bacterial tends to be binocular with a mucopurulent discharge.

✓ Even if it's "just" viral, do a fluorescein examination to rule out other signs of irritation that warrant more aggressive treatment.

REFERENCES

Mahmood AR, Narang AT. Diagnosis and management of the acute red eye. *Emerg Med Clin North Am.* 2008;26:35-55.

Tintinalli JE, Stapczynski JS, Ma OJ, et al, eds. *Tintinalli's Emergency Medicine: A Comprehensive Study Guide.* 8th ed. New York, NY: McGraw-Hill; 2012: 1543-1579.

Trobe JD. *The Physician's Guide to Eye Care.* 4th ed. San Francisco, CA: American Academy of Ophthalmology; 2012:81-83.

151. The correct answer is B, Instruct him to use analgesics and sialagogues.

Why is this the correct answer?

The patient has symptoms consistent with sialolithiasis, which occurs when a salivary gland stone gets stuck in the salivary duct. The obstruction most commonly occurs in the submandibular gland (80%), followed by the parotid gland. Salivary gland stones are almost always unilateral in presentation and usually consist of calcium carbonate or calcium phosphate. They are most likely to be symptomatic in middle-aged men. Sometimes, the stone can be milked out of the duct, which resolves the symptoms. If not, as long as the patient does not have any signs of an underlying infection with the obstruction, the only therapy needed in the emergency department is analgesia and sialagogues (like lemon drops) to help promote passage of the stone. If the stone does not pass, the patient should follow up with an ENT specialist.

Why are the other choices wrong?

Without any signs of infection, antibiotics are not indicated. Passage of the stone will resolve the symptoms.

The diagnosis is made based primarily on clinical examination. Computed tomography of the face, along with emergent ENT consultation, is needed only if there is suspicion for an abscess. This patient is afebrile and has no other clinical signs of an overlying infection.

Since there are no signs of an abscess, incision and drainage is not indicated. If a patient with salivary gland stones does have an abscess, ENT consultation is prudent to determine the next treatment steps.

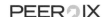

PEER REVIEW

✓ Sialolithiasis most commonly presents in middle-aged men in the submandibular gland.

✓ Assuming no other signs of infection, initial treatment is to promote passage of the obstructing stone.

✓ If there are signs of overlying infection, antibiotics and close ENT follow-up are indicated.

REFERENCES

Butt F, Yuan-Shin F. Benign Diseases of the Salivary Glands. In: Lalwani AK, eds. *CURRENT Diagnosis & Treatment in Otolaryngology—Head & Neck Surgery.* 3rd ed. New York, NY: McGraw-Hill; 2012. http://accessmedicine.mhmedical.com/content.aspx?bookid=386&sectionid=39944053. Accessed May 18, 2017.

Tintinalli JE, Stapczynski JS, Ma OJ, et al, eds. *Tintinalli's Emergency Medicine: A Comprehensive Study Guide.* 8th ed. New York, NY: McGraw-Hill; 2012: 1585-1591.

152. The correct answer is C, Order basic metabolic panel, consider starting hydrochlorothiazide, and arrange for outpatient follow-up.

Why is this the correct answer?

Focused laboratory testing can be useful in certain patient populations. In this patient with essentially asymptomatic hypertension, laboratory testing for renal dysfunction is potentially of value. He has no primary care doctor and likely can be considered to have difficulty in obtaining short-term medical follow-up. In fact, a level C recommendation in the ACEP clinical policy on hypertension suggests that, in patients with "poor follow-up," emergency physicians may order laboratory testing to search for renal dysfunction, as is the likely case here. Another level C recommendation suggests that, in this same subset of patients, emergency physicians may start long-term blood pressure control therapy; hydrochlorothiazide is a reasonable choice for this black male until he can arrange for follow-up. And, of course, a referral for outpatient follow-up is very appropriate.

Why are the other choices wrong?

A hypertensive emergency is characterized not just by a blood pressure reading, but by markedly elevated blood pressure plus end-organ damage. There is no evidence that the patient in this case has end-organ damage, so inpatient management is not warranted.

Prochlorperazine and diphenhydramine are standard treatments for migraine headache. The classic features of migraine headache are throbbing, unilateral pain, often with nausea, vomiting, photophobia, or phonophobia. The headache described by the patient in this case does not match this list of features, so migraine is unlikely.

Laboratory testing that includes a CBC, basic metabolic panel and, urinalysis is likely excessive in this scenario. Urinalysis alone is not a very useful determination of renal function. Focused laboratory testing, however, can be useful in certain patient populations. In this patient, investigation for potential renal dysfunction can be of value; it can be done at follow-up with a primary care doctor or in the emergency department at the time of presentation. Again, the justification is that the patient has no primary care doctor and might have difficulty obtaining short-term medical follow-up. This approach in this particular patient is consistent with the recommendation on laboratory testing for renal dysfunction in patients with "poor follow-up."

PEER REVIEW

✓ In general, you don't have to lower the blood pressure of patients with asymptomatic hypertension in the emergency department, especially those known to have essential hypertension.

✓ Hypertensive emergency is defined by evidence of end-organ effect, not by a definitive blood pressure reading.

REFERENCES

Marx JA, Hockberger RS, Walls RM, eds. *Rosen's Emergency Medicine: Concepts and Clinical Practice*. 8th ed. St. Louis, MO: Elsevier; 2014: 1113-1123.

Wolf SJ, Lo B, Shih, Rd, et al. *Clinical Policy: Critical Issues in the Evaluation and Management of Adult Patients in the Emergency Department With Asymptomatic Elevated Blood Pressure*. Ann Emerg Med. 2013;62:59-68.

153. The correct answer is A, Allergic rhinitis.

Why is this the correct answer?

The patient is presenting with symptoms consistent with allergic rhinitis, a diagnosis that is primarily clinical. Patients with allergic rhinitis tend to have other atopic medical conditions such as asthma and eczema. Treatment involves removing any precipitating allergens such as pollen or pets. Allergic rhinitis is treated with antihistamine. For more severe cases, inhaled or systemic steroids might be indicated.

Why are the other choices wrong?

The patient has no sinus tenderness, facial pain, or fever and has not had symptoms for more than 10 days, so bacterial sinusitis is unlikely. The use of antibiotics in sinusitis is controversial, as there is mixed evidence that it improves outcomes.

Nasal foreign body is unlikely since the patient is an adult. With a nasal foreign body, symptoms are more likely to be unilateral. Treatment for nasal foreign body is removal, either emergently if there are signs of airway compromise or electively in the emergency department or by an ENT specialist. Button batteries in the nose must be removed immediately.

The patient has no fever, cough, sore throat, or myalgias, so URI is unlikely at this time. Most URIs are viral and require only supportive therapy.

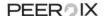

PEER REVIEW

✓ Patients with allergic rhinitis typically have a history of other atopic conditions.
✓ If you're treating a patient with allergic rhinitis, prescribe an antihistamine and tell the patient to remove or stay away from any possible allergens.

REFERENCES
Kishiyama JL. Disorders of the Immune System. In: Hammer GD, McPhee SJ, eds. *Pathophysiology of Disease: An Introduction to Clinical Medicine*. 7th ed. New York, NY: McGraw-Hill; 2013. http://accessmedicine.mhmedical.com/content.aspx?bookid=961&sectionid=53555684. Accessed May 18, 2017.
Tintinalli JE, Stapczynski JS, Ma OJ, et al, eds.*Tintinalli's Emergency Medicine: A Comprehensive Study Guide*. 8th ed. New York, NY: McGraw-Hill; 2012: 1591-1598.

154. The correct answer is B, Gram-positive cocci in clusters.

Why is this the correct answer?

Considering the patient's fever and the pus-like appearance of the shoulder synovial fluid, it is likely the patient has septic arthritis. The most common cause of septic arthritis is *Staphylococcus aureus*, which typically appears as a gram-positive cocci collecting in grape-like clusters. Other bacteria that can be found in septic arthritis include Group *A Streptococcus*, *Streptococcus pneumoniae*, and, rarely, *Neisseria gonorrhoeae* (a gram-negative diplococci). Patients with septic arthritis typically present with fever, joint swelling and pain, and limited range of motion in the affected joint, which is almost always monoarticular. Elevated ESR and C-reactive protein levels are suggestive of infection. Septic arthritis, especially in children, is not an obvious diagnosis, and clinicians must be cautious about performing arthrocentesis. One set of clinical criteria is the Kocher criteria, which were developed retrospectively to estimate the risk for septic arthritis of the hip in children. But a definitive clinical diagnosis can be made only from a synovial culture, which must be obtained by arthrocentesis. A Gram stain of the synovial fluid might reveal the causal bacteria but is more likely to show only WBCs. The synovial fluid drawn from the septic shoulder is turbid and purulent and has a low viscosity, low glucose, and 30,000 or more WBCs/cm^3, most of which is polynucleated cells.

Why are the other choices wrong?

Gram-negative diplococci are the typical appearance of *Neisseria* species. *N. gonorrhoeae* can cause a migratory polyarthritis associated with a vesicular or pustular rash. It can also, rarely, cause a septic monoarthritis, usually in the knee, wrist, or ankle.

Needle-shaped negatively birefringent crystals are caused by the precipitation of monosodium urate in the synovial fluid. This is the cause of gout and typically affects the first metatarsal phalangeal joint but can occur as a monoarthritis in other joints, including the ankle, knee, and elbow.

Rhomboid-shaped positively birefringent crystals are caused by the precipitation of calcium pyrophosphate crystals and are seen in pseudogout.

PEER POINT

Another type of septic arthritis is found in the hip in children. These are the Kocher criteria for estimating the risk for septic arthritis of the hip in children.

- Fever of 38.5°C (101.3°F) or higher
- Inability to bear weight on the affected side
- ESR more than 40 mm/hr
- WBC count above 12,000 cells/mm^3

With one criterion present, the risk of septic arthritis is only 3%. With all four criteria present, the risk is 99%.

PEER REVIEW

✓ The most common bacteria in septic arthritis is *Staphylococcus aureus*.

✓ Fever, joint swelling, and restricted range of motion are the classic triad for septic arthritis.

✓ Needle-shaped negatively birefringent crystals are caused by urate in gout, and rhomboid-shaped positively birefringent crystals are calcium pyrophosphate in pseudogout.

REFERENCES

Adams JG, Barton ED, Collings J, et al, eds. *Emergency Medicine*. Philadelphia, PA: Saunders; 2008: 929-943.

Marx JA, Hockberger RS, Walls RM, eds. *Rosen's Emergency Medicine: Concepts and Clinical Practice*. 8th ed. St. Louis, MO: Elsevier; 2014: 1831-1850.

155. The correct answer is C, Instill a cycloplegic eye drop, and tell the patient to see an ophthalmologist in 24 to 48 hours.

Why is this the correct answer?

The diagnosis in this case is iritis or anterior uveitis, inflammation of the anterior segment of the uvea and the ciliary muscle. The key finding is cells seen on slit lamp examination, which differentiates iritis from uveitis. The photophobia is caused by ciliary spasm, so a cycloplegic agent (cyclopentolate, tropicamide) should be given to help with pain relief. Complications can include vision loss, so patients with iritis should follow up with an ophthalmologist in 24 to 48 hours for reassessment. Prednisolone drops should be started only after consultation with ophthalmology. The clinical presentation of anterior uveitis includes periocular pain, photophobia, blurred vision, ciliary flush, and a small or irregularly shaped pupil. Slit lamp examination findings include floating particles in the anterior chamber and turbidity in the aqueous humor. Anterior uveitis is an autoimmune response. It can be isolated or develop in association with seronegative spondyloarthropathies (herpes simplex, herpes zoster, sarcoidosis, Bechet disease). It also has been associated with malignancy and ulcerative colitis. Before making the diagnosis of iritis, it is important to rule out trauma and other foreign bodies on initial evaluation.

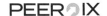

Why are the other choices wrong?

A 1-week course of ophthalmic antibiotics would be the appropriate treatment for a corneal abrasion. But in this case, a corneal abrasion is unlikely given the negative fluorescein examination. However, it is important to do the fluorescein examination to rule out an abrasion given that the patient complains of eye pain.

Reassurance and discharge would be appropriate if the diagnosis were subconjunctival hemorrhage. Although the patient has injection of the conjunctiva, no signs of frank hemorrhage are noted. Patients with subconjunctival hemorrhage have no symptoms other than the hemorrhage itself, which usually is caused by a sudden increase in venous pressure due to a Valsalva maneuver.

Emergent ophthalmology consultation is the right action for patients with retinal detachment, who should be treated immediately. Although the patient complains of blurry vision and acuity has been affected, no visual field cuts were found on examination. Additionally, retinal detachments do not typically cause pain.

PEER REVIEW

- ✓ A good slit lamp examination with fluorescein stain is essential to the diagnosis of eye emergencies.
- ✓ Be sure to document visual acuities.
- ✓ If you're treating a patient with iritis, coordinate follow-up care with ophthalmology.

REFERENCES

Greenberg RD, Daniel KJ. Eye Emergencies. In: Stone C, Humphries RL, eds. *CURRENT Diagnosis & Treatment Emergency Medicine*. 7th ed. New York, NY: McGraw-Hill; 2011. http://accessmedicine.mhmedical.com/content. aspx?bookid=385&sectionid=40357247. Accessed May 18, 2017.

Tintinalli JE, Stapczynski JS, Ma OJ, et al, eds. *Tintinalli's Emergency Medicine: A Comprehensive Study Guide*. 8th ed. New York, NY: McGraw-Hill; 2012: 1563.

Trobe JD. *The Physician's Guide to Eye Care*. 4th ed. San Francisco, CA: American Academy of Ophthalmology; 2012:67-68.

156. The correct answer is C, Perform rapid sequence intubation.

Why is this the correct answer?

In this case, given the concerns for burns and edema of the oropharynx, emergent rapid sequence intubation is clinically indicated as the next intervention. It is prudent to establish a definitive airway as early as possible; as edema worsens, securing an airway becomes increasingly difficult. Once the airway is secured, checking carboxyhemoglobin levels with ABG analysis is important, as carbon monoxide poisoning might also be a concern. Humidified oxygen should be continued. The primary concern here is a ventilation issue, not an oxygenation issue, so vital signs are likely to be well compensated immediately before the loss of a tenuous airway. In addition to burns of the face or perioral region, other indications for rapid intubation include acute respiratory distress, worsening hoarseness, stridor, altered mental status with respiratory depression, circumferential neck burns, and supraglottic edema as seen by fiber optic examination.

Why are the other choices wrong?

Fluid resuscitation is important for any losses resulting from burns but must be done carefully. Overly aggressive fluid resuscitation can lead to acute respiratory distress syndrome and pulmonary edema, so hemodynamic monitoring should be used in conjunction with fluid resuscitation efforts. In this case, however, without significant cutaneous burns, the patient does not need fluid resuscitation.

An xray of the neck might be warranted in a patient whose hoarseness has a likely infectious cause, but that is not the case here. An xray of the neck in a burn patient does not clearly show the airway edema. In this patient's case, obtaining plain films, even at the bedside, delays the definitive airway management the patient needs.

Although albuterol treatments would help with the patient's breathing, they would not address his upper airway edema and might delay definitive treatment.

PEER REVIEW

✓ Patients with inhalational burns can decompensate quickly, so rapid endotracheal intubation is indicated.

✓ Once an airway is secured, check for inhalational toxins, especially those with reversible causes.

✓ Vital signs can be falsely reassuring for an impending airway compromise.

REFERENCES

Olson KR. *Poisoning & Drug Overdose.* 6th ed. New York, NY: McGraw-Hill; 2012. http://accessmedicine.mhmedical.com.foyer. swmed.edu/content.aspx?bookid=391&sectionid=42069956. Accessed May 17, 2017.

Tintinalli JE, Stapczynski JS, Ma OJ, et al, eds. *Tintinalli's Emergency Medicine: A Comprehensive Study Guide.* 8th ed. New York, NY: McGraw-Hill; 2012: 1398-1405.

157. The correct answer is A, Autoantibodies against the nicotinic acetylcholine receptors.

Why is this the correct answer?

Myasthenia gravis is an autoimmune neuromuscular disorder that affects voluntary muscles. The underlying cause of myasthenia gravis is autoantibody formation to the nicotinic acetylcholine receptors on the motor endplate of nerve fibers. These autoantibodies reduce the number of acetylcholine receptors and their function in spite of the fact that the nerve anatomy appears normal. The result is muscle weakness and fatigability. Common presenting complaints of patients with myasthenia include proximal muscle weakness that worsens over the course of the day, ptosis, and diplopia. Patients who present with these vision issues

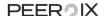

should undergo a workup for myasthenia gravis. Although it is rare, patients can initially present in acute myasthenic crisis with weakness of the respiratory muscles. Other causes of myasthenic crisis include infection and missed medication doses. Respiratory failure is the most common cause of death among patients with myasthenia. If the patient requires intubation, paralytic medications should be used with caution due to concern for prolonged effects. It is imperative to keep myasthenia gravis on the differential diagnosis when a patient presents to the emergency department with proximal muscle weakness, ptosis, and diplopia so appropriate diagnostic studies can be ordered. Diagnosis is made using a combination of blood tests, electromyelographic testing, and an edrophonium or ice bag test. Both administration of edrophonium, an acetylcholinesterase inhibitor, and application of an ice bag should improve ptosis in patients with myasthenia. These tests should be performed in consultation with a neurology service. Once recognized, myasthenia gravis is treated with cholinesterase inhibitors such as pyridostigmine and neostigmine to help prolong the effects of acetylcholine at the neuromuscular junction. Other possible treatments include thymectomy if a thymoma is present and immunomodulatory therapy such as intravenous immunoglobulin or plasmapheresis. These are both controversial. Myasthenic crisis is the severe form of myasthenia gravis in which the respiratory muscles become so weak that respiratory failure ensues. It is important to recognize the respiratory distress and promptly treat it with ventilatory support.

Why are the other choices wrong?

Lewy bodies are cellular cytoplasmic inclusions within brain cells. They are thought to be the cause of Parkinson disease. Classic symptoms of Parkinson disease include cogwheel rigidity, resting tremor, and bradykinesia or akinesia.

Neurotropic enteroviruses cause poliomyelitis, which is uncommon in the United States but still endemic in the developing world. Individuals who become symptomatic often have symptoms like viral meningitis then develop significant paralysis without sensory loss.

Upper and lower motor neuron degeneration is the cause of amyotrophic lateral sclerosis, also known as Lou Gehrig disease. The motor neuron degeneration leads to rapidly progressive weakness and atrophy of the muscles. Both upper and lower motor neuron involvement is found, with loss of reflexes and spasticity.

PEER POINT

Drugs to avoid in myasthenia gravis

- Steroids: Adrenocorticotropic hormone, methylprednisolone, prednisone
- Anticonvulsants: Phenytoin, ethosuximide, trimethadione, paraldehyde, magnesium sulfate, barbiturates, lithium
- Antimalarials: Chloroquine, quinine
- Intravenous fluids: Sodium lactate solution

- Antibiotics: Aminoglycosides, fluoroquinolones, neomycin, streptomycin, kanamycin, gentamicin, tobramycin, dihydrostreptomycin, amikacin, polymyxin A, polymyxin B, sulfonamides, viomycin, colistimethate, lincomycin, clindamycin, tetracycline, oxytetracycline, rolitetracycline, macrolides, metronidazole
- Psychotropics: Chlorpromazine, lithium carbonate, amitriptyline, droperidol, haloperidol, imipramine
- Antirheumatics: d-Penicillamine, colchicine, chloroquine
- Cardiovascular: Quinidine, procainamide, beta blockers (propranolol, oxprenolol, practolol, pindolol, sotalol), lidocaine, trimethaphan; magnesium; calcium channel blockers (verapamil)
- Local anesthetics: Lidocaine, procaine,
- Analgesics: Narcotics (morphine, hydromorphone, codeine, Pantopon, meperidine)
- Endocrine: Thyroid replacement
- Eye drops: Timolol, echothiophate
- Others: Amantadine, diphenhydramine, emetine, diuretics, muscle relaxants, central nervous system depressants, respiratory depressants, sedatives, procaine, phenothiazines
- Neuromuscular blocking agents: Tubocurarine, pancuronium, rocuronium, gallamine, dimethyl tubocurarine, succinylcholine, decamethonium

From *Tintinalli's Emergency Medicine*, Table 173–1.

PEER REVIEW

✓ Myasthenia gravis is an autoimmune disease that causes proximal muscle weakness, ptosis, and double vision.

✓ The symptoms of myasthenia gravis get worse throughout the course of the day.

✓ Respiratory failure is a common cause of death in myasthenia gravis and should be promptly recognized and managed appropriately.

REFERENCES

Marx JA, Hockberger RS, Walls RM, eds. *Rosen's Emergency Medicine: Concepts and Clinical Practice*. 8th ed. St. Louis, MO: Elsevier; 2014: 1441-1446.

Tintinalli JE, Stapczynski JS, Ma OJ, et al, eds. *Tintinalli's Emergency Medicine: A Comprehensive Study Guide*. 8th ed. New York, NY: McGraw-Hill; 2012:1185-1192.

158. The correct answer is D, Perform a capillary blood glucose check.

Why is this the correct answer?

Any patient who presents with altered mental status should have a capillary blood glucose level checked as part of the initial assessment. This is a high-yield, minimally invasive test that can be performed rapidly at the bedside and provides immediately actionable information. Even when the cause of altered mental status appears obvious such as in cases of trauma, stroke, or overdose, hypoglycemia should still be ruled out. This can prevent more expensive invasive and time-consuming interventions.

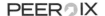

Why are the other choices wrong?

In most patients, even in known or suspected benzodiazepine overdose, empiric treatment with flumazenil should be avoided. Flumazenil is a selective central benzodiazepine antagonist. Seizure activity can occur after administration of flumazenil to patients who are physically dependent on benzodiazepines. Furthermore, due to adverse effects of cerebral hemodynamics, flumazenil is contraindicated in patients with possible increased intracranial pressure.

Significant opioid toxicity typically manifests with respiratory depression. This patient is cooperative and breathing at a normal rate with good oxygenation. Administration of naloxone, a competitive antagonist at opioid receptors, is probably unnecessary and might precipitate withdrawal symptoms. In this case, diagnosing hypoglycemia is a higher priority.

Emergency physicians should have a low threshold for performing head CT on patients with altered mental status in the setting of possible trauma. In this case, the patient was found down and cannot give a reliable history. Unless additional history becomes available that clearly rules out head trauma, she should probably undergo CT scanning, but not before having her blood glucose level measured.

PEER REVIEW

✓ Always rule out hypoglycemia in patients with altered mental status.
✓ Don't use flumazenil in patients with suspected increased intracranial pressure.
✓ Consider naloxone in patients with respiratory depression in the setting of suspected opioid overdose.

REFERENCES
Tintinalli JE, Stapczynski JS, Ma OJ, et al, eds. *Tintinalli's Emergency Medicine: A Comprehensive Study Guide*. 8th ed. New York, NY: McGraw-Hill; 2012: 1237-1240, 1251-1255.

159. The correct answer is A, Bacterial tracheitis.

Why is this the correct answer?

The most likely diagnosis in this case is bacterial tracheitis, a secondary bacterial infection following a viral URI. High fever and a toxic appearance are commonly associated with the airway symptoms. Other names for this disease process are membranous laryngotracheobronchitis, pseudomembranous croup, and bacterial croup. It is relatively uncommon (4-8/1,000,000 children), and the average patient age is between 5 and 8 years. The most common pathogen in bacterial tracheitis is *Staphylococcus aureus*, followed by *Streptococcus pneumoniae* and *Streptococcus pyogenes*, *Haemophilus influenzae*, and *Moraxella catarrhalis*. If bacterial tracheitis is suspected, emergent ENT consultation is warranted; mortality rates can be as high as 20%. Endoscopy is the diagnostic method of choice, and intubation under controlled circumstances might be needed to control a tenuous airway. Given the narrowing of the airway, a smaller-than-anticipated endotracheal tube might be needed. Given the copious drainage from the larynx, intubation might require advanced airway techniques and tried-and-true classics like looking for air bubbles. Emergency department management also includes initiation of antibiotic therapy. The initial antibiotic choice is ampicillin-sulbactam combined with clindamycin and a third-generation cephalosporin. Vancomycin should be added if MRSA is a concern.

Why are the other choices wrong?

Bronchiolitis is a lower respiratory tract infection most commonly seen in children younger than 2 years. Children with bronchiolitis do not usually present with stridor or lethargy. It is most commonly caused by respiratory syncytial virus. These patients also tend to have more nasal congestion, cough, and wheezing.

Pneumonia does not tend to present with stridor. If in doubt, a chest xray can differentiate between the two since air-space disease on radiography and the absence of stridor point more to pneumonia.

Viral laryngotracheobronchitis, or croup, tends to present in slightly younger patients (6 months to 3 years) and with a less toxic appearance than does bacterial tracheitis. A barky or brassy cough is the classic sign of croup. Bacterial tracheitis can present across a broader age range than croup.

PEER REVIEW

✓ Bacterial tracheitis is uncommon but emergent, so get an immediate ENT consultation.
✓ Croup follows a more benign viral URI course than bacterial tracheitis does.
✓ If you're treating a patient with suspected bacterial tracheitis, start antibiotics empirically even before confirming the diagnosis with endoscopy.

REFERENCES
Kuo CY, Parikh SR. Bacterial tracheitis. Pediatr Rev. 2014;35(11):497-499.
Schafermeyer RW, Tenenbein M, Macias CG, et al, eds. *Strange and Schafermeyer's Pediatric Emergency Medicine*. 4th ed. New York, NY: McGraw-Hill; 2015: 212.
Tintinalli JE, Stapczynski JS, Ma OJ, et al, eds. *Tintinalli's Emergency Medicine: A Comprehensive Study Guide*. 8th ed. New York, NY: McGraw-Hill; 2012: 1562;835-842.

160. The correct answer is A, Excessive ultrafiltration.

Why is this the correct answer?

Hemodialysis treatments remove fluid and filter electrolytes and toxins from the blood, with approximately 1 to 3 L taken off per hour over a 4-hour period. As a result of these extreme and rapid fluid shifts, hypotension is a common complication of hemodialysis, occurring in about 50% of treatments. The most common cause for hypotension during hemodialysis is excessive ultrafiltration, essentially taking off too much fluid too quickly, often related to underestimation

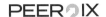

of the patient's ideal blood volume. This occurs most often toward the end of the dialysis session. In most situations, hypotension associated with hemodialysis resolves on its own or after small volume infusions of saline. When it does not resolve, the patient should be sent to the emergency department for testing and treatment.

Why are the other choices wrong?

A GI bleed should be suspected if a patient has melena, hematochezia, or hematemesis; the patient in this case did not. Hemodialysis can cause transient thrombocytopenia, and renal failure alone can lead to platelet dysfunction. If GI bleed is suspected, DDAVP can be used to reverse the platelet dysfunction.

A screening ECG should be performed on any patient who presents to the emergency department with hypotension associated with hemodialysis. Myocardial infarction should be considered in this differential, and the patient should be asked about cardiac symptoms. The patient in this case did not report cardiovascular symptoms. Another critical cardiac diagnosis to consider in patients with peridialytic hypotension is cardiac tamponade, which can be diagnosed using bedside echocardiography.

A patient with renal failure is predisposed to infection due to immunosuppression. If the patient has fever or infectious symptoms, renal failure should be considered. If the patient has an indwelling line present for dialysis, it should be considered as a source for infection. Hypotension from pre-existing hypovolemia from causes such as sepsis is more likely to occur when the dialysis session is just starting.

PEER POINT

The differential diagnosis of peridialytic hypotension

- Excessive ultrafiltration
- Predialytic volume loss (GI losses, decreased oral intake)
- Intradialytic volume loss (tube and hemodialyzer blood losses)
- Postdialytic volume loss (vascular access blood loss)
- Medication effects (antihypertensives, opiates)
- Decreased vascular tone (sepsis, food, dialysate temperature >37°C or 98.6°F)
- Cardiac dysfunction (left ventricular hypertrophy, ischemia, hypoxia, arrhythmia, pericardial tamponade)
- Pericardial disease (effusion, tamponade)

This is Table 90-3 from *Tintinalli* 8e, Copyright© McGraw-Hill Education, used with permission. www.accessemergencymedicine.com

PEER REVIEW

- ✓ Hypotension associated with hemodialysis is common, occurring about half the time.
- ✓ The differential for hypotension associated with dialysis is broad, but the most common cause is excessive ultrafiltration.
- ✓ If you're treating a patient with hemodialysis-related hypotension, focus your history taking and examinations on the common causes.

REFERENCES

Marx JA, Hockberger RS, Walls RM, eds. *Rosen's Emergency Medicine: Concepts and Clinical Practice.* 8th ed. St. Louis, MO: Elsevier; 2014: 1636-1651.

Tintinalli JE, Stapczynski JS, Ma OJ, et al, eds. *Tintinalli's Emergency Medicine: A Comprehensive Study Guide.* 8th ed. New York, NY: McGraw-Hill; 2012: 584-589.

161. The correct answer is C, Oral antiplatelet therapy and intravenous heparin bolus.

Why is this the correct answer?

The diagnostic criteria for STEMI include the following:

- Two contiguous leads with ST-segment elevation of more than 2 mm in leads V2 and V3, or
- More than 1 mm in all other leads

The patient in this case is experiencing a STEMI and is waiting to undergo PCI. Before the procedure, the patient should ideally receive several medications, including an oral antiplatelet agent and anticoagulant therapy. Oral ticagrelor or prasugrel, the preferred antiplatelet agents, should be administered as a loading dose. Although not a specific choice in this scenario, aspirin is a highly effective antiplatelet agent in STEMI; it significantly reduces mortality rates. Intravenous heparin bolus is the preferred anticoagulant therapy when patients are treated with primary PCI.

Why are the other choices wrong?

Alteplase is a recombinant tissue plasminogen activator that acts as a fibrinolytic agent in the treatment of STEMI. Fibrinolysis would be preferred over PCI for this patient only if it were going to take more than 60 minutes for him to undergo PCI from first medical contact. But the time to therapy in this case is within the PCI window due to the patient's early acute MI presentation: he is being prepared to undergo emergent PCI in the next 20 to 25 minutes, which makes PCI preferred over fibrinolytic therapy.

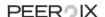

Avoiding beta blockers and administering benzodiazepines might be appropriate if the patient were suspected of having cocaine-induced chest pain. In cocaine-induced MI, the cardiac ischemia is primarily via coronary spasm. Administering beta blockers might exacerbate coronary spasm and result in worsening ischemia. Furthermore, beta blockers can improve outcome, but the appropriate time to administration is within the initial 24 hours of infarction; postponing beta blocker administration to later in the first hospital day in most STEMI patients is appropriate due to the potential adverse effects seen early in the course of acute MI.

Although an intravenous heparin bolus is appropriate in this scenario, the oral ibuprofen is contraindicated. Ibuprofen is an NSAID, and with the exception of aspirin, NSAIDs have been associated with increased adverse cardiovascular events. They should be avoided in patients with acute MI.

PEER POINT

Fibrinolysis or PCI?

Fibrinolytic therapy is preferred over PCI in STEMI management only if PCI can't be performed within an appropriate timeframe. That timeframe is based on the time from onset of infarction, as follows:

- If the time from onset of infarction is less than 2 hours, PCI should be performed within 60 minutes.
- If the time from onset of infarction is between 2 and 3 hours, PCI should be performed within 60 to 120 minutes.
- If the time from onset of infarction is between 3 and 12 hours, PCI should be performed within 120 minutes. If PCI cannot be performed within this time frame and the patient is a candidate for fibrinolytic therapy, a fibrinolytic agent should be administrated.

PEER REVIEW

- ✓ What should you give a patient with acute STEMI who is waiting for PCI? Aspirin, pain control, antiplatelet therapy, and anticoagulation.
- ✓ Diagnostic ECG criteria for STEMI: two contiguous leads with ST-segment elevation of more than 2 mm in leads V2 and V3 or more than 1 mm in all other leads.

REFERENCES

Marx JA, Hockberger RS, Walls RM, eds. *Rosen's Emergency Medicine: Concepts and Clinical Practice*. 8th ed. St. Louis, MO: Elsevier; 2014:997-1033.

O'Connor RE, Al Ali AS, Brady WJ, et al: Part 9: Acute Coronary Syndromes—2015 American Heart Association Guidelines Update for Cardiopulmonary Resuscitation and Emergency Cardiovascular Care. *Circulation*. 2015;132:s483-500.

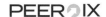

162. The correct answer is B, Fingerstick blood glucose.

Why is this the correct answer?

Balanoposthitis is inflammation of the glans penis and foreskin. It occurs in approximately 6% of uncircumcised males. Recurrent episodes of balanoposthitis should raise the concern for occult diabetes, so this patient should be screened using a fingerstick blood glucose test. Balanoposthitis is most commonly caused by poor hygiene or candidal infection. Patients who are found to have balanoposthitis should be treated with topical antifungals such as nystatin. If the inflammation is more severe, topical steroids such as hydrocortisone 0.5% may be considered to add to the regimen, or oral fluconazole. If there is concern for concomitant cellulitis, treatment with a first-generation cephalosporin is appropriate. Circumcision might be considered in patients with recurrent episodes, so appropriate urology follow-up should be arranged.

Why are the other choices wrong?

A CBC would be indicated if the examination had revealed evidence of an associated cellulitis or deeper space infection. The WBC count in these situations can function as a screening tool.

The diagnosis of urethritis caused by chlamydia or gonorrhea is supported by penile discharge or dysuria, neither of which this patient describes. Therefore, urethral cultures are not indicated.

If the patient had complained of dysuria, flank pain, or urinary frequency, urinalysis would be an appropriate choice; UTI is generally rare in young men.

PEER REVIEW

- ✓ Balanoposthitis is most commonly caused by poor hygiene or a fungal infection.
- ✓ Diagnostic tip: recurrent episodes of balanoposthitis can be the sole presenting symptom of diabetes mellitus.
- ✓ If you suspect diabetes mellitus, screen for it with a fingerstick blood glucose measurement.

REFERENCES

Marx JA, Hockberger RS, Walls RM, eds. *Rosen's Emergency Medicine: Concepts and Clinical Practice.* 8th ed. St. Louis, MO: Elsevier; 2014: 2206-2207.

Tintinalli JE, Stapczynski JS, Ma OJ, et al, eds. *Tintinalli's Emergency Medicine: A Comprehensive Study Guide.* 8th ed. New York, NY: McGraw-Hill; 2012: 603-605.

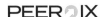

163. The correct answer is D, Thiamine.

Why is this the correct answer?

Wernicke encephalopathy is a medical emergency with a 10% to 20% mortality rate. It is caused by thiamine (vitamin B1) deficiency and potentially also related to a deficient or less active transketolase enzyme, which is thiamine dependent. It classically presents in a patient with malnutrition or chronic alcohol abuse, with oculomotor abnormalities (nystagmus being the most common), ataxia, and confusion or altered mental status. Wernicke encephalopathy is a clinical diagnosis, and it is difficult to recognize; the symptoms can closely overlap those of acute alcohol intoxication. If Wernicke encephalopathy is suspected, thiamine may be administered intravenously. Prior teaching that it should be administered before treating hypoglycemia with glucose-containing solution has been debunked; it is now thought that acute treatment of hypoglycemia does not precipitate Wernicke encephalopathy.

Why are the other choices wrong?

Vitamin B12 (cyanocobalamin) deficiency occurs mainly in individuals who are unable to absorb the B12 complex such as those who have had colorectal surgery or pernicious anemia. Patients who are strict vegetarians can also develop a deficiency because vitamin B12 is found mainly in meat, milk, and eggs. Common symptoms of B12 deficiency include megaloblastic anemia, paresthesias, and psychiatric symptoms such as depression.

Folic acid (vitamin B9) is a B vitamin that is important for RBC production and fetal development. Folate deficiency can also be present in patients with malnutrition and chronic alcoholism. A macrocytic anemia can be present with folate deficiency.

Riboflavin is vitamin B2. It is a key element to help maintain vision. Riboflavin deficiency is rare.

PEER REVIEW

- ✓ Wernicke encephalopathy is caused by thiamine (vitamin B1) deficiency.
- ✓ Clinical presentation of Wernicke encephalopathy: ataxia, oculomotor abnormalities, and confusion.
- ✓ If you're treating a patient with Wernicke encephalopathy, go with intravenous thiamine.
- ✓ Acute treatment of hypoglycemia does not cause Wernicke encephalopathy.

REFERENCES

Marx JA, Hockberger RS, Walls RM, eds. *Rosen's Emergency Medicine: Concepts and Clinical Practice*. 8th ed. St. Louis, MO: Elsevier; 2014: 2378-2394.

Tintinalli JE, Stapczynski JS, Ma OJ, et al, eds. *Tintinalli's Emergency Medicine: A Comprehensive Study Guide*. 8th ed. New York, NY: McGraw-Hill; 2012: 1341-1345.

164. The correct answer is A, *Campylobacter jejuni*.

Why is this the correct answer?

The clinical presentation in this case is most consistent with the diagnosis of Miller Fisher syndrome, which is closely related to Guillain-Barré syndrome (GBS). It is an acute ascending paralysis thought to be caused by autoimmune-mediated demyelination. Patients with GBS experience a symmetric ascending paralysis that begins shortly after an acute upper respiratory or viral illness. In particular *Campylobacter jejuni*, which causes diarrhea, is associated with the Miller Fisher variant GBS. These patients present with ataxia, ophthalmoplegia, and areflexia. Physical examination reveals either weakened or absent reflexes in addition to the motor weakness. A key initial test in patients presenting with GBS is a forced vital capacity (FVC) measurement, as respiratory compromise can lead to significant illness and death. The normal vital capacity range is 60 to 70 mL/kg, and an FVC result of 20 mL/kg is associated with respiratory compromise. Patients with diminished FVC require close monitoring and ICU admission. Lumbar puncture in patients with GBS reveals elevated protein levels and a low WBC count, less than 10 cells/mm3 with a mononuclear predominance. In patients with an elevated WBC count in the CSF, alternative diagnoses such as HIV, Lyme disease, and bacterial meningitis should be considered. Electrodiagnostic testing also is used in later evaluation, although not in the emergency department. It reveals demyelination in patients with GBS. In addition to close monitoring of respiratory status, patients with GBS should be treated with intravenous immunoglobulin. Steroids are no longer recommended. Recovery times range from weeks to years.

Why are the other choices wrong?

E. coli infection can cause GI symptoms but has not been found to be linked to GBS — and some types of *E. coli* cause bloody diarrhea.

Meningitis can be associated with neurologic symptoms such as altered mental status, but it would be rare to have ascending paralysis and areflexia as presenting symptoms.

S. pneumoniae infection can cause upper respiratory symptoms and pneumonia or meningitis. There is no clear association between *S. pneumoniae* and GBS. There is, however, a known association between *mycoplasma pneumoniae* and other viral illnesses that cause upper respiratory infection symptoms and GBS.

PEER REVIEW

- ✓ Guillain-Barré syndrome presents with a symmetric ascending paralysis. It is frequently preceded by either an upper respiratory or a diarrheal illness.
- ✓ Patients with Guillain-Barré syndrome have motor weakness and either hyporeflexia or areflexia on examination.

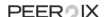

✓ If you're treating a patient with suspected (or known) Guillain-Barré syndrome, assess respiratory status right away by measuring forced vital capacity; results help you determine whether to go with intubation or close monitoring.

REFERENCES

Marx JA, Hockberger RS, Walls RM, eds. *Rosen's Emergency Medicine: Concepts and Clinical Practice*. 8th ed. St. Louis, MO: Elsevier; 2014: 1428-1440.

Tintinalli JE, Stapczynski JS, Ma OJ, et al, eds. *Tintinalli's Emergency Medicine: A Comprehensive Study Guide*. 8th ed. New York, NY: McGraw-Hill; 2012: 1178-1185.

165. The correct answer is C, Otic antibiotics for 10 to 14 days and ENT follow-up in 2 to 3 weeks.

Why is this the correct answer?

Either barotrauma or acute otitis media can result in a perforated tympanic membrane. Perforations tend to heal within a few weeks. After a 10- to 14-day course of otic antibiotics, patients should follow up in 2 to 3 weeks with an ENT specialist to evaluate for healing and ongoing hearing loss. If the tympanic membrane has not healed in 3 to 6 months, surgical repair might be needed. As long as the perforation exists, exposure to water in the auditory canal should be limited.

Why are the other choices wrong?

Warm water irrigation is a home remedy for cerumen removal. It should be avoided as long as the perforated tympanic membrane is healing. The ear must be kept dry except for otic antibiotics.

Systemic antibiotics are less effective in the treatment of a ruptured tympanic membrane, according to a recent Cochrane review.

A patient with a perforated tympanic membrane might have transient vertigo, but in light of no other persistent neurologic findings, head CT is not indicated. The likelihood of an underlying neurologic process is small.

PEER REVIEW

✓ Classic findings for perforated tympanic membrane: pain before perforation, then suddenly it feels better.
✓ Prescribe otic antibiotics only if you're concerned about an underlying infection.
✓ Perforated tympanic membrane resulting from barotrauma does not require antibiotic therapy.

REFERENCES

Hay WW Jr., Levin MJ. *Current Diagnosis & Treatment: Pediatrics*. 23rd ed. New York, NY: McGraw-Hill; 2016: http://accessmedicine.mhmedical.com/content.aspx?bookid=1795&sectionid=125740558. Accessed May 18, 2017.

Macfadyen CA1, Acuin JM, Gamble C. Systemic antibiotics versus topical treatments for chronically discharging ears with underlying eardrum perforations. *Cochrane Database Syst Rev.* 2006;(1):CD005608.

Tintinalli JE, Stapczynski JS, Ma OJ, et al, eds. *Tintinalli's Emergency Medicine: A Comprehensive Study Guide*. 8th ed. New York, NY: McGraw-Hill; 2012: 1579-1585.

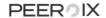

166. The correct answer is B, First 2 days.

Why is this the correct answer?

Originally, TIA was defined as stroke symptoms lasting fewer than 24 hours. Recently, the definition has been changed to reflect a lack of acute infarction identified on neuroimaging such as MRI. Patients who experience a TIA are at risk for future stroke, with the greatest risk in the first 2 days. Of the 10% of people who have a stroke in the 90 days following a TIA, 50% have it within the first 48 hours. Tools to assess risk have been suggested. One of these, the ABCD2 score, can be used to help approximate a patient's risk for stroke following a TIA, although it is less accurate than hoped. Although it can provide basic guidelines regarding patient risk, it should be viewed as only one factor in determining if a patient presenting with TIA requires further expedited workups; it should not be relied on to determine if a patient can be safely discharged from the emergency department. Patients who present to the emergency department on the same day they experience a TIA should generally be admitted to the hospital under the care of a neurologist. Expedited workup should include MRI, carotid assessment, telemetry monitoring, and possible echocardiogram. A subset of patients — those who have access and the ability to seek out and obtain expeditious care and additional diagnostic testing — can be discharged with detailed return precautions after arrangements are made for close outpatient follow-up. Outpatient testing should include carotid Doppler ultrasonography, MRI/MRA, and an echocardiogram. Antiplatelet therapy should be considered in consultation with a neurologist.

Why are the other choices wrong?

If a patient has recurrent symptoms within the first hour of TIA resolution, the event would likely be classified as an infarct rather than as a TIA.

The risk for stroke following a TIA diminishes after 48 hours. As the time progresses following TIA symptoms, patients are at less risk for stroke. In turn, 1 week out from a TIA, there is less risk than in the initial 2 days prior.

Over a period of 90 days following a TIA, the overall risk for stroke is approximately 10%. However, 50% of these events occur within the first 2 days. Thirty days following TIA symptoms is not the highest risk period for stroke.

PEER POINT

Return precautions for patients discharged after evaluation for TIA

Neurologic symptoms, including

- Slurred speech
- Facial droop
- Unilateral weakness
- Dizziness or unsteady gait

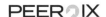

PEER REVIEW

- ✓ One definition of TIA: resolved stroke symptoms without any evidence of tissue damage or infarction on neuroimaging.
- ✓ Many patients with TIA should be admitted for expedited workup and monitoring given the high risk of future stroke.
- ✓ When is a person who had a TIA at highest risk for stroke? Within the first 48 hours.

REFERENCES

Marx JA, Hockberger RS, Walls RM, eds. *Rosen's Emergency Medicine: Concepts and Clinical Practice.* 8th ed. St. Louis, MO: Elsevier; 2014: 1362-1374.

Tintinalli JE, Stapczynski JS, Ma OJ, et al, eds. *Tintinalli's Emergency Medicine: A Comprehensive Study Guide.* 8th ed. New York, NY: McGraw-Hill; 2012: 1142-1155.

167. The correct answer is C, Myocardial ischemia.

Why is this the correct answer?

The most common cause of polymorphic ventricular tachycardia (VT) is myocardial ischemia, in contrast to monomorphic VT, which can also be seen in the setting of myocardial ischemia but is most often secondary to a re-entrant mechanism through scarred myocardium (chronic forms of ischemic heart disease). In the acute phase of an MI, polymorphic VT and ventricular fibrillation are more common than monomorphic VT. Although re-entry might still be a factor in the etiology of polymorphic VT during acute ischemia, abnormal automaticity is a more likely mechanism. Patients presenting with polymorphic VT should be considered candidates for urgent revascularization therapy due to the high incidence of ischemia. Both monomorphic and polymorphic VT involve an ectopic pacemaker originating within or below the bundle of His. In monomorphic VT, the QRS complexes in one lead have the same morphology. In polymorphic VT, the QRS complexes have different morphologies in one lead.

Why are the other choices wrong?

An inherited reduction in cardiac sodium activity is seen in Brugada syndrome. This syndrome can lead to a polymorphic VT. However, myocardial ischemia is the most common underlying cause of polymorphic VT.

Electrolyte abnormalities can exacerbate the tendency toward ventricular ectopy, thus leading to polymorphic VT. However, the most common underlying cause of polymorphic VT is acute myocardial ischemia. It is still prudent to correct any electrolyte abnormalities that might be present.

A re-entrant mechanism through scarred myocardium is the most frequent etiology underlying monomorphic VT and is commonly seen in the chronic phase after an MI. The likelihood of ventricular arrhythmia in a patient with coronary artery disease is directly related to the extent of myocardial damage and scarring.

PEER POINT

ECG changes in polymorphic VT and monomorphic VT

- The most common cause of polymorphic VT (top) is myocardial ischemia. Consider urgent revascularization once the patient's condition is stabilized.
- The most common cause of monomorphic VT (bottom) is a re-entrant mechanism through scarred myocardium.

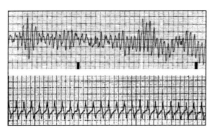

PEER Point 16

PEER REVIEW

✓ Consider any patient presenting with polymorphic VT as a possible ACS patient and a potential urgent revascularization candidate.

✓ Monomorphic VT often develops secondary to a re-entrant mechanism related to scarred myocardium — in other words, in a patient who had an MI in the past.

✓ Polymorphic VT in a patient with acute ischemia is likely secondary to abnormal automaticity.

REFERENCES

Crawford MH. *CURRENT Diagnosis & Treatment: Cardiology.* 3rd ed. Philadelphia, PA: Elsevier; 2010:847-859.

Roberts-Thomson KC, Lau DH, Sanders P. The diagnosis and management of ventricular arrhythmias. *Nat Rev Cardiol.* 2011;8(6):311-321.

168. The correct answer is B, Labetalol.

Why is this the correct answer?

This presentation is concerning for acute stroke, and given that the patient presented so soon after symptom onset, evaluation and treatment should occur expeditiously. The initial focus of treatment should be on blood pressure management: a blood pressure higher than 185 systolic or 110 diastolic is a contraindication to tPA administration. Recommended therapy for initial blood pressure management is labetalol 10 to 20 mg IV or nicardipine infusion starting at 5 mg/hour. These medications generally can be titrated for a slow and reliable lowering of the blood pressure and have less effect on cerebral blood vessels. If this patient's blood pressure cannot be lowered to the parameters specified above, she

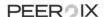

is not a candidate to receive tPA. It is important to not lower the patient's blood pressure too much, as it might result in decreased cerebral perfusion and worsening stroke symptoms. It is important to note that, if the blood pressure cannot be lowered using these initial interventions, the patient is not eligible to receive tPA.

Why are the other choices wrong?

Diltiazem is a calcium channel blocker; it can lower blood pressure as well as heart rate. It should be avoided when trying to lower blood pressure in acute ischemic stroke because it can cause a precipitous decrease that can worsen stroke symptoms. Diltiazem is most commonly used in the emergency department for rate control in patients presenting with narrow-complex tachyarrhythmias such as atrial fibrillation and atrial flutter.

Metoprolol is a beta blocker and has both inotropic and chronotropic effects. It should be avoided in acute ischemic stroke because it can cause a sudden decrease in blood pressure, and that worsens cerebral perfusion and in turn stroke symptoms.

Nitroprusside can be used following the administration of tPA if the blood pressure is not adequately controlled with either labetalol or nicardipine. Nitroprusside can also have greater effects on the diastolic blood pressure and should be used if it remains higher than 140 mm Hg. But it is not a first-line agent for treatment of hypertension before administration of tPA because of the risk of a rapid decrease in blood pressure.

PEER REVIEW

- ✓ Don't use tPA if a patient's blood pressure is higher than 185 systolic or 110 diastolic.
- ✓ First-line treatment for lowering blood pressure before tPA administration is labetalol or nicardipine.

REFERENCES

Marx JA, Hockberger RS, Walls RM, eds. *Rosen's Emergency Medicine: Concepts and Clinical Practice*. 8th ed. St. Louis, MO: Elsevier; 2014: 1363-1374.

Tintinalli JE, Stapczynski JS, Ma OJ, et al, eds. *Tintinalli's Emergency Medicine: A Comprehensive Study Guide*. 8th ed. New York, NY: McGraw-Hill; 2012: 1142-1155.

169. The correct answer is D, Pyogenic granuloma.

Why is this the correct answer?

Pyogenic granuloma is the commonly used term for the vascular lesion depicted in this case. In pregnant patients, it might be referred to as granuloma gravidarum. Neither name is accurate, however, as this benign collection of capillaries is not granulomatous, purulent, or infective; lobular capillary hemangioma is a better term. It develops as a result of minor skin (or in this case, mucosal) trauma in about one-third of patients, most commonly in children, pregnant women, and younger adults, and most commonly on the hands or other extremities. The appearance is usually shiny and bright red; the lesion bleeds easily and briskly when touched. In fact, bleeding is usually the impetus for seeking care in the emergency department. Suggested interventions to treat the bleeding include pressure, suturing, and silver nitrate (although not on the face). In pregnant patients, this type of hemangioma can resolve spontaneously after delivery. For this reason, unless the lesion is actively bleeding, conservative management and waiting until the postpartum period are prudent. But in general, patients should be referred for biopsy and histology to evaluate for other more serious causes and for definitive treatment. Recurrence rate can be as high as 40% if nonsurgical means are used for removal.

Why are the other choices wrong?

Gingivitis presents as more diffuse irritation of the gingiva. A focal lesion is not consistent with this presentation.

Melanomas can be discolored, but they tend to be brown, and they are not as large as this lesion is. The "ABCDE Checklist" is a tool for remembering the diagnostic criteria of a melanoma: Asymmetry, Border, Color, Diameter/Difference, Elevation/ Evolving.

A periodontal abscess is a pus-filled cavity. This lesion is vascular, not an abscess.

PEER REVIEW

✓ Pregnant patients can develop vascular abnormalities with minor trauma, and they can spontaneously resolve.
✓ If you're treating a patient who has a so-called pyogenic granuloma, treat active bleeding and refer for testing and definitive treatment.

REFERENCES
Knoop KJ, Stack LB, Storrow AB, et al. *The Atlas of Emergency Medicine.* 4th ed. New York, NY: McGraw-Hill; 2016: 380.
Roberts JR, Custalow CB, Thomsen TW, eds. *Roberts and Hedges' Clinical Procedures in Emergency Medicine.* 6th ed. Philadelphia, PA: Elsevier; 2014: 714.
Tintinalli JE, Stapczynski JS, Ma OJ, et al, eds. *Tintinalli's Emergency Medicine: A Comprehensive Study Guide.* 8th ed. New York, NY: McGraw-Hill; 2012: 1680.

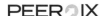

170. The correct answer is A, Administer one dose of acetazolamide 500 mg IV or PO.

Why is this the correct answer?

Acute angle-closure glaucoma is a medical emergency. The goal of treatment is to quickly lower the intraocular pressure, and instillation of timolol is the correct initial action. The American Academy of Ophthalmology recommends administering one dose of acetazolamide 500 mg IV or PO in addition to the timolol. Intravenous administration of mannitol is one way to lower the pressure, but it must be carefully administered in patients with low blood pressure. Other appropriate treatments include apraclonidine 1% drops and pilocarpine 1% to 2% drops every 15 minutes. Pilocarpine is effective only after the intraocular pressure has decreased so that the pupil can constrict and pull the iris away from the angle to promote drainage of the aqueous humor. After the pressure has been lowered, the ophthalmologist might perform laser iridectomy. In the situation described in this question, emergent ophthalmology consultation is needed to provide definitive treatment and minimize the risk of permanent vision loss.

Why are the other choices wrong?

Pilocarpine is part of the overall emergency management of acute angle-closure glaucoma, but it is effective only after the intraocular pressure has been lowered. The patient needs to be treated with another medication first to accomplish this.

Continuing the timolol drops and waiting for the desired response without consulting ophthalmology delays definitive treatment. Medical treatment should be initiated by the emergency physician at the same time ophthalmology is consulted to evaluate the patient and provide definitive treatment.

The patient cannot be discharged before the pressure has been lowered given the risk of permanent vision loss. Acute angle-closure glaucoma is a time-sensitive emergency that requires quick evaluation by an ophthalmologist.

PEER REVIEW

- ✓ Acute angle-closure glaucoma is a medical emergency that requires emergent ophthalmology consultation.
- ✓ The key in initial medical management is to first lower the intraocular pressures then constrict the pupil to promote drainage.

REFERENCES

Riordan-Eva P, Cunningham ET. *Vaughn & Ashbury's General Ophthalmology.* 18th ed. New York, NY: McGraw-Hill; 2011: http://accessmedicine.mhmedical.com/content.aspx?bookid=387&sectionid=40229328. Accessed May 16, 2017.

Tintinalli JE, Stapczynski JS, Ma OJ, et al, eds. *Tintinalli's Emergency Medicine: A Comprehensive Study Guide.* 8th ed. New York, NY: McGraw-Hill; 2012: 1572-1574.

Trobe JD. *The Physician's Guide to Eye Care.* 4th ed. San Francisco, CA: American Academy of Ophthalmology; 2012:68-71.

171. The correct answer is B, Left ventricular aneurysm.

A left ventricular (LV) aneurysm is a focal area of infarcted myocardium that bulges outward during both systole and diastole. The ECG changes associated with LV aneurysm, as seen in this case, are typically ST-segment elevation in the anterior leads (V1-V5) with accompanying Q waves. It can be difficult to distinguish LV aneurysm from anterior MI; however, the presence of Q waves typically reveals a completed anterior infarction. Approximately 10% to 30% of patients who survive an acute MI develop a left ventricular aneurysm. Patients with large LV aneurysms can present with dyspnea that often has persisted from the time of infarction. The prevalence of LV aneurysm appears to have declined with the improved reperfusion treatment of acute MI. Patients who experience acute MI without prompt or appropriate therapy can have a completed infarction with a large amount of infarcted myocardium; these patients can then develop a ventricular aneurysm. Most LV aneurysms are anterolateral near the apex of the heart and are the result of complete occlusion of the left anterior descending (LAD) artery. Small and moderate-sized aneurysms are often associated with no symptoms, although the patient might experience angina in other portions of adjacent myocardium.

Why are the other choices wrong?

Late post-MI myopericarditis, often referred to as Dressler syndrome, typically presents with pleuritic chest pain, fever, leukocytosis, and pericardial friction rub. It usually occurs a few weeks after large acute MI. Typical ECG findings are similar to pericarditis with diffuse ST-segment elevation and PR segment depression without reciprocal change of both the PR and ST segments. Of course, not all cases of myopericarditis demonstrate these classic ECG abnormalities.

The electrocardiographic pattern of left ventricular hypertrophy (LVH) frequently has repolarization abnormalities, which include ST-segment elevation and depression as well as T-wave abnormalities. Approximately 75% to 80% of patients with electrocardiographic LVH have these ST-segment and T-wave abnormalities, termed the strain pattern. Electrocardiographic LVH should be considered if the sum of the S wave in lead V1 or V2 and the R wave in lead V5 or V6 is greater than 35 mm in a patient older than 35 years.

In this patient, STEMI is less likely both clinically and electrocardiographically. He has had persistent dyspnea for 2 weeks without apparent change in the pattern; thus no new major event appears to be occurring. Regarding the ECG, the prominent Q waves with ST-segment elevation suggest possible aneurysm. Also, a comparison of the height of the T wave to that of the QRS complex can also assist in this distinction. With LV aneurysm, the T wave is often small or flattened compared to a prominent QRS complex in the configuration of a Q wave. With STEMI, the T wave is often quite prominent and near equal to equal in amplitude to the accompanying QRS complex.

PEER POINT

Important ECG findings in left ventricular aneurysm

A shows samples of the ST-segment elevation, and B shows a comparison of ST-segment elevation associated with LVA (left) and STEMI (right).

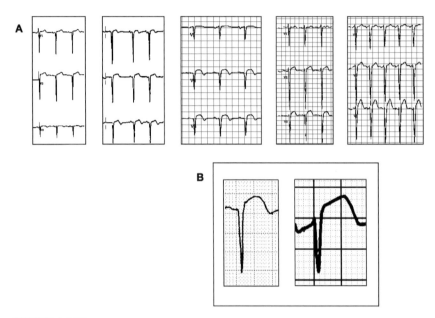

PEER Point 17

PEER REVIEW

✓ Persistent ST-segment elevation with prominent Q waves in anterior leads is suggestive of left ventricular aneurysm.

✓ A T wave-to-QRS amplitude ratio greater than 0.36 is suggestive of left ventricular aneurysm.

✓ Left ventricular hypertrophy can be determined by summing the voltage of the S wave in V1 or V2 with R wave in V5 or V6.

✓ The ST-segment elevation of MI is more frequently convex compared to concave changes seen in pericarditis, LV aneurysm, and left ventricular hypertrophy.

REFERENCES

Marx JA, Hockberger RS, Walls RM, eds. *Rosen's Emergency Medicine: Concepts and Clinical Practice*. 8th ed. St. Louis, MO: Elsevier; 2014:997-1033.

Mattu A, Brady WJ, et al (eds). *Cardiovascular Emergencies*. Dallas, TX: American College of Emergency Physicians Publishing; 2014: 11-35.

O'Connor RE, Al Ali AS, Brady WJ, et al. Part 9: Acute Coronary Syndromes—2015 American Heart Association Guidelines Update for Cardiopulmonary Resuscitation and Emergency Cardiovascular Care. *Circulation*. 2015;132(18 Suppl 2):S483-500.

172. The correct answer is B, Fibrinolytic agents.

Why is this the correct answer?

This patient's presentation should raise suspicion for an aortic dissection given his symptoms. The ECG demonstrates sinus rhythm with significant ST-segment elevation in leads III and AVF as well as ST-segment depression in leads I and AVL likely resulting from an inferior STEMI involving the right coronary artery. The ST depression in leads V1-2-3 are consistent with reciprocal changes. Administering fibrinolytic agents to a patient with a dissection would have catastrophic consequences, including cardiac tamponade and death. The following features of this presentation suggest aortic dissection:

- Tearing chest pain radiating to the back
- History of poorly treated hypertension
- Extremely elevated blood pressure
- Upper extremity paresthesia (any manifestation of additional organ system involvement)

Any one of these features is not particularly suggestive of aortic dissection but, when considered from the entire perspective, should make the treating clinician consider aortic dissection. Inferior wall STEMI coexists with approximately 3% of dissections due to the proximal aortic injury and involvement of the coronary arteries, usually the right coronary artery. This occurs with the retrograde expansion of the Aortic dissection plane into the right coronary cusp and hence clipping off the ostium of the RCA, as the mechanism behind inferior STEMI in this setting. Therefore, the presence of STEMI on the ECG (here, ST-segment elevation in leads III and aVF) does not rule out a dissection. Additionally, 15% of aortic dissections present with some signs of ischemia on the ECG. This patient should undergo more imaging such as chest radiography and/or CT angiography. If the patient has an aortic dissection, treatment should focus on reducing blood pressure and decreasing heart rate. Lowering the heart rate decreases shear force on the aorta. A type A dissection (proximal dissection) such as this one involving the ascending aorta requires emergent surgical treatment. Type B dissections involving the distal segment of the thoracic aorta can be managed medically.

Why are the other choices wrong?

Beta-blocking agents are the mainstay of medical therapy for aortic dissection and are certainly not contraindicated in this situation. They lower both blood pressure and heart rate effectively. They should be used even in normotensive patients to achieve a heart rate of 60. Beta blockers can be used to control blood pressure in patients with an acute STEMI without dissection as well.

Pain control also is not contraindicated for this patient. In fact, it is important in the management of all patients with aortic dissection. Achieving adequate pain control for patients with either STEMI or aortic dissection with morphine or other narcotics limits sympathetic tone, thus lowering blood pressure and heart rate.

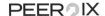

Nitrates also are not contraindicated in this case. They can be used to reduce blood pressure in patients with aortic dissection and STEMI. They can cause reflex tachycardia and, especially in patients with dissection, should be used with a beta blocker to subvert this effect. Nitroprusside is a more effective arterial dilator than nitroglycerin, so it generally is the nitrate of choice in dissection.

PEER REVIEW

✓ Aortic dissections can involve the coronary arteries and create a STEMI pattern on ECG.

✓ Hypertension is a risk factor for aortic dissection.

✓ Beta blockers are an important part of the medical treatment for aortic dissection.

REFERENCES

Marx JA, Hockberger RS, Walls RM, eds. *Rosen's Emergency Medicine: Concepts and Clinical Practice*. 8th ed. St. Louis, MO: Elsevier; 2014:1124-1128.

Tintinalli JE, Stapczynski JS, Ma OJ, et al, eds. *Tintinalli's Emergency Medicine: A Comprehensive Study Guide*. 8th ed. New York, NY: McGraw-Hill; 2012: 412-415.

173. The correct answer is B, Anovulatory cycles.

Why is this the correct answer?

Endometrial cancer is the most common cancer of the female pelvic organs. It is eventually diagnosed in approximately 10% of patients with postmenopausal bleeding. Prolonged exposure to high levels of estrogen and a thickened endometrium contribute to the development of this neoplasm. Therefore, obesity, nulliparity, a longer period of fertility (early menarche/late menopause), and anovulatory cycles are risk factors for endometrial cancer. When evaluating a patient with postmenopausal bleeding, the first step is to determine the exact source of the blood. It could be coming from the urethra due to a urinary tract infection, from the vagina due to atrophy or tear, from the rectum due to lower gastrointestinal bleeding, or from the uterus. Any postmenopausal woman presenting with blood from the uterus should be referred for an endometrial biopsy to rule out endometrial cancer.

Why are the other choices wrong?

Patients with anorexia tend to lack cycles and lack the high estrogen levels more commonly seen in obese women.

Multiparity is a protective factor for endometrial cancer; women who never have children (nulliparity) have more exposure to hormonal stimulation of the endometrial lining.

Having multiple sexual partners exposes a woman to more strains of human papillomavirus and is a risk factor for cervical cancer, not endometrial cancer. Commercial sex workers are at high risk for cervical cancer. Celibate women are more likely to get endometrial cancer.

PEER REVIEW

✓ Obesity, nulliparity, early menarche/late menopause, and anovulatory cycles are risk factors for endometrial cancer.

✓ Postmenopausal women with uterine bleeding should be referred for an endometrial biopsy.

✓ Localizing the source (vagina, uterus, urethra, rectum) of the bleeding is the first step in evaluating postmenopausal bleeding.

REFERENCES

Adams JG, Barton ED, Collings J, et al, eds. *Emergency Medicine*. Philadelphia, PA: Saunders; 2008: 1069-1078.

Marx JA, Hockberger RS, Walls RM, eds. *Rosen's Emergency Medicine: Concepts and Clinical Practice*. 8th ed. St. Louis, MO: Elsevier; 2014: 273-277.

174. The correct answer is D, Rapid ventricular response.

Why is this the correct answer?

The ECG demonstrates an irregularly irregular narrow-complex rhythm consistent with atrial fibrillation (AF) with rapid ventricular response (RVR). The typical heart rate in a patient with AF, unaffected by medications and other active diseases, is approximately 170 bpm. An extremely rapid ventricular response, as shown in this case, is a very common reason for a patient with AF to present with other difficulties like fatigue, weakness, palpitations, and shortness of breath. Atrial fibrillation with RVR can produce difficulty via several mechanisms, including reduced time for ventricular filling (resulting in decreased systemic perfusion) and altered myocardial perfusion (resulting in myocardial ischemia and further cardiac decompensation). The primary task of the emergency physician in most presentations like this one is rate control, which can be achieved by judicious administration of an intravenous fluid bolus and atrioventricular node blocking agents such as a calcium channel blocker or a beta-adrenergic antagonist. Rhythm conversion is a second goal and can be addressed if the patient is unstable due to the rapid AF rate or if cardioversion is medically appropriate for other reasons.

Why are the other choices wrong?

Thrombus formation can occur in the atrial chambers due to the sluggish blood flow generally occurring after 48 hours. If the thrombus passes into the ventricle, it can pass into systemic circulation and cause stroke or ischemic viscera or extremity. But thrombus formation does not usually cause the generalized symptoms of fatigue and diffuse weakness.

A common finding in patients with AF is left atrial enlargement. This characteristic can lead to recurrent episodes of AF but does not directly lead to the symptoms of fatigue and generalized weakness. With AF, the atria do not contract in an organized manner due to the dysrhythmia, not due to the enlarged size, thus reducing ventricular filling and systemic perfusion.

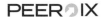
Myocardial ischemia can certainly cause patient intolerance and decline due to AF. But it usually occurs in addition to other pathophysiologic issues such as the rapid rate and is rarely the primary reason for patient decompensation. This ECG does not show any obvious signs of ischemia, which might be seen with ST-segment depression or inverted T waves.

PEER REVIEW

- ✓ An irregularly irregular narrow complex tachycardia is the classic ECG finding for atrial fibrillation.
- ✓ The cause of symptoms such as weakness in AF is generally the reduced time for ventricular filling resulting in decreased systemic perfusion.
- ✓ The primary management goal for rapid AF is rate control. It can be achieved with careful use of an intravenous fluid bolus and a calcium channel blocker or beta-adrenergic antagonist.
- ✓ Patient decompensation in AF with RVR isn't always caused primarily by the rhythm disorder, so be sure to consider the total patient presentation so you can provide appropriate therapy and avoid unnecessary or dangerous treatment.

REFERENCES

Link MS, Berkow LC, Kudenchuk PJ, et al. Part 7: adult advanced cardiovascular life support: 2015 American Heart Association Guidelines Update for Cardiopulmonary Resuscitation and Emergency Cardiovascular Care. *Circulation*. 2015; 132(suppl 2):S444–S464.

Winters ME, Bond MC, DeBlieux P, et al (eds). *Emergency Department Resuscitation of the Critically Ill*. Dallas, TX: American College of Emergency Physician Publishing; 2011: 51-68.

175. The correct answer is D, Irrigate the site with saline, and refer the patient for dental follow-up.

Why is this the correct answer?

Postextraction alveolar osteitis, also known as dry socket, occurs in about 30% of impacted third molar (wisdom teeth) extractions. The etiology is a displacement of the clot from the socket that exposes the alveolar bone and results in a local osteomyelitis. In most cases, all that is needed is irrigation of the socket with chlorhexidine 0.12% oral rinse or warmed normal saline. Patients often need analgesia, either with an NSAID or an opiate or regional anesthesia. If there are signs of infection, antibiotics are warranted, either penicillin VK or clindamycin for penicillin-allergic patients. All patients should be referred back to the dentist who performed the procedure for follow-up.

Why are the other choices wrong?

Closing the dry socket with sutures is not the right course of action. It does not treat the underlying osteomyelitis, and it increases the risk of an abscess formation.

Discharging this patient on oral antibiotics alone is not correct treatment either, especially since he does not have any signs of local or systemic infection.

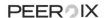
Care should be initiated in the emergency department before the patient is referred back to the dentist. If the socket is not irrigated, the risk of worsening infection might increase in the days prior to follow-up.

PEER REVIEW

✓ Dry socket is a common complication after the extraction of impacted wisdom teeth.

✓ Gentle irrigation is the best initial treatment for dry socket in the emergency department before patients are referred back to their dentists for follow-up care.

REFERENCES

Buttaravoli P, Leffler SM. *Minor Emergencies*. 3rd ed. Philadelphia, PA: Elsevier; 2012:183-184.

Tintinalli JE, Stapczynski JS, Ma OJ, et al, eds. *Tintinalli's Emergency Medicine: A Comprehensive Study Guide*. 8th ed. New York, NY: McGraw-Hill; 2012: 1598-1613.

176. The correct answer is A, Adenosine.

Why is this the correct answer?

The rhythm strip reveals a regular narrow QRS complex tachycardia at a rate of approximately 200 bpm. The differential diagnosis of this dysrhythmias includes atrioventricular nodal re-entrant tachycardia (AVNRT, also known as paroxysmal supraventricular tachycardia), atrial flutter, atrial tachycardia, and Wolff-Parkinson-White syndrome (WPW) atrioventricular re-entrant tachycardia (AVRT). With the patient's history of WPW, this is the most likely diagnosis, and adenosine is the most appropriate first choice due to its rapid onset of action and short half-life. The WPW syndrome is complicated by three different dysrhythmias, atrioventricular reentrant tachycardia (AVRT), both narrow (orthodromic) and wide (antidromic) QRS complex varieties, and atrial fibrillation. Of the three dysrhythmias, the orthodromic AVRT is the least concerning WPW presentations; this rhythm can be managed with AV node blocking agents such as adenosine, calcium channel blockers, and bet-adrenergic antagonists. The other two rhythm presentations are much more malignant and cannot be treated with AV node blocking medications; the preferred treatments for these two rhythms are intravenous procainamide and/or electrical cardioversion. Again, the dysrhythmia encountered in this case is orthodromic AVRT and is managed appropriately with adenosine. Conduction of the impulse is antegrade through the AV node and retrograde via the accessory pathway. The intraventricular conduction pathway is used, thus the QRS complex is narrow. Reducing impulse conduction through the AV node likely interrupts the conduction loop and assists in dysrhythmia termination. Any of the agents listed above can be used in this WPW rhythm presentation, but adenosine is the most appropriate first choice.

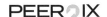

Why are the other choices wrong?

Diltiazem is a potent AV node blocking agent and is an appropriate treatment for this narrow QRS complex tachycardia associated with WPW — the orthodromic AVRT — but adenosine represents the first choice. The other two dysrhythmias of WPW are wide complex (antidromic) AVRT and atrial fibrillation; AV node blocking agents are not appropriate in their treatment and should not be administered.

Like diltiazem, esmolol can be used in this scenario, but adenosine is the first choice.

Procainamide can be used to treat any of the three WPW rhythm presentations, but adenosine is the best first choice for the narrow complex AVRT that is not causing hemodynamic instability.

PEER REVIEW

✓ Narrow-complex tachycardia in Wolff-Parkinson-White syndrome (orthodromic AVRT) can be treated with AV node blocking agents.

✓ You can't conclusively distinguish PSVT (AVNRT) from orthodromic AVRT in WPW until you can analyze a postconversion ECG in sinus rhythm with subsequent demonstration of the classic triad of WPW findings.

REFERENCES

Link MS, Berkow LC, Kudenchuk PJ, et al. Part 7: adult advanced cardiovascular life support: 2015 American Heart Association Guidelines Update for Cardiopulmonary Resuscitation and Emergency Cardiovascular Care. *Circulation*. 2015; 132(suppl 2):S444–S464.

Tintinalli JE, Stapczynski JS, Ma OJ, et al, eds. *Tintinalli's Emergency Medicine: A Comprehensive Study Guide*. 8th ed. New York, NY: McGraw-Hill; 2012: 112-134.

177. The correct answer is D, Oral aspirin therapy with serial troponin measurement and 12-lead ECG sampling.

Why is this the correct answer?

Patients with suspected ACS and an entirely normal ECG who are hemodynamically stable have a very low rate of acute MI, ranging from 1% to 3%. Thus management decisions should be based on the total presentation, considering all the features of the patient's data, observing the patient's response to treatment, and reassessing the clinical picture and risk factors. A patient who is stable, does not develop concerning issues during the emergency department stay, has a negative workup with normal serial troponins and ECGs, and who does not exhibit signs of worrisome alternative diagnoses can be safely discharged and referred to either a primary care physician or cardiologist for further evaluation. In this setting (stable patient with initially negative evaluation), oral aspirin is the most appropriate therapy.

Why are the other choices wrong?

In a stable patient with an initially negative evaluation who has remained hemodynamically stable during a period of observation and reassessment, administering antiplatelet and anticoagulant agents in the emergency department is excessive; of course, this statement does not apply to oral aspirin therapy. The early use of exercise stress testing (emphasis on "early") likely is not the most appropriate evaluation strategy in a patient such as the one in the case who has a concerning but stable ACS presentation.

Again, the heparin and clopidogrel are not necessary given that the patient is stable. But monitoring with serial troponin measurements and 12-lead ECG sampling is appropriate for this nondiagnostic chest pain presentation.

Aspirin is one of the most appropriate initial therapies in suspected ACS; it has significant abilities to favorably affect mortality rates. But without serial troponin measurements and 12-lead ECG sampling, early exercise stress testing at this point in the patient's care is not the most appropriate evaluation strategy for a concerning but stable ACS presentation.

PEER REVIEW

- ✓ If you're treating a patient and concerned about ACS, consider the whole presentation: the history, risk issues, examination, ECG, serum markers, other study results, and emergency department course.
- ✓ A normal or minimally abnormal (nonspecific) ECG does not rule out ACS by itself, particularly early in the course.

REFERENCES

Marx JA, Hockberger RS, Walls RM, eds. *Rosen's Emergency Medicine: Concepts and Clinical Practice*. 8th ed. St. Louis, MO: Elsevier; 2014: 997-1033.

Mattu A, Brady WJ, et al (eds). *Cardiovascular Emergencies*. Dallas, TX: American College of Emergency Physicians Publishing; 2014: 11-35.

O'Connor RE, Al Ali AS, Brady WJ, et al. Part 9: Acute Coronary Syndromes—2015 American Heart Association Guidelines Update for Cardiopulmonary Resuscitation and Emergency Cardiovascular Care. *Circulation*. 2015;132:s483-500.

178. The correct answer is B, Cavernous sinus thrombosis.

Why is this the correct answer?

Cavernous sinus thrombosis is a known complication after infections of the head and neck. Given that cranial nerves III, IV, V1, and V2 run along the wall of the cavernous sinus, they can be affected as a result of an infection. Most infectious etiologies in cavernous sinus thrombosis are from *Staphylococcus* or *Streptococcus* species. In a patient with fever, headache, and vision changes, cavernous sinus thrombosis must be considered. The patient might also complain of chills, lethargy, nausea, or vomiting. Blood cultures, CBC, and coagulation studies (PT and PTT) should be ordered, as well as CT of the head and orbits with contrast. Parenteral antibiotic treatment should be started with gram-positive coverage (nafcillin plus a

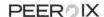

third-generation cephalosporin or vancomycin if concerned for MRSA). The patient should be admitted with neurology and ophthalmology consultations. A classic rare finding is weakness of cranial nerve VI — abducens palsy.

Why are the other choices wrong?

Acute angle-closure glaucoma typically presents with findings of a hazy cornea with a fixed pupil. This patient's cornea is clear on examination.

Temporal arteritis can present with unilateral headache and vision changes, but it is rare in patients younger than 50 years. An ESR greater than 50 and temporal artery biopsy confirm the diagnosis.

A transient ischemic attack is unlikely given the patient's age, sex, and lack of history of other neurologic presentations. Her fever and headache also suggest another diagnosis.

PEER REVIEW

✓ Cavernous sinus thrombosis is a rare complication, but it can occur after head and neck infections.

✓ The key to minimizing poor outcomes in cavernous sinus thrombosis is early antibiotic administration.

REFERENCES

Hall JB, Schmidt GA, Wood LDH. *Principles of Critical Care*. 3rd ed. New York, NY: McGraw-Hill; 2005: 801-814.

Stone CK, Humphries RL. *CURRENT Diagnosis & Treatment Emergency Medicine*. 7th ed. New York, NY: McGraw-Hill; 2011: 489-512.

Tintinalli JE, Stapczynski JS, Ma OJ, et al, eds. *Tintinalli's Emergency Medicine: A Comprehensive Study Guide*. 8th ed. New York, NY: McGraw-Hill; 2012: 1579-1585.

179. The correct answer is D, Pericardiocentesis.

Why is this the correct answer?

Pericardial effusion is an abnormal accumulation of fluid in the pericardial space, and in this case, it is evident on the echocardiogram. The patient has hypotension with this large circumferential pericardial effusion, a presentation most consistent with pericardial tamponade. Pericardiocentesis is indicated in the emergency department to remove the fluid in this unstable patient. The pericardial space has a limited volume. With the accumulation of fluid, intrapericardial pressure increases and can negatively impact cardiac function, ultimately reducing cardiac output and producing systemic hypoperfusion. Slowly accumulating pericardial effusions cause hemodynamic compromise less often than those that develop more rapidly. Several diseases can produce pericardial effusions: rheumatologic disorders, chest malignancies, atypical infectious disorders such as tuberculosis, perforation of cardiac chambers, and proximal aortic dissection, among others. And as seen in this case, echocardiography is usually very helpful in establishing the diagnosis.

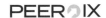

Why are the other choices wrong?

Although chest tube placement is a very reasonable intervention in pneumothorax and hemothorax, it has no utility in the resolution of a pericardial effusion.

Emergent CT angiography of the aorta to assess for aortic dissection is another consideration in a patient with dyspnea and hypotension; proximal aortic dissection can present with pericardial effusion with or without tamponade. But the patient in this case does not have chest pain, so she is not likely experiencing an aortic dissection. Instead, her condition should be stabilized, and pericardiocentesis is likely the most appropriate initial intervention.

In certain rare circumstances, establishing central venous access to measure central venous pressures is indicated. However, in this case, with a presentation consistent with pericardial effusion with tamponade, both the diagnosis and the treatment goals are obvious.

PEER REVIEW

- ✓ Pericardial effusions that accumulate slowly cause hemodynamic compromise less often than the ones that develop fast.
- ✓ Echocardiography is usually very helpful in establishing the diagnosis of pericardial effusion.
- ✓ Which disorders cause pericardial effusions? Rheumatologic disorders, chest malignancies, some atypical infectious like tuberculosis, cardiac chamber perforation, and proximal aortic dissection, to name a few.

REFERENCES

Marx JA, Hockberger RS, Walls RM, eds. *Rosen's Emergency Medicine: Concepts and Clinical Practice*. 8th ed. St. Louis, MO: Elsevier; 2014:1091-1105.

Tintinalli JE, Stapczynski JS, Ma OJ, et al, eds. *Tintinalli's Emergency Medicine: A Comprehensive Study Guide*. 8th ed. New York, NY: McGraw-Hill; 2012: 412-415.

180. The correct answer is C, Thoracentesis.

Why is this the correct answer?

The bedside ultrasound image shows a large pleural effusion, seen as a hypoechoic area above the diaphragm. Thoracentesis is the indicated treatment to remove the fluid in the patient's pleural space in order to improve her oxygenation and relieve her dyspnea. Although thoracentesis is not frequently performed in the emergency department, it is indicated to relieve dyspnea associated with a large effusion. Other indications include suspected pleural space infection and new effusion without a clear clinical diagnosis. After the pleural effusion is removed, the patient's lung should reexpand, and her oxygenation and ventilation should improve.

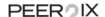

Why are the other choices wrong?

Needle decompression of the chest wall with a large-bore needle is the initial treatment for suspected tension pneumothorax. In a patient with a pneumothorax, breath sounds are absent over the involved lung, and the chest wall is tympanitic to percussion. An ultrasound examination would show absence of lung sliding and would not show fluid in the chest cavity. Needle decompression has no role in the management of a pleural effusion.

Pericardiocentesis is the initial treatment for pericardial tamponade. The classic signs of pericardial tamponade are hypotension, muffled heart sounds, and distended neck veins. An ultrasound examination would show fluid in the pericardial sac surrounding the heart. As with needle decompression, pericardiocentesis has no role in the management of a pleural effusion.

Thoracostomy is used in the treatment of pneumothorax, hemothorax, and empyema. Placing a chest tube in this case would evacuate the pleural fluid that is causing the dyspnea, but it is much more invasive than thoracentesis and is thus not indicated.

PEER REVIEW

✓ What are the indications for thoracentesis? Relief of dyspnea associated with a large effusion, suspected pleural space infection, and new effusion without a clear clinical diagnosis.

REFERENCES

Roberts JR, Custalow CB, Thomsen TW, eds. Roberts and Hedges' *Clinical Procedures in Emergency Medicine*. 6th ed. Philadelphia, PA: Elsevier; 2014: 173-188.

Tintinalli JE, Stapczynski JS, Ma OJ, et al, eds. *Tintinalli's Emergency Medicine: A Comprehensive Study Guide*. 8th ed. New York, NY: McGraw-Hill; 2012: 434-436.

181. The correct answer is C, Procainamide 1 g IV.

Why is this the correct answer?

This ECG shows monomorphic ventricular tachycardia (VT) in a patient who is currently hemodynamically stable. Initial treatment for stable sustained monomorphic VT is generally intravenous administration of antiarrhythmic agents (including procainamide, amiodarone, sotalol, or lidocaine) or synchronized cardioversion. Procainamide and amiodarone are considered the first-line antiarrhythmic agents in stable VT. Procainamide is a Class Ia antiarrhythmic agent administered at a rate of 25 to 50 mg/min IV with a maximum dose of 17 mg/kg. It should not be used in patients with acute MI, long QT interval, or significant left ventricular dysfunction. Amiodarone is the antiarrhythmic agent of choice in stable monomorphic VT when the patient has an acute MI or severe left ventricular dysfunction. Sotalol is a nonselective beta blocker with Class III antiarrhythmic properties that is also used in stable VT but should not be given in patients with a long QT interval. Lidocaine is a second-line therapy in stable VT. Synchronized cardioversion may be considered in any patient with sustained VT and is the treatment of choice in unstable VT.

Why are the other choices wrong?

Calcium-channel blockers such as diltiazem and verapamil are not recommended in the acute treatment of stable (or unstable) VT or to aid in the diagnosis of a wide-complex tachycardia. Although they can be effective in rhythm conversion, these medications can cause serious adverse events such as severe hypotension.

Magnesium is the initial treatment of choice in the polymorphic VT torsades de pointes. It is unlikely to be of use in a patient with monomorphic VT with a normal QT interval.

Unsynchronized cardioversion, or defibrillation, is used in pulseless VT or ventricular fibrillation arrest or where the defibrillator is unable to synch in an unstable patient. Electrical cardioversion in stable patients should be synchronized.

PEER POINT

Potential treatments for stable sustained monomorphic VT

- Procainamide
- Amiodarone
- Sotalol
- Lidocaine
- Overdrive pacing
- Synchronized cardioversion

PEER REVIEW

- ✓ Treat stable VT with intravenous antiarrhythmic agents or synchronized cardioversion, and consider the need for procedural sedation.
- ✓ First-line antiarrhythmic agents for stable VT include amiodarone and procainamide.
- ✓ Don't use procainamide and sotalol in patients with a prolonged QT interval.

REFERENCES

Silvers SM, White RD, Yannopoulos D, Donnino MW. Part 7: adult advanced cardiovascular life support: 2015 American Heart Association Guidelines Update for Cardiopulmonary Resuscitation and Emergency Cardiovascular Care. *Circulation.* 2015; 132(suppl 2):S444–S464.

Tintinalli JE, Stapczynski JS, Ma OJ, et al, eds. *Tintinalli's Emergency Medicine: A Comprehensive Study Guide.* 8th ed. New York, NY: McGraw-Hill; 2012: 112-134.

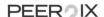

182. The correct answer is A, Back pain.

Why is this the correct answer?

Back pain is a common emergency department presentation, and it is vital to distinguish between uncomplicated musculoskeletal symptoms and those suggesting more serious disease. The patient in this case has some concerning red-flag symptoms for more ominous pathology: perianal paresthesias, urinary incontinence or retention, fecal incontinence, and sciatica. Spinal epidural abscess is the likely cause of this patient's compression syndrome. Risk factors for epidural abscess include intravenous drug use, chronic renal insufficiency, diabetes, immunocompromised state, and recent invasive spinal procedures. The classic triad of back pain, fever, and neurologic deficit occurs in a minority of patients, with back pain being the most common presenting symptom (present in 70% to 90% of cases). The imaging modality of choice is MRI, as laboratory tests often reveal nonspecific findings such as an elevated WBC count, ESR, or C-reactive protein. *Staphylococcus aureus* is the most common bacterial cause of spinal epidural abscess, and MRSA (methicillin-resistant *Staphylococcus aureus*) should always be considered. If epidural abscess is confirmed, intravenous antibiotic therapy and an emergent neurosurgical consultation are indicated. Vancomycin plus ceftazidime or cefepime is the first-line antibiotic choice.

Why are the other choices wrong?

Fever, either reported or subjective, along with back pain and neurologic symptoms, supports the diagnosis of epidural abscess; however, it is not the most common presenting complaint. Other potential diagnoses in patients who present with fever and back pain include discitis and vertebral osteomyelitis.

Motor weakness can be present in patients with nerve root compression as well as those with spinal cord compression. Alone, without other red-flag symptoms such as urinary or fecal incontinence or perianal paresthesias, motor weakness does not specifically support the diagnosis of spinal epidural abscess. Generally, if motor weakness is present, the patient should undergo neurosurgical intervention.

Patients who present with back pain should be queried regarding the presence or absence of urinary retention symptoms. Urinary retention should raise suspicion for spinal cord compression due to either mechanical causes or infection such as an abscess.

PEER REVIEW

✓ Risk factors for spinal epidural abscess: intravenous drug use, chronic renal insufficiency, diabetes, immunocompromised, recent invasive spinal procedures.

✓ The classically taught triad of fever, back pain, and neurologic symptoms is present in only a small percentage of patients with spinal epidural abscess.

✓ Back pain is the most common presenting symptom in spinal epidural abscess.

✓ If you're treating a patient with spinal epidural abscess, get an emergent neurosurgical consult and start intravenous antibiotics.

REFERENCES

Marx JA, Hockberger RS, Walls RM, eds. *Rosen's Emergency Medicine: Concepts and Clinical Practice.* 8th ed. St. Louis, MO: Elsevier; 2014: 643-655.

Tintinalli JE, Stapczynski JS, Ma OJ, et al, eds. *Tintinalli's Emergency Medicine: A Comprehensive Study Guide.* 8th ed. New York, NY: McGraw-Hill; 2012: 1192-1199.

183. The correct answer is C, Multiple alcohol-related injuries in the past year.

Why is this the correct answer?

The recurrent use of alcohol in situations where it is physically hazardous is one of the DSM-5 criteria for alcohol use disorder. The fact that this patient continues to drink despite sustaining multiple injuries should raise concern that he suffers from this disorder. The other answer choices presented are signs of acute alcohol intoxication but are not necessarily indicative of alcohol addiction. Other criteria for the diagnosis of alcohol use disorder include tolerance, in which the individual requires increasing amounts of alcohol to achieve the same effect, and withdrawal. Patients with alcohol use disorder might also continue to drink despite negative social and professional consequences and failure to achieve major role obligations at home and work. They might also crave alcohol and spend prolonged amounts of time and effort obtaining alcohol. Alcohol use disorder can be categorized as mild, moderate, or severe, depending on the number of symptoms present. As far as an emergency department intervention, it has been shown that a brief negotiated interview with the patient summarizing options to help stop drinking is successful in reducing hazard-related drinking.

Why are the other choices wrong?

Involuntary jerking of the eyeballs becomes more pronounced as persons become intoxicated, and the horizontal gaze nystagmus test is commonly used to determine whether someone has acute alcohol intoxication. But it does not indicate whether a person has an alcohol use disorder.

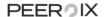

Many people exhibit problematic psychological or behavior changes after drinking alcohol such as inappropriate sexual behavior, labile mood, poor judgment, and aggressive behavior. But these behaviors do not on their own indicate alcohol use disorder.

Other signs and symptoms of alcohol intoxication include:
- Slurred speech
- Unsteady gait
- Coma or stupor
- Incoordination
- Memory impairment

PEER REVIEW

✓ Persons who have an alcohol use disorder continue to drink despite negative social and professional consequences.

✓ Nystagmus and slurred speech are signs of alcohol intoxication.

✓ If you're treating a patient you think might have an alcohol use disorder, talk to him or her about the options to get help.

REFERENCES

American Psychiatric Association: Diagnostic and Statistical Manual of Mental Disorders. 5th ed. Washington, DC: American Psychiatric Association, 2013.

Tintinalli JE, Stapczynski JS, Ma OJ, et al, eds. *Tintinalli's Emergency Medicine: A Comprehensive Study Guide.* 8th ed. New York, NY: McGraw-Hill; 2012: 1976-1982.

184. The correct answer is C, Her husband was killed in a car crash 2 days earlier.

Why is this the correct answer?

Conversion disorder, also known as functional neurologic symptom disorder, psychogenic disorder, hysterical neurosis, or pseudoneurologic syndrome, is a type of somatoform disorder involving persistent physical symptoms with no identifiable physical cause. Although identification of a stressor is not absolutely necessary to make the diagnosis, the disorder is often associated with a recent trauma or stressor, which certainly applies to the patient in this case. It is also important to note that the diagnosis should be based on the entire clinical picture and not on a single finding. Furthermore, it is of primary importance that an organic cause be first ruled out. As such, the diagnosis is rarely made in the emergency department and should be considered with an abundance of caution. Conversion disorder must involve one or more motor or sensory symptoms that are incompatible with recognized neurologic or medical conditions. The symptoms of conversion disorder are produced unconsciously, in contrast to factitious disorder or malingering, and this can be difficult to tease out in the emergency department.

Why is this the correct answer?

A lack of concern by a patient about his or her situation, known as la belle indifférence, has been associated with conversion disorder, but it is not specific and should not be used to make the diagnosis. In the past, this sign was thought to be a hallmark of the disorder, but it actually can be seen just as often in patients with organic disease.

Inconsistent effort can be associated with a variety of conditions such as radiculopathy and can occur secondary to individual variation. In fact, use of its presence to make the diagnosis of conversion disorder has been identified as a factor in erroneous diagnosis.

Although the presence of back pain or trauma in this patient would make an organic etiology more likely, that alone is insufficient to suspect conversion disorder. More information to rule out an organic medical condition is needed.

PEER REVIEW

✓ If you're treating a patient who has a motor or sensory deficit and you can't identify a physical cause, consider conversion disorder.
✓ Conversion disorder is typically associated with a recent stressor.
✓ La belle indifférence can be seen with both conversion disorder and organic illness.

REFERENCES

American Psychiatric Association: Diagnostic and Statistical Manual of Mental Disorders, 5th ed. Washington, DC: American Psychiatric Association, 2013. Section on Somatic Symptom and Related Disorders.

Tintinalli JE, Stapczynski JS, Ma OJ, et al, eds. *Tintinalli's Emergency Medicine: A Comprehensive Study Guide*. 8th ed. New York, NY: McGraw-Hill; 2012: 1951-1952.

185. The correct answer is D, Cocaine-induced psychosis symptoms can persist for several weeks.

Why is this the correct answer?

Although most incidents of substance-induced and medication-induced psychosis resolve shortly after discontinuation of the offending agent, some substances have been reported to cause persistent psychosis for several weeks after cessation of use. These include cocaine, amphetamines, and phencyclidine, often worse with higher doses. Other symptoms include agitation, aggression, and confusion. The psychosis induced by cocaine is often a paranoia regarding being monitored, followed, or watched for drug use, and this can help distinguish psychosis from schizophrenia.

Why are the other choices wrong?

Alcohol-induced psychotic disorder generally occurs in patients with underlying moderate or severe alcohol addiction (alcohol use disorder) after prolonged, heavy intake of alcohol. Hallucinations are common in this patient group, but they are

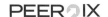

typically auditory. Although some drugs such as cocaine can cause psychosis within minutes of use, alcohol-induced psychosis typically develops over a period of days to weeks of heavy use. A separate alcohol-related condition is Korsakoff psychosis, which involves memory impairment, apathy, and confabulation.

Formication is sometimes referred to as a tactile hallucination: it is the feeling of bugs crawling on or under the skin. It can be seen with amphetamine-induced or cocaine-induced psychotic disorder. Patients can present with significant skin excoriations.

Cannabis-induced psychotic disorder usually involves severe anxiety, emotional lability, and persecutory delusions. The onset can be rapid after high-dose usage and typically resolves within a few days. It is much less likely in amphetamine use.

PEER REVIEW

✓ Alcohol-induced psychosis occurs in moderate to severe alcohol use disorder after prolonged periods of heavy drinking.
✓ Psychoses induced by medications can happen right away or days or weeks later, depending on the offending agent.

REFERENCES

American Psychiatric Association: Diagnostic and Statistical Manual of Mental Disorders. 5th ed. Washington, DC: American Psychiatric Association, 2013.

Hoffman RS, Howland MA, Lewin NA, et al. *Goldfrank's Toxicologic Emergencies.* 10th ed. New York, NY: McGraw-Hill; 2010:1054-1063.

Marx JA, Hockberger RS, Walls RM, eds. *Rosen's Emergency Medicine: Concepts and Clinical Practice.* 8th ed. St. Louis, MO: Elsevier; 2014: 2378-2394.

Tintinalli J, Benegal V. Psychosis among substance users. *Curr Opin Psychiatry.* 2006;19(3):239-245. Available at: http://www.medscape.com/viewarticle/528487_5. Accessed October 8, 2016.

186. The correct answer is A, Germ cell tumor.

Why is this the correct answer?

Testicular cancer (a germ cell tumor) presents with a painless and unilateral mass. Some patients also describe a fullness, tugging, or a heavy sensation in the testis. On examination, a firm mass is palpated; the mass cannot be transilluminated. In this patient, the positive hCG test supports the diagnosis of a germ cell tumor; this marker is secreted by the cancer cells in some of the germ cell tumors found in testicular cancer. The remainder of the physical examination should focus on lymphadenopathy (especially inguinal and supraclavicular), the abdomen, and gynecomastia. It is important to note that the diagnosis of testicular mass can be complicated by a concomitant hydrocele or acute hemorrhage into the tumor. Additional emergency department workup for patients with suspected testicular carcinoma or testicular mass includes ultrasound examination and urgent urologic referral. There is an increased incidence of testicular cancer among patients with undescended testes. Most testicular tumors are of germ cell origin, divided between seminomas and other mixed tumors.

Why are the other choices wrong?

A hydrocele, a collection of fluid around the tunica vaginalis more common on the right side, can be associated with a tumor. The area of the hydrocele should transilluminate on examination. Hydroceles generally resolve by 2 years of age without intervention.

The most common cancers that metastasize to the testes include lymphoma, leukemia, and lung cancer. Patients with lung cancer generally have supraclavicular lymphadenopathy or pulmonary symptoms.

Orchitis is inflammation of the testis and is commonly associated with viral infections such as Epstein-Barr virus or mumps. Orchitis is rare and presents with painful and enlarged testes.

PEER REVIEW

✓ Testicular cancer presents as a painless testicular mass that does not transilluminate on examination.
✓ Germ cell tumors secrete hCG, so a clinical suspicion can be investigated by ordering a quantitative hCG level.
✓ Urgent ultrasonography examination and urology referral are indicated in patients who present with testicular mass.

REFERENCES

Marx JA, Hockberger RS, Walls RM, eds. *Rosen's Emergency Medicine: Concepts and Clinical Practice*. 8th ed. St. Louis, MO: Elsevier; 2014: 2205-2223.

Tintinalli JE, Stapczynski JS, Ma OJ, et al, eds. *Tintinalli's Emergency Medicine: A Comprehensive Study Guide*. 8th ed. New York, NY: McGraw-Hill; 2012: 601-609.

187. The correct answer is D, Older than 75 years.

Why is this the correct answer?

According to the National Center for Health Statistics, the U.S. suicide rate rose 24% over a 15-year period ending in 2014. Although there were sharp increases among women 45 to 64 years old and girls 10 to 14 years old, the largest suicide rate is still in men older than 75 years. Although suicide risk must be assessed on an individual basis, various risk factors have been identified. The SAD PERSONS scale, originally published in 1983 and since modified and adapted, is a helpful tool to assess a patient's suicide risk according to patient characteristics such as sex, age, depression, previous attempt, social factors, and more. Patients with depression and suicidal ideation frequently present to the emergency department. Indeed, one of the most important tasks for the emergency physician in assessing a patient with depression is to assess for suicidality. Although females do attempt suicide more frequently than males, males are four times more likely to complete suicide. Another key factor on the scale is sickness, in particular, chronic, debilitating, or severe illness. Other notable risk factors include concomitant substance abuse, lack of a spouse, previous suicide

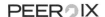

attempts, access to firearms, and previous history of childhood abuse. Adults with a history of childhood maltreatment have been found to be 25 times more likely to attempt suicide than those without such a history.

Why are the other choices wrong?

Organized plan is another of the factors of the SAD PERSONS scale, and the implication is that a person who has a plan is more likely to carry it out than is someone who does not.

Sex is another factor on the scale. Although the gap has narrowed over the past decade, men are still far more likely to complete suicide than women.

Persons who are married and who have other forms of social support are less likely to complete a suicide attempt.

PEER POINT

SAD PERSONS Scale

Developed by Patterson (1983) and modified by Hockberger and Rothstein (1988)

S = Sex (male)

A = Age (<19 or >45)

D = Depression or hopelessness; admits to depression or decreased concentration, appetite, sleep, libido

P = Previous suicide attempt; previous attempts or psychiatric care; previous inpatient or outpatient psychiatric care

E = Ethanol abuse; excessive alcohol or drug use; stigmata of chronic addiction or recent frequent use

R = Rational thinking loss; organic brain syndrome or psychosis

S = Social supports lacking; separated, divorced, or widowed

O = Organized plan; organized or serious attempt; well-thought-out plan or "life-threatening" presentation

N = No spouse; no social supports; no close family, friends, job, or active religious affiliation

S = Sickness (chronic debilitating disease); stated future intent; determined to repeat attempt or ambivalent

PEER REVIEW

- ✓ Assess for suicidality in the evaluation of depressed patients.
- ✓ Elderly white men are at highest risk of successfully committing suicide.
- ✓ History of childhood abuse is a significant risk factor for suicide.

REFERENCES

Hockberger RS, Rothstein RJ. Assessment of suicide potential by nonpsychiatrists using the SAD PERSONS scale. *J Emerg Med.* 1988;6:99-107.

Tintinalli JE, Stapczynski JS, Ma OJ, et al, eds. *Tintinalli's Emergency Medicine: A Comprehensive Study Guide.* 8th ed. New York, NY: McGraw-Hill; 2012: 1963-1969.

Zun L, Chepenik LG, Mallory MNS. *Behavioral Emergencies for the Emergency Physician.* Cambridge, NY: Cambridge; 2013: 60.

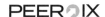

188. The correct answer is D, Tracheoesophageal fistula.

Why is this the correct answer?

A tracheoesophageal fistula is an anatomical defect, an abnormal channel that connects the trachea and the esophagus. It can affect the tolerance of feeding or even secretions in neonates. A congenital fistula is most often associated with esophageal atresia (85%), and because of this combination, patients present for evaluation early in the neonatal period. The most common type of tracheoesophageal fistula is the H type, so named because the shape formed from the anatomic positioning from the esophagus to the trachea is an H.

Why are the other choices wrong?

An esophageal web is a congenital membrane that often allows liquids but not solid foods to pass. As such, this condition does not become an issue until solid foods are introduced.

Gastroesophageal reflux disease (GERD) is an extremely common condition, especially in premature neonates. It presents with emesis after feeds and can be severe enough to lead to aspiration issues, esophageal disorders (including inflammation, stricture, or ulceration), or even nutritional issues that result in failure to thrive. It often requires no medical intervention and resolves as the child grows. It is characterized by multiple small bouts of emesis, also known as "wet burps." In contrast, the tracheoesophageal fistula presents with episodes of respiratory distress after a feed.

A Meckel diverticulum is ectopic gastric tissue that is found in only 2% of the population and becomes an issue in only 2% of those who have it. It generally presents with a history of GI bleeding but can manifest as intussusception or even peritonitis from perforation.

PEER REVIEW

- ✓ If you're treating a patient younger than 3 months who has choking and gagging episodes, consider a congenital malformation of the esophagus.
- ✓ Gastroesophageal reflux disease is common, especially in premature neonates, but is often outgrown.
- ✓ How can you tell it's gastroesophageal reflux disease? Multiple bouts of spit up or wet burps soon after feeds.

REFERENCES

Fleisher GR, Ludwig S, et al, eds. *Textbook of Pediatric Emergency Medicine*. 6th ed. Philadelphia, PA: Lippincott, Williams & Wilkins; 2010: 1298; 1529.

Wolfson AB, Hendey GW, Ling LJ, et al, eds. *Harwood-Nuss' Clinical Practice of Emergency Medicine*. 6th ed. Philadelphia, PA: Lippincott, Williams & Wilkins; 2014: 1069-1070.

189. The correct answer is C, Nearly all demonstrate a high tolerance to pain.

Why is this the correct answer?

Excited delirium syndrome (ExDS), previously referred to as agitated delirium, is a unique syndrome that can be identified by the presence of a distinctive group of behavioral and clinical characteristics. It is associated with altered mental status due to delirium along with severe aggressiveness or excitement. One characteristic demonstrated by nearly all patients is pain tolerance, along with tachypnea, sweating, agitation, and tactile hyperthermia. Due to their extreme combativeness, many patients with ExDS are first encountered by law enforcement and EMS personnel. Excited delirium syndrome has become well known to the public because of its association with sudden death in patients in police custody.

Why are the other choices wrong?

Approximately 11% (not 50%) of patients with ExDS experience sudden death. When sudden death occurs, it is typically following physical control measures, and there is no clear anatomic cause found on autopsy. Some features associated with death include male gender, suspected or known stimulant drug abuse, nudity, unusual physical strength, and cardiopulmonary collapse immediately following a struggle.

Most patients with ExDS exhibit tactile hyperthermia, not hypothermia.

Although stimulants such as cocaine, methamphetamine, and PCP have been associated with ExDS, opiates have not. Benzodiazepines are helpful in the management of ExDS patients; they have not been thought to be a cause of the syndrome.

PEER POINT

Features most frequently associated with excited delirium syndrome, from ACEP "White Paper Report on Excited Delirium Syndrome"

- Pain tolerance
- Tachypnea
- Sweating
- Agitation
- Tactile hyperthermia
- Police noncompliance
- Lack of tiring
- Unusual strength
- Inappropriately clothed
- Mirror or glass attraction

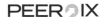

PEER REVIEW

✓ Excited delirium syndrome is associated with altered mental status, delirium, and aggressiveness.

✓ Nearly all patients with excited delirium syndrome exhibit high pain tolerance.

✓ Benzodiazepines are a good first-line therapy for the management of excited delirium syndrome, especially if the source of agitation is thought to be stimulant drug use.

REFERENCES

ACEP Excited Delirium Task Force. *White Paper Report on Excited Delirium Syndrome*. Dallas, TX: American College of Emergency Physicians. September 10, 2009.

Zun L, Chepenik LG, Mallory MNS. *Behavioral Emergencies for the Emergency Physician*. Cambridge, NY: Cambridge; 2013: 125-131.

190. The correct answer is B, Increased efficacy in treating negative symptoms.

Why is this the correct answer?

The atypical antipsychotic agents, which are mostly newer medications than the typical antipsychotic agents, more specifically target dopamine receptors or inhibit serotonin reuptake. They are also more effective in managing the negative symptoms of psychoses such as affective flattening or blunting (a reduction of the external signs of emotion), alogia (decreased speech), and poverty of speech.

Why are the other choices wrong?

Because of the improved receptor specificity of the atypical over the typical antipsychotic medications, some of the adverse effects such as sedation, QTc interval prolongation, tardive dyskinesia, and extrapyramidal symptoms are reduced but not totally eliminated. Both classes of medications are associated with hypotension, typically orthostatic, which is thought to be related to adrenergic and anticholinergic blockade. This can usually be easily managed with intravenous fluids.

Neuroleptic malignant syndrome is a rare reaction to both typical and atypical neuroleptic medications characterized by rigidity, confusion, autonomic instability, and fever; it is considered a medical emergency with a high rate of morbidity and mortality.

The U.S. Food and Drug Administration has placed a black box warning on both typical and atypical antipsychotic agents for their use in managing agitation in elderly patients with dementia, as chronic use of these medications in this population has been linked to increased rates of cardiovascular and cerebrovascular events and mortality.

PEER POINT

From the U.S. Food & Drug Administration

Atypical antipsychotic drugs

- Aripiprazole (marketed as Abilify)
- Asenapine maleate (marketed as Saphris)
- Clozapine (marketed as Clozaril)
- Iloperidone (marketed as Fanapt)
- Lurasidone (marketed as Latuda)
- Olanzapine (marketed as Zyprexa)
- Olanzapine/Fluoxetine (marketed as Symbyax)
- Paliperidone (marketed as Invega)
- Quetiapine (marketed as Seroquel)
- Risperidone (marketed as Risperdal)
- Ziprasidone (marketed as Geodon)

PEER REVIEW

✓ Patients who take atypical antipsychotic medications experience fewer movement and muscle control side effects than they would if they took the typical medications.

✓ Atypical antipsychotic agents manage the negative symptoms of psychosis more effectively.

✓ Neuroleptic malignant syndrome is a rare reaction, but it's associated with both typical and atypical antipsychotic medications and high morbidity and mortality rates.

REFERENCES

Tintinalli JE, Stapczynski JS, Ma OJ, et al, eds. *Tintinalli's Emergency Medicine: A Comprehensive Study Guide*. 8th ed. New York, NY: McGraw-Hill; 2012: 1969-1972.

Wolfson AB, Hendey GW, Ling LJ, et al, eds. *Harwood-Nuss' Clinical Practice of Emergency Medicine*. 6th ed. Philadelphia, PA: Lippincott, Williams & Wilkins; 2014: 806-808.

191. The correct answer is B, Driveline.

Why is this the correct answer?

Infection is a common adverse event following placement of a left ventricular assist device (LVAD), occurring in approximately 40% of patients. Infection most often occurs between 2 weeks and 2 months after implantation. The various sites of LVAD-related infection include the incision site, pump pocket, driveline, and the various cannulas. The driveline is the most common site of infection. This line exits the chest wall protected by a skin seal and is thus most susceptible to infection. Empiric antibiotic therapy should cover both staphylococcal species as well as various gram-negative organisms, including *Pseudomonas*.

Why are the other choices wrong?

The various cannulas of the LVAD circuit can be involved in the infectious process, but they are not the most common site of infection.

The site of the incision is also susceptible to infection, but it is not the most common site of infection following LVAD placement.

The pump pocket is the second most common area of infection. The driveline goes into the pump, which is contained within a pocket in the chest wall.

PEER REVIEW

✓ The most common location for infection in LVAD is most commonly the driveline, and then the pump pocket.

REFERENCES

Birks EJ, Tansley PD, Hardy, J et al. Left ventricular assist device and drug therapy for the reversal of heart failure. *N Engl J Med.* 2006;355:1873–1884.

Kovala CE, Rakitab R; AST Infectious Diseases Community of Practice. Ventricular assist device related infections and solid organ transplantation. *Am J Transplant.* 2013;13: 348–354.

Rose EA, Gelijns AC, Moskowitz AJ et al: Long-Term Use of a Left Ventricular Assist Device for End-Stage Heart Failure. *N Engl J Med.* 2001; 345:1435-1443.

192. The correct answer is D, Transthoracic echocardiography.

Why is this the correct answer?

The ECG demonstrates left ventricular hypertrophy, and Q waves in leads I and aVL are all characteristic and highly suggestive of hypertrophic cardiomyopathy. Such findings should prompt ordering of transthoracic echocardiography to confirm the diagnosis; furthermore, exercise restriction and cardiology referral should also be considered. Hypertrophic cardiomyopathy is an autosomal-dominant disease characterized by disorganized cardiac cell arrangement, asymmetric hypertrophy of the ventricular septum, and malformations of the mitral valve leaflets. These structural abnormalities can lead to fatal tachyarrhythmias and ventricular outflow obstruction. Hypertrophic cardiomyopathy is the single most common cardiac cause of death in young athletes. Patients might present with activity-induced shortness of breath, near syncope, syncope, chest pain, palpitations, and even sudden death. In addition to strenuous activity or exertion, other "hyperadrenergic" states can precipitate arrhythmia, including extreme emotions (anger, fright). Thus the consideration of adrenergically related syncope is a more appropriate screening process than simply exertional syncope. The most specific ECG findings in hypertrophic cardiomyopathy are deep, narrow Q waves in the lateral leads (I, aVL, V5, V6). The most common, however, are large-amplitude QRS complexes consistent with left ventricular hypertrophy and associated ST-segment and T-segment changes in the precordial leads. Other ECG findings might include high-voltage R waves in V1 and V2 and deep narrow Q waves in the inferior leads

(II, III, aVF). In the 12-lead ECG from this case, note the presence of prominent R waves and ST-segment elevation in the right to midprecordial leads and Q waves in the lateral leads. The lateral Q waves are very specific in the correct clinical setting for hypertrophic cardiomyopathy. Beta blockers, which are the mainstay of therapy, decrease the effect of catecholamines on the outflow gradient.

Why are the other choices wrong?

In a stable patient who had a syncopal episode and does not have any respiratory abnormalities, a chest xray has limited value.

Similarly, CT scanning of the head has limited utility in the syncope patient who has no neurologic concerns.

Coronary CT angiography is useful in some chest pain patients suspected of coronary abnormalities, but it has no value in the initial evaluation of the syncope patient.

PEER REVIEW

✓ Hypertrophic cardiomyopathy is the most common cause of sudden cardiac death in young athletes.
✓ The most specific ECG findings of hypertrophic cardiomyopathy are deep, narrow Q waves in the lateral leads.
✓ Consider adrenergically mediated syncope as a possible suggestion of the presence of hypertrophic cardiomyopathy.

REFERENCES
Brady WJ, Truwit JD. *Critical Decisions in Emergency and Acute Care Electrocardiography*. Blackwell Publishing, Ltd.; 2009: 43-44.
Tintinalli JE, Stapczynski JS, Ma OJ, et al, eds. *Tintinalli's Emergency Medicine: A Comprehensive Study Guide*. 8th ed. New York, NY: McGraw-Hill; 2012: 112-134.

193. The correct answer is D, Immediate transfer for primary PCI.

Why is this the correct answer?

Patients with STEMI and cardiogenic shock or severe heart failure initially seen at non–PCI-capable hospitals should be transferred for cardiac catheterization and revascularization as soon as possible regardless of time delay from STEMI onset. The patient in this case is hypotensive and has pulmonary edema. His ECG shows significant anterolateral ST-segment elevation. He is demonstrating signs of cardiogenic shock and severe heart failure, and transfer for PCI can be achieved in less than 120 minutes, so he should be transferred immediately. Immediate transfer to a PCI center is also recommended for patients without shock if the symptoms have been present for fewer than 12 hours and the first provider contact-to-balloon time is expected to be less than 120 minutes. In general, transfer for primary PCI, the preferred strategy in STEMI, is indicated in STEMI patients but is related to the total STEMI duration time. Early in STEMI, the recommended time to reperfusion therapy is quite short — if the duration of the STEMI is less than 2 hours, PCI should be initiated in 60 minutes or less, and if the duration of the STEMI is 2 to 3 hours, PCI should be initiated within 120 minutes. Later in STEMI time course, longer time periods are allowed — after 3 hours of STEMI, PCI should be initiated within 120 minutes.

Why are the other choices wrong?

Emergency coronary artery bypass grafting within 6 hours of symptom onset may be considered in patients with STEMI who do not have cardiogenic shock and are not candidates for PCI or fibrinolytic therapy (IIbC). The patient in this case is demonstrating signs of shock.

In the absence of contraindications, fibrinolytic therapy should be started for patients with STEMI and onset of ischemic symptoms within the previous 12 hours when it is anticipated that primary PCI cannot be performed in a timely manner. In the absence of contraindications and when PCI is not available, fibrinolytic therapy is reasonable for patients with STEMI if there is clinical or ECG evidence of ongoing ischemia within 12 to 24 hours of symptom onset and a large area of myocardium at risk or hemodynamic instability (IIaC). But this approach is not the intervention for the patient in this case, who is very sick and can undergo PCI within the acceptable timeframe.

Multiple studies have investigated the role of facilitated PCI (full-dose or partial-dose fibrinolysis followed by immediate transfer to a PCI-capable facility for PCI) in the management of STEMI. In general, this reperfusion strategy has failed to show a benefit when giving full-dose or partial-dose fibrinolytic agents with planned PCI within 90 to 120 minutes as compared to PCI alone. Thus it is not recommended.

PEER REVIEW

- ✓ The preferred strategy in STEMI is PCI, but whether it should be done depends on how long the STEMI has been underway and how long it will take to get the procedure started.
- ✓ What is "in a timely manner" when it comes to transferring a STEMI patient for PCI? If the duration of the STEMI is less than 2 hours, PCI should be initiated in 60 minutes or less. If it's 2 to 3 hours, PCI should be initiated within 120 minutes.
- ✓ Cardiogenic shock + STEMI = immediate transfer for primary PCI; this is a very sick patient, and fibrinolysis has little outcome-altering benefit.
- ✓ If you're treating a STEMI patient who has been resuscitated from cardiac arrest, strongly consider PCI.

REFERENCES

Marx JA, Hockberger RS, Walls RM, eds. *Rosen's Emergency Medicine: Concepts and Clinical Practice*. 8th ed. St. Louis, MO: Elsevier; 2014: 997-1032.

O'Connor RE, Al Ali AS, Brady WJ, et al: Part 9: Acute Coronary Syndromes—2015 American Heart Association Guidelines Update for Cardiopulmonary Resuscitation and Emergency Cardiovascular Care. *Circulation*. 2015;132:S483-S500.

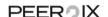
194. The correct answer is C, Necrotizing enterocolitis.

Why is this the correct answer?

The radiograph demonstrates pneumatosis intestinalis, or air within the bowel wall. This is a hallmark finding of necrotizing enterocolitis (NEC), but up to one third of patients with this condition do not have this finding. Necrotizing enterocolitis can be seen in premature and full-term neonates, usually within the first 1 to 2 weeks of life. Concerning clinical signs include a toxic appearance, lethargy or somnolence, a distended abdomen, and hematochezia. In general, emergency physicians should have a heightened suspicion for abdominal illness in the evaluation of any neonate or young infant presenting with decreased activity or failure to thrive.

Why are the other choices wrong?

Gastroesophageal reflux, although common, is rarely a cause of abdominal pain and bloody stools in neonates. It is more commonly associated with vomiting and possibly failure to thrive.

Intussusception is an abdominal emergency that involves invagination of a section of bowel into the next section, with potential disruption of blood flow that could ultimately lead to necrosis. The classic triad presentation is intermittent, colicky abdominal pain (followed by periods of sleepiness), emesis, and bloody stools, but this triad is present in less than half of those with the disease. Intussusception rarely presents in children younger than 5 months or older than early school age. A radiograph might show a filling defect corresponding to the area of invaginated bowel.

Volvulus is a surgical emergency; any bilious vomiting in a neonate warrants immediate evaluation. Radiographs might not show signs of obstruction in this age group (air/fluid levels, paucity of gas in the distal bowel). A high clinical suspicion might be confirmed with an upper GI series, which can then delineate the location of the volvulus.

PEER REVIEW

- ✓ Necrotizing enterocolitis can develop in both preterm and full-term neonates.
- ✓ Pneumatosis intestinalis, gas within the bowel wall, is a hallmark finding for necrotizing enterocolitis.
- ✓ What are the concerning clinical signs for necrotizing enterocolitis? Toxic appearance, lethargy/somnolence, distended abdomen, and hematochezia.
- ✓ Suspect abdominal illness in any neonate or young infant with decreased activity or failure to thrive.

REFERENCES

Fleisher GR, Ludwig S, et al, eds. *Textbook of Pediatric Emergency Medicine*. 6th ed. Philadelphia, PA: Lippincott, Williams & Wilkins; 2010: 575.

Wolfson AB, Hendey GW, Ling LJ, et al, eds. *Harwood-Nuss' Clinical Practice of Emergency Medicine*. 6th ed. Philadelphia, PA: Lippincott, Williams & Wilkins; 2014: 1125.

195. The correct answer is D, Vancomycin.

Why is this the correct answer?

Vancomycin is the most appropriate initial antibiotic choice for the emergency department treatment of suspected infective endocarditis. *Staphylococcus aureus* is the most common causative pathogen (over 30% of cases) in all types of infective endocarditis, and vancomycin provides excellent antibiotic coverage. It also is the drug of choice for MRSA infections. Use of combination antibiotic therapy is generally recommended for endocarditis, but vancomycin is the most appropriate first-line antibiotic for an emergency physician to start while considering the possible etiology and assistance from infectious disease consultation. Most patients with endocarditis have either predisposing cardiac abnormalities (prosthetic valve, mitral valve prolapse, bicuspid aortic valve, calcific aortic stenosis) or risk factors for disease (Injected drug use, indwelling catheters, poor dental hygiene, HIV). A history of intravenous drug abuse puts a patient at even higher risk of *S. aureus* infection (>50% cases). The diagnosis of infective endocarditis can be made using the modified Duke Criteria (sensitivity >90%), which involves the identification of two major criteria or one major and three minor criteria or five minor criteria.

Why are the other choices wrong?

Cefepime is a cephalosporin commonly used in the treatment of pneumonia, febrile neutropenia, UTIs, skin infections, and as an adjunct in the treatment of intraabdominal infections. It covers *S. aureus* infection, but studies indicate that its potential effectiveness against a MRSA infection lies in combination with another antimicrobial. For that reason, it is not a good empiric choice for endocarditis, and certainly not a better choice than vancomycin.

Gentamicin is an aminoglycoside and often a first-line choice against infections with gram-negative organisms such as *Pseudomonas aeruginosa, Proteus, Escherichia coli, Klebsiella, Enterobacter, Serratia,* and *Citrobacter,* as well as gram-positive staphylococcal infections. But like moxifloxacin, gentamicin does not provide adequate antistaphylococcal coverage for suspected infective endocarditis. Gentamicin is part of the treatment regimen for some types of infective endocarditis but in combination with another antibiotic such as penicillin, nafcillin, or ceftriaxone. In recent years, MRSA infection has become resistant to gentamicin.

Moxifloxacin is a fluoroquinolone that has good coverage for streptococcal species and variable susceptibility with MRSA, but it does not provide adequate antistaphylococcal coverage for suspected infective endocarditis. It is typically used in the treatment of community-acquired pneumonia, as well as skin infections, some abdominal infections, and bacterial bronchitis and sinusitis.

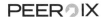

PEER POINT

Duke criteria for infective endocarditis

Look for two major criteria or one major and three minor criteria or five minor criteria

Major

- Positive blood culture (two separate blood cultures)
- Typical infective endocarditis microorganism (*S. aureus* or *enterococci*, or *Streptococcus bovis*, viridans, or HACEK group [*Haemophilus*, *Actinobacillus*, *Cardiobacterium*, *Eikenella*, and *Kingella*])

OR

- Microorganisms consistent with infective endocarditis from persistently positive blood cultures
- Positive cardiac involvement on echocardiogram (vegetations, abscess, new prosthetic valve dehiscence, or new valvular regurgitation)
- Positive ECG

Minor

- Predisposing heart condition or prior intravenous drug use
- Fever
- Vascular phenomena (septic emboli, Janeway lesions, etc.)
- Immunologic phenomena (glomerulonephritis, Osler nodes, Roth spots, rheumatic fever)
- Microbiologic evidence (positive blood culture not meeting major criteria)

PEER REVIEW

- ✓ Vancomycin is the most appropriate empiric antibiotic choice for suspected infective endocarditis.
- ✓ The most common pathogen causing infective endocarditis is *Staphylococcus aureus*.
- ✓ Infective endocarditis is most commonly associated with either predisposing cardiac abnormalities or risk factors of disease such as intravenous drug abuse, HIV, indwelling catheters, and poor dental hygiene.
- ✓ The Duke Criteria have a sensitivity higher than 90% for the diagnosis of infective endocarditis.

REFERENCES

Gilbert DN, Chambers HF, Eliopoulous GM, et al, eds. The Sanford Guide to Antimicrobial Therapy 2015. 2015: 72-76.

Infective Endocarditis in Adults: Diagnosis, Antimicrobial Therapy, and Management of Complications (AHA) (Endorsed by IDSA). *Circulation*. 2015;132:1 -53. http://circ.ahajournals.org/content/circulationaha/early/2015/09/15/CIR.0000000000000296.full. pdf

Marx JA, Hockberger RS, Walls RM, eds. *Rosen's Emergency Medicine: Concepts and Clinical Practice*. 8th ed. St. Louis, MO: Elsevier; 2014: 1106-1112.

Mattu A, Brady WJ, et al (eds). *Cardiovascular Emergencies*. Dallas, TX: American College of Emergency Physicians Publishing; 2014: 209-226.

196. The correct answer is B, Presence of diaphoresis.

Why is this the correct answer?

The presence of diaphoresis, while not diagnostic of ACS, is strongly suggestive of ACS and presents a high likelihood for it. Of course, when taking a history and performing a physical examination, the emergency physician should investigate other explanations for diaphoresis, including hypoglycemia, high environmental temperature, anxiety, medications, and so on. In the approach to a patient with suspected acute coronary ischemia, the emergency physician has to consider many factors of the history and examination — how the patient describes his or her symptoms, what the patient's medical history is, whether there is a family history of cardiovascular disease, what clues the ECG provides, what abnormalities are noted in cardiac markers, and often more. The high likelihood features of ACS, in addition to diaphoresis, include chest pain that is similar to the patient's prior anginal chest pain, known coronary artery disease, a history of MI, mitral regurgitation, hypotension, pulmonary edema, new ST-segment elevation greater than or equal to 1 mm or T-wave inversion in multiple anatomically oriented leads, and elevated cardiac serum markers.

Why are the other choices wrong?

If a patient presents with classic risk factors for coronary artery disease such as a medical history of hypertension, diabetes mellitus, or hyperlipidemia; a family history of MI before age 50 years; and smoking, the emergency physician should, of course, consider ACS. But these features are not the most suggestive of acute coronary ischemia, and are not even high likelihood features for ACS. They represent, at most, intermediate likelihood features.

Recent cocaine use is a low likelihood finding for acute MI.

Although T-wave flattening is an abnormal ECG finding, it has a low likelihood for ACS.

PEER REVIEW

✓ Diaphoresis is strongly suggestive of ACS.

✓ Clinical features — in addition to diaphoresis — associated with a high likelihood for ACS: chest pain, mitral regurgitation, hypotension, pulmonary edema, elevated cardiac serum markers.

✓ The ECG features on the ACS high likelihood list: new ST-segment elevation greater than or equal to 1 mm or T-wave inversion in multiple anatomically oriented leads.

✓ High likelihood features of ACS from a patient's history: previous MI, known coronary artery disease.

REFERENCES

Marx JA, Hockberger RS, Walls RM, eds. *Rosen's Emergency Medicine: Concepts and Clinical Practice.* 8th ed. St. Louis, MO: Elsevier; 2014: 997-1033.

Mattu A, Brady WJ, et al (eds). *Cardiovascular Emergencies.* Dallas, TX: American College of Emergency Physicians Publishing; 2014: 11-35.

O'Connor RE, Al Ali AS, Brady WJ, et al: Part 9: Acute Coronary Syndromes—2015 American Heart Association Guidelines Update for Cardiopulmonary Resuscitation and Emergency Cardiovascular Care. *Circulation.* 2015;132:S483-500.

197. The correct answer is A, Abnormal sensation of the finger pad of the second finger.

Why is this the correct answer?

Carpal tunnel syndrome (CTS), or median mononeuropathy, is the most common entrapment neuropathy in the United States. Symptoms are generally unilateral and are worsened by repetitive use such as typing at work all day. Carpal tunnel syndrome is commonly associated with pregnancy, obesity, diabetes mellitus, and renal failure. In patients with bilateral symptoms, CTS usually is related to systemic illness. When examining a patient with suspected CTS, it is important to remember that the median nerve causes numbness involving the palm and palmar surface of the first three fingers, then splits at the fourth digit and supplies only the radial aspect of that finger, generally leaving sensation of the ulnar side of the fourth finger and the fifth finger intact. Sensory findings generally precede motor symptoms, and the most sensitive examination finding is an alteration in sensation to the distal tuft of the index finger. Initial treatment for CTS is application of a wrist splint and instructions to the patient to reduce activities that make the condition worse. Patients should be referred for surgical follow-up; a surgeon or other specialist would consider steroid injections or surgical management if wrist splinting fails to resolve the symptoms.

Why are the other choices wrong?

The Phalen maneuver is conducted by having the patient hold his or her wrists in the flexed position with the hands touching each other on the dorsal surface. If CTS is present, the patient should experience tingling in the distribution of the median nerve. However, this test has been found to be not sensitive or specific in determining who should be referred for electrodiagnostic testing.

The Tinel test, another approach to diagnosing CTS, is positive when percussion over the median nerve causes tingling in the hand in the distribution of the median nerve. Similar to the Phalen maneuver, it has been found to be not sensitive or specific in determining who should be referred for electrodiagnostic testing.

A patient with CTS might demonstrate weakened grip strength on examination, but this is not the most sensitive finding. It is important to remember that sensory findings generally precede motor symptoms.

PEER POINT

Color blocking to show innervation of the hand

Purple indicates median nerve distribution (yellow, ulnar; red, radial)

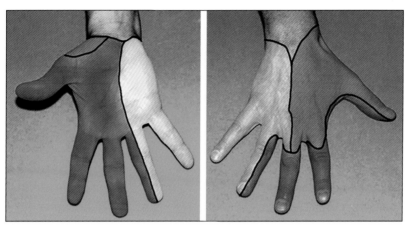

PEER Point 18

PEER REVIEW

✓ Characteristic feature of carpal tunnel syndrome: paresthesias of the first three digits of the hand and the dorsal aspect of the fourth.

✓ The Tinel sign and the Phalen maneuver are neither sensitive nor specific for carpal tunnel syndrome.

✓ How do you treat carpal tunnel syndrome? Initially, splint the wrist in a neutral position and tell the patient to stop doing what makes it hurt. If this doesn't resolve it, the patient should follow up with a surgeon.

REFERENCES

Marx JA, Hockberger RS, Walls RM, eds. *Rosen's Emergency Medicine: Concepts and Clinical Practice.* 8th ed. St. Louis, MO: Elsevier; 2014: 1428-1440.

Tintinalli JE, Stapczynski JS, Ma OJ, et al, eds. *Tintinalli's Emergency Medicine: A Comprehensive Study Guide.* 8th ed. New York, NY: McGraw-Hill; 2012: 1178-1185.

198. The correct answer is B, Infuse unfractionated heparin while waiting for results of CT angiography.

Why is this the correct answer?

The concern for PE in this patient begins with her symptoms of pleuritic chest pain and shortness of breath. Applying the Wells criteria puts her in the high-risk category for PE: alternative diagnosis less likely than PE, 3 points; heart rate over 100, 1.5 points; suspected DVT, 3 points; and active malignancy, 1 point, for a total of 8.5. Given this high pretest probability for PE, initiating empiric treatment with heparin while waiting for confirmation of the diagnosis is a reasonable approach. She has no major contraindications to anticoagulation, and the delay for CT angiography can be several hours in a busy emergency department. Studies have shown that unfractionated heparin and low-molecular-weight heparin have the same efficacy. Low-molecular-weight heparin has fewer bleeding complications but should not be used in patients with renal insufficiency or those at the extremes of weight. The Wells criteria are as follows:

- Suspected DVT, 3 points
- Alternative diagnosis less likely than PE, 3 points
- Heart rate higher than 100 beats/min, 1.5 point
- Prior venous thromboembolism, 1.5 points
- Immobilization within prior 4 weeks, 1.5 point
- Active malignancy, 1 point
- Hemoptysis, 1 point

High risk is a score higher than 6. A score of 2 to 6 reflects moderate risk for PE, and a score lower than 2 is low risk.

Why are the other choices wrong?

Fibrinolytic agents are indicated for hemodynamically unstable patients and/or patients with a large clot burden, but this patient is normotensive and not hypoxic. In hemodynamically unstable patients with known PE, fibrinolysis is potentially indicated. If PE is suspected but not yet diagnosed, there is insufficient data to support the empiric use of fibrinolytic agents.

This patient has a high pretest probability for PE, and the D-dimer is not useful in ruling out PE in this situation. A D-dimer can be used to rule out PE in patients with a low pretest probability for PE. Additionally, in patients who have had symptoms longer than 3 days, the sensitivity of the D-dimer can decrease because the half-life is less than 8 hours.

Surgical embolectomy is indicated for patients with severe refractory hypotension or with very large clot burden, which this patient does not have.

PEER POINT

ECG changes in PE: right bundle branch block, T-wave inversion, and S1Q3T3 pattern

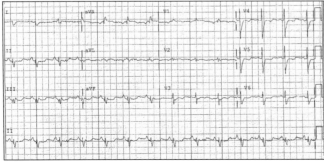

PEER Point 19

PEER REVIEW

✓ You should start heparin in patients with a high pretest probability for PE while waiting for confirmatory test results.

✓ A negative D-dimer is useful to rule out PE in low probability patients but not in patients with a high pretest probability.

✓ Fibrinolytic agents are indicated for hemodynamically unstable patients with PE.

REFERENCES

Marx JA, Hockberger RS, Walls RM, eds. *Rosen's Emergency Medicine: Concepts and Clinical Practice.* 8th ed. St. Louis, MO: Elsevier; 2014: 1157-1169.

Tintinalli JE, Stapczynski JS, Ma OJ, et al, eds. *Tintinalli's Emergency Medicine: A Comprehensive Study Guide.* 8th ed. New York, NY: McGraw-Hill; 2012: 388-399.

199. The correct answer is D, Most tobacco-related conditions are caused by the non-nicotine components of tobacco.

Why is this the correct answer?

Smoking, according to the Surgeon General of the United States, is one of the greatest public health catastrophes of the 20th century. Fortunately, nicotine replacement products, first approved by the U.S. Food & Drug Administration in 1984, are effective at relieving nicotine withdrawal symptoms and weaning smokers off cigarettes. Using "nicotine to treat a nicotine addiction" is counterintuitive to many patients, and one strategy is to explain that most of the medical consequences of tobacco use are related to tars, carbon monoxide, and other non-nicotine components. According to the National Institute on Drug Abuse, nicotine replacement products generally provide users with lower overall nicotine levels than does tobacco, have little abuse potential, and, as mentioned, do not contain the carcinogens and gases associated with tobacco smoke. The success of nicotine replacement therapy, whether in the form of a patch, gum, spray, or inhaler, is enhanced with behavioral treatment.

Why is this the correct answer?

Nicotine withdrawal can occur when a smoker stops smoking and when a person trying to quit smoking stops using a nicotine replacement product such as a patch. Symptoms include irritability, headaches, increased appetite, depression, and trouble sleeping. Withdrawal symptoms peak 2 to 3 days after the last use.

Nicotine absorption or ingestion can lead to clinically significant overdoses resulting in GI, cardiovascular, respiratory, and neurologic toxicity. Manifestations include tremor, bronchorrhea, bradycardia, arrhythmias, seizures, respiratory failure, coma, and even death. Nicotine poisoning can occur in children after ingestion of as little as one cigarette.

Long-term use of nicotine replacement products does not appear to cause medical harm.

PEER REVIEW

✓ Most illnesses associated with smoking are related to the non-nicotine components of cigarettes.

✓ Nicotine overdose can result in significant clinical toxicity.

✓ If you're counseling a patient about smoking cessation, remember that nicotine replacement therapy is more effective when combined with behavioral therapy.

REFERENCES

American Psychiatric Association: Diagnostic and Statistical Manual of Mental Disorders. 5th ed. Washington, DC: American Psychiatric Association, 2013.

National Institute on Drug Abuse. Are there effective treatments for tobacco addiction? NIDA website. Available at: https://www. drugabuse.gov/publications/research-reports/tobacco/are-there-effective-treatments-tobacco-addiction. Accessed October 9, 2016.

Tintinalli JE, Stapczynski JS, Ma OJ, et al, eds. *Tintinalli's Emergency Medicine: A Comprehensive Study Guide.* 8th ed. New York, NY: McGraw-Hill; 2012: 1280-1284.

200. The correct answer is B, Physicians are immune from legal retaliation by parents.

Why is this the correct answer?

Although the details of the specific legal requirements for reporting suspected child abuse and neglect vary by state, all states require physicians to report any suspected abuse or neglect to a legal authority. Furthermore, as mandatory reporters, physicians are granted complete immunity from legal retaliation by parents for reporting their suspicions. These protections exist specifically so that physicians do not hesitate to report abuse or neglect that they cannot definitively prove. Nearly 1 million cases of suspected child maltreatment are reported each year in the United States. Of those, the vast majority involve general neglect. The second most prevalent form of maltreatment involves physical abuse, followed by sexual abuse, psychological maltreatment, and medical neglect.

Why are the other choices wrong?

Although physicians might be hesitant to report abuse or neglect without definitive proof, they are nonetheless legally required to do so. It is not the role of physicians to provide legal proof of abuse; they must merely report their suspicions in a clear and objective manner.

All states consider physicians to be mandatory reporters of suspected child abuse and neglect. It is not optional.

Any suspected child maltreatment should be reported, including all forms of abuse and neglect.

PEER REVIEW

✓ Emergency physicians are mandatory reporters of suspected child maltreatment.

✓ You don't have to be absolutely certain before you report suspected abuse.

✓ There are many forms of child maltreatment, including physical and sexual abuse, general neglect, and medical neglect.

REFERENCES

Marx JA, Hockberger RS, Walls RM, eds. *Rosen's Emergency Medicine: Concepts and Clinical Practice*. 8th ed. St. Louis, MO: Elsevier; 2014: 845-854.

Tintinalli JE, Stapczynski JS, Ma OJ, et al, eds. *Tintinalli's Emergency Medicine: A Comprehensive Study Guide*. 8th ed. New York, NY: McGraw-Hill; 2012: 999-1006.

201. The correct answer is D, Pregnancy.

Why is this the correct answer?

Intimate partner violence (IPV), previously known as spousal abuse or domestic violence, occurs across all gender, ethnic, racial, and socioeconomic categories. Up to 45% of women report assault or abuse during pregnancy, and those who suffer abuse during pregnancy are also at increased risk for postnatal abuse. Furthermore, pregnant assault victims are three times more likely than nonpregnant women to be admitted to the hospital. The American Medical Association and The Joint Commission recommend screening all emergency department patients for IPV. Risk factors include female sex, low income level, separated status (as opposed to married or divorced), and age 18 to 24 years. In females 1 to 34 years old, homicide is one of the top five leading causes of death. Of note, nearly half of IPV homicide victims visited a health care provider within 1 year of their deaths. Since the 1970s, there actually has been a steady decline in the rate of homicides attributed to IPV. This decline might be related to improvements in the health, social service, and criminal justice systems, as well as to changing social constructs that more openly address family violence.

Why are the other choices wrong?

Although emergency department clinicians and providers should always have the potential for IPV on their radar, there are certain injury patterns that should increase suspicion. These include injuries suggestive of a defensive posture, multiple injuries in various stages of healing, central injury pattern, and injury type and extent inconsistent with the patient's explanation. Two acute extremity fractures is not necessarily indicative of IPV.

If the relationship status of the couple is separated, rather than divorced or married, the risk for IPV is higher.

Previous IPV is a risk factor for future IPV. There is a typical cycle to IPV: tension building, followed by escalation to abuse, followed by a "honeymoon" phase. Over time, the time intervals between episodes of abuse become shorter. In nearly three-

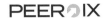

quarters of IPV homicide cases, the death is the end result of an escalating pattern of IPV in the household. The presence of weapons in the home, or a history of threats of murder or previous threat or actual use of weapons, is associated with increased risk of homicide.

PEER REVIEW

✓ Homicide attributed to intimate partner violence is a leading cause of death in females younger than 35 years.

✓ Pregnant patients are at increased risk of intimate partner violence.

✓ The presence of weapons in the home increases the risk of homicide by intimate partner violence.

REFERENCES

Marx JA, Hockberger RS, Walls RM, eds. *Rosen's Emergency Medicine: Concepts and Clinical Practice.* 8th ed. St. Louis, MO: Elsevier; 2014: 872-884.

Tintinalli JE, Stapczynski JS, Ma OJ, et al, eds. *Tintinalli's Emergency Medicine: A Comprehensive Study Guide.* 8th ed. New York, NY: McGraw-Hill; 2012: 1988-1991.

202. The correct answer is B, Chest compressions, electrical defibrillation, basic airway management.

Why is this the correct answer?

In cardiac arrest, the initial rhythm provides important information to guide management. The rhythm shown for this patient is ventricular fibrillation, a shockable rhythm. Electrical defibrillation is the most appropriate intervention and should be performed as early as possible after resuscitation is initiated. Chest compressions are, of course, a priority in early management. Studies have shown that basic airway management (bag-valve mask) is appropriate while prioritizing compressions and defibrillation. The four cardiac arrest rhythm scenarios are:

• Ventricular fibrillation (VF)

• Pulseless ventricular tachycardia (VT)

• Pulseless electrical activity (PEA)

• Asystole

Two of the four, VF (again, as shown in the case) and pulseless VT, are considered shockable rhythms, meaning that electrical defibrillation is the most appropriate intervention and should be provided as early as possible after initiation of resuscitation. In VF (and pulseless VT), electrical defibrillation and chest compressions are the priorities in early management. The nonshockable rhythms are PEA and asystole; electrical defibrillation is not indicated in these two rhythm scenarios. In all four cardiac arrest scenarios, appropriate chest compressions are indicated. Intravenous fluids, cardioactive medications, and airway management are additional priorities. If possible, identification of the underlying or causative issue is important so that additional therapy can be tailored to the situation.

Why are the other choices wrong?

Cardioactive medications should become a management priority only after maximizing chest compressions and defibrillation in patients with pulseless VF or VT. Transvenous pacing, which is a laborious procedure not easily done while chest compressions are ongoing, is unlikely to benefit the patient and is not indicated.

Additional therapies such as definitive airway management with orotracheal intubation are important after the patient is stabilized but must not detract from the first steps in management — chest compressions and defibrillation.

Transcutaneous pacing is unlikely to benefit the patient and is not indicated.

PEER POINT

The four cardiac arrest rhythms

Asystole, not shockable

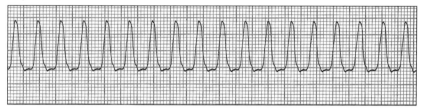

PEER Point 20

Pulseless electrical activity, not shockable

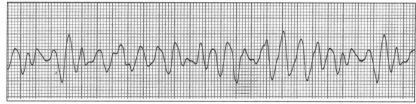

PEER Point 21

Ventricular fibrillation, shockable

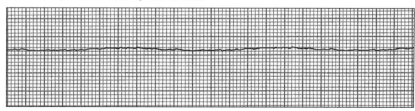

PEER Point 22

Ventricular tachycardia, shockable

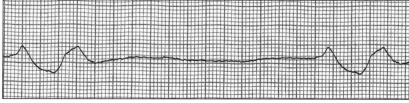

PEER Point 23

✓ High-quality chest compressions and electrical defibrillation are very important in the treatment of cardiac arrest manifesting with pulseless VT or VF.

✓ Invasive airway management and cardioactive medications can be important interventions in all four cardiac arrest rhythm presentations but should not detract from chest compressions and defibrillation for VT and VF.

REFERENCES

Adams JG, Barton ED, Collings J, et al, eds. *Emergency Medicine: Clinical Essentials.* 2nd ed. Philadelphia, PA: Saunders; 2013: 55-71.

Link MS, Berkow LC, Kudenchuk PJ, et al. Part 7: adult advanced cardiovascular life support: 2015 American Heart Association Guidelines Update for Cardiopulmonary Resuscitation and Emergency Cardiovascular Care. *Circulation.* 2015; 132(suppl 2):S444–S464.

203. The correct answer is A, Not necessary if more than 96 hours have elapsed.

Why is this the correct answer?

If performed more than 72 hours after a sexual assault, a forensic examination is unlikely to produce useful forensic evidence. Therefore, most authorities do not recommend performing a forensic examination if more than 72 hours have elapsed. There is variation among states, some of which allow for evidence collection up to 96 hours. It is important for all emergency department clinicians and providers to know the policy of the states where they practice. An emergency department evaluation might still be needed, including a physical examination and pelvic examination, depending on the circumstances, but evidence specifically for forensic purposes cannot be used if there is more than a 96-hour delay from assault to examination. In the United States, sexual assault has a case rate of 27.3 per 100,000, and 18.3% of women report having been raped in their lifetimes. Up to 22.2% of males have experienced sexual assault.

Why are the other choices wrong?

When they initially present to the emergency department, victims of sexual assault might not have decided whether they want to file a police report. Although the forensic evidence kit is used to collect evidence to use in a criminal case, many hospitals allow for collection and storage of the kit until the patient decides whether to file a police report. Of note, the chain of custody must be strictly maintained; the kit cannot be left unattended. If the kit is to be stored until the police are able to accept it, it should be kept in a locked refrigerator.

The ACEP Clinical Policy on management of patients presenting after sexual assault states that "specially trained, nonphysician medical personnel should be allowed to perform evidentiary examinations in jurisdictions in which evidence collected in such a manner is admissible in criminal cases." In many emergency departments, the examination can be performed by a certified Sexual Assault Nurse Examiner (SANE) or a Sexual Assault Forensic Examiner (SAFE).

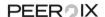

It is not necessary to perform the entire forensic evidence kit in every circumstance. The collection of evidence should be tailored to the specifics of the assault.

PEER REVIEW

✓ It is not necessary to perform a sexual assault examination more than 96 hours after an assault.

✓ A physician or any other specially trained provider may perform the sexual assault forensic examination.

✓ Sexual assaults account for 10% of all assault-related emergency department visits by female patients.

REFERENCES

Marx JA, Hockberger RS, Walls RM, eds. *Rosen's Emergency Medicine: Concepts and Clinical Practice*. 8th ed. St. Louis, MO: Elsevier; 2014: 855-871.

Tintinalli JE, Stapczynski JS, Ma OJ, et al, eds. *Tintinalli's Emergency Medicine: A Comprehensive Study Guide*. 8th ed. New York, NY: McGraw-Hill; 2012: 1983-1988.

204. The correct answer is B, Intravenous haloperidol.

Why is this the correct answer?

A patient such as the one in this case who has overused cocaine develops abnormalities that are typical of the sympathomimetic toxic syndrome: hypertension, hyperthermia, tachycardia, tachypnea. Any of these disorders can harm the patient, but evidence suggests that the hyperthermia is the most critical. Giving this patient haloperidol or some other antipsychotic medication such as droperidol or chlorpromazine would lower the seizure threshold and might cause dysrhythmia and worsen the hyperthermia. Instead, it is appropriate to provide sedative medications to help decrease the sympathetic outflow, thus resolving the tachycardia and hypertension.

Why are the other choices wrong?

Hyperthermia in cocaine-toxic patients must be rapidly identified and treated. Untreated, it leads to multisystem organ failure and death. Not only should active and passive cooling not be avoided, both measures are indicated. Cooling blankets alone are likely to be inadequate. Other measures, including cold intravenous fluids, ice packs, and muscle relaxation with benzodiazepines (to prevent generation of further hyperthermia), should be used.

Intravenous benzodiazepines are a mainstay of treatment for cocaine toxicity. They provide sedation and temperature reduction and decrease excessive neural and autonomic stimulation. Both lorazepam and diazepam can be titrated with repeated doses to achieve improvement in vital signs and symptomatic relief. Benzodiazepines also are the first-line therapy for cocaine-induced seizures, although additional antiepileptic medications might be required.

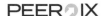

Intravenous fluids should not be avoided in cocaine toxicity. Patients with cocaine-induced rhabdomyolysis should be aggressively resuscitated with intravenous fluids. This helps reduce further renal injury and maintain urine output.

PEER REVIEW

✓ Patients with cocaine and other stimulant toxicity exhibit sympathetic symptoms, including tachycardia, hypertension, and hyperthermia.

✓ When you're treating a patient with cocaine toxicity, monitor vital signs and provide sedation.

✓ Hyperthermia related to cocaine toxicity is associated with significant morbidity and mortality rates and should be managed aggressively.

REFERENCES

Hoffman RS, Howland MA, Lewin NA, et al, eds. *Goldfrank's Toxicologic Emergencies*. 10th ed. New York, NY: McGraw-Hill; 2015: 1054-1063.

Marx JA, Hockberger RS, Walls RM, eds. *Rosen's Emergency Medicine: Concepts and Clinical Practice*. 8th ed. St. Louis, MO: Elsevier; 2014: 1999-2006.

Tintinalli JE, Stapczynski JS, Ma OJ, et al, eds. *Tintinalli's Emergency Medicine: A Comprehensive Study Guide*. 8th ed. New York, NY: McGraw-Hill; 2012: 1256-1260.

205. The correct answer is C, Disclosure of psychotherapy notes for use in insurance billing.

Why is this the correct answer?

The purpose of the Health Insurance Portability and Accountability Act of 1996, or HIPAA, is to provide for the protection of confidential health information. Under the act, protected health information, or PHI, may not be disclosed outside of the entity holding the information without the patient's written authorization except in certain circumstances. In general, PHI needed for treatment, operations, and payment does not require specific written consent. One exception is for psychotherapy notes, which typically cannot be disclosed without consent except in cases of treatment, specific legal matters, and if there is a significant public safety concern.

Why are the other choices wrong?

Disclosure of PHI is allowed, without written consent for the purpose of treatment. Treatment includes the management, provision, and coordination of health care and health care-related services, including coordination with consultants and referrals. There are also exceptions for payment and for use in operations such as quality improvement, employee evaluation and credentialing, and auditing programs.

Individual patient confidentiality concerns must be weighed against the general health and well-being of the population. With that in mind, HIPAA does not mandate written authorization for the purpose of public health reporting, which includes things like communicable diseases, vital statistics, and other public safety concerns.

The release of PHI for the purposes of a workers' compensation claim is allowed under HIPAA without written authorization.

PEER REVIEW

✓ The law we know as HIPAA was enacted to protect confidential patient health information.

✓ Disclosure of personal health information, except under specifically defined circumstances, requires written patient authorization.

✓ Personal health information may be released without written authorization, in general, when used for purposes of treatment, operations, or payment.

REFERENCES

Strauss RW, Mayer TA, eds. *Emergency Department Management*. New York, NY: McGraw-Hill; 2014: 637-642.

Tintinalli JE, Stapczynski JS, Ma OJ, et al, eds. *Tintinalli's Emergency Medicine: A Comprehensive Study Guide*. 8th ed. New York, NY: McGraw-Hill; 2012: 2030-2041.

206. The correct answer is B, Close monitoring with admission to a setting with cardiac monitoring capabilities.

Why is this the correct answer?

Third-degree heart block, or complete heart block, is characterized by the absence of AV conduction — all atrial impulses to the ventricles are blocked. The diagnosis is made by recognizing the characteristic ECG features — no association of P wave with QRS complexes, an atrial rate greater than the ventricular rate (which is regular), wide QRS complexes (usually), and narrow QRS complexes (occasionally) — and relating them to the patient presentation. In this case, the patient's syncopal episode and dyspnea and bradycardia on presentation are consistent with the diagnosis. Definitive management is placement of an implanted pacemaker. Correct initial emergency department management involves ruling out correctable causes such as electrolyte abnormality, monitoring the patient's condition closely, and admitting her to a unit where she can undergo cardiac monitoring. Typically, an escape pacemaker paces the ventricles at rate that is slower than the atrial rate. The QRS interval is either narrow or wide, depending on whether the escape pacemaker is at the AV node or infranodal, respectively. Complete heart block is associated with acute ischemia (inferior and anterior STEMI) leading to structural heart disease, medication adverse effect (digitalis, beta blockers, calcium channel blockers), and other conditions such as Lyme disease.

Why are the other choices wrong?

Administration of atropine in this setting is unlikely to produce benefit. In addition, the rhythm diagnosis is third-degree heart block; this presentation requires admission to the hospital for monitoring and further management.

Discharge from the hospital is not appropriate for the vast majority of patients with third-degree heart block even after a period of observation. Admission for further evaluation and management is correct, especially since this patient had an associated syncopal episode with her dysrhythmia.

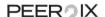

Initial evaluation and management of this patient might include the placement of transcutaneous pacing pads in case she has another episode of syncope. However, transcutaneous pacing does not need to be started: she is currently asymptomatic, and her blood pressure is currently normal.

PEER REVIEW

✓ If you're treating a patient with third-degree heart block who is lightheaded, having chest tightness, or has syncope, admit that patient to a monitored bed.

✓ Third-degree heart block can be caused by ischemia, medications, or conditions such as Lyme disease.

REFERENCES

Link MS, Berkow LC, Kudenchuk PJ, et al. Part 7: adult advanced cardiovascular life support: 2015 American Heart Association Guidelines Update for Cardiopulmonary Resuscitation and Emergency Cardiovascular Care. *Circulation.* 2015; 132(Suppl 2):S444–S464.

Tintinalli JE, Stapczynski JS, Ma OJ, et al, eds. *Tintinalli's Emergency Medicine: A Comprehensive Study Guide.* 8th ed. New York, NY: McGraw-Hill; 2012: 112-134.

207. The correct answer is B, No, the first clinician's failure to diagnose was not the cause of the patient's harm.

Why is this the correct answer?

In order for the standard of negligence to be met in a medical liability case, a plaintiff must not only show that the standard of care was breached, but that that breach was the cause of harm or injury to the patient. In this case, the patient's bad outcome was the indirect result of his underlying medical problem (acute appendicitis) and not a result of the failure to diagnose it correctly. For a negligence claim to be successful, all four components of negligence must occur, as follows:

- The provider must have a duty to care for the patient.
- There must a breach of duty, that is, the standard of care is not met.
- An injury or harm must occur.
- The failure to meet the standard of care must be the cause of injury In this case, it could be argued that the standard of care was not met. However, failure to meet the standard of care alone is not sufficient to prove negligence.

Why are the other choices wrong?

In general, the standard of care is what a reasonable physician in the same specialty would do under similar circumstances. This is most often defined by expert witnesses. A breach of the standard of care is one factor necessary for medical negligence to occur, but the other components must occur as well.

A bad outcome alone is insufficient grounds for a medical negligence claim. A successful claim requires that the standard of care was not met and that this breach directly resulted in harm to the patient. Furthermore, the cause must be shown to be proximate (there must be a direct temporal relationship between the negligence and the injury) and actual (the negligence must directly cause the injury).

Medical negligence requires that a physician has a duty to care for the patient, that is, that a doctor-patient relationship has been established. This relationship is clearly established when a clinician treats a patient in the emergency department but can also be established in other ways such as giving medical advice over the telephone or even by providing informal medical advice to persons who are not patients. Even if the patient subsequently seeks care in another emergency department, the physician-patient relationship in this case has already been established.

PEER REVIEW

- ✓ The four required legal components of negligence are duty, breach of duty, injury or harm, and causation.
- ✓ A duty to care for a patient exists when the physician-patient relationship is established.
- ✓ Causation for medical negligence must be proximate and actual.

REFERENCES

Strauss RW, Mayer TA, eds. *Emergency Department Management*. New York, NY: McGraw-Hill; 2014: 671-678.

Wolfson AB, Hendey GW, Ling LJ, et al, eds. *Harwood-Nuss' Clinical Practice of Emergency Medicine*. 6th ed. Philadelphia, PA: Lippincott, Williams & Wilkins; 2014: 1579.

208. The correct answer is A, Developing a system to report and track errors and near misses.

Why is this the correct answer?

High-reliability organizations address errors and near misses by identifying and tracking them and by implementing processes to prevent similar mistakes in the future. Before errors can be addressed, they must be identified and measured. High-reliability organizations have a robust system in place for reporting and tracking errors — they have an error-reporting chart or some other kind of tool that is accessible to everyone throughout the department. Clinicians and providers should be familiar with and feel comfortable using the reporting system; they must know they will not be punished for using it. Once errors are being effectively tracked, they can be analyzed; patterns can be assessed. In a culture of safety, all staff members feel they are part of the team and have a stake in error reduction. As part of this, it is critical to involve them in the process of analyzing errors and improving system processes. For this to occur, errors must be visible and should not be kept secret from staff (after ensuring individual patient and provider confidentiality). One approach to creating such a system, described by Espinosa and Nolan, is built on prevention, identification, and mitigation. Some situations are known to be high risk for errors. These situations can be identified ahead of time, and systems can be put into place to prevent and mitigate associated problems. Some of these high-risk situations involve specific medical complaints that have been associated with malpractice cases such as chest pain or acute MI. Other high-risk situations include patient handoffs and seasonal illness surges.

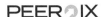

Why are the other choices wrong?

Although it might be tempting to pin blame for errors on individual providers, this typically does very little to improve overall patient safety in a complex health care system. In fact, studies of human error in complex systems have shown that only about 15% of errors are related to individuals, while 85% are related to flawed system processes.

Sometimes it is appropriate to discipline providers for egregious errors, but a culture of safety is present more often in an environment where individuals feel comfortable reporting errors without undue fear of personal repercussions.

Again, in a culture of safety, all staff members feel they have a stake in error reduction. This works only if errors are not kept secret from staff (after ensuring necessary confidentiality).

PEER POINT

Elements of an error reporting chart

- Record number
- Incident
- Category
- Results
- Recommended improvements

PEER REVIEW

- ✓ Creating a culture of safety and becoming a high reliability organization starts with error reduction.
- ✓ Clinicians, providers, and staff should feel comfortable reporting errors without fear of punishment.
- ✓ All staff members are stakeholders in any mission to improve patient safety.

REFERENCES

Nolan TW. System changes to improve patient safety. *BMJ.* 2000;320(7237):771-773.
Strauss RW, Mayer TA, eds. *Emergency Department Management.* New York, NY: McGraw-Hill; 2014: 38-44.

209. The correct answer is A, Cardiotocography.

Why is this the correct answer?

Cardiotocography is a type of electronic fetal monitoring (EFM) used to monitor and record fetal heartbeats and uterine contractions. Both external and internal EFM devices are available, but because the internal device is used only after membranes have ruptured, it is not indicated for use in the emergency department. Studies show that EFM is a sensitive marker for diagnosing placental abruption quite early, which can be missed by both pelvic and ultrasound examinations. The fetal heart rate is determined by ultrasound, and uterine contractions are measured by a tocodynamometer. A normal fetal heart rate is between 120 and 160 beats/min; indicators of fetal distress include late decelerations and persistent drop in fetal heart rate (<120 bpm) during contractions. Prolonged fetal bradycardia indicates distress and the need for delivery. Fetal distress detected by EFM might be the earliest sign of impending shock. Even nominal injuries can result in fetal harm and death. For any viable pregnancy (>20 weeks), continuous EFM should be performed for at least 4 hours to assess for fetal heart rate abnormalities, uterine contractions, bleeding, or uterine tenderness. Patients can be safely discharged with appropriate instructions if there are fewer than three (some references say four) contractions per hour for 4 hours.

Why are the other choices wrong?

Kleihauer-Betke testing is used to measure the amount of fetal hemoglobin transferred to the mother's bloodstream to quantify fetal-maternal hemorrhage. This is performed in Rhesus-negative (Rh-) mothers to determine the required dose of Rho(D) immune globulin needed to inhibit formation of Rh antibodies in the mother and prevent Rh disease with future pregnancies. This test determines if there is blood transfer, which could occur in trauma, but does not assess the fetus for distress.

Pelvic, speculum, and bimanual examinations should not be performed on patients presenting with vaginal bleeding in the third trimester until after an ultrasound examination has been performed to rule out placenta previa to prevent catastrophic bleeding. A pelvic examination can be useful to determine the etiology of the problem but does not measure the distress of the fetus.

Ultrasound examination is very useful in the third trimester and provides lots of information, for example, size of the fetus, age, activity or demise, location of the placenta, and amniotic fluid volume. But ultrasound can be insensitive to life-threatening conditions such as placental abruption and uterine rupture and is not a good tool for assessing fetal distress.\

PEER REVIEW

✓ Monitoring for fetal distress requires at least 4 hours of cardiotocography or electronic fetal monitoring.
✓ Fetal bradycardia (<120 bpm) is a strong indicator of distress.
✓ Patients with fewer than three contractions per hour for 4 hours can be safely discharged.

REFERENCES

Marx JA, Hockberger RS, Walls RM, eds. *Rosen's Emergency Medicine: Concepts and Clinical Practice*. 8th ed. St. Louis, MO: Elsevier; 2014: 296-304.

Tintinalli JE, Stapczynski JS, Ma OJ, et al, eds. *Tintinalli's Emergency Medicine: A Comprehensive Study Guide*. 8th ed. New York, NY: McGraw-Hill; 2012: 1692-1695.

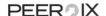

210. The correct answer is D, Paramyxovirus.

Why is this the correct answer?

Mumps is caused by paramyxovirus, and it is characterized by fever and swelling of the salivary glands (parotitis). After approximately 1 week of illness, orchitis might develop. Orchitis is a bacterial or viral infection of the testes that presents with swelling and pain of the affected testis with associated discoloration of the scrotum. When orchitis is associated with mumps, it is generally unilateral, so it rarely causes infertility. Although mumps is one of the most common causes of orchitis in postpubertal males, other etiologies include *Escherichia coli, Klebsiella pneumoniae, Pseudomonas aeruginosa*, Epstein-Barr virus, and arbovirus. It is important to distinguish orchitis from other causes of testicular pain such as testicular torsion and epididymitis. In female patients, mumps can also lead to oophoritis, or infection of the ovary. The MMR vaccine (measles, mumps, rubella) should offer protection against paramyxovirus infection, but there is a growing number of individuals in the United States who are not vaccinated, and vaccination rates vary in developing countries.

Why are the other choices wrong?

Adenoviruses can cause many different illnesses, including bladder inflammation and infection, but they are more commonly implicated in minor respiratory illnesses. Severe illness associated with adenovirus is usually limited to infants and young children and persons with existing immunocompromise or cardiac or respiratory disease.

Chlamydia trachomatis is a common genitourinary infection that is transmitted sexually. Chlamydial infections can present with penile discharge and dysuria in male patients. They can cause testicular pain with swelling (orchitis) and epididymitis. In addition, it can cause conjunctivitis and a rash, although not pharyngitis or parotitis as described in this patient. In female patients, *C. trachomatis* infection presents with vaginal discharge, and in the case of ascending infection, lower abdominal pain and symptoms of pelvic inflammatory disease.

Haemophilus ducreyi is a sexually transmitted infection with a common presentation of painful genital ulcers and large swollen lymph nodes. The lymphadenopathy is found near the infection, in the inguinal nodes, not the nodes of the neck or face. This infection is rare in the United States but common in many other parts of the world such as Africa and Asia.

PEER REVIEW

- ✓ Mumps is caused by paramyxovirus.
- ✓ The classic presentation of mumps infection is fever, parotitis, and then delayed orchitis.
- ✓ Orchitis resulting from mumps is generally unilateral, so infertility is a less likely outcome.

REFERENCES

Centers for Disease Control and Prevention. Adenoviruses. CDC website. https://www.cdc.gov/adenovirus/index.html. Accessed September 15, 2016.

Marx JA, Hockberger RS, Walls RM, eds. *Rosen's Emergency Medicine: Concepts and Clinical Practice.* 8th ed. St. Louis, MO: Elsevier; 2014: 2205-2223.

Tintinalli JE, Stapczynski JS, Ma OJ, et al, eds. *Tintinalli's Emergency Medicine: A Comprehensive Study Guide.* 8th ed. New York, NY: McGraw-Hill; 2012: 601-609.

211. The correct answer is A, Asking the family a few questions to gauge what they understand about the situation.

Why is this the correct answer?

Delivery of bad news, particularly the news that someone's loved one has died, can be one of the most difficult and emotionally challenging aspects of emergency medicine. Various frameworks like the GRIEV_ING mnemonic have been created to guide practitioners. Prior to delivering the news, it is helpful for the emergency physician to first determine how much the family understands about the situation. This can be accomplished by asking a simple question or two such as, "Tell me what you know about what happened today." The information gleaned from this can help the physician to see the event as the family is seeing it and adjust the conversation accordingly.

Why are the other choices wrong?

In delivering bad news, it is important to convey information clearly, in plain language, and without medical jargon. Euphemisms such as "he moved on to a better place," while perhaps making the delivery less stressful for the physician, might confuse the family. It is better to be clear and use the words "dead" or "died."

As the physician who last cared for the patient, the onus is on the emergency practitioner to have this difficult conversation. It should not be delegated to other clinicians or providers.

Although rapidly disengaging from the situation helps insulate the physician from stress, it potentially increases stress for the family. Rather, it is important to give the family time to absorb the information and the opportunity to ask questions.

PEER POINT

The GRIEV_ING mnemonic, from Hobgood et al

G = Gather; gather the family; ensure that all members are present.

R = Resources; call for support resources available to assist the family with their grief, i.e., chaplain services, ministers, family, and friends.

I = Identify; identify yourself, identify the deceased or injured patient by name, and identify the state of knowledge of the family relative to the events of the day.

E = Educate; briefly educate the family as to the events that have occurred in the emergency department, educate them about the current state of their loved one.

V = Verify; verify that their family member has died. Be clear. Use the words "dead" or "died."

_ = space; give the family personal space and time for an emotional moment; allow the family time to absorb the information.

I = Inquire; ask if there are any questions, and answer them all.

N = Nuts and bolts; inquire about organ donation, funeral services, and personal belongings. Offer the family the opportunity to view the body.

G = Give; give them your card and access information. Offer to answer any questions that may arise later. Always return their call.

PEER REVIEW

✓ Delivering bad news is a stressful task, but learning and following a structured approach is helpful and effective.

✓ Ask a couple of simple questions to determine how much the family understands about the situation before delivering bad news.

REFERENCES

Hobgood C, Harward D, Newton K, et al. The educational intervention "GRIEV_ING" improves the death notification skills of residents. *Acad Emerg Med.* 2005;12(4):296-301. Available at: http://onlinelibrary.wiley.com/doi/10.1197/j.aem.2004.12.008/epdf. Accessed October 20, 2016.

Marx JA, Hockberger RS, Walls RM, eds. *Rosen's Emergency Medicine: Concepts and Clinical Practice.* 8th ed. St. Louis, MO: Elsevier; 2014: 2518.

Tintinalli JE, Stapczynski JS, Ma OJ, et al, eds. *Tintinalli's Emergency Medicine: A Comprehensive Study Guide.* 8th ed. New York, NY: McGraw-Hill; 2012: 2017-2020.

212. The correct answer is D, Verbal deescalation.

Why is this the correct answer?

Whatever technique is used to diffuse a potentially violent patient encounter or subdue an aggressive patient, the first objective is to ensure the safety of the patient, staff, and other persons nearby. Recommended approaches are typically stepwise, starting with verbal deescalation, followed by a show of force, pharmacologic management, and finally, physical restraint. In one study of verbal deescalation of agitated patients, researchers suggest a three-step approach: first, engage the patient verbally; second, establish a collaborative relationship; and third, deescalate the patient's agitated or aggressive state verbally. These authors suggest that the initial attempt to engage the patient is a verbal loop: the clinician hears the patient out, circles back to something the patient said that he or she can validate or agree with, then tells the patient what he or she or the staff wants to happen next, whether that is for the patient to sit down or take a medication or something else. The authors use the term loop because this initial conversation might require many repetitions, but if it is effective, other measures such as chemical and physical restraints might be avoided. Attitude and body language are key factors in the success of verbal deescalation attempts; other considerations include respecting personal space, avoiding provocation, being concise, setting clear limits, offering choices and optimism, and listening closely to what the patient says.

Why are the other choices wrong?

Physical restraint might become necessary in the management of an agitated or aggressive patient after verbal and pharmacologic strategies fail. The patient should be restrained in the supine position or on a side. The head of the bed should be slightly elevated to prevent aspiration. While the patient is in restraints, frequent monitoring should be performed to prevent injury, and clinical efforts should focus on removing the restraints as soon as safely possible. It is never appropriate to restrain a patient in a prone position. The technique of securing a patient's legs to his or her hands while the patient is in a prone position, known as a hog-tie, has been linked to positional asphyxia and death.

Many classes of medication are available for sedation. Typical antipsychotics (haloperidol) and atypical antipsychotics (olanzapine) are used frequently. Clinicians should keep in mind that these medications have many potential adverse effects, including QT interval prolongation and increased risk of death in elderly persons. Benzodiazepines, including lorazepam, are also used often and to good effect for pharmacologic restraint. These should be considered if verbal deescalation and a show of force fail.

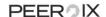

A show of force involves surrounding the patient with numerous security and emergency department personnel to demonstrate that aggressive behavior is not tolerated. This is considered the patient's last chance to calm down before more aggressive techniques such as sedation and physical restraint are used. A show of force is an appropriate next step if verbal deescalation fails.

PEER REVIEW

✓ Never hog-tie or physically restrain a patient in a prone position.

✓ You can diffuse a potentially violent patient situation in a stepwise manner: verbal deescalation, show of force, sedation, physical restraint.

✓ Sometimes you have to use physical restraint when other techniques don't work.

REFERENCES

Richmond JS, Berlin JS, Fishkind AB, et al. Verbal de-escalation of the agitated patient: consensus statement of the American Association for Emergency Psychiatry Project BETA De-escalation Workgroup. *West J Emerg Med.* 2012;13(1):17-25.

Tintinalli JE, Stapczynski JS, Ma OJ, et al, eds. *Tintinalli's Emergency Medicine: A Comprehensive Study Guide.* 8th ed. New York, NY: McGraw-Hill; 2012: 1952-1958.

Zun L, Chepenik LG, Mallory MNS. *Behavioral Emergencies for the Emergency Physician.* Cambridge, NY: Cambridge; 2013: 170.

213. The correct answer is A, Dopamine.

Why is this the correct answer?

The ECG shows polymorphic wide-complex tachycardia consistent with ventricular fibrillation (VF). First-line treatments for VF include amiodarone and defibrillation. When they are attempted without effect (refractory VF, electrical storm), other treatment approaches can be attempted. There are many to choose from, although compared to the other drugs listed, dopamine is a poor choice due to its proarrhythmic effect. Dopamine is a beta-1 agonist and to lesser extent an alpha-1 agonist. It increases sinoatrial nodal conduction and is known to induce narrow-complex tachyarrhythmia such as atrial fibrillation as well as increased ventricular ectopy. And although dopamine is less well studied in humans, it has been shown to induce ventricular tachyarrhythmias as well. In a patient presenting with refractory VF, this is not the best choice to convert the arrhythmia to a perfusing rhythm or to maintain cardiac output if the rhythm can be converted.

Why are the other choices wrong?

Epinephrine is a potent beta-agonist even more so than dopamine. Like dopamine there is potential for this medication to worsen VF. However, epinephrine, although not proved to improve survival after cardiac arrest, is a mainstay of ACLS and can be used accordingly.

Lidocaine was once first-line treatment for ventricular tachyarrhythmia along with electrical defibrillation. More recently amiodarone has been shown to be more effective and has replaced lidocaine as first-line medical therapy. However, in a patient refractory to amiodarone, lidocaine is a viable option. Other potential second-line therapies for persisting ventricular tachyarrhythmias are propranolol or esmolol (beta blockade decreases sympathetic outflow and raises the fibrillation threshold just as dopamine lowers this threshold), isoproterenol, or quinidine (this agent is specifically useful for Brugada syndrome).

Magnesium is used to treat a specific subset of ventricular tachycardias. It is known to be beneficial in torsades de pointes, long QT-interval-associated ventricular tachycardia, digitalis toxicity, and post-MI ventricular arrhythmia. Although it might not be curative in this case, the risk of inducing further arrhythmias is very low; it should be considered for all patients presenting in ventricular arrhythmia because of its potential benefit and low risk.

PEER REVIEW

- ✓ Electrical storm? Possible treatments after first-line therapy for VF fails include lidocaine, isoproterenol, and propranolol or esmolol.
- ✓ Dopamine has a proarrhythmic effect, so don't use it to treat electrical storm or refractory ventricular arrhythmia.

REFERENCES
Eifling M, Razavi M, Massumi A. The evaluation and management of electrical storm. *Tex Heart Inst J.* 2011;38(2):111-121.
Tintinalli JE, Stapczynski JS, Ma OJ, et al, eds. *Tintinalli's Emergency Medicine: A Comprehensive Study Guide.* 8th ed. New York, NY: McGraw-Hill; 2012: 160-167.

214. The correct answer is D, Prepare to perform lateral canthotomy.

Why is this the correct answer?

In this case, the patient presentation is classic for retrobulbar hemorrhage: a history of blunt trauma to the eye followed by symptoms of worsening vision, proptosis, and increased intraocular pressure. Retrobulbar hemorrhage is an ocular emergency, and an ophthalmologist should be consulted immediately. If the ophthalmologist is unavailable and the patient has intraocular pressure higher than 40 mm Hg, the emergency physician should perform a lateral canthotomy. This procedure decreases the pressure on the blood flow to the optic nerve and can be vision saving. It is also important to consider other causes of a retrobulbar hematoma such as coagulopathy and thrombocytopenia.

Why are the other choices wrong?

Outpatient management is inappropriate in this scenario because retrobulbar hemorrhage is a true ocular emergency requiring immediate intervention.

Pilocarpine and timolol drops are used to treat acute angle-closure glaucoma, which can also increase intraocular pressure. Pilocarpine constricts the pupil, opening the trabecular complex, and timolol decreases aqueous humor production. Both medications effectively lower intraocular pressure but have no role in the treatment of increased intraocular pressure from a retrobulbar hematoma.

Ocular massage may be considered to treat central retinal artery occlusion (CRAO), which can cause acute vision changes. However, there is no evidence for or against performing this maneuver in CRAO, and the ophthalmologist should be involved if this diagnosis is suspected. Ocular massage has no role in the treatment of retrobulbar hematoma and could worsen an associated open globe injury.

PEER POINT

Paper clips bent to use as eyelid retractors

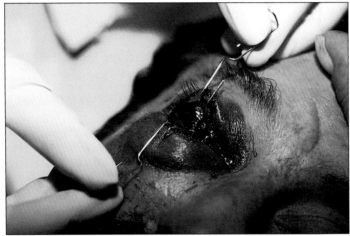

PEER Point 24

PEER REVIEW

✓ Remember to include retrobulbar hematoma in the differential diagnosis for ocular trauma.

✓ If you're treating a patient with retrobulbar hemorrhage, consider lateral canthotomy when intraocular pressure is higher than 40 mm Hg.

REFERENCES
Roberts JR, Hedges JR, eds. *Clinical Procedures in Emergency Medicine.* 6th ed. St. Louis, MO: WB Saunders; 2013: 1293-1295.
Tintinalli JE, Stapczynski JS, Ma OJ, et al, eds. *Tintinalli's Emergency Medicine: A Comprehensive Study Guide.* 8th ed. New York, NY: McGraw-Hill; 2012: 1566-1570.

215. The correct answer is B, If the cause remains untreated, he might become comatose or die.

Why is this the correct answer?

This patient is suffering from delirium, which is characterized by an acute-onset disturbance in awareness and attention and associated with mood lability and agitation. If the underlying cause of his delirium — which might be infection, medication toxicity, alcohol intoxication, urinary retention, trauma, CNS disturbance, or a number of other conditions — remains untreated, it might progress to stupor, coma, seizures, and even death. The three main types of delirium are hyperactive, hypoactive, and mixed. A patient who is agitated such as the one in this case or combative is in the hyperactive category. Patients in the hypoactive category are more subdued and seem drowsy; they are more common than those who are agitated, and their conditions are more likely to be misdiagnosed. Patients with suggestive histories or abnormal physical examination findings should have medical illness excluded as a cause or contributing factor of their altered mental status. Patients without a prior psychiatric history should undergo a thorough medical evaluation, including vital sign assessment with pulse oximetry and, in select patients, blood glucose measurement. Overall, patients who are at the highest risk for having a medical condition causing a psychiatric presentation are elderly patients and those who are substance abusers, those with pre-existing medical conditions, and those without a previous psychiatric illness. Studies indicate that 22% to 76% of patients with delirium die during the hospital admission.

Why are the other choices wrong?

Delirium is associated with increased risk of lasting cognitive deficits, increased hospital length of stay, and increased risk of hospitalization.

Hospitalization for delirium is predictive of multiple poor outcomes, including discharge to long-term care facilities. It is also predictive of functional decline and long-term cognitive deficits.

Delirium is more likely to be seen in patients with hearing impairment (not visual impairment), patients with dementia, and those less functional in their activities of daily living.

PEER REVIEW

✓ Delirium is characterized by an acute onset of confusion and inattention and can be associated with mood lability and agitation.
✓ Delirium is an independent risk factor for death.
✓ Delirium is predictive of numerous poor outcomes in hospitalized patients.

REFERENCES

Diagnostic and Statistical Manual of Mental Disorders: DSM-5. 5th ed. Washington, D.C.: American Psychiatric Association; 2013. http://dx.doi.org.foyer.swmed.edu/10.1176/appi.books.9780890425596.dsm17. Accessed May 26, 2017.

Gower LEJ, O'Keefe Gatewood M, Kang CE. Emergency department management of delirium in the elderly. *West J Emerg Med.* 2012;13(2): 194-201.

Han JH, Zimmerman EE, Cutler N, et al. Delirium in older emergency department patients: recognition, risk factors, and psychomotor subtypes. *Acad Emerg Med.* 2009;16(3):193-200.

Tintinalli JE, Stapczynski JS, Ma OJ, et al, eds. *Tintinalli's Emergency Medicine: A Comprehensive Study Guide.* 8th ed. New York, NY: McGraw-Hill; 2012: 1941-1952;1958-1963.

216. The correct answer is C, Intravenous diazepam.

Why is this the correct answer?

The patient in this case is showing signs consistent with delirium associated with LSD intoxication. Benzodiazepines such as lorazepam or diazepam, administered orally or intravenously, can be helpful in hallucinogen toxicity for the management of agitation and delirium. In fact, benzodiazepines alone are often sufficient to control the associated hypertension and tachycardia. They also are first-line therapy for treatment of hallucinogen-induced seizures. The effects of LSD begin to manifest about 30 minutes after ingestion; they peak at 4 hours and generally last 8 to 12 hours. Patients can present with sympathomimetic stimulation, including tachycardia, hyperthermia, and hypertension. They might have facial flushing, piloerection, increased muscle tension, and hyperreflexia. Large overdoses can result in seizures, coma, coagulopathy, and respiratory failure. "Bad trips," or dysphoric reactions, are more common with LSD than with other hallucinogens like *Psilocybe cubensis* mushrooms.

Why are the other choices wrong?

Gastric decontamination is rarely indicated after hallucinogen ingestion. Most substances in this class are rapidly absorbed, and patients typically do not present until several hours after ingestion. Although the patient in this case is showing signs consistent with LSD intoxication, activated charcoal is of little benefit. Some consideration can be given to using activated charcoal if the hallucinogen ingestion is known to be within the previous hour or in cases of delayed gastric emptying such as with anticholinergic poisoning.

Intravenous bicarbonate is used for treatment of substances that cause similar symptoms (including dysrhythmias) by changing the pH to treat cardiac conduction disorders. With LSD, this mechanism is not a useful treatment.

Naloxone, a competitive opioid antagonist, is used in the management of opioid overdoses to reduce respiratory depression. This patient is not exhibiting symptoms of opioid overdose. There is no indication for naloxone in LSD intoxication.

PEER REVIEW

✓ Patients with LSD intoxication might present with sympathomimetic stimulation.
✓ Most hallucinogens are rapidly absorbed and do not require gastric decontamination.
✓ Large overdoses of hallucinogens can result in coma, seizure, and death.

REFERENCES

Marx JA, Hockberger RS, Walls RM, eds. *Rosen's Emergency Medicine: Concepts and Clinical Practice*. 8th ed. St. Louis, MO: Elsevier; 2014: 2015-2023.

Tintinalli JE, Stapczynski JS, Ma OJ, et al, eds. *Tintinalli's Emergency Medicine: A Comprehensive Study Guide*. 8th ed. New York, NY: McGraw-Hill; 2012: 1260-1265.

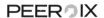

217. The correct answer is A, Factitious disorder by proxy.

Why is this the correct answer?

Factitious disorder by proxy (FDBP), previously termed Munchausen by proxy, is a disorder in which a caregiver fakes the illness of a child or, less frequently, an elderly person he or she cares for so as to receive attention. It is the most likely diagnosis in this case because the presentation matches many of the typical signs — multiple medical evaluations with extensive testing; symptoms that do not correlate to test results; symptoms that are reported but rarely seen by medical personnel; symptoms that resolve during hospitalization but return after the patient is discharged home; and symptoms that do not fit any specific disease or signs and symptoms. In the case of children, it is more common for the caregiver responsible for faking the illness to be the mother. Often the caregiver is involved in health care and has medical knowledge and appears to dote on the child, which can make factitious disorder by proxy difficult to diagnose. It is imperative that an organic cause for the presenting complaint be sought, but once that has been done, and if the symptomatology persists, the diagnosis of factitious disorder by proxy should be considered.

Why are the other choices wrong?

Idiopathic thrombocytopenic purpura (ITP) is a disorder of decreased platelet count and is the most common platelet disorder in children. Severe bleeding is rare, so ITP often presents with unexplained bruising and petechiae with clinical findings of prolonged epistaxis, gum bleeding, or even bloody urine but rarely with bloody stools.

Milk protein allergy often manifests as colitis with loose, mucoid stools, possibly with blood mixed into the stool. It is a reasonable diagnosis to consider, but in this case, extensive testing has already been performed and has yielded negative results, making milk protein allergy unlikely.

Rectal fissure is a common cause of blood found in a child's stool. It is often associated with constipation or very firm stools. But it is not likely the cause in this case because a rectal examination was performed and was negative.

PEER REVIEW

✓ Rectal fissures are the most common cause of bloody stools in pediatric patients, especially in infants.

✓ Clues to factitious disorder by proxy: several medical evaluations without a diagnosis, symptoms that resolve during hospitalization and recur when the patient returns home, symptoms that do not match test results or any disease.

✓ The most common causes of blood in the stool change with the age of the child.

REFERENCES

Fleisher GR, Ludwig S, et al, eds. *Textbook of Pediatric Emergency Medicine.* 6th ed. Philadelphia, PA: Lippincott, Williams & Wilkins; 2010: 875-877; 1656-1700.

Wolfson AB, Hendey GW, Ling LJ, et al, eds. *Harwood-Nuss' Clinical Practice of Emergency Medicine.* 6th ed. Philadelphia, PA: Lippincott, Williams & Wilkins; 2014: 812-815; 1297-1302.

218. The correct answer is C, Oral contraceptive.

Why is this the correct answer?

The emergency physician's role in treating women who present with acute pelvic pain suspected to be caused by endometriosis is to rule out other causes, provide pain relief, and refer patients for gynecology follow-up and definitive treatment. For a patient like the one in this case, who has a history of endometriosis, after NSAIDs, oral contraceptive pills are the next logical step in treatment — unless contraindicated — until she can follow up with a gynecologist. If symptoms can be relatively controlled, the patient may be discharged with close follow-up. Endometriosis is a chronic condition, and the diagnosis typically is not made in the emergency department, but it should be suspected in women who present with vague pelvic pain, dysmenorrhea, and/or dyspareunia in the absence of other objective findings. More severe symptoms might require admission for further management and evaluation. Ultrasonography or MRI can help make the diagnosis, but definitive diagnosis usually requires surgical exploration.

Why are the other choices wrong?

Gonadotropin-releasing hormone agonists such as leuprolide acetate have been found in many studies to help relieve pain associated with endometriosis; however, this approach is part of an ongoing treatment plan prescribed and followed by a gynecologist after pain management with NSAIDs and oral contraceptive pills.

Medroxyprogesterone acetate is indicated for more severe symptoms related to endometriosis but is not usually administered through the emergency department. It is usually prescribed by a gynecologist as part of an ongoing treatment plan.

Narcotic pain relievers might help acutely but do not treat the underlying source of the patient's pain. They should be used only as a medication of last resort.

PEER REVIEW

- ✓ Suspect endometriosis in women with vague pelvic pain, dysmenorrhea, and/or dyspareunia in the absence of other objective findings.
- ✓ If you're treating a patient with endometriosis who can't get pain relief with NSAIDs, try oral contraceptive pills and refer her for outpatient gynecology care.

REFERENCES

Hamilton C, Stany M, Gregory W, et al. Gynecology. In: Brunicardi F, Andersen DK, Billiar TR, et al, eds. *Schwartz's Principles of Surgery*. 10th ed. New York, NY: McGraw-Hill; 2015. http://accessmedicine.mhmedical.com/content. aspx?bookid=980&sectionid=59610883. Accessed May 18, 2017.

Tintinalli JE, Stapczynski JS, Ma OJ, et al, eds. *Tintinalli's Emergency Medicine: A Comprehensive Study Guide*. 8th ed. New York, NY: McGraw-Hill; 2012: 625-628.

219. The correct answer is A, ABO incompatibility.

Why is this the correct answer?

When considering the possible causes of jaundice, time of onset is a crucial branch point: it provides clues to the underlying cause and its severity. Jaundice in the first 24 hours of life is an ominous finding. These patients are more likely to develop severe jaundice that could progress to kernicterus (hyperbilirubinemia-induced encephalitis). The factors that place a patient at high risk include a total bilirubin at discharge in a high-risk zone, gestational age of 35 to 36 weeks, jaundice in the first 24 hours, sibling who required phototherapy, ABO/hemolytic disease, breastfeeding but poor growth/feeding, and East Asian or Mediterranean ancestry. Hemolytic disease not only can lead to jaundice but also to anemia, which can affect the patient's hemodynamic stability. A Coombs test can detect maternal IgG antibodies on the baby's RBCs; it should be included in the evaluation of this patient, as should testing for hemoglobin, liver function, a total and fractionated bilirubin, and possibly blood typing for the patient and mother if this information is unknown.

Why are the other choices wrong?

Jaundice is 3 to 6 times more likely in a breastfed child than in one who is bottle fed. Breast milk jaundice has two stages: early and late (early is considered within the first week of life, while late is considered starting in the first week, peaking by 2 weeks, and then resolving by 3 months). Early breast milk jaundice is likely related to the decreased volume and/or frequency of feeds. This can lead to dehydration and thus delayed meconium passage. It may also be related to the decreased enterohepatic recirculation and immaturity of the liver in these children. Treatment for early breast milk jaundice is geared toward improving hydration (increase feeds to more than 10/day; possibly supplementing with formula (not water or dextrose/H20) while continuing to breastfeed. Late breast milk jaundice is believed to be caused by properties of the breast milk (beta-glucuronidase, nonesterified fatty acids), which seem to decrease bilirubin metabolism. Treatment for late breast milk jaundice is to temporarily withhold breast feeding (the mother is advised to continue to pump). The bilirubin level should decline rapidly in 48 hours with this approach. Bilirubin levels, in general, peak on days 6 to 14. Jaundice develops in 30% of heathy breastfed infants. Phototherapy is used to decrease the rise of total bilirubin in any neonate of any gestational age. It should be used when the rate of rise is greater than 5 mg/dL per 24-hour period or when advised to do so using either the bilirubin nomogram or bilirubin calculator.

Familial nonhemolytic jaundice, also known as Gilbert disease, is a hereditary disorder that leads to decreased bilirubin metabolism. It is not common in neonates but is often found in older children and adults.

Physiologic jaundice is related to the polycythemia of newborns as well as the immaturity of the liver, leading to an elevated conjugated bilirubinemia. This peaks between days 3 and 5 and resolves spontaneously by 14 days of life.

PEER POINT

What causes jaundice in neonatal patients, by age

Younger than 24 hours

- Hemolytic disease of newborn: ABO, Rh, minor blood group incompatibility
- Infections: TORCH infections, malaria
- G-6PD deficiency

24 to 72 hours

- Physiologic (resolves spontaneously in <1 week)
- Hemorrhagic breakdown (cephalohematoma, etc.)
- Sepsis
- Polycythemia
- Increased enterohepatic circulation

Older than 72 hours

- Sepsis
- Metabolic disease
- Neonatal hepatitis
- Extrahepatic biliary atresia
- Breast milk jaundice

PEER REVIEW

- ✓ Jaundice in the first 24 hours of life is concerning — evaluate it thoroughly.
- ✓ Physiologic jaundice peaks between days 3 and 5 and resolves on its own by the second week of life.
- ✓ Treatment of jaundice depends on the level and cause of the condition.

REFERENCES

Fleisher GR, Ludwig S, et al, eds. *Textbook of Pediatric Emergency Medicine*. 6th ed. Philadelphia, PA: Lippincott, Williams & Wilkins; 2010: 996-997.

Sidberry GK, Iannone R, eds. *The Harriet Lane Handbook: A Manual for Pediatric House Officers*. 15th ed. St. Louis, MO: Mosby; 2000: 257-258.

Wolfson AB, Hendey GW, Ling LJ, et al, eds. *Harwood-Nuss' Clinical Practice of Emergency Medicine*. 6th ed. Philadelphia, PA: Lippincott, Williams & Wilkins; 2014: 553; 1099-1103.

220. The correct answer is A, Communication of medication orders by radio from an emergency physician to a paramedic.

Why is this the correct answer?

Online medical direction, also known as online medical control or command, or direct medical control or oversight, is the real-time provision of orders or direction from a medical command physician (typically an emergency physician) to a paramedic or EMT concurrent with prehospital patient care. This medical direction can be provided via radio, telephone, or, in select cases, by a physician on scene.

Depending on the design of the particular EMS system, online command might be given by someone at the destination hospital or from a centralized location. Although the person giving direct medical control need not be the EMS agency's medical director, it is important for that person to have an understanding of his or her EMS system, the protocols that are in place, and the capabilities of the EMS agency. It is unhelpful for the EMS crew to receive orders to start medications they do not carry or to perform procedures that are outside of their scope of practice. Although most EMS agencies follow specific patient care protocols, there are times when orders or advice from a physician can be invaluable to the crew and their patient.

Why are the other choices wrong?

In contrast with direct medical control, indirect or offline medical control involves activities such as protocol development and revision, quality assurance and improvement, and personnel education that do not occur concurrently with patient care. Although EMS agencies typically follow specific patient care protocols, usually driven by chief complaint, these protocols vary widely by system. Some states require statewide protocols, and others provide only recommended protocols. Still other states provide no protocols at all and leave protocol development and revision up to individual medical directors.

High-functioning EMS systems have continuous quality assurance and improvement systems in place as part of their offline medical control program. It is the role of the EMS medical director to oversee the medical components of such programs, typically in coordination with dedicated personnel from the EMS agency. This can involve chart audits, call reviews, and other initiatives.

As with any other area of medicine, retrospective case review in invaluable for paramedic education and remediation. Perhaps the largest offline medical command role for the EMS medical director is to review calls and provide feedback to crew members.

PEER REVIEW

- ✓ Online or direct medical control involves real-time medical direction to paramedics and EMTs.
- ✓ Medical directors are responsible for leading quality assurance and improvement initiatives in EMS.
- ✓ Medical command physicians must be familiar with their EMS systems and their associated protocols and capabilities.

REFERENCES

Marx JA, Hockberger RS, Walls RM, eds. *Rosen's Emergency Medicine: Concepts and Clinical Practice*. 8th ed. St. Louis, MO: Elsevier; 2014: 2433-2441.

Tintinalli JE, Stapczynski JS, Ma OJ, et al, eds. *Tintinalli's Emergency Medicine: A Comprehensive Study Guide*. 8th ed. New York, NY: McGraw-Hill; 2012: 1-3.

221. The correct answer is C, Begin norepinephrine continuous infusion.

Why is this the correct answer?

The patient in this case is presenting in septic shock; MAP is less than 65 mm Hg despite adequate (30 mL/kg) isotonic crystalloid resuscitation. He has evidence of organ hypoperfusion and dysfunction (elevated lactate and inadequate urine output [<0.5 mL/kg/hr]). (Alternative indicators of organ hypoperfusion include altered mental status and a mixed venous oxygen saturation of less than 70%.) At this point in his therapy, it is most reasonable to initiate vasopressor medications. Either norepinephrine or dopamine are listed in various guidelines, but evidence suggests norepinephrine is preferable because of a higher rate of all cause mortality and arrhythmias with dopamine. Early goal-directed therapy was based on the belief that a strict protocol-based treatment was the best approach to managing sepsis. However, the ProCESS trial in 2014 and other similar studies have since demonstrated three keys to the management of sepsis:

- Early recognition of sepsis
- Early antimicrobial therapy
- Adequate fluid hydration

Why are the other choices wrong?

The use of stress-dose intravenous steroids in septic shock is controversial, with conflicting study results. It is considered only in septic shock refractory to multiple vasopressors.

Initiating dopamine could be considered in this patient, but in septic shock, norepinephrine is the preferred agent.

Fluid resuscitation should continue in this patient to achieve ventricular filling, and more fluid might be indicated. However, he remains hypotensive with evidence of organ hypoperfusion, so vasopressors should be initiated.

PEER POINT

Keys to the management of sepsis

- Empiric antibiotic therapy
- Adequate fluid resuscitation — measure adequacy by response to vital signs, ultrasound measurement of jugular vein diameter, and/or central venous pressure measurement
- Initiation of vasopressors if MAP remains below 65 mm Hg
- Serial measurements of serum lactate — the goal is to reduce it by 10% within 1 to 2 hours

PEER REVIEW

✓ Norepinephrine is the preferred vasopressor in septic shock.

✓ Elevated lactate level, decreased urine output, and a low mixed venous oxygen saturation are signs of organ hypoperfusion.

✓ Septic shock is defined as evidence of infection, persistent hypotension of a MAP less than 65 mm Hg despite fluid resuscitation, and a serum lactate level greater than 2 mmol/L.

REFERENCES

Adams JG, Barton ED, Collings JL, et al, eds. *Emergency Medicine: Clinical Essentials.* 2nd ed. Philadelphia, PA: Elsevier; 2013: 1454-1457.e1.

Marx JA, Hockberger RS, Walls RM, eds. *Rosen's Emergency Medicine: Concepts and Clinical Practice.* 8th ed. St. Louis, MO: Elsevier; 2014: 67-74.e1.

222. The correct answer is A, Cardiac MRI.

Why is this the correct answer?

Approximately 10% of patients with myocarditis display fulminant myocarditis at the time of presentation. This condition is characterized by an abrupt-onset myocarditis with development of overt heart failure within days to weeks of a viral illness. The presumptive diagnosis is made clinically, but the most effective diagnostic test is indium contrast-enhanced cardiac MRI. This diagnostic modality identifies myocardial cells damaged by a virus and is becoming the gold standard diagnostic test; some studies demonstrate diagnostic accuracy as high as 78%. Patients with fulminant myocarditis typically have favorable recoveries after presenting in extremis, which is not frequently the case in patients with more indolent myocarditis. The ECG changes in myocarditis are typically nonspecific and can range from sinus tachycardia to diffuse ST-segment elevation and PR-interval depression as illustrated in myopericarditis. The ECG changes in myocarditis also can frequently mimic STEMI, so myocarditis should be kept on the differential for a patient who presents with atypical prodromal symptoms and ECG changes. Parvovirus B-19 is a frequently recognized pathogen in myocarditis and has been identified in 11% to 56% of patients with myocarditis and in 10% to 51% of patients with diastolic cardiomyopathy. Parvovirus has been shown to infect the endothelium alone and causes a significant up-regulation of the innate immune system, which can lead to a broad spectrum of myocarditis. Patients with fulminant myocarditis frequently present with significant hemodynamic compromise and frequently require pressor support, ECMO, or intra-aortic balloon pump to maintain perfusion. Young patients presenting with atypical chest pain or findings of acute heart failure with a viral prodrome should be considered to have myocarditis.

Why are the other choices wrong?

Echocardiography reveals diffuse global hypokinesia, normal or small ventricular size, and ventricular wall thickening, which is likely due to myocardial inflammation and edema. Decreased left ventricular ejection fraction is often seen, but none of these symptoms is definitive for the diagnosis of myocarditis.

In patients with fulminant myocarditis, myocardial biopsy typically reveals diffuse myocarditis in fewer than 50% of the cases. With myocarditis, there is a sporadic myocardial inflammation in acute disease. Myocardial biopsy was previously considered the gold standard, but it is now understood that cardiac tissue has inconsistent injury patterns, which limits accurate sampling with biopsy.

Positive viral titers might support the presumption of a viral cause for the myositis that is causing the patient's symptoms. Positive viral titers do not, in isolation, provide a definitive diagnostic finding.

PEER REVIEW

- ✓ If you're treating a child or a young adult who has signs of heart failure and a viral prodrome, consider myocarditis.
- ✓ Frequently observed ECG changes associated with myopericarditis: sinus tachycardia or diffuse ST-segment elevation with PR-interval depression.
- ✓ Most cases of myocarditis go undiagnosed.
- ✓ Endocardial biopsy has limited diagnostic value in acute myocarditis because of sporadic myocardial inflammation.

REFERENCES

Brady WJ, Ferguson J, Perron A. Myocarditis. *Emerg Med Clin* NA. 2004;22:865-885.2.

Marx JA, Hockberger RS, Walls RM, eds. *Rosen's Emergency Medicine: Concepts and Clinical Practice*. 8th ed. St. Louis, MO: Elsevier; 2014: 1091-1105.

Mattu A, Brady WJ, et al (eds). *Cardiovascular Emergencies*. Dallas, TX: American College of Emergency Physicians Publishing; 2014: 209-226.

223. The correct answer is B, No further evaluation is necessary.

Why is this the correct answer?

Based on the pulmonary embolism rule-out criteria—the PERC rule—this patient with anxiety has a pretest probability of having PE that is less than 1.8%. Ordering a D-dimer is more likely to result in a false-positive result, leading to more testing and unnecessary radiation exposure. The absence of tachycardia or hypoxia in a patient younger than 50 years is reassuring; patients with anxiety or panic attacks often present with tachycardia and tachypnea. She is further at low risk for PE because she has no symptoms of DVT, no history of thromboembolic disease, no use of oral hormones, no hemoptysis, and no history of surgery, trauma, or prolonged immobilization.

Why are the other choices wrong?

A D-dimer is useful for ruling out thrombosis when it is negative, but unfortunately a positive result is very nonspecific: its sensitivity in venothrombotic disease is 94% to 98%, and specificity is only 50% to 60%. When used in the lowest-risk patients, it leads to unnecessary testing and therefore unnecessary radiation exposure and expense.

Overall, the best test for ruling in PE is CT angiography of the chest. It has a sensitivity of 83% to 86% and a specificity of 96%. But it is not necessary in this patient because she has a low pretest probability.

Doppler ultrasonographic imaging of the lower extremity is a good alternative for identifying thromboembolic disease in a patient with suspected PE. If a DVT is found, the treatment for the DVT is identical to that for PE. It can be done at the bedside and does not involve radiation. Unfortunately, negative Doppler ultrasonography does not effectively rule out PE.

PEER POINT

Pulmonary Embolism Rule-Out Criteria (PERC Rule)

Pulmonary embolism can be reliably excluded clinically if all of the following are met:

- Age <50
- Oxygen saturation >95%
- Heart rate <100
- No unilateral leg swelling
- No hemoptysis
- No prior DVT or PE
- No recent surgery or trauma
- No hormone use

PEER REVIEW

- ✓ Patients who meet none of the PE rule-out criteria have a 1.8% pretest probability of PE and are unlikely to require further evaluation for that disease.
- ✓ A negative D-dimer in a patient with low or moderate risk of PE reliably excludes the disease.
- ✓ Tachycardia and tachypnea are common with anxiety and panic attacks.

REFERENCES

Adams JG, Barton ED, Collings JL, et al, eds. *Emergency Medicine: Clinical Essentials.* 2nd ed. Philadelphia, PA: Elsevier; 2013: 602-610.e1.

Kline JA, Mitchell AM, Kabrhel C, Richman PB, Courtney DM. Clinical criteria to prevent unnecessary diagnostic testing in emergency department patients with suspected pulmonary embolism. *J Thromb Haemost.* 2004;2(8):1247–1255.

Marx JA, Hockberger RS, Walls RM, eds. *Rosen's Emergency Medicine: Concepts and Clinical Practice.* 8th ed. St. Louis, MO: Elsevier; 2014: 1157-1169.e1.

Tintinalli JE, Stapczynski JS, Ma OJ, et al, eds. *Tintinalli's Emergency Medicine: A Comprehensive Study Guide.* 8th ed. New York, NY: McGraw-Hill; 2012: 388-399.

224. The correct answer is A, Blood cultures.

Why is this the correct answer?

This patient likely has endocarditis, and the two most definitive tests for this disease are blood cultures (from at least two different venipuncture sites) and echocardiography. These are the two major Duke criteria and, if results of both tests are positive, indicate a definitive diagnosis of infective endocarditis. The minor Duke criteria are a predisposing factor (such as intravenous drug use), fever above 38°C (100.4°F), evidence of septic emboli (such as Janeway lesions, Osler nodes, or, as in this case, splinter hemorrhages), and a single positive blood culture. With two positive blood cultures, the patient has one major criterion and at least two minor criteria, providing good evidence of endocarditis. An echocardiogram, preferably transesophageal, would be an appropriate next step: it is more sensitive (>90%) for valve disease than is a transthoracic echocardiogram (only about 60%).

Why are the other choices wrong?

A chest xray might reveal evidence of septic emboli with scattered infiltrates in the lungs, but it is unlikely to be diagnostic in a case of infective endocarditis.

Influenza is an important consideration when evaluating a patient with a fever and no clear localizing signs. This patient had a more protracted course and is less symptomatic than most patients with influenza.

Lyme disease is an important consideration when evaluating a patient with a chronic fever and no clear localizing signs. Most patients with Lyme disease are more symptomatic, especially with muscle aches, joint pain, and possible target-lesion rash.

PEER POINT

Modified Duke criteria for endocarditis
- Two major or
- One major and three minor or
- Five minor

Major Criteria
- Persistently positive blood cultures (two sets 1 hr apart or 12 hr apart) for a typical organism
- Positive echocardiogram for vegetation, root abscess, or dehiscence of prosthetic valve

Minor Criteria
- Fever
- Presence of a predisposing valvular condition or intravenous drug abuse
- Vascular phenomenon such as emboli to organs or the brain, hemorrhages in the mucous membranes around the eyes
- Immunologic phenomenon such as glomerulonephritis, Osler Nodes, and rheumatoid fever
- Positive blood cultures that do not meet the strict definitions of a major criterion

PEER REVIEW

✓ The most common cause of endocarditis is *Staphylococcus aureus* infection.

✓ Transesophageal echocardiography is more sensitive for valve disease than is a transthoracic echocardiogram.

✓ The two major Duke criteria are two positive blood cultures and echocardiographic evidence of valve vegetations.

REFERENCES

Marx JA, Hockberger RS, Walls RM, eds. *Rosen's Emergency Medicine: Concepts and Clinical Practice*. 8th ed. St. Louis, MO: Elsevier; 2014: 1106-1112.e1.

Tintinalli JE, Stapczynski JS, Ma OJ, et al, eds. *Tintinalli's Emergency Medicine: A Comprehensive Study Guide*. 8th ed. New York, NY: McGraw-Hill; 2012: 1057-1061.

225. The correct answer is A, Brugada syndrome.

Why is this the correct answer?

Brugada syndrome is a genetic disorder that causes abnormal sodium channel function. The classic ECG findings with Brugada syndrome, which appear on this patient's ECG, include an incomplete RBBB pattern and ST-segment elevations in leads V1 and V2. Death resulting from Brugada syndrome is related to subsequent polymorphic ventricular tachycardia or ventricular fibrillation. Patients commonly have a family history of sudden death or cardiac syncope without structural heart disease. Management in the emergency department includes cardiac monitoring with admission for further monitoring and cardiology consultation; Brugada syndrome is associated with a high risk of death. Ultimate treatment includes placement of an automatic implanted cardiac cardioverter-defibrillator. The ECG findings can often be normal at the time of evaluation in the emergency department, so any patient with a family history of sudden death should be referred for further evaluation and provocative testing.

Why are the other choices wrong?

The ECG findings in prolonged QT syndrome are notable for significant prolongation of the QT interval. The syndrome causes increased susceptibility to polymorphic ventricular tachycardia. The QT interval in this patient's ECG is normal.

Third-degree AV block (complete heart block) is noted with dissociation of P waves from QRS complexes. A ventricular rate of less than 60 is noted; the specific rate and QRS complex morphologies are dependent on the level of the block (nodal versus infranodal). The PR intervals are normal and regular on this ECG and show no evidence of heart block.

Wolff-Parkinson-White syndrome can also lead to syncope and, extremely rarely, sudden cardiac death. The associated ECG changes, while the patient is in normal sinus rhythm, are classically shortened PR interval, delta wave, and minimally widened QRS complex — none of which is present in this patient.

PEER REVIEW

✓ Classic ECG findings of Brugada syndrome: incomplete right bundle branch block and ST-segment elevation of V1 and V2.

✓ There's a high risk of ventricular tachycardia, ventricular fibrillation, and sudden death with Brugada syndrome, so if you see it, admit the patient for cardiac monitoring and consultation for placement of an implanted defibrillator.

✓ If you're treating a patient who had a syncopal episode and who also has a family history of sudden death, refer that patient for provocative testing even if the initial ECG doesn't suggest Brugada syndrome.

REFERENCES

Mattu A, Brady WJ, et al (eds). *Cardiovascular Emergencies*. Dallas, TX: American College of Emergency Physicians Publishing; 2014: 11-35.

Tintinalli JE, Stapczynski JS, Ma OJ, et al, eds. *Tintinalli's Emergency Medicine: A Comprehensive Study Guide*. 8th ed. New York, NY: McGraw-Hill; 2012: 112-134.

226. The correct answer is C, Serum lactate measurement.

Why is this the correct answer?

This patient presentation is concerning for sepsis. In addition to aggressive fluid hydration and antibiotic therapy, an important next step is to measure the patient's serum lactate level. This finding is an important marker to evaluate his prognosis. A primary goal of therapy is to lower the serum lactate level by 10% within a couple of hours. Sepsis was previously defined as the presence of infection in a patient with the systemic inflammatory response syndrome, or SIRS. In February 2016, the Third International Consensus Definitions for Sepsis and Septic Shock (Sepsis-3) were published: sepsis is now defined as organ dysfunction due to an infection, and organ dysfunction is defined by a qSOFA score of 2 or more. The qSOFA, or quick SOFA, score is a modified version of a complicated scoring tool used in intensive care. Patients who have two or more of the following clinical criteria are likely to have a high mortality rates from infection: hypotension less than 100 mm Hg, altered mental status (Glasgow Coma Scale score <15), or tachypnea greater than 21 bpm. Sepsis-3 further defines septic shock as persistent hypotension requiring vasopressors to maintain a MAP greater than 65 mm Hg and a lactate greater than 2 mmol/L.

Why are the other choices wrong?

The patient requires aggressive fluid hydration (not cautious maintenance) to maintain a MAP greater than 65 mm Hg. Although excessive hydration can lead to pulmonary edema, especially in patients with congestive heart failure, this patient should get 2 L of crystalloid and reassessment of his volume status.

Hypothermia, rather than fever, is a common reaction to infection, especially in patients at the extremes of age. This patient's low temperature should be interpreted as an indicator of his severe infection rather than an environmental hypothermia.

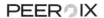

Urine and blood culture results might be useful in this patient's care a couple of days after the initial encounter, but they do not benefit the patient immediately. The initial assessment and stabilization take priority.

PEER POINT

Using the qSOFA score, high-risk patients have two or more of the following:

- Hypotension: systolic blood pressure less than or equal to 100 mm Hg
- Altered mental status: a Glasgow Coma Scale score less than 15
- Tachypnea: respiratory rate greater than or equal to 22

PEER REVIEW

- ✓ To meet the criteria for sepsis, a patient should have the presence of infection and elevation of the qSOFA score.
- ✓ To meet the criteria for septic shock, the patient should have persistent hypotension requiring vasopressors and a lactate greater than 2 mmol/L.
- ✓ Initial therapy should consist of fluid hydration, antibiotic treatment, and a goal of lowering the lactate level 10% within a couple of hours.

REFERENCES

Marx JA, Hockberger RS, Walls RM, eds. *Rosen's Emergency Medicine: Concepts and Clinical Practice.* 8th ed. St. Louis, MO: Elsevier; 2014: 1864-1873.

Singer M, Deutschman CS, Seymour C, et al. The Third International Consensus Definitions for Sepsis and Septic Shock (Sepsis-3). *JAMA.* 2016;315(8):801-810. doi:10.1001/jama.2016.0287.

Tintinalli JE, Stapczynski JS, Ma OJ, et al, eds. *Tintinalli's Emergency Medicine: A Comprehensive Study Guide.* 8th ed. New York, NY: McGraw-Hill; 2012: 1021-1029.

227. The correct answer is C, Monitor for 3 hours in the emergency department.

Why is this the correct answer?

Emergency department treatment of laryngotracheobronchitis, or croup, as described in the case, includes administration of nebulized epinephrine and corticosteroids. Discharge home after treatment has been demonstrated to be safe in well-appearing patients with normal vital signs and no stridor, no retractions, no hypoxia, and access to close follow-up. But because the effects of inhaled epinephrine on respiratory vasoconstriction persist for 2 to 3 hours, investigators recommend at least 3 hours of observation to ensure no recurrence of stridor. Use of racemic epinephrine or L-epinephrine is safe and efficacious.

Why are the other choices wrong?

Hospitalization for treatment of croup is infrequently needed. After administration of corticosteroids and inhaled epinephrine in the emergency department, factors that support the need for admission include persistence of stridor at rest, persistence of respiratory distress, hypoxia, young age (<6 months), high fever, and poor access to close follow-up.

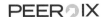

Discharge home immediately following inhaled epinephrine therapy is inappropriate: its effects last for about 2 hours, so monitoring the patient for at least this long — 3 hours is often recommended — is necessary to ensure no recurrence of symptoms. Discharge home after corticosteroids, inhaled epinephrine, and an appropriate emergency department monitoring period is appropriate in a well-appearing patient with none of the following: hypoxia, tachycardia, tachypnea, retractions, or stridor.

Albuterol has no role in the treatment of croup and can worsen airway edema through its beta-mediated vasodilatory effects on the respiratory mucosa.

PEER REVIEW

- ✓ You may discharge a well-appearing patient with croup after treatment and a 3-hour monitoring period if there's no recurrence of respiratory symptoms.
- ✓ It takes about 2 hours for the effects of inhaled epinephrine to wear off, so don't discharge a patient with croup right after treatment.
- ✓ There's no role for albuterol in the management of croup.

REFERENCES

Marx JA, Hockberger RS, Walls RM, eds. *Rosen's Emergency Medicine: Concepts and Clinical Practice.* 8th ed. St. Louis, MO: Elsevier; 2014: 2112-2114.

Tintinalli JE, Stapczynski JS, Ma OJ, et al, eds. *Tintinalli's Emergency Medicine: A Comprehensive Study Guide.* 8th ed. New York, NY: McGraw-Hill; 2012: 793-802.

228. The correct answer is B, CT scan of the orbits.

Why is this the correct answer?

Although different symptoms suggest that a patient has postseptal (orbital) cellulitis rather than preseptal (periorbital) cellulitis, a CT scan of the orbits is required to make the diagnosis. Obtaining an MRI is also an option. In general, preseptal cellulitis is seen in patients younger than 10 years and usually originates with URIs in the sinuses or eyelids. However, similar symptoms can be seen in postseptal cellulitis, which classically is characterized by pain with extraocular movement and proptosis in significant infections. Patients with mild preseptal cellulitis can be treated as outpatients with oral antibiotics. In contrast, patients with postseptal cellulitis require admission for intravenous antibiotic therapy and management by an ophthalmologist.

Why are the other choices wrong?

Blood cultures do not definitively rule in one disease process over the other.

Erythrocyte sedimentation rate is not a specific test to differentiate between the two types of infection.

Although some studies suggest that ocular ultrasonography can help diagnose orbital cellulitis, CT is still the definitive imaging modality.

PEER REVIEW

✓ Preseptal and postseptal orbital cellulitis have overlapping clinical symptoms, so get CT or MRI of the orbits.

✓ Patients with postseptal cellulitis should be admitted for intravenous antibiotic treatment and management by ophthalmology.

✓ Patients with mild preseptal cellulitis can be discharged on oral antibiotics.

REFERENCES

Sullivan JH. Orbit. In: Riordan-Eva P, Cunningham ET, Jr, eds. *Vaughan & Asbury's General Ophthalmology*. 18th ed. New York, NY: McGraw-Hill; 2011. http://accessmedicine.mhmedical.com/content.aspx?bookid=387&sectionid=40229330. Accessed May 16, 2017.

Tintinalli JE, Stapczynski JS, Ma OJ, et al, eds. *Tintinalli's Emergency Medicine: A Comprehensive Study Guide*. 8th ed. New York, NY: McGraw-Hill; 2012: 1558-1563.

Trobe JD. *The Physician's Guide to Eye Care*. 4th ed. San Francisco, CA: American Academy of Ophthalmology; 2012:63-64.

229. The correct answer is D, Pantoprazole and ciprofloxacin.

Why is this the correct answer?

Patients who have cirrhosis and present with upper GI bleeding not attributed to varices should receive proton pump inhibitors (PPIs) in addition to prophylactic antibiotics to address immunocompromise. Patients with cirrhosis have an increased risk of translocation of gut bacteria in the setting of acute bleeding. Antibiotic prophylaxis is associated with reduced mortality rates, decreased bacterial infection, lowered risk of rebleeding, and shortened length of hospitalization. Standard antibiotic choices include ciprofloxacin 400 mg IV or ceftriaxone 1 g IV. The delivery of a PPI is aimed at increasing gastric pH to allow for clot formation. It is shown to reduce the need for surgical intervention and hospital length of stay. The PPI of choice is omeprazole 80 mg bolus IV followed by an infusion of 8 mg/hr.

Why are the other choices wrong?

Vasopressor agents such as dopamine might be required in severe cases of GI bleeding. However, volume and blood resuscitation should be the initial therapy provided. Vasopressin is a pressor of choice for reducing splanchnic blood flow and portal hypertension.

Vasopressor agents such as norepinephrine might be required in severe cases of GI bleeding. However, volume and blood resuscitation should be the initial therapy provided. Vasopressin is a pressor of choice for reducing splanchnic blood flow and portal hypertension. The question indicates the patient had a recent endoscopy showing ulcers, and since varices are not mentioned, splanchnic vasoconstrictors such as octreotide are not indicated.

Octreotide, a somatostatin analogue and splanchnic vasoconstrictor, is indicated in patients with variceal bleeding. In this patient, with a history of a recent endoscopy showing only ulcers but not known varices, splanchnic vasoconstrictors are not indicated.

PEER REVIEW

✓ If a patient with acute GI bleeding also has cirrhosis, start antibiotic prophylaxis.

✓ Proton pump inhibitors are recommended for patients with nonvariceal bleeding from peptic ulcers.

✓ If you're treating a patient with hepatic decompensation, octreotide is indicated for variceal bleeding — but not for any other form of GI bleeding.

REFERENCES

Barkun AN, et al. International Consensus Recommendations on the Management of Patients with Nonvariceal Upper Gastrointestinal Bleeding. *Ann Intern Med.* 2010; 152(2):101-13. doi: 10.7326/0003-4819-152-2-201001190-00009.

Marx JA, Hockberger RS, Walls RM, eds. *Rosen's Emergency Medicine: Concepts and Clinical Practice.* 8th ed. St. Louis, MO: Elsevier; 2014: 248-252.

Tintinalli JE, Stapczynski JS, Ma OJ, et al, eds. *Tintinalli's Emergency Medicine: A Comprehensive Study Guide.* 8th ed. New York, NY: McGraw-Hill; 2012: 505.

UptoDate, http://www.uptodate.com/contents/approach-to-acute-upper-gastrointestinal-bleeding-in-adults#H9942856, paragraph on Somatostatin and its Analogues.

230. The correct answer is C, Perform synchronized cardioversion if dysrhythmia recurs; admit to CCU.

Why is this the correct answer?

In this case, the patient is experiencing recurrent episodes of polymorphic ventricular tachycardia (VT) in a configuration that suggests torsades de pointes (TdP). Management in a patient with sustained perfusion as indicated by having a pulse includes treatment or correction of any inciting event, close monitoring, and cardioversion of any sustained, compromising episode of TdP. Caution is needed: TdP has a tendency to frequently recur. Patients with this dysrhythmia should be admitted to a CCU for further monitoring and treatment. Morphologically, VT is separated into two basic subtypes, monomorphic and polymorphic. Torsades de pointes is one particular form of polymorphic VT that occurs in the setting of abnormal ventricular repolarization (manifested by prolongation of the QTc interval beyond 450 msec while in a supraventricular rhythm) and the characteristic pattern of the TdP (progressively increasing/decreasing QRS complex amplitude, as noted in the ECG). Of course, a determination of the QTc interval while in this dysrhythmia is not possible. In this case, the dysrhythmia with its characteristic TdP features and a prolonged QTc interval can be seen in normal sinus rhythm, thus revealing the diagnosis. Torsades de pointes occurs in the setting of electrolyte abnormality (particularly hypokalemia and hypomagnesemia), medication adverse effect (agents that prolong the QT interval), congenital issues, ACS, and other less common issues. Management in cardiac arrest is similar to that of VT in general but with attention to electrolyte issues, if possible.

Why are the other choices wrong?

This patient should be closely monitored, so discharging him, even if he is asymptomatic during his emergency department stay, is not appropriate. Electrical cardioversion should be considered if the dysrhythmia recurs, but only if it is sustained and compromising. Laboratory testing is important, particularly considering electrolytes and troponin. Admission to the hospital is almost always required in this presentation.

Again, close monitoring is needed, as well as admission to the hospital for further observation and treatment. Procainamide is an excellent antiarrhythmic agent but should not be used here because it can prolong the QT interval (which is already abnormally long). In addition, while the stated dose is appropriate, the time of infusion is much too rapid. Procainamide, if given too rapidly, can precipitate hypotension. More appropriately, this medication is administered over 45 to 60 minutes.

As noted above, determination of electrolytes and correction of any significant abnormality is a treatment goal. In addition, if ACS abnormalities are noted, treatment is appropriate; if electrical therapy is needed for an unstable rhythm with a pulse, synchronized cardioversion is appropriate (electrical defibrillation is not appropriate for these situations).

PEER REVIEW

✓ Torsades de pointes is a polymorphic ventricular tachycardia with an abnormally prolonged QTc interval on baseline ECG.
✓ Manage torsades de pointes in cardiac arrest pretty much the same way you manage any VT arrest presentation — if it occurs with a pulse, pay attention to inciting events and optimize oxygenation, ventilation, and perfusion.
✓ Don't use procainamide in patients with torsades de pointes.

REFERENCES

Tintinalli JE, Stapczynski JS, Ma OJ, et al, eds. *Tintinalli's Emergency Medicine: A Comprehensive Study Guide*. 8th ed. New York, NY: McGraw-Hill; 2012: 332-348.

Winters ME, Bond MC, DeBlieux P, et al (eds). *Emergency Department Resuscitation of the Critically Ill*. 2nd ed. Dallas, TX: American College of Emergency Physician Publishing; 2016: 51-68.

231. The correct answer is B, Give oral antibiotics.

Why is this the correct answer?

In this case, the concern is a periodontal infection that has extended into the buccal space but without evidence of systemic infection. The initial treatment is oral antibiotics, either penicillin V or clindamycin. Chlorhexidine gluconate 0.12% rinse is an alternative, but it is expensive and not always covered by insurance. The underlying etiology of the patient's symptoms is usually dental caries and poor dental hygiene, so a follow-up appointment with a dentist is indicated.

Why are the other choices wrong?

Although the patient might eventually require a tooth extraction, it rarely needs to be performed in the emergency department. Most dentists prefer that the patient start a course of antibiotics before extraction.

There is rarely a discrete fluid collection in a periodontal infection, so incision and drainage is unlikely to enhance management. If in doubt, an ultrasound examination can be performed to look for a hypoechoic area.

For the same reason that incision and drainage is unlikely to be successful, aspiration is unlikely to result in improved outcomes.

PEER REVIEW

✓ Periodontal infection, even if indurated, rarely requires emergent drainage.

✓ First-line treatment for periodontal infection: penicillin or clindamycin.

✓ Close follow-up with a dentist is indicated for patients with periodontal infection.

REFERENCES

Knoop KJ, Stack LB, Storrow AB, et al, eds. *The Atlas of Emergency Medicine*. 4th ed. New York, NY: McGraw-Hill; 2016: 135-163.

Laudenbach JM, Simon Z. Common Dental and Periodontal Diseases: Evaluation and Management. *Med Clin N Am*. 2014;98: 1239-1260.

Tintinalli JE, Stapczynski JS, Ma OJ, et al, eds. *Tintinalli's Emergency Medicine: A Comprehensive Study Guide*. 8th ed. New York, NY: McGraw-Hill; 2012: 1598-1613.

232. The correct answer is B, Branchial cleft cyst.

Why is this the correct answer?

Branchial cysts, sinuses, and fistulas are produced by abnormal development of the branchial arches and clefts, and this patient's presentation is consistent with a branchial cleft cyst. Most children who present with these neck masses are younger than 5 years old, and the masses can occur spontaneously. Patients are usually well appearing with no difficulties with breathing or swallowing. The second branchial cleft is the most common site of origin (95%). If there are no signs of an underlying infection, outpatient excision by an otolaryngologist is the definitive treatment.

Why are the other choices wrong?

This patient has no signs of an underlying infection, so an abscess is unlikely. If he had signs of an infection, ENT consultation would be suggested. Given the location, if there were an infection, incision and drainage might be indicated.

Hemangiomas typically present in the first 2 to 4 weeks of life and last until 9 to 10 months of age. After this, they tend to get smaller. They are usually mobile and soft and have a blue tint. Given the patient's age and no signs of discoloration, a hemangioma is not likely.

Because the mass is not midline, a thyroid mass is unlikely. Additionally, the patient does not demonstrate any signs of hyperthyroidism or hypothyroidism.

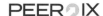

PEER REVIEW

✓ In children, branchial cleft cysts can show up suddenly as a neck mass and prompt a visit to the emergency department.

✓ Branchial cleft cysts can look troubling, but they're usually benign, and outpatient referral to an ENT is appropriate disposition.

REFERENCES

Brown KD, Banuchi V, Selesnick SH, et al. Diseases of the External Ear. In: Lalwani AK, eds. *CURRENT Diagnosis & Treatment in Otolaryngology—Head & Neck Surgery*. 3rd ed. New York, NY: McGraw-Hill; 2012. http://accessmedicine.mhmedical.com/content.aspx?bookid=386&sectionid=39944089. Accessed May 18, 2017.

Schafermeyer RW, Tenenbein M, Macias CG, et al, eds. *Pediatric Emergency Medicine*. 4th ed. New York, NY: McGraw-Hill; 2015: 40-44.

Tintinalli JE, Stapczynski JS, Ma OJ, et al, eds. *Tintinalli's Emergency Medicine: A Comprehensive Study Guide*. 8th ed. New York, NY: McGraw-Hill; 2012: 786-793.

233. The correct answer is C, Roseola infantum.

Why is this the correct answer?

Roseola infantum, or exanthema subitum, is a common acute febrile illness in children 6 months to 3 years old. It is caused by human herpes virus 6. It is characterized by a high spiking fever that lasts 3 to 5 days with additional nonspecific symptoms then defervescence. Next is the sudden onset of a rash often described as pink and maculopapular that blanches to touch and is typically located on the neck, trunk, and buttocks and occasionally on the face and extremities. The rash normally fades after 2 days and is treated with only supportive care. Occasionally, due to the rapid and elevated nature of the febrile portion of this disease, roseola can cause febrile seizures.

Why are the other choices wrong?

Erythema infectiosum, or fifth disease, is a viral exanthema. It is caused by parvovirus B19 and is commonly seen in pediatric patients 5 to 15 years old during the spring. The rash begins as a diffuse erythema on the cheeks (not on the trunk, as it did in this case) with circumoral pallor and subsequent development of a maculopapular rash on the trunk and limbs. After 4 to 5 days, the facial rash resolves, while the body rash clears centrally over the course of 1 week, leaving a lacy appearance. Management is supportive care. Complications include recurrence over the next 3 weeks, arthralgias in teenagers, fetal anomalies in pregnant women, and aplastic crisis in those with sickle cell anemia.

Measles is a highly contagious myxovirus. Its prevalence has decreased due to vaccinations, but it has had a resurgence in recent years in unvaccinated communities; it often presents in winter or spring months. Measles is characterized by a more systemically ill patient with upper respiratory symptoms of cough, coryza, conjunctivitis, and pathognomonic findings of small white to blue spots on a red base seen in the buccal mucosa known as Koplik spots. The rash begins on the face; the spots rapidly blend into each other then spread down the body with often fine desquamation and resolution into a copper rash. Treatment is supportive, but complications include pneumonia, encephalitis, and years later subacute sclerosing panencephalitis.

Rubella, or German measles, is a less commonly seen (again, because of vaccinations) viral exanthema. It is characterized by a prodrome of 1 to 5 days of fever, malaise, sore throat, and suboccipital, posterior auricular or posterior cervical lymphadenopathy. The rash begins as a pink, irregular, maculopapular exanthema starting on the face and progressing down the body, eventually reaching the lower extremities and ultimately coalescing throughout. Small petechiae on the soft palate, or Forchheimer spots, are occasionally present but can be nonspecific. The treatment is supportive.

PEER POINT

A mnemonic for the five most common pediatric rashes

- **Really** — Rubella
- **Red** — Roseola
- **Munchkins** — Measles
- **Scare** — Scarlet fever
- **Parents** — Parvovirus B19

PEER REVIEW

✓ Roseola has high spiking fevers then a nondescript rash.
✓ Rubella has a rash that moves from head to toe with fever and soft palate petechiae.
✓ Measles has Koplik spots and spreads head to toe with confluence.

REFERENCES

Marx JA, Hockberger RS, Walls RM, eds. *Rosen's Emergency Medicine: Concepts and Clinical Practice*. 8th ed. St. Louis, MO: Elsevier; 2014: 1676-1692.

Tintinalli JE, Stapczynski JS, Ma OJ, et al, eds. *Tintinalli's Emergency Medicine: A Comprehensive Study Guide*. 8th ed. New York, NY: McGraw-Hill; 2012: 881-888.

234. The correct answer is B, Lesions in three or more dermatomes.

Why is this the correct answer?

Herpes zoster is the reactivation of the dormant varicella-zoster virus that causes a painful vesicular rash in a dermatomal distribution. The rash characteristically involves one dermatome and is unilateral. Involvement of three or more dermatomes, known as disseminated zoster, should raise the question of an underlying immunocompromised state, perhaps HIV/AIDS, lymphoproliferative disorder, chronic immunosuppressant therapy, or organ transplant. Healthy people can have reactivation of herpes zoster and, in fact, one in every three persons has zoster at some point in life. Incidence increases with age and is most common in patients older than 60 years. If an immunocompromised state is not already known, further investigation is warranted.

Why are the other choices wrong?

Zoster lesions can become superinfected with bacterial pathogens in both immunocompetent and immunocompromised hosts, often as a result of excoriation and skin breakage. Treatment should include appropriate antibiotic therapy in addition to antiviral therapy.

Vesicles in the auditory canal suggest herpes zoster oticus, or Ramsay-Hunt syndrome, and can occur in an immunocompetent host. The characteristic triad includes vesicles in the auditory canal, unilateral facial paralysis, and ear pain. Treatment involves oral steroids in addition to antiviral medication.

Zoster vesicles on the tip of the nose, also known as Hutchinson sign, represent reactivation of the virus along the nasociliary branch of the trigeminal nerve. The nasociliary branch also innervates the cornea and should therefore prompt the physician to evaluate the eye for herpes zoster ophthalmicus. Reactivation along any trigeminal distribution can occur in immunocompetent hosts. Treatment involves topical ophthalmic steroids in addition to antiviral medication.

PEER REVIEW

- ✓ Herpes zoster causes a characteristic painful vesicular rash in a dermatomal distribution.
- ✓ About one in three healthy persons suffers from herpes zoster at some point.
- ✓ Does the patient have a rash involving three or more dermatomes? This might be a clue to underlying immunocompromise.

REFERENCES

Adour KK. Otological complications of herpes zoster. *Ann Neurol.* 1994;35 Suppl:S62.

Centers for Disease Control and Prevention. About shingles (herpes zoster). CDC website. http://www.cdc.gov/shingles/about/index.html. Accessed August 16, 2016.

Pavan-Langston D. Herpes zoster ophthalmicus. *Neurology.* 1995;45(12 Suppl 8):S50.

Tintinalli JE, Stapczynski JS, Ma OJ, et al, eds. *Tintinalli's Emergency Medicine: A Comprehensive Study Guide.* 8th ed. New York, NY: McGraw-Hill; 2012: 1039-1047.

235. The correct answer is C, Single dose of both azithromycin and ceftriaxone.

Why is this the correct answer?

Cervicitis is inflammation of the cervix. Acute cervicitis is typically infectious, and *Chlamydia trachomatis* is the most commonly identified organism, followed by *Neisseria gonorrhoeae*. Given that coinfection is common, CDC guidelines recommend treating for both without waiting for confirmatory testing. Treatment consists of azithromycin 1 g PO for *C. trachomatis* and ceftriaxone 250 mg IM for *N. gonorrhoeae*. Prompt treatment is essential to prevent the spread of infection to sexual partners and to prevent development of more significant infection (pelvic inflammatory disease [PID], tubo-ovarian abscess, endometritis) and long-term sequelae (ectopic pregnancy, infertility). This is especially important with patients who present to emergency departments because follow-up is uncertain.

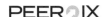

Why are the other choices wrong?

Waiting for confirmatory test results might seem appropriate; however, many women are asymptomatic with chlamydia cervicitis so treatment without culture results is recommended. Annual screening for *C. trachomatis* is currently recommended for all sexually active women 25 years old and younger. Annual screening is also recommended in women older than 25 with new and/or multiple sexual partners, incarcerated women, and pregnant women. Annual screening for males is currently not recommended.

A single dose of azithromycin alone is appropriate treatment for *C. trachomatis* but not for *N. gonorrhoeae*, which is a common coinfectant. Again, current CDC guidelines call for treating both *C. trachomatis* and *N. gonorrhoeae* without confirmatory testing. Dual treatment is a convenient option in the emergency department because a single dose is curative. This also makes adherence a nonissue.

A single dose of ceftriaxone with 14 days of doxycycline and metronidazole is the appropriate treatment for PID. The patient described does not have signs or symptoms of PID. Although pelvic examination in patients with PID commonly reveals cervical erythema, these patients also typically have adnexal or uterine tenderness. Additionally, systemic symptoms are common, including malaise, nausea/vomiting, and fever. In the absence of these additional signs and symptoms or suspicion for PID, simple cervicitis can be treated with a single dose of ceftriaxone and azithromycin, rather than a 14-day course of antibiotics.

PEER REVIEW

- ✓ If a patient's history or examination suggests cervicitis, go ahead and treat it in the emergency department before test results come back.
- ✓ *Chlamydia* and *N. gonorrhoeae* are often coinfectants in cervicitis, so pick antibiotics to cover both.
- ✓ Single-dose therapy with azithromycin (1 g PO) and ceftriaxone (250 mg IM) cures cervicitis.

REFERENCES
Tintinalli JE, Stapczynski JS, Ma OJ, et al, eds. *Tintinalli's Emergency Medicine: A Comprehensive Study Guide*. 8th ed. New York, NY: McGraw-Hill; 2012: 668-672, 1007-1017.

236. The correct answer is B, Heavy bedding during sleep.

Why is this the correct answer?

Sudden unexpected infant death (SUID) is the third leading cause of infant death and is most common in babies 2 to 4 months old. It has been associated with prone sleeping, sleeping on a soft surface, maternal smoking during or after pregnancy, overheating from heavy bedding or clothing, late or no prenatal care, young maternal age, prematurity, low birth weight, and male sex. The incidence of SUID is also notably higher (2 to 3 times) in black and Native American populations. Although the rate of SUID has been decreasing as a result of many initiatives, the "Back to Sleep" and "Safe to Sleep" campaigns among them, SUID remains an important medical issue, and emergency physicians must stay abreast of the common causes. The Centers for Disease Control and Prevention (CDC) defines SUID as death of an infant less than 1 year of age that occurs suddenly and unexpectedly, and whose cause of death is not immediately obvious before investigation. Statistics from the CDC indicate that, in 2014, 3,490 infants in the United States died suddenly and unexpectedly. Emergency physicians are often tasked not only with the resuscitation of the critically ill child but also with investigating the possible causes of death in those infants who die.

Why are the other choices wrong?

Soft bedding, not firm, is associated with SUID. Current recommendations also warn against the use of fluffy blankets, pillows, bumper pads, wedges, and more.

Pet ownership has no association with SUID but can be related to tick exposure and certain types of dermatologic issues.

Prone, not supine, sleeping is associated with SUID. The American Academy of Pediatrics reports that many deaths occur when babies who are used to sleeping supine at home are placed prone to sleep by another caregiver.

PEER REVIEW

- ✓ Sudden unexpected infant death is the third leading cause of infant mortality and is most common between 2 and 4 months of life.
- ✓ Factors associated with sudden unexpected infant death: prone sleeping, sleeping on a soft surface, maternal smoking during or after pregnancy, overheating from heavy bedding or clothing, late or no prenatal care, young maternal age, prematurity, low birth weight, male sex.
- ✓ Sudden unexpected infant death is more common among black and Native American infants.

REFERENCES

Centers for Disease Control and Prevention. About SUID and SIDS. CDC website. http://www.cdc.gov/sids/aboutsuidandsids.htm. Accessed August 14, 2016.

Fleisher GR, Ludwig S, et al, eds. *Textbook of Pediatric Emergency Medicine.* 6th ed. Philadelphia, PA: Lippincott, Williams & Wilkins; 2010:161-163.

Wolfson AB, Hendey GW, Ling LJ, et al, eds. *Harwood-Nuss' Clinical Practice of Emergency Medicine.* 6th ed. Philadelphia, PA: Lippincott, Williams & Wilkins; 2014: 1137-1141; 1307-1308.

237. The correct answer is D, 3.0 uncuffed endotracheal tube.

Why is this the correct answer?

The current recommendation is that endotracheal tubes (ETTs) should be cuffed for all pediatric intubations except for those involving neonates. Endotracheal tube sizing is based on the age of a child except for neonates; sizes are weight based in neonates. For a premature newborn, a 2.5 ETT is recommended because this is

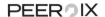

the smallest size available. For a baby weighing 1.6 kg to 3 kg or more, a 3.0 ETT is appropriate. Treatment of the meconium-stained baby has changed dramatically in the past few years. Routine intubation with endotracheal suctioning is no longer recommended for these patients. Only in the depressed child with meconium staining should intubation with suctioning be performed. Acrocyanosis can persist for 24 to 48 hours and is not an indicator of hypoxia but is rather related to blood flow and vasoconstriction.

Why are the other choices wrong?

Neither the 2.5 nor the 3.0 cuffed tube is the right choice for intubating the newborn patient in this case. Recommendations of the American Heart Association call for the use of uncuffed tubes in newborns and cuffed tubes in all other pediatric patients.

The 2.5 uncuffed ETT is the smallest available and is the right choice for a premature newborn but not for a full-term infant like the one described in the case.

Acrocyanosis can persist for 24 to 48 hours and is not a sign of hypoxia.

PEER REVIEW

✓ Only neonates should be intubated with an uncuffed ETT.
✓ Tracheal suctioning should be performed only on a meconium-stained newborn with respiratory depression.

REFERENCES

de Caen AR, Berg MD, Chameides L, et al. Part 12: pediatric advanced life support: 2015 American Heart Association Guidelines Update for Cardiopulmonary Resuscitation and Emergency Cardiovascular Care. *Circulation*. 2015;132(suppl 2):S526–S542. Available at: http://circ.ahajournals.org/content/132/18_suppl_2/S543. Accessed October 12, 2016.

Fleisher GR, Ludwig S, et al, eds. *Textbook of Pediatric Emergency Medicine*. 6th ed. Philadelphia, PA: Lippincott, Williams & Wilkins; 2010: 32-45.

Wolfson AB, Hendey GW, Ling LJ, et al, eds. *Harwood-Nuss' Clinical Practice of Emergency Medicine*. 6th ed. Philadelphia, PA: Lippincott, Williams & Wilkins; 2014: 12-24.

238. The correct answer is B, Herniated disc between L5 and S1.

Why is this the correct answer?

This patient has developed a herniated lumbar disc causing radiculopathy. Based on the physical examination, the affected spinal levels must be L5 and S1, so a disc herniation in this region explains the findings. Most patients with herniated spinal discs recover with medical and physical therapy; operative repair should be avoided. Two elements of the examination contribute to pinpointing the spinal level of the pathology: deep tendon reflexes and skin dermatomes. Deep tendon reflexes correspond to certain spinal levels; the biceps reflex is mediated by C5-C6, the patella reflex by L2-L4, and the ankle jerk by L5-S1. Spinal levels can also be identified by loss of sensation along dermatomes. In the case of this patient, the

L5 dermatome runs along the lateral side of the leg and wraps around to include the toes. The S1 dermatome runs mostly along the back of the leg and wraps into the plantar surface of the foot. Because spinal nerves emerge from the vertebral column and extend inferiorly, herniating spinal discs press on the spinal levels above the level of origin (for example, an L5 herniated disc presses on spinal nerves from L4). Not every patient with back pain should be subjected to imaging, but it is indicated in certain situations. Red flags from the history that indicate the need for imaging include fever, weight loss, incontinence, elderly, intravenous drug use, and a history of cancer or aneurysm. When a neurosurgical emergency is suspected (cauda equina syndrome or spinal cord compression), the MRI is the imaging modality of choice.

Why are the other choices wrong?

A large broad-based disc or mass pressing on the terminal fibers of the spinal cord (the cauda equina) causes the cauda equina syndrome: a loss of sensation in sacral dermatomes between the legs and in the perineum (saddle anesthesia) and a loss of bowel or bladder continence. This patient has localized, distal neurologic abnormalities and no bowel or bladder symptoms.

A lytic lesion, suggesting a neoplasm, is a possible cause of this patient's back pain. But a lesion compressing the L2 nerve root would lead to a decreased patella reflex and anesthesia along the thigh into the medial leg. This patient's examination points to a lesion at the L5-S1 level.

A lesion compressing the L2 nerve root would lead to a decreased patellar reflex and anesthesia along the thigh into the medial leg. This patient's examination points to a lesion at the L5-S1 level.

PEER POINT

Levels of the spine with corresponding dermatomes and reflexes

- C5-C6 — Lateral surface of upper extremity — Biceps or brachioradialis
- C7 — Middle finger — Triceps
- L2-L4 — Thigh into medial leg — Patella
- S1 — Lateral foot — Ankle

Physical examination findings in low back pain that indicate a need for imaging

- Decreased rectal tone — Possible cauda equina syndrome
- Identified level of sensory loss — Spinal cord compression
- Asymmetrical pulses or blood pressure — Suggestive of vascular emergency
- Fever in the context of midline spine pain — Concern for spinal epidural abscess or osteomyelitis
- Herniated lumbar disc on MRI

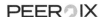
PEER REVIEW

✓ Worrisome low back pain: an asymmetrical pulse or BP might be a sign of vascular emergency.

✓ Deep tendon reflexes and skin dermatomes can help pinpoint the level of spine pathology in patients with low back pain.

✓ Low back pain red flags: fever, weight loss, incontinence, elderly, intravenous drug use, and a history of cancer or aneurysm.

REFERENCES

Adams JG, Barton ED, Collings JL, et al, eds. *Emergency Medicine: Clinical Essentials.* 2nd ed. Philadelphia, PA: Elsevier; 2013: 645-660.e1.

Marx JA, Hockberger RS, Walls RM, eds. *Rosen's Emergency Medicine: Concepts and Clinical Practice.* 8th ed. St. Louis, MO: Elsevier; 2014: 278-284.e1.

239. The correct answer is C, Needle decompression of chest.

Why is this the correct answer?

This patient has pulseless electrical activity (PEA). Given the past medical history of cystic fibrosis and the "H's" and "T's" of PEA, decompression of the bilateral lungs should be performed. There should be a strong suspicion that the cause of the patient's cardiac arrest is respiratory in nature because of the history of cystic fibrosis (CF) and the fact that she was being treated for respiratory difficulties prior to the event. Pneumothorax is a common complication of CF (the second most common cause of chest pain in these patients) and occurs much more commonly than in the general public (up to 3.5% of CF patients develop a spontaneous pneumothorax, and there is a 20% recurrence rate). Given the high rate of spontaneous disease, the patient with pulseless electrical activity should be assessed and if found, treated rapidly for a tension pneumothorax. If the patient is already intubated, the mnemonic, DOPE — Displacement of the endotracheal tube, Obstruction within the endotracheal tube, Pneumothorax, and Equipment malfunction — can point to causes for acute respiratory decompensation. This is especially true in the intubated patient who is being moved from one position to another, for example, from a prehospital stretcher to an emergency department stretcher.

Why are the other choices wrong?

Even though access is an important component of CPR, central line placement would not be a life-saving procedure in this patient.

A cricothyrotomy is not warranted in this patient, as there is no indication of upper airway obstruction (such as would be found in a patient with acute anaphylaxis or foreign body obstruction). Patients with cystic fibrosis do have an increase in mucus production, but this causes lower airway obstruction, not upper airway obstruction.

The same can be said for peripheral intravenous access. The patient is in cardiopulmonary arrest. Although a tenet of care is to obtain venous access, the crucial aspect in this case is to quickly address the potential cause for the arrest. Given the patient's clinical presentation, a tension pneumothorax is the likely cause and should be addressed.

PEER POINT

Remember your H's and T's — the causes of cardiac arrest

5 H's

- Hypovolemia or hemorrhage
- Hypoxia
- Hydrogen ion (acidosis)
- Hypokalemia or hyperkalemia
- Hypothermia

5 T's

- Trauma, tablets (overdose)
- Tamponade (cardiac)
- Thrombosis (coronary)
- Tension pneumothorax
- Thrombosis (PE)

PEER REVIEW

✓ What's the best initial approach to acute cardiopulmonary arrest? Start by considering the current illness and past medical history.

✓ Use DOPE to run through the possible causes of respiratory decompensation in an intubated patient — Displacement of the endotracheal tube, Obstruction within the endotracheal tube, Pneumothorax, and Equipment malfunction.

REFERENCES

Fleisher GR, Ludwig S, et al, eds. *Textbook of Pediatric Emergency Medicine*. 6th ed. Philadelphia, PA: Lippincott, Williams & Wilkins; 2010: 1091-1098.

Tintinalli JE, Stapczynski JS, Ma OJ, et al, eds. *Tintinalli's Emergency Medicine: A Comprehensive Study Guide*. 8th ed. New York, NY: McGraw-Hill; 2012: 160-167.

Wolfson AB, Hendey GW, Ling LJ, et al, eds. *Harwood-Nuss' Clinical Practice of Emergency Medicine*. 6th ed. Philadelphia, PA: Lippincott, Williams & Wilkins; 2014: 434-436, 1224-1230.

240. The correct answer is C, Hypocarbia, cerebral vasoconstriction.

Why is this the correct answer?

Psychiatric illnesses, most commonly major depressive disorder and generalized anxiety disorder, can be associated with symptoms of syncope. Hyperventilation as a result of these disorders causes a blowing off of carbon dioxide resulting in hypocarbia. This respiratory alkalosis leads to constriction of the cerebral blood vessels. The vasoconstriction can lead to lightheadedness with resultant syncope if the patient concurrently performs a Valsalva maneuver or has been standing for a prolonged period of time. The alkalosis can also result in constriction of peripheral blood vessels contributing to the tingling feeling in the hands and feet. A thorough medical workup for organic causes of the syncopal event should be initiated before diagnosing a psychiatric syncope.

Why are the other choices wrong?

Hyperventilation leads to hypocarbia, not hypercarbia. Hypercarbia occurs in respiratory acidosis from decreased volume or rate of breathing. Hyperventilation leads to hypocarbia, not hypercarbia. But hypercarbia from respiratory acidosis can cause minimal cerebral vasodilation. Hypocarbia from respiratory alkalosis is associated with cerebral vasoconstriction and decreased cerebral blood flow.

PEER POINT

Causes of syncope, with examples

- Hyperventilation leads to hypocarbia and respiratory alkalosis, with cerebral vasoconstriction.
- Cardiac — Arrhythmias, myxoma, aortic dissection, myocardial infarction
- Neurologic — Subclavian stenosis, transient ischemic attack
- Orthostatic — Dehydration, medications
- Psychiatric — Hyperventilation
- Reflex-mediated — Vasovagal, cough, micturition

PEER REVIEW

- ✓ Vasoconstriction leads to presyncope/syncope and symptoms of peripheral tingling.
- ✓ Psychogenic syncope is a diagnosis of exclusion and requires a careful history, physical examination, and medical workup.

REFERENCES

Marx JA, Hockberger RS, Walls RM, eds. *Rosen's Emergency Medicine: Concepts and Clinical Practice.* 8th ed. St. Louis, MO: Elsevier; 2014: 339-367.e4.

Tintinalli JE, Stapczynski JS, Ma OJ, et al, eds. *Tintinalli's Emergency Medicine: A Comprehensive Study Guide.* 8th ed. New York, NY: McGraw-Hill; 2012: 360-365.

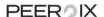

241. The correct answer is A, Extra-abdominal disorders such as pneumonia can result in abdominal pain.

Why is this the correct answer?

Extra-abdominal disorders commonly present with abdominal pain. In some cases, the pathology is simply close to the diaphragm or peritoneum and stimulates the somatic innervation, resulting in sharp, easily localized abdominal pain. Pneumonia in a lower lobe is a good example. In other cases, the pathology results in visceral pain, a dull, poorly localized pain associated with autonomic symptoms; this is the case with inferior MIs presenting as epigastric discomfort. Another well-described phenomenon obscuring the source of pain in the abdomen or torso is the concept of referred pain. With referred pain, the nerves of the same spinal level as the noxious stimulus are triggered, causing perceived pain in the corresponding dermatome. For example, diaphragmatic irritation from blood in the right upper quadrant causes right shoulder pain. Irritation of foregut structures such as the stomach and esophagus results in pain in the epigastric region. Pain in midgut structures such as the small intestine and appendix stimulates nerves, and that results in periumbilical pain. Hindgut organ pain, including pain in the sigmoid colon and rectum, results in lower abdominal pain. Other examples of extra-abdominal conditions presenting as abdominal pain include herpes zoster infection affecting an abdominal dermatome, testicular torsion causing flank or lower abdominal pain, diabetic ketoacidosis causing generalized abdominal pain frequently associated with vomiting, and the well-known phenomenon in children of somatization of many complaints to the abdomen (especially sore throats, headaches, and stress).

Why are the other choices wrong?

Irritation of the peritoneum causes sharp, well-localized visceral pain, not dull and poorly localized pain.

Distention of abdominal organs results in visceral pain, not somatic pain.

Visceral pain from irritation of the colon manifests as lower, not upper, abdominal pain.

PEER POINT

Extra-abdominal disorders and how they manifest as abdominal pain

- Black widow spider bite — Severe abdominal pain associated with rigidity
- Diabetic ketoacidosis — Generalized abdominal pain
- Herpes zoster infection — Sharp pain across one side into back
- MI and unstable angina — Epigastric pain associated with autonomic symptoms
- Pharyngitis — Generalized abdominal pain in children
- Pneumonia — Sharp upper abdominal or flank pain
- Porphyria — Episodic attacks of generalized pain
- Testicular torsion — Flank or lower abdominal pain

PEER REVIEW

✓ Somatic pain is caused by stimulation of the peritoneum and is sharp and well localized.

✓ Visceral pain is caused by stretching of the visceral nerves surrounding organs and is poorly localized, dull, and associated with autonomic symptoms such as nausea or diaphoresis.

✓ Abdominal pain may result from extra-abdominal disorders causing pain adjacent to abdominal structures or causing referred pain that manifests in an abdominal location.

REFERENCES

Marx JA, Hockberger RS, Walls RM, eds. *Rosen's Emergency Medicine: Concepts and Clinical Practice*. 8th ed. St. Louis, MO: Elsevier; 2014: 223-231.e1.

Tintinalli JE, Stapczynski JS, Ma OJ, et al, eds. *Tintinalli's Emergency Medicine: A Comprehensive Study Guide*. 8th ed. New York, NY: McGraw-Hill; 2012: 481-489.

242. The correct answer is C, Right internal jugular vein.

Why is this the correct answer?

Emergency pacing is indicated for unstable bradycardias, unstable high-degree AV blockades, and overdrive pacing of torsades de pointes and ventricular tachycardia. Transvenous pacemakers are placed using specialized central line kits and are typically inserted through either the right internal jugular vein or left subclavian vein due to the more direct route of passage to the heart. Inserting a transvenous pacemaker follows the same initial steps as central line insertion. After the catheter is in place, a special pacing wire is passed through the central line introducer and advanced approximately 10 cm. The distal balloon is inflated, and the wire is advanced until it reaches the apex of the right ventricle. Proper placement can be confirmed by following ECG tracings, fluoroscopy, or cardiac ultrasonography. Once in place, the pacemaker should be set to demand mode at 80 to 100 beats per minute, and the output dial should be increased until capture. Once capture is obtained, the output dial should be lowered until capture is lost, and then it should be set at 1.5 to 2 times the minimal threshold output required for capture. Complications include cardiac dysrhythmias, myocardial perforation, catheter dislodgment, and circuit failure, as well as those complications known to occur with central venous access. The presence of a prosthetic tricuspid valve is an absolute contraindication to transvenous pacing.

Why are the other choices wrong?

The right external jugular vein has a short course before joining the right internal jugular vein. It is often used for peripheral access; however, it is not used for transvenous pacing.

The right femoral vein may be used for transvenous pacing, but is not preferred due to the difficulty of accessing the right ventricle when entering the right atrium from the inferior vena cava.

The right subclavian vein may be used for transvenous pacing, but involves entering the superior vena cava at a bifurcation, which significantly increases the likelihood of pacemaker wire misplacement. Thus the left subclavian vein and right internal vein are preferred for access when possible.

PEER REVIEW

✓ Preferred access sites for placing a transvenous pacemaker: right internal jugular vein and left subclavian vein.

✓ Once capture is obtained, decrease the output dial to 1.5 to 2 times the minimal threshold necessary for capture.

REFERENCES

Roberts JR, Hedges JR, eds. *Clinical Procedures in Emergency Medicine*. 6th ed. St. Louis, Mo: WB Saunders; 2013: 277-293.

Tintinalli JE, Stapczynski JS, Ma OJ, et al, eds. *Tintinalli's Emergency Medicine: A Comprehensive Study Guide*. 8th ed. New York, NY: McGraw-Hill; 2012: 218.

243. The correct answer is A, Check the patient's electrolyte levels and replenish them as needed.

Why is this the correct answer?

Patients with eating disorders, including anorexia nervosa and bulimia nervosa, frequently develop electrolyte abnormalities. Hypokalemia is common, particularly in patients who purge, and should be treated with potassium repletion. Elevated bicarbonate (>35 mEq/L) and low potassium levels (<3 mEq/L) in young and otherwise healthy patients should raise suspicion for purging behavior. Patients with anorexia might present with the restrictive subtype, which involves simply minimizing caloric intake, binge/purge subtype, or a combination of the two. There is some crossover between anorexia and bulimia. In fact, up to half of all patients with anorexia eventually develop bulimia.

Why are the other choices wrong?

Pharmacotherapy for this patient is best determined in consultation with a psychiatrist. Bupropion is contraindicated in patients with eating disorders: it can lower seizure threshold in those with electrolyte abnormalities and can also lead to worsening weight loss. Other antidepressants such as the SSRIs might have some benefit in treating bulimia and can be helpful in treating comorbid symptoms of anxiety and depression.

Intravenous fluids should be given cautiously in this patient. Many patients like her develop heart muscle atrophy, and excessive fluid administration can result in pulmonary edema and signs of heart failure.

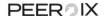

Malnourished patients with anorexia nervosa typically have lower than normal blood pressure (<90 mm Hg systolic) and heart rate (<60 bpm). Although the patient in this scenario might indeed be dehydrated and require oral or intravenous hydration, overly aggressive resuscitation with vasopressors is not indicated.

PEER REVIEW

✓ If you're treating a patient who has an eating disorder, suspect electrolyte abnormalities.

✓ Patients with anorexia nervosa often have chronic asymptomatic hypotension — they don't need aggressive blood pressure treatment in the emergency department.

✓ Another caution on patients with eating disorders: getting too aggressive with intravenous hydration can result in pulmonary edema and heart failure.

✓ Patients with eating disorders shouldn't be taking bupropion.

REFERENCES

Tintinalli JE, Stapczynski JS, Ma OJ, et al, eds. *Tintinalli's Emergency Medicine: A Comprehensive Study Guide.* 8th ed. New York, NY: McGraw-Hill; 2012: 1973-1976.

Zun L, Chepenik LG, Mallory MNS. *Behavioral Emergencies for the Emergency Physician.* Cambridge, NY: Cambridge; 2013: Chapter 19 ("Acute Care of Eating Disorders").

244. The correct answer is B, Cesarean delivery.

Why is this the correct answer?

This patient is suffering from endometritis, a polymicrobial infection of the uterus following delivery. Risk factors for its development include retained products of conception or placenta, cesarean delivery, young maternal age, premature rupture of membranes, frequent vaginal examinations, and the use of intrauterine monitoring devices. The history of a cesarean delivery is the risk factor most frequently associated with endometritis, which might be associated with a concomitant wound infection. Complications of endometritis include parametrial abscesses, pelvic abscesses, and septic thrombophlebitis of the pelvic veins. Obese and diabetic patients are at risk for developing necrotizing fasciitis of the pelvis if their infections are not controlled aggressively. Endometritis typically begins 3 to 5 days following delivery and is characterized by foul lochia, fever, pelvic pain, and uterine tenderness. The ultrasonographic examination can be normal, or it can show a thickened endometrium with increased vascularity. In severe cases, gas might be identified within the uterus. In all but the mildest of cases, these patients should be treated as inpatients with intravenous, broad-spectrum antibiotics (typically, third-generation cephalosporins or clindamycin plus gentamicin).

Why are the other choices wrong?

Younger maternal age and lower socioeconomic status are risk factors for endometritis.

Internal fetal monitors, any instrumentation, and repeated digital examinations are risk factors for the development of endometritis.

Any condition that prolongs the period of exposure of the unprotected endometrium to the vaginal canal can lead to endometritis such as the premature rupture of membranes and a prolonged period of active labor.

PEER REVIEW

✓ Endometritis develops a few days after delivery with fever, pelvic pain, uterine tenderness, and foul-smelling lochia.

✓ Endometritis is a polymicrobial infection that should be treated with broad-spectrum antibiotics, usually including beta-lactam antibiotics.

REFERENCES

Adams JG, Barton ED, Collings JL, et al, eds. *Emergency Medicine: Clinical Essentials.* 2nd ed. Philadelphia, PA: Elsevier; 2013: 1061-1068.e1.

Tintinalli JE, Stapczynski JS, Ma OJ, et al, eds. *Tintinalli's Emergency Medicine: A Comprehensive Study Guide.* 8th ed. New York, NY: McGraw-Hill; 2012: 644-652.

245. The correct answer is D, Wait-and-see prescription for antibiotics.

Why is this the correct answer?

The patient has symptoms consistent with acute otitis media. He is a candidate for a "wait-and-see" prescription for an antibiotic if his symptoms do not improve in 48 to 72 hours. He meets the criteria for "wait and see" including age ≥ to 2 years old, unilateral infection, symptoms for fewer than 48 hours, and temperature is less than 39°C. Assuming there are no contraindications, amoxicillin (90 mg/kg/day PO for 5 to 10 days) is the first-line treatment. Amoxicillin-clavulanate is appropriate if the patient has failed a course of amoxicillin. Cephalosporins like cefdinir or cefuroxime or clindamycin are appropriate in penicillin-allergic patients. *Streptococcus pneumoniae* is the most common bacterial organism, although most cases are viral.

Why are the other choices wrong?

Given the tympanic membrane visualized, antipyretics alone are not sufficient if there is no improvement within 48 to 72 hours. Complications from untreated bacterial otitis media include mastoiditis and hearing complications.

If the wait-and-see approach fails, the patient should complete a course of antibiotics. Referral to an ENT for possible tympanostomy should only occur after repeated episodes of otitis media.

Immediate use of antibiotics has been shown not to improve outcomes when using these criteria. In addition, there is an increased risk of diarrhea and antibiotic resistance for those who take antibiotics.

✓ The wait-and-see approach to antibiotic administration in acute otitis media in children is safe when patients meet certain criteria.

✓ Wait-and-see has been found to cut in half the use of antibiotics with no worse outcomes.

REFERENCES

Friedman NR, Scholes MA, Yoon PJ, et al. Ear, Nose, & Throat. In: Hay WW, Jr., Levin MJ, Deterding RR, et al, eds. *CURRENT Diagnosis & Treatment: Pediatrics*. 22nd ed. New York, NY: McGraw-Hill; 2013. http://accessmedicine.mhmedical.com/content. aspx?bookid=1016&sectionid=6159776. Accessed May 18, 2017.

Tintinalli JE, Stapczynski JS, Ma OJ, et al, eds. *Tintinalli's Emergency Medicine: A Comprehensive Study Guide*. 8th ed. New York, NY: McGraw-Hill; 2012: 757-764.

246. The correct answer is C, Send a urine sample for *Chlamydia trachomatis* and *Neisseria gonorrhoeae* PCR assay.

Why is this the correct answer?

Among patients in the United States, urethritis is most commonly caused by infection with *Chlamydia trachomatis*. The most sensitive and specific test for *C. trachomatis* is a nucleic acid amplification technique (NAAT) such as the polymerase chain reaction (PCR) assay. Because infection with *N. gonorrhoeae* often accompanies infection with *C. trachomatis*, if one is considered, the other must be as well. The NAAT is not quite as sensitive for *N. gonorrhoeae* as it is for chlamydial infection, but the yield is still vastly improved over the traditional chocolate agar or Thayer-Martin culture medium. In men, the symptoms of chlamydial infection — dysuria with urethritis or epididymitis — appear 1 to 3 weeks after exposure. In women, the infection is asymptomatic in up to 75% of cases, so the Centers for Disease Control recommends the screening of asymptomatic women as a public health measure. Samples may be obtained from the urethra in women, but endocervical samples have a higher yield. Treatment consists of azithromycin 1 g PO for chlamydial infection and ceftriaxone 250 mg IM for gonorrhea. Widespread resistance to quinolones and other agents in *N. gonorrhoeae* severely limits the options for oral therapy. Gonorrhea can also cause pharyngitis or proctitis. Generally, the symptoms of these two infections are indistinguishable, and coinfection is common.

Why are the other choices wrong?

Because of the availability of NAATs for testing of patients' urine, it is not necessary to obtain samples from men from inside the urethra. This is unnecessarily painful. Furthermore, cell cultures for *C. trachomatis* are difficult to perform and are unreliable. Also, the proper medium for *N. gonorrhoeae* is the chocolate agar or Thayer-Martin agar, not the standard blood agar.

Detection via latex agglutination testing of *C. trachomatis* and *N. gonorrhoeae* in the pharynx is possible for patients who have engaged in oral-genital contact. But if they have not, the best test is a PCR assay, as with testing patient's urine.

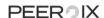

A urinalysis with microscopic examination and culture is appropriate for patients with dysuria when a urinary tract infection is suspected. That is a reasonable initial step in this patient's evaluation, but the presence of urethral discharge ("drip") is strongly suspicious for urethritis caused by *C. trachomatis* or *N. gonorrhoeae*. A standard urine culture does not grow either of these organisms.

PEER REVIEW

✓ The nucleic acid amplification technique, or NAAT, is the best test for *C. trachomatis* and *N. gonorrhoeae*, and in men, it works with a urine sample.

✓ Up to 75% of women with chlamydial infection are asymptomatic.

✓ If you're treating a chlamydial infection with azithromycin, add ceftriaxone parenterally to treat gonorrhea.

REFERENCES

Marx JA, Hockberger RS, Walls RM, eds. *Rosen's Emergency Medicine: Concepts and Clinical Practice.* 8th ed. St. Louis, MO: Elsevier; 2014: 1312-1325.e1.

Tintinalli JE, Stapczynski JS, Ma OJ, et al, eds. *Tintinalli's Emergency Medicine: A Comprehensive Study Guide.* 8th ed. New York, NY: McGraw-Hill; 2012: 1007-1017.

247. The correct answer is A, Apply a long-leg splint to the left leg and arrange follow-up care.

Why is this the correct answer?

Toddler fracture is a very common injury in children who have recently began to walk (toddlers). Emergency department treatment is largely supportive, usually placement of a long-leg splint. The mechanism of injury described by the father is consistent with findings on the xray, so there is no specific reason to suspect child abuse. This type of fracture, considered to be a subset of childhood accidental spiral tibia (CAST) fractures, occurs in young children from those just beginning to walk to those older than 7 years. The mean age for it is 50 months, just over 4 years. It is a fracture of the tibia diaphysis and usually occurs in the distal third but can extend into the midshaft. Spiral fractures of the proximal third of the tibia or of the femur are less likely to be accidental and should prompt consideration of abuse. A toddler fracture can be radiographically obscure at initial presentation. If this fracture is suspected because the patient is not walking but xrays are negative, repeat the films in 7 to 10 days: the fracture might be more evident then. The patient might benefit from splinting of the extremity in the interim.

Why are the other choices wrong?

Percutaneous pins are used to secure the epiphyseal (growth) plate to the diaphysis in unstable Salter-Harris fractures. This patient's injury is limited to the diaphysis; the epiphyseal plate is not involved.

The higher types of Salter-Harris fractures carry a worse prognosis for normal bone development and might need more aggressive treatment. Also, supracondylar fractures require immediate operative management. But toddler fractures are generally benign and may be treated conservatively.

Spiral fractures can result from child abuse, from a perpetrator twisting the victim's arm or leg. But spiral fractures of the tibia in a toddler, given the appropriate context, are very common and do not always warrant suspicion of abuse. Again, spiral fractures of the proximal third of the tibia or of the femur are more likely the result of abuse.

PEER REVIEW

✓ What is a CAST fracture? Childhood accidental spiral tibia–spiral fractures of the tibia diaphysis common in children who are new at walking.
✓ Toddler fractures are generally benign, so you can treat them conservatively in the emergency department with a long-leg splint.
✓ So which leg fractures in kids warrant suspicion of abuse? Spiral fractures of the proximal tibia and of the femur, and leg fractures in infants who aren't walking yet.

REFERENCES

Adams JG, Barton ED, Collings JL, et al, eds. *Emergency Medicine: Clinical Essentials.* 2nd ed. Philadelphia, PA: Elsevier; 2013: 204-208.e1.

Schafermeyer RW, Tenenbein M, Macias CG, et al, eds. *Pediatric Emergency Medicine.* 4th ed. New York, NY: McGraw-Hill; 2015: 189-195.

Tintinalli JE, Stapczynski JS, Ma OJ, et al, eds. *Tintinalli's Emergency Medicine: A Comprehensive Study Guide.* 8th ed. New York, NY: McGraw-Hill; 2012: 915-934.

248. The correct answer is A, Administer an opioid and a benzodiazepine to relieve his symptoms.

Why is this the correct answer?

Although both inpatient and outpatient hospice services are widely available, the emergency department is frequently the default location for end-of-life care. Emergency practitioners can do a notable service to their patients by providing relief of painful and uncomfortable symptoms toward the end of life. In many cases, opioid analgesia is appropriate for pain relief, and benzodiazepines can help alleviate anxiety and dyspnea symptoms. Emergency clinicians must be aware of issues specific to patients at the end of life and be comfortable providing not only life-sustaining treatment but also palliative care. Early in the encounter with a patient at the end of life, the emergency physician should talk with the patient and family to learn what the goals of care are — what the patient's wishes are, how those wishes have been communicated or documented, what the patient and family expect from the encounter, what therapeutic and palliative options are available, what the likely outcome of treatment is, and overall, what the overall trajectory of the patient's current condition is. Many hospitals have a palliative care team available for consultation. Palliative care should be thought of as any other consulting service

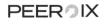

that can provide specialized expertise to assist with patient care. Although palliative care is more generally considered to be in the domain of the inpatient services, there are situations in which it is appropriate to engage these experts in the emergency department to assist with medical decision making, symptomatic treatment, and disposition planning.

Why are the other choices wrong?

Although it might be reasonable to withhold certain treatments and to provide others, such decisions should be made with the patient's comfort and expressed wishes in mind and after consulting with the patient and family. So, while it might be reasonable to withhold antibiotics in this situation, it is more important to determine the patient's specific goals of care. It is important in a case like this to determine whether the patient and family are comfortable with treating the pneumonia while withholding more aggressive measures like CPR and intubation.

The POLST form — Physician Orders for Life-Sustaining Treatment — is a standardized physician order designed to stay with the patient across inpatient and outpatient settings. It has become increasingly popular and widespread over the past several years and was designed to address deficiencies in the advance directive process. However, a POLST form is not required for a physician to act in accordance with a patient's wishes. Whenever possible, care providers should discuss goals of care with the patient and family. Even at the end of life, many patients are clear minded enough to express their wishes in a way that is much more helpful than simply relying on a document such as a DNR order or living will.

Do-not-resuscitate (DNR) orders take various forms, and it is incumbent on the emergency physician to parse each DNR order's specific nuances. In many cases, "do not resuscitate" is not synonymous with "do nothing." Many patients at the end of their lives might have a desire to receive medical care if it is directed toward a reversible condition or symptom.

PEER REVIEW

- ✓ The emergency department is increasingly becoming a location for end-of-life and palliative care.
- ✓ Palliative care consultation is frequently available and appropriate in the emergency department.
- ✓ When possible, care providers should discuss the goals of care with patients and families.

REFERENCES

Marx JA, Hockberger RS, Walls RM, eds. *Rosen's Emergency Medicine: Concepts and Clinical Practice*. 8th ed. St. Louis, MO: Elsevier; 2014: 2518.

Tintinalli JE, Stapczynski JS, Ma OJ, et al, eds. *Tintinalli's Emergency Medicine: A Comprehensive Study Guide*. 8th ed. New York, NY: McGraw-Hill; 2012: 2013-2017.

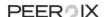

249. The correct answer is D, Wrap the toe in a dry, bulky dressing and discharge.

Why is this the correct answer?

Gangrene occurs when there is insufficient blood supply to affected tissues. In this case, the patient has dry gangrene, which is defined as necrotic tissue without secondary bacterial infection. Dry gangrene is not a surgical emergency. Treatment is application of bulky dressings to protect the affected tissues and prevent the development of wet gangrene. Diabetic persons, those with advanced atherosclerotic disease, and elderly persons are most at risk. Ultimately, this patient needs surgical evaluation for revascularization or debridement of the affected extremity. Given that her symptoms are chronic, she is nontoxic, and she has no acute vascular compromise or infection, her care can be coordinated on an urgent outpatient basis. In contrast, wet gangrene (gangrenous tissue with evidence of infection) is treated with broad-spectrum intravenous antibiotics, emergent surgical consultation, and immediate debridement of affected tissue.

Why are the other choices wrong?

Hyperbaric oxygen is a controversial treatment for diabetic foot infections. It has no role in the acute management of either dry gangrene or wet gangrene.

Dry gangrene, by definition, is not an infection, so oral antibiotic therapy is not part of the treatment. If infection of the gangrenous tissue were suspected, oral antibiotics and outpatient follow-up would be inappropriate. Appropriate care of dry gangrene is important to prevent conversion from uninfected dry gangrene to infected wet gangrene.

Intravenous vancomycin and piperacillin-tazobactam with emergent surgical consultation is the treatment of choice for wet gangrene. Patients at risk for wet gangrene are often prone to polymicrobial infections, and broad-spectrum antibiotics should be used. Bacterial species commonly implicated in wet gangrene include *Staphylococcus*, *Streptococcus*, *Pseudomonas*, and anaerobic bacteria. Aggressive antibiotic treatment and early debridement followed by revascularization can help prevent progression of the disease and maximize limb salvage.

PEER REVIEW

- ✓ Gangrene is tissue that died as a result of disrupted blood supply.
- ✓ Chronic dry gangrene is not a surgical emergency and is treated with protective dressings.
- ✓ Wet gangrene is an infection of gangrenous tissue and is a surgical emergency. Treat it with broad-spectrum antibiotics and prompt surgical consultation.

REFERENCES

Marx JA, Hockberger RS, Walls RM, eds. *Rosen's Emergency Medicine: Concepts and Clinical Practice*. 8th ed. St. Louis, MO: Elsevier; 2014: 1809-1830.

Tintinalli JE, Stapczynski JS, Ma OJ, et al, eds. *Tintinalli's Emergency Medicine: A Comprehensive Study Guide*. 8th ed. New York, NY: McGraw-Hill; 2012: 1029-1039.

250. The correct answer is C, Lorazepam.

Why is this the correct answer?

This patient's complicated presentation is a combination of cocaine intoxication and out-of-control diabetes (and possibly diabetic ketoacidosis). Her abnormal vital signs are due to adrenergic stimulation from the cocaine, physiologic response to hypovolemia and dehydration, and respiratory compensation for metabolic acidosis. The treatment of choice for the symptoms of cocaine intoxication is a benzodiazepine such as lorazepam or diazepam. Cocaine is a sympathomimetic that blocks the reuptake of sympathetic neurotransmitters. It induces vasoconstriction via alpha-adrenergic stimulation and has sodium channel blocking properties (class I antiarrhythmics). Clinically, cocaine causes hypertension, tachycardia, palpitations, anxiety, diaphoresis, and mydriasis. The sodium channel blockade can lead to ventricular wide-complex tachyarrhythmias. Because cocaine causes alpha-agonist and beta-agonist stimulation, the use of beta-blocking medications in acute cocaine intoxication has been associated with rapidly elevated blood pressure due to unopposed alpha stimulation. Wide-complex arrhythmias should be treated with sodium bicarbonate to counter the sodium channel blockade. Chest pain from cocaine intoxication is usually relieved by nitroglycerin. Phentolamine, an alpha-blocking medication, may be considered for refractory vasoconstriction. Patients who are attempting to smuggle packets of cocaine in their bowels (body packers) are at risk for dramatic and severe overdoses if packets rupture.

Why are the other choices wrong?

Haloperidol can contribute to the risk of a tachyarrhythmia and also lowers the seizure threshold. It and other antipsychotic medications should be avoided in cocaine intoxication.

Lidocaine is a Class Ib antiarrhythmic drug, indicating that it has sodium channel-blocking properties. It is contraindicated in cocaine toxicity because it can potentiate the development of a wide-complex tachycardia, potentiate cocaine toxicity, and decrease seizure threshold.

Metoprolol, a "cardioselective" beta blocker, is relatively contraindicated in acute cocaine intoxication because of the risk of unopposed alpha stimulation. Although the risk of this complication has been questioned by some authors, other broader-acting adrenergic antagonists are a better choice.

PEER REVIEW

✓ The treatment of choice for the symptoms of cocaine and methamphetamine intoxication is a benzodiazepine.

✓ Cocaine has sodium channel-blocking properties that can lead to ventricular wide-complex tachyarrhythmias.

✓ Nitroglycerin or phentolamine may be given for severe vasoconstriction and chest pain associated with cocaine intoxication.

REFERENCES

Adams JG, Barton ED, Collings JL, et al, eds. *Emergency Medicine: Clinical Essentials*. 2nd ed. Philadelphia, PA: Elsevier; 2013: 1280-1285.e1.

Tintinalli JE, Stapczynski JS, Ma OJ, et al, eds. *Tintinalli's Emergency Medicine: A Comprehensive Study Guide*. 8th ed. New York, NY: McGraw-Hill; 2012: 1256-1260.

251. The correct answer is C, Posterior reversible encephalopathy syndrome.

Why is this the correct answer?

The posterior reversible encephalopathy syndrome (PRES) was first described in 1996 and is characterized by seizures, altered mental status, hypertension, and vision changes. It is associated with bilateral white matter changes in the posterior temporal and occipital lobes, which are most easily seen on MRI. Patients with PRES are typically those who are prone to sharp spikes in blood pressure, as seen in eclampsia and kidney disease, and those on immunosuppressive therapy such as those with autoimmune disease and transplanted organs. Patients with diabetes and malignancies are also as risk to develop PRES. Patients with this condition typically have days of fluctuating symptoms (hence the term reversible) before presentation. The onset of seizures is the most common presenting sign. Computed tomography usually does not show an abnormality, but if it does, the changes are seen bilaterally in the posterior brain. This is a stark difference from ischemic strokes, which are unilateral, in a single vascular distribution. Magnetic resonance imaging of the brain is a more reliable way to see the characteristic posterior white matter changes in PRES. Treatment consists of the usual antiepileptic treatments for seizures, including benzodiazepines and fosphenytoin or phenobarbital. The hypertension should be managed in the same way any hypertensive emergency is, with intravenous calcium channel blockers or beta blockers.

Why are the other choices wrong?

An adrenergic agonist overdose might be associated with tachycardia, hypertension, and seizures, but patients are unlikely to have normal pupils. A patient who is acutely intoxicated with an adrenergic agonist is more likely to be diaphoretic with dilated pupils.

A basilar artery aneurysm can be associated with vertigo and vision disturbances and could be more likely to develop in a patient with hypertension; however, a basilar artery aneurysm is not necessarily associated with seizures and is very unlikely to present with bilateral lesions.

Sheehan syndrome is the ischemic necrosis of the pituitary gland that can develop following maternal hemorrhage and hypotension in the peripartum period. It leads to hypopituitarism, hypothyroidism, adrenal insufficiency, and amenorrhea. Patients with Sheehan syndrome can initially be asymptomatic; the condition is identified after the patient develops difficulty breastfeeding (agalactorrhea) or amenorrhea.

PEER REVIEW

✓ Posterior reversible encephalopathy syndrome, or PRES, is characterized by seizures, altered mental status, hypertension, and vision changes.

✓ You can see the bilateral white matter changes associated with PRES most easily using MRI.

✓ Treat PRES with antiepileptic medications and emergent lowering of elevated blood pressure.

REFERENCES

Adams JG, Barton ED, Collings JL, et al, eds. *Emergency Medicine: Clinical Essentials.* 2nd ed. Philadelphia, PA: Elsevier; 2013: 1061-1068.e1.

Tintinalli JE, Stapczynski JS, Ma OJ, et al, eds. *Tintinalli's Emergency Medicine: A Comprehensive Study Guide.* 8th ed. New York, NY: McGraw-Hill; 2012: 399-409.

252. The correct answer is D, Midline vertical incision from pubic symphysis to xiphoid process.

Why is this the correct answer?

Understanding the indications and gaining competence in the technique for performing resuscitative hysterotomy (perimortem cesarean delivery) are crucial for emergency physicians. The midline vertical incision from pubic symphysis to just below the xiphoid process is the most rapid and safe technique for a perimortem cesarean delivery. A single vertical incision is made vertically using a #10 scalpel through the abdominal wall to the peritoneum; then the blade is reflected inferiorly, and then a small vertical incision is made through the inferior uterine body. After that, the incision is extended using bandage scissors vertically to the fundus. The indication for the procedure is maternal cardiac arrest (greater than 24 weeks' gestation) with resuscitation efforts of less than 5 minutes. A recent case series identified that resuscitation times up to 10 to 11 minutes might also result in a survivable outcome for the mother and neonate. Gestational age can be approximated by measuring from the pubic symphysis to the apex of the uterus, 1 inch for every week of gestation. If the apex of the uterus is at the level of the umbilicus, this approximates 20 weeks' gestational age.

Why are the other choices wrong?

The high transverse incision is not indicated for perimortem cesarean delivery and can result in injury to the neonate.

The low transverse incision is a more time-consuming approach; thus it is not the preferred technique in perimortem scenarios. However, the low transverse incision is the preferred technique in nonperimortem conditions.

Similarly, the midline vertical incision from pubic symphysis to umbilicus might be large enough for a second trimester fetus, but most texts and experts indicate that an emergency physician not familiar with surgical delivery should use the larger incision.

PEER POINT

Remember 24 and 4 for perimortem cesarean delivery

- 24 weeks' gestational age (above level of umbilicus) and
- Start the procedure within 4 minutes (optimally) of arrest

PEER REVIEW

✓ When should you perform perimortem cesarean delivery? Maternal cardiac arrest at greater than 24 weeks' gestation.

✓ The mother and neonate are most likely to survive when perimortem cesarean delivery is performed less than 5 minutes after maternal arrest.

✓ To perform perimortem cesarean delivery, make the incision vertically from the pubic symphysis to the umbilicus.

REFERENCES

Einav S, Kaufman N, Sela HY. Maternal cardiac arrest and perimortem caesarean delivery: evidence or expert-based? *Resuscitation.* 83:10 (2012): 1191-1200.

Marx JA, Hockberger RS, Walls RM, eds. *Rosen's Emergency Medicine: Concepts and Clinical Practice.* 8th ed. St. Louis, MO: Elsevier; 2014: 303-304.

Roberts JR, Hedges JR, eds. *Clinical Procedures in Emergency Medicine.* 6th ed. St. Louis, Mo: WB Saunders; 2013: 1175-1177.

253. The correct answer is D, Milking the tube backward.

Why is this the correct answer?

When a gastrostomy tube gets clogged with accumulated feeding solution and medications, cleaning it can be difficult. Milking the tube backward is a safe technique that removes some of the thick material. This alone might resolve the clog and make the tube patent again. Additional techniques might be required to open up the tube, but this is a good and safe first step. If all techniques fail, the tube must be exchanged.

Why are the other choices wrong?

Inserting a guidewire or a stylet might be a safe way to clear the proximal portion of a clogged gastrostomy tube. But it should not be advanced in the subcutaneous portion of the tube because it might puncture the tube and injure the patient or create a leak.

A commercial tube declogger is commonly used after the proximal portion of the tube is milked backwards. It is inserted into the clog repeatedly and moved back and forth until the clog is removed and fluid flows freely. Generally, the tube is milked backward first to remove as much of the clog as possible before deploying the commercial declogger.

High-pressure irrigation is not the best technique to try first to remove a clot in a gastrostomy feeding tube. Although this technique is frequently used after milking

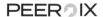

the tube, it must be used with caution: high-pressure irrigation is associated with tube rupture and subsequent internal leakage. After high-pressure irrigation is used, the tube should be radiographically interrogated with contrast media to check its integrity.

PEER REVIEW

✓ Milking the proximal portion of the tube to remove as much of the clog as possible is the first technique used to troubleshoot a clogged feeding tube.

✓ Subsequent techniques include insertion of a guide wire or stylet, used of a commercial declogger, use of a Fogarty arterial embolectomy catheter, irrigation with carbonated beverages, or high-pressure irrigation.

REFERENCES

Roberts JR, Hedges JR, eds. *Clinical Procedures in Emergency Medicine.* 6th ed. St. Louis, Mo: WB Saunders; 2013: 820-830.e6.

Tintinalli JE, Stapczynski JS, Ma OJ, et al, eds. *Tintinalli's Emergency Medicine: A Comprehensive Study Guide.* 8th ed. New York, NY: McGraw-Hill; 2012: 566-567.

254. The correct answer is B, Deferoxamine.

Why is this the correct answer?

The patient in this case is in the third of four phases of iron toxicity, and he requires treatment for both the shock state and the hepatic injury. Decontamination should be performed with chelation using deferoxamine. Phase 1 of iron toxicity is characterized by vomiting and diarrhea as the iron has a direct effect on the gastric mucosa. If the toxicity is severe enough, the patient can present with signs of shock and bloody vomiting or diarrhea associated with metabolic acidosis. In phase 2, there is resolution of the GI symptoms. This phase can last for 6 to 24 hours, and patients treated during this phase often have a complete recovery. It is during this phase that the iron begins to injure the liver itself, which can lead to the signs and symptoms of phase 3. In phase 3, there is more acidosis associated with seizures or shock status, and there are signs of hepatic failure with alteration in gluconeogenesis. Jaundice and elevated transaminases develop during this phase. Phase 4 occurs in those who survive the iron ingestion and are at risk of developing pyloric stenosis. Most toxic iron incidents are the result of prenatal vitamin ingestion. These tablets have a high concentration of elemental iron. Toxicity can occur with doses as low as 20 mg/kg, and ingestion of 50 mg/kg or more is likely to lead to symptoms of toxicity.

Why are the other choices wrong?

Activated charcoal is not effective in GI decontamination of iron toxicity. Iron is a substance to which charcoal does not bind.

Ipecac is no longer recommended for the management of ingested poisonings.

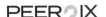

Vitamin B6, pyridoxine, should be used as an antidote for isoniazid toxicity, not iron toxicity.

PEER POINT

The C-PHAILS mnemonic for recalling the substances charcoal does not bind

- **C**austics
- **P**esticides
- **H**ydrocarbons
- **A**lcohols
- **I**ron
- **L**ithium
- **S**olvents

PEER REVIEW

✓ There are different phases of iron ingestion, each with different clinical signs and symptoms.

✓ Always consider toxic ingestion when you evaluate children presenting in extremis.

✓ Deferoxamine is the antidote used to chelate iron toxicity.

REFERENCES

Fleisher GR, Ludwig S, et al, eds. *Textbook of Pediatric Emergency Medicine.* 6th ed. Philadelphia, PA: Lippincott, Williams & Wilkins; 2010: 1198-1200.

Wolfson AB, Hendey GW, Ling LJ, et al, eds. *Harwood-Nuss' Clinical Practice of Emergency Medicine.* 6th ed. Philadelphia, PA: Lippincott, Williams & Wilkins; 2014: 1428-1431.

255. The correct answer is B, Direct laryngoscopy.

Why is this the correct answer?

Direct laryngoscopy is the traditional first-line approach in emergent airway management. There are no contraindications to the use of direct laryngoscopy. Its use in an unconscious patient with a bloody airway is recommended because it can be performed successfully in both unconscious patients and those with blood or vomit in the oropharynx. However, in this case, the person performing the procedure should keep the cervical spine stabilized in the neutral position given the neck trauma. A gum elastic bougie is a helpful airway adjunct to use with direct laryngoscopy. It has an angled tip that helps with insertion when the larynx cannot be fully visualized.

Why are the other choices wrong?

Blind nasotracheal intubation is a maneuver that is rarely used today because there are safer, more successful advanced airway techniques. Blind nasotracheal intubation can be used in dyspneic, awake patients who are cooperative and is contraindicated in unconscious patients.

Fiberoptic laryngoscopy can be particularly helpful with predictably difficult intubations due to anatomic limitations such as limited mouth opening, upper airway swelling due to infection or angioedema, and limited cervical spine mobility. Fiberoptic laryngoscopy requires time to set up, and a patient who is spontaneously breathing is relatively contraindicated if the airway contains blood or vomit because the scope gets occluded.

Video laryngoscopy improves glottic views and has demonstrated superior first-pass success compared to direct laryngoscopy, particularly in obese patients or those with limited neck mobility. However, video laryngoscopy should be avoided if blood or vomit might be occluding the camera.

PEER REVIEW

✓ Video and fiberoptic laryngoscopy are especially helpful in the management of patients who have difficult airways because of anatomic abnormalities.
✓ But keep in mind that video and fiberoptic laryngoscopy are relatively contraindicated if the airway contains blood or vomit.

REFERENCES

Roberts JR, Hedges JR, eds. *Clinical Procedures in Emergency Medicine*. 6th ed. St. Louis, Mo: WB Saunders; 2013: 66-101.

Tintinalli JE, Stapczynski JS, Ma OJ, et al, eds. *Tintinalli's Emergency Medicine: A Comprehensive Study Guide*. 8th ed. New York, NY: McGraw-Hill; 2012: 183-192.

256. The correct answer is B, Doxycycline.

Why is this the correct answer?

Rocky Mountain spotted fever (RMSF) is a tickborne illness caused by *Rickettsia rickettsii*. Doxycycline is the treatment of choice for all age groups and should be initiated within 5 days of symptom onset without waiting for confirmatory testing. Although tetracyclines are typically avoided in children younger than 8 years, new studies have shown a lack of permanent dental staining that was previously thought to occur with use in pediatric patients. Additionally, doxycycline has been shown to be superior over other antibiotics for the treatment of RMSF and should be given as soon as clinically suspected. Doxycycline should be given for at least 3 days after fever subsides, often 7 to 14 days. Contrary to its name, most (60%) cases are reported in the following five states: Arkansas, Missouri, North

Carolina, Oklahoma, and Tennessee. Common symptoms include fever, rash, headache, myalgias, abdominal pain, and vomiting. The rash is described as small macules starting on extremities, including palms or soles (or both), and spreading to the torso and later becoming petechial. In severe cases, the illness can cause a vasculitis, multiorgan system failure, and even death. Early treatment improves outcomes, especially in pediatric patients, who are five times more likely to die from RMSF than adults are.

Why are the other choices wrong?

Chloramphenicol is sometimes used to treat RMSF in pregnant patients with a mild course of illness or in patients with life-threatening allergies to doxycycline. Chloramphenicol should not be given routinely, however, as there is an increased mortality rate compared to doxycycline. Additionally, there is no oral form available in the United States, and it has some severe side effects, including aplastic anemia and gray baby syndrome.

Supportive care is encouraged, especially in patients with severe illness with multiorgan system failure. However, supportive care alone is insufficient for the treatment of RMSF. Doxycycline must be given as soon as clinically suspected because a delay in treatment leads to increased morbidity and mortality rates.

Trimethoprim-sulfamethoxazole should not be used to treat RMSF because it is less effective than doxycycline and because sulfa drugs can worsen infection.

PEER POINT

From the CDC, annual reported incidence (per million population) for Rocky Mountain spotted fever in the United States in 2010

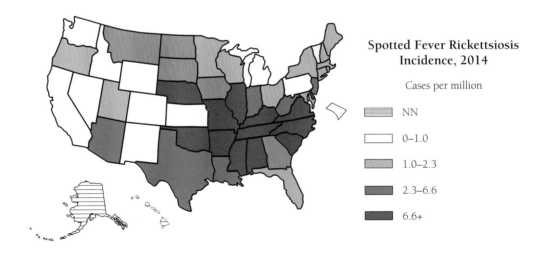

PEER REVIEW

✓ Symptoms of Rocky Mountain spotted fever: fever, myalgias, headache, abdominal pain, and a macular rash that starts on the extremities, spreads to the torso, and later becomes petechial.

✓ Don't wait for test results to come back — early diagnosis and treatment of Rocky Mountain spotted fever are required to prevent fatal outcomes.

✓ Treatment of choice for Rocky Mountain spotted fever is doxycycline even in pediatric patients.

REFERENCES

Centers for Disease Control and Prevention. Rocky Mountain spotted fever (RMSF). CDC website. Available at: http://www.cdc.gov/rmsf/index.html. Accessed August 17, 2016.

Tintinalli JE, Stapczynski JS, Ma OJ, et al, eds. *Tintinalli's Emergency Medicine: A Comprehensive Study Guide.* 8th ed. New York, NY: McGraw-Hill; 2012: 183-192.

Todd SR, Dahlgren FS, Traeger MS, et al. No visible dental staining in children treated with doxycycline for suspected Rocky Mountain Spotted Fever. *J Pediatr.* 2015;166(5):1246-1251.

257. The correct answer is C, Toddler who woke up in the same room as a bat.

Why is this the correct answer?

Rabies postexposure prophylaxis (PEP) is indicated for individuals who are bitten or experience other mucous membrane exposure to a bat. Sometimes patients are unsure or unaware that they have been bitten by a bat, such as might be the case with a small child or with someone who was sleeping at the time. These cases should be considered equivalent to a known exposure. Other high-risk exposures requiring immediate PEP include bites or other mucous membrane exposures from raccoons, skunks, and foxes. If the animal can be captured, PEP can be started on the patient until definitive testing can be obtained on the animal. The PEP process has three steps. First is early and aggressive irrigation of the wound with soap, water, and povidone-iodine solution. Second, human rabies immune globulin (HRIG) is administered surrounding the wound. Third, human diploid cell vaccine is administered away from the HRIG and repeated on days 3, 7, and 14 with a dose at day 28 if the patient is immunocompromised.

Why are the other choices wrong?

There has never been a reported case of human rabies as a result of a bite from farm livestock. But if there is a question, the clinician should contact an infectious disease specialist or the CDC to discuss the case.

In the case of a bite from a domestic dog or cat, the animal can be quarantined and observed for 10 days for behavior suggestive of rabies. If suspicious behavior is identified, the animal can be killed and tested, and PEP can be initiated pending the results. If the dog or cat cannot be quarantined for 10 days, the clinician should review local public health guidelines and act accordingly; recommendations vary among states, depending on local prevalence of disease.

Rabies is spread through the saliva of an infected animal. A person who has general contact with a rabid animal or a high-risk animal is not considered at risk if he or she knows there was no animal saliva exposure to mucous membranes. Exposure to animal blood, urine, or feces also does not create risk for contracting rabies. Other insignificant exposures are bites from birds, reptiles, or rodents. Being able to differentiate the risk of exposure is crucial for an emergency physician, as it is estimated that 30% to 60% of PEP is avoidable.

PEER REVIEW

✓ High-risk animals for rabies in the United States: bats, foxes, raccoons, and skunks.

✓ Dogs are the most common carriers of rabies outside of the United States.

✓ When in doubt about rabies postexposure prophylaxis, contact your local public health department.

✓ When in doubt about rabies exposure, treat the patient according to the instructions for prophylaxis.

REFERENCES

Centers for Disease Control and Prevention. Rabies vaccine. CDC website. Available at: https://www.cdc.gov/rabies/medical_care/vaccine.html. Accessed May 23, 2017.

Marx JA, Hockberger RS, Walls RM, eds. *Rosen's Emergency Medicine: Concepts and Clinical Practice.* 8th ed. St. Louis, MO: Elsevier; 2014: 1693-1717.

Tintinalli JE, Stapczynski JS, Ma OJ, et al, eds. *Tintinalli's Emergency Medicine: A Comprehensive Study Guide.* 8th ed. New York, NY: McGraw-Hill; 2012: 1029-1038.

258. The correct answer is D, L4-L5.

Why is this the correct answer?

Lumbar puncture in an infant should be performed at the L4-L5 or L5-S1 interspace levels. This is necessary to avoid damaging the spinal cord because, in an infant, the spinal cord ends at the L3 vertebral body level. Lumbar puncture in adults and children may be performed at higher levels, from the L2-L3 interspace downward. Positioning for lumbar puncture commonly involves placing the patient in the lateral recumbent position and allows for the measurement of opening pressure using a monometer. The L4 spinous process is located at the intersection of the patient's midline and a line connecting the posterior-superior iliac crests. Special attention is required when positioning an infant to make sure that hyperflexion of the neck does not result in airway occlusion. Correction of severe thrombocytopenia (<20 x 103) or elevated INR (>1.4) should be carefully considered before performing a lumbar puncture.

Why are the other choices wrong?

The L1-L2 interspace is not a recommended location to enter when performing a lumbar puncture in any patient, neither pediatric nor adult, due to the presence of the spinal cord. The spinal cord ends as distal as the L2 level in about one third of adults.

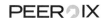

The L2-L3 interspace is an acceptable location to enter when performing a lumbar puncture in children and adults but not in infants.

Again, the L3-L4 interspace is an acceptable location to enter when performing a lumbar puncture in children and adults but not in infants.

PEER POINT

The conus medullaris ends at …

- L2-L3 in infants
- L1-L2 in adults

PEER REVIEW

✓ The appropriate interspace levels for lumbar puncture in an infant are L4-L5 and L5-S1.

✓ The appropriate interspace levels for lumbar puncture in adults and children are L2-L3 and below.

✓ You should avoid neck hyperflexion in all patients, but especially in infants because the airway can be compromised.

REFERENCES

Marx JA, Hockberger RS, Walls RM, eds. *Rosen's Emergency Medicine: Concepts and Clinical Practice.* 8th ed. St. Louis, MO: Elsevier; 2014: 2226-2227.

Roberts JR, Hedges JR, eds. *Clinical Procedures in Emergency Medicine.* 6th ed. St. Louis, MO: WB Saunders; 2013: 1221-1227.

259. The correct answer is A, Bilateral DVT ultrasound.

Why is this the correct answer?

The differential diagnosis for shortness of breath in a pregnant patient is wide, but in this case, PE is the most likely underlying disorder. Compressive ultrasonography has been found to have a sensitivity of 97% and a specificity of 94% for the diagnosis of symptomatic proximal DVT in the general population. The test has no radiation exposure and no known risks to mother or fetus. It is reasonable to start with a bilateral lower-extremity ultrasound examination, and if this test is positive, to treat for venous thromboembolism. If the ultrasound is negative, however, further testing is warranted for evaluation of suspected PE. Negative DVT ultrasonography with a positive D-dimer warrants follow-up ultrasound examination and D-dimer in the following week if the primary concern is for DVT, but further testing for PE is warranted with a negative ultrasound examination and a high suspicion for PE. Chest xrays are often normal in PE, but unilateral basilar atelectasis, pleural-based wedge-shaped area of infiltrate (Hampton hump), or unilateral oligemia (Westermark sign) is suggestive. Chest xray often shows an alternative diagnosis.

Why are the other choices wrong?

Using CT pulmonary angiography exposes patients to the maximum amount of radiation, and in the case of a pregnant woman, this is not the right choice. It confers an increase in breast cancer risk over 1% and causes exposure to the fetus with amounts that increase with gestational age. If the DVT ultrasound is negative and there is still concern for PE, CT pulmonary angiography can be used, but V/Q scanning is also appropriate.

Point-of-care ultrasonography is indicated to evaluate cardiac functioning, and it can reveal elevated right heart pressures. But formal imaging using echocardiography is best to assess for the right heart strain of a large PE. In the majority of cases, including this case, however, with no signs of obstructive shock or heart strain, there are no significant findings, and thus the study is not warranted.

Magnetic resonance imaging is both sensitive and specific for many patients and is safer for pregnant patients. However, results are inconclusive in 30% of patients, so it has not become an accepted study in the assessment of PE.

PEER REVIEW

✓ Compressive ultrasonography is highly sensitive and specific for symptomatic proximal DVT and safe in pregnant patients.
✓ Echocardiography is the best test to find the right heart strain of a big PE, but if there aren't any signs of obstruction, it's not warranted in a lot of patients.

REFERENCES

Marx JA, Hockberger RS, Walls RM, eds. *Rosen's Emergency Medicine: Concepts and Clinical Practice*. 8th ed. St. Louis, MO: Elsevier; 2014: 1157-1169.

Revel MP, Sanchez O, Couchon S, et al. Diagnostic accuracy of magnetic resonance imaging for an acute pulmonary embolism: results of the 'IRM-EP' study. *J Thromb Haemost*. 2012;10(5):743-750.

Tintinalli JE, Stapczynski JS, Ma OJ, et al, eds. *Tintinalli's Emergency Medicine: A Comprehensive Study Guide*. 8th ed. New York, NY: McGraw-Hill; 2012: 1496-1500.

260. The correct answer is B, Deep posterior leg compartment pressure 15 mm Hg lower than diastolic BP.

Why is this the correct answer?

It is difficult to define compartment syndrome on the basis of any one specific intracompartmental pressure reading; however, ischemia generally occurs when the compartment pressure increases to within 20 mm Hg of the patient's diastolic pressure. Compartment syndrome is suggested when the delta pressure (diastolic pressure minus compartment pressure) is less than 30 mm Hg. Because tissue perfusion is due to the difference between arterial blood pressure and the pressure of venous return, the closer the compartment pressure comes to the arterial blood pressure, the more likely compartment pressure is to develop.

Why are the other choices wrong?

A normal compartment pressure is somewhere between 0 and 10 mm Hg. Patients can tolerate pressures up to 30 mm Hg or even higher without signs of compartment syndrome. The absolute number depends on multiple factors, including the current injury and presence of shock as well as pre-existing vascular disease and duration of pressure.

Distal pulses, skin temperature, color, and capillary refill are actually poor indicators of compartment syndrome, contrary to what is commonly taught. The pressure to cause a compartment syndrome is well below systemic arterial pressure. In this patient, loss of pulses would more likely be due to an arterial injury than to a compartment syndrome.

Ongoing pain is consistent with and highly sensitive for compartment syndrome, but it is a relatively nonspecific finding and can also be attributed to a fracture or muscle injury; it is not diagnostic for compartment syndrome. Most concerning is pain that is clearly out of proportion to the injury or findings. This pain is usually poorly localized, deep, and worsened by passive stretching of the muscles. Patients can have ongoing and increasing analgesia requirements. Other findings include tense or tight muscles on palpation and decreased sensation or hypothesia in the distribution of nerves running through the compartment.

PEER REVIEW

✓ Unless there's an arterial injury, compartment syndrome initially presents with normal pulses.
✓ Pain with compartment syndrome is characterized as deep, poorly localized, burning, and severe.
✓ Loss of pulses is uncommon in acute compartment syndrome: the pressure of the tissues does not exceed that of the arterial pressure.

REFERENCES

Marx JA, Hockberger RS, Walls RM, eds. *Rosen's Emergency Medicine: Concepts and Clinical Practice*. 8th ed. St. Louis, MO: Elsevier; 2014: 521–523

Tintinalli JE, Stapczynski JS, Ma OJ, et al, eds. *Tintinalli's Emergency Medicine: A Comprehensive Study Guide*. 8th ed. New York, NY: McGraw-Hill; 2012: Chapter 278.

261. The correct answer is B, Boerhaave syndrome.

Why is this the correct answer?

Boerhaave syndrome is a life-threatening full-thickness perforation of the esophagus from a rapid rise in esophageal pressure. Iatrogenic perforation from endoscopy is an increasingly common etiology, but it can result from any straining Valsalva maneuver or weakening of the esophageal mucosa (forceful vomiting, coughing, heavy lifting, childbirth, foreign body or caustic ingestion, esophagitis, cancer, or trauma). The patient's history of marijuana use with several episodes of vomiting is consistent with cannabinoid hyperemesis syndrome. Boerhaave syndrome classically results in sudden, severe, and unrelenting chest pain that might radiate to the neck, back, shoulders, and abdomen. Thirty percent of patients might develop emphysema in the mediastinal or cervical areas, resulting in crepitus on palpation or a Hamman crunch on auscultation. It is important to note that mediastinal emphysema can take time to develop, and its absence does not necessarily rule out perforation.

Why are the other choices wrong?

The presentation of Boerhaave syndrome can be clinically challenging and might mimic other conditions. Although acute MI should be considered in a patient who presents with chest pain, it is unlikely given the other aspects of the complaint.

The patient in this question has a trigger for powerful emesis with evidence for laryngeal involvement. Peptic ulcer disease can produce vomiting with bloody emesis but usually has a relationship with food and body position. Perforation caused by an ulcer can produce severe pain, but this would usually not ascend into the neck or shoulders.

Pain from PE is not associated with episodes of forceful vomiting. Perforation of the lower esophagus can cause a pneumothorax, but this would not be a primary presentation of spontaneous pneumothorax.

PEER REVIEW

- ✓ Boerhaave syndrome is a full-thickness perforation of the esophagus.
- ✓ Esophageal perforation can present with sudden, severe, unrelenting chest pain.
- ✓ Sometimes esophageal perforation is associated with subcutaneous emphysema due to pneumomediastinum.

REFERENCES

Marx JA, Hockberger RS, Walls RM, eds. *Rosen's Emergency Medicine: Concepts and Clinical Practice*. 8th ed. St. Louis, MO: Elsevier; 2014: 244, 1172-1173.

Tintinalli JE, Stapczynski JS, Ma OJ, et al, eds. *Tintinalli's Emergency Medicine: A Comprehensive Study Guide*. 8th ed. New York, NY: McGraw-Hill; 2012: 508-514.

262. The correct answer is D, Uterine prolapse.

Why is this the correct answer?

With uterine prolapse, patients typically complain of a pelvic pressure, worse with standing up or bearing down. The symptoms get better when the patient lies down. On pelvic examination, the uterus is seen coming down into the center of the vagina. Risk factors include increased age, parity, obesity, and past surgery. For mild symptoms, patients are treated as outpatients with nonoperative techniques such as pelvic exercises, weight loss, and pelvic pessaries. More severe symptoms might require surgical repair.

Why are the other choices wrong?

A cystocele is a form of pelvic relaxation in which the bladder wall prolapses down through the anterior wall of the vagina. Symptoms include urinary incontinence or difficulty emptying the bladder.

A prolapsed fibroid or leiomyoma is a firm mass that can prolapse through the cervix into the vagina, but it usually requires visualization with a speculum.

Rectoceles occur when the rectum herniates into the posterior aspect of the vaginal vault. It occurs especially when the patient bears down to have a bowel movement. Symptoms include fecal incontinence and discharge or drainage with protruding rectum.

PEER REVIEW

✓ Pelvic organ prolapse is common in older women with high parity and obesity.
✓ The type of prolapse can be differentiated on pelvic examination.
✓ Treatment for uterine prolapse is primarily outpatient, depending on the severity of the prolapse and related symptoms.

REFERENCES

Knoop KJ, Stack LB, Storrow AB, et al. *The Atlas of Emergency Medicine*. 4th ed. New York, NY: McGraw-Hill; 2016: 249-283. Access online on March 13, 2015 at http://accessmedicine.mhmedical.com/content.aspx?bookid=351§ionid=39619709&jumpsectionID=39621490&Resultclick=2.

Marx JA, Hockberger RS, Walls RM, eds. *Rosen's Emergency Medicine: Concepts and Clinical Practice*. 8th ed. St. Louis, MO: Elsevier; 2014: 1276-1289.

263. The correct answer is C, Early consultation with a hand specialist.

Why is this the correct answer?

Patients who present with seemingly innocuous findings after high-pressure injection injury can see their conditions rapidly deteriorate. Early consultation is critical to allow for timely surgical decompression and debridement. Less viscous substances can penetrate deeper with less pressure, leading to worsened outcomes. Paint and paint thinners produce a large and early inflammatory response, and the rate of associated amputation is high. Even when patients present soon after injury and with little pain and minimal other findings, prompt consultation with a hand specialist is recommended. Symptoms can develop and progress rapidly to inflammation and swelling and to ischemia and tissue death. Getting the consultation with a hand specialist right away helps prevent delayed surgical management when it is necessary.

Why are the other choices wrong?

Initial emergency department management of an injection injury generally consists of pain control, radiographs, splinting, intravenous administration of antibiotics, and tetanus prophylaxis. However, these are not high-risk injuries for tetanus, and prophylaxis, even if indicated, does not need to be performed immediately. In fact,

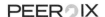

none of the emergency department interventions, outside of pain control, is likely as important as recognition of the potential severity of the injury and early consultation with a hand specialist.

The proper way to clean puncture wounds remains debatable, but in this case, no amount of cleansing in the emergency department is likely to make a difference in outcome. The concern with injection wounds is not the superficial puncture but the deep penetration of substances that can lead to increased compartment pressures as well as a robust inflammatory response.

Digital blocks are excellent tools to relieve pain and provide anesthesia without distorting the field during wound repair. However, in this case, increased compartment pressures in the finger might lead to tissue ischemia. Injecting an anesthetic agent into the tissue planes and finger compartments can increase the pressure and worsen the injury. There might also be theoretical concerns related to difficulty following the physical examination. In patients with injuries such as the one in this question, systemic pain control using intravenous administration is a better choice.

PEER REVIEW

✓ Recognition and early consultation are the cornerstones of managing a high-pressure injection injury.

✓ Don't use digital blocks in high-pressure injection injuries. They might increase intracompartmental and tissue pressure and worsen ischemia.

✓ Initial management of a high-pressure wound: pain control, splinting, elevation, intravenous antibiotics, and tetanus prophylaxis.

REFERENCES

Marx JA, Hockberger RS, Walls RM, eds. *Rosen's Emergency Medicine: Concepts and Clinical Practice*. 8th ed. St. Louis, MO: Elsevier; 2014:

Tintinalli JE, Stapczynski JS, Ma OJ, et al, eds. *Tintinalli's Emergency Medicine: A Comprehensive Study Guide*. 8th ed. New York, NY: McGraw-Hill; 2012: 1801.

264. The correct answer is A, CT angiography of the neck.

Why is this the correct answer?

In a stable patient, CT angiography is a highly accurate test to diagnose injuries to the vascular structure, obtain a general assessment of injury to the other underlying structures, and visualize the trajectory of the wound. In the past, it was thought that the sensitivity might be lower for aerodigestive tract injuries, but significant injuries are generally found by performing serial physical examinations or endoscopy when necessary. Newer studies with multidetector CT angiography show a high sensitivity and specificity for screening when used in conjunction with a good physical examination. Sometimes the findings of vascular injury are obvious, especially in

Zone II, the area of the neck between the angle of the mandible and the cricoid cartilage. These "hard" findings include, for example, active bleeding, neurologic deficit, stridor, or expanding hematoma. But in many cases, an injury presents with occult or minor or "soft" findings such as nonexpanding hematoma, minor change in voice, or pain. Although the physical examination is highly sensitive for vascular injury, a missed carotid artery injury can have significant consequences. A patient with an undiagnosed injury to the aerodigestive tract can develop infection, abscess, or sepsis, while an unappreciated carotid injury could develop, including pseudoaneurysm, embolus and stroke, or delayed hemorrhage.

Why are the other choices wrong?

Computed tomography angiography can show many GI tract injuries and can help rule them out as well, so it should be done first to assess the important vascular structures and identify any aerodigestive tract injuries. If concern remains, CT angiography may be followed by a more specific esophageal workup.

When a patient has a hard finding or instability, airway control and surgical management are the correct initial approach. In the past, stable Zone II injuries without a hard finding were routinely explored in the operating room. But this approach has fallen out of favor due to a high negative exploration rate with its attendant morbidity. Although surgical exploration is still an option in hospitals that do not have the necessary radiology resources or staffing to perform serial examinations, CT angiography is a much faster and highly accurate diagnostic study for identifying life-threatening and otherwise concerning injuries.

Although serial examinations have been used in patients with very low concern for injury, the patient in this case has several soft or otherwise concerning findings that make it difficult to rule out an occult injury. In addition to a hematoma, he has changes to his voice and possibly some dysphonia. So CT angiography done immediately is the better choice than 12 hours of observation.

PEER REVIEW

- ✓ Mandatory surgical exploration of Zone II penetrating neck wounds is no longer universally recommended.
- ✓ Computed tomography angiography of the neck is highly sensitive and specific for vascular injury to the carotid vessels.
- ✓ Hard signs of vascular injury that require surgical intervention: active pulsatile bleeding, expanding hematomas, focal neurologic deficits.

REFERENCES

Legome E, Shockley LW. *Trauma: A Comprehensive Emergency Medicine Approach.* 1st ed. New York, NY: Cambridge University Press; 2011:129-143.

Tintinalli JE, Stapczynski JS, Ma OJ, et al, eds. *Tintinalli's Emergency Medicine: A Comprehensive Study Guide.* 8th ed. New York, NY: McGraw-Hill; 2012: 1736-1737.

265. The correct answer is D, Yes, because it lacks the capacity to care for the patient.

Why is this the correct answer?

The Emergency Medical Treatment and Labor Act, or EMTALA, requires that hospitals capable of caring for patients with emergency medical conditions (EMCs) accept transfers from facilities without those capabilities. However, whether the receiving hospital has the "specialized capabilities or facilities" to treat the patient depends on various factors, including available space and physician expertise. For example, a hospital would not be required to accept a transfer of a critical patient if it had no open ICU beds or had just sustained a catastrophic power loss. Similarly, if the hospital in this case does not have a qualified physician available to treat the patient, it may decline the transfer. However, if the receiving hospital would be able to accommodate the patient by creating capacity by, for example, calling in another vascular surgeon, particularly if it has done this in the past, then it would be expected to accept the transfer.

Why are the other choices wrong?

The law requires only that hospitals accept "appropriate" transfers. If the receiving hospital does not have the facilities or capabilities to care for the patient, it may decline a transfer. Furthermore, if the referring hospital has the capability to care for the patient's EMC, then the receiving hospital may refuse the transfer. However, hospitals may not refuse a patient with an EMC that they are capable of taking care of for other reasons such as lack of insurance, physician convenience, or location of the referring facility (as long as the referring facility is within the boundaries of the United States).

Capacity is dependent on the resources that are available at the time of transfer. A hospital should not accept a patient in transfer if it is unable to provide appropriate care and doing so would not be in the patient's best interest. Having an appropriate specialist on staff is irrelevant if that provider is not available at the time he or she is needed.

It is not illegal to transfer unstable patients. In fact, the transfer requirements of EMTALA apply only to unstable patients. The statute specifically requires that unstable patients be transferred when the referring facility is not able to stabilize them and when the benefits of the transfer outweigh the risks.

PEER REVIEW

- ✓ EMTALA transfer requirements apply only to unstable patients.
- ✓ Hospitals are required to accept transfer of patients with emergency medical conditions if they are capable of caring for them.
- ✓ Hospitals may not refuse transfers for reasons of money or convenience.

REFERENCES

Bitterman RA. *EMTALA: Providing Emergency Care Under Federal Law*. Irving, TX: American College of Emergency Physicians, 2001; 103-117.

Strauss RW, Mayer TA. Strauss and Mayer's *Emergency Department Management*. New York, NY: McGraw-Hill; 2014:613.

266. The correct answer is D, Topical corticosteroid and antibiotic solution.

Why is this the correct answer?

The normal tympanic membrane, erythematous ear canal, and tender pinna and tragus indicate that this patient has otitis externa. Topical treatment such as a corticosteroid-antibiotic combination solution is the correct approach. Otitis externa is most commonly caused by *Pseudomonas aeruginosa* and *Staphylococcus aureus*, usually following conditions that alter the normal external ear canal flora. Warm temperatures and exposure to moisture increase the risk for otitis externa, hence the common name "swimmer's ear." Direct trauma to the ear such as use of a cotton-tipped applicator for cleaning can also precipitate otitis externa. Again, the treatment for otitis externa is primarily topical. Although steroid-antibiotic combination drops are most commonly used, simple acidifying therapy with boric acid or acetic acid also is effective. The key is to get the drops to the canal where they are needed. If the ear canal is so swollen that it is closed, putting a cotton wick into the canal helps get the drops deeper toward the tympanic membrane. Malignant otitis externa, or necrotizing otitis externa, is an aggressive form of the disease occurring in immunocompromised hosts, usually patients with diabetes. It is caused by *P. aeruginosa* and characterized by local invasion of infection into the skull and underlying structures. Complications include meningitis and cerebral abscesses.

Why are the other choices wrong?

Oral beta-lactam antibiotics are the primary therapy for acute otitis media. The sine qua non of acute otitis media is a bulging, nonmobile tympanic membrane.

Oral corticosteroids and acyclovir are used to treat Ramsay-Hunt syndrome, which is herpes zoster infection of a cranial nerve associated with the ear. The same therapy is recommended for Bell palsy, which is also thought to be caused by a herpes virus.

Surgical debridement is not recommended for most cases of otitis externa but could become necessary in necrotizing otitis externa that fails to respond to prolonged antibiotic therapy.

PEER POINT

Ear infections along with common causes and first-line therapy

- Acute otitis media — *S. pneumoniae, H. influenzae, Moraxella catarrhalis* — Oral beta-lactam antibiotics
- Malignant otitis externa — *P. aeruginosa* — Oral ciprofloxacin
- Otitis externa — *P. aeruginosa, S. aureus* — Topical antibiotic-corticosteroid solution
- Ramsay-Hunt syndrome — Herpes zoster oticus — Oral acyclovir, corticosteroids

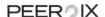

PEER REVIEW

✓ Treatment for otitis externa: topical antibiotic-corticosteroid combinations or simple acidifying therapies.

✓ Malignant otitis externa is an aggressive, invasive infection of the skull most often seen in patients with diabetes.

✓ Bell palsy and Ramsay-Hunt syndrome, both aural conditions caused by herpes viruses, are treated with antiviral medications and steroids.

REFERENCES

Adams JG, Barton ED, Collings JL, et al, eds. *Emergency Medicine: Clinical Essentials*. 2nd ed. Philadelphia, PA: Elsevier; 2013: 226-235.e1.

Marx JA, Hockberger RS, Walls RM, eds. *Rosen's Emergency Medicine: Concepts and Clinical Practice*. 8th ed. St. Louis, MO: Elsevier; 2014: 931-940.e2.

267. The correct answer is C, It can result in higher patient satisfaction scores.

Why is this the correct answer?

Emergency department observation units, also referred to as clinical decision units, short stay units, or rapid diagnostic treatment units, are designed to provide active patient care services for a period of less than 24 hours. Studies have shown that patients placed in observation units have increased satisfaction scores as compared with those admitted to the hospital. They also tend to have shorter lengths of stay, decreased costs, and better or comparable clinical outcomes. Additionally, they are useful for patients with some level of diagnostic uncertainty after their initial emergency department evaluation who will benefit from an extended period of observation and management until they can either be safely discharged home or have been determined to require admission. Some of these critical diagnostic syndromes include chest pain, abdominal pain, syncope, trauma, GI bleeding, and other conditions.

Why are the other choices wrong?

Patients who are observed in the emergency department and subsequently admitted to the hospital are covered by inpatient payment codes. However, if a patient is observed and then discharged home, the service is typically covered not by an inpatient code but by a composite payment code that covers both the observation and emergency department visit.

Observation units should not be used as holding units for the hospital, which are simply a location for passively holding admitted patients until inpatient beds can be made available. Observation units are ideal for patients with conditions that can be treated over a short enough period of time that they do not require a full hospital admission.

Health care payers appreciate considerable cost savings, ranging from $1,000 to $3,000 per patient, with use of an observation unit rather than full hospital admission. These cost savings have been shown in studies of numerous conditions, ranging from asthma to chest pain to croup. However, this does not necessarily translate into increased hospital revenue. Indeed, because observation units tend to improve resource utilization, the hospital might not benefit from the increased revenue it might generate from an inpatient admission.

PEER POINT

Good things an observation unit can do for an emergency department

- Prevent unnecessary admissions, thus improving cost effectiveness and saving the hospital money
- Improve diagnostic accuracy — a patient with a challenging presentation like abdominal pain, chest pain, TIA, or seizure isn't discharged until the physician is confident it's safe to do so
- Improve treatment success — a patient who might fail an acute trial of clinical therapy, for asthma or acute heart failure may be treated and reassessed for improvement
- Increase patient satisfaction

PEER REVIEW

✓ Emergency department observation units help improve diagnostic accuracy and therapeutic outcomes.
✓ Observation units have been demonstrated to lower health care costs, improve patient safety and satisfaction, and shorten hospital length of stay.

REFERENCES

Marx JA, Hockberger RS, Walls RM, eds. *Rosen's Emergency Medicine: Concepts and Clinical Practice*. 8th ed. St. Louis, MO: Elsevier; 2014: 2481-2491.
Strauss RW, Mayer TA. Strauss and Mayer's *Emergency Department Management*. New York, NY: McGraw-Hill; 2014:242.

268. The correct answer is B, Elliptical.

Why is this the correct answer?

The conditions under which excision of an external thrombosed hemorrhoid is indicated include acute onset (within 48 to 72 hrs) and the need to relieve pain and prevent skin tags (which can become infected). Of the four types of incision listed, the best one for evacuating the clot is the elliptical incision. An elliptical incision allows for adequate clot removal without the need for sutures post procedure. The first step is to infiltrate the area with a local anesthetic agent. Next, an elliptical incision is made directed radially from the anal orifice. The edges are then excised and the clot removed with forceps. If needed, the area can be packed gently with gauze. Patients require re-evaluation if pain or bleeding persists longer than 48 hours. Complications of this procedure include bleeding, infection, perianal skin tag, incomplete evacuation, and premature closure. Contraindications include

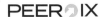

immunocompromise, pregnancy, portal hypertension, and coagulopathy. The procedure also is contraindicated in pediatric patients. Patients require referral for hemorrhoidectomy (definitive care). Internal hemorrhoids are above the dentate line and lack sensory innervation. Prolapsed and nonreducible internal hemorrhoids, hemorrhoids with severe bleeding, and hemorrhoids causing intractable pain are indications for emergent surgical consultation.

Why are the other choices wrong?

A circumferential incision requires complete excision of the epidermis of the hemorrhoid. Due to an extensive incision, the area often requires sutures for approximation. This leads to an increased complication rate (bleeding, infection) given the proximity of the veins at the anal verge.

Linear incisions are often inadequate for clot removal. Additionally, they have been associated with an elevated rate of rethrombosis.

Stellate or other incisions to attempt to temporarily deroof the thrombosis have similar complications to linear incisions, namely rethrombosis. The optimal exposure of the thrombosis (or multiple clots) is to completely expose the area with an elliptical excision of the overlying epidermis and to allow healing by secondary intention.

PEER REVIEW

✓ An elliptical incision is best to evacuate a thrombosed hemorrhoid and minimize complications.

✓ Why not a simple or linear incision for a thrombosed hemorrhoid? It's associated with a significant rate of rethrombosis.

REFERENCES

Roberts JR, Hedges JR, eds. *Clinical Procedures in Emergency Medicine*. 6th ed. St. Louis, Mo: WB Saunders; 2013: 883-885.e6.

Tintinalli JE, Stapczynski JS, Ma OJ, et al, eds. *Tintinalli's Emergency Medicine: A Comprehensive Study Guide*. 8th ed. New York, NY: McGraw-Hill; 2012: 548-549.

269. The correct answer is C, Leukemia.

Why is this the correct answer?

Pediatric oncologic disease can present with symptoms similar to many other less severe illnesses, but it should be considered in the differential in patients presenting with fever without source, multiple systemic symptoms (pain), adenopathy, or findings of a blood line disorder (petechiae). In this case, the combination of fever, petechiae, and organomegaly make leukemia a likely diagnosis. Of all childhood cancers, leukemia is the most common. Among pediatric patients from birth to 14 years old, leukemia accounts for 29% of all cancer diagnoses. More than 95% of pediatric leukemia presentations are acute, and acute lymphoblastic leukemia accounts for most of them.

Why are the other choices wrong?

Idiopathic thrombocytopenic purpura (ITP) is the most common pediatric platelet disorder and often presents clinically with petechiae or bruising without other significant clinical findings. Symptoms can include bleeding from the nose or mouth, blood in the urine, and heavy bleeding in a menstruating female. Intracranial hemorrhage can be life-threatening with this disorder, but it is rare with a platelet count above 20,000 without significant trauma. Typically, patients with ITP presents with acute onset of significant bruising with or without trauma; fever is not typically associated with presentation.

Infectious mononucleosis is a viral illness that presents with exudative pharyngitis, regional or diffuse lymphadenopathy, and malaise; organomegaly can be present, as well. Petechiae are not a common finding with mononucleosis, making this diagnosis less likely. The heterophile-agglutination test for mononucleosis can be falsely negative in children younger than 7 years.

Sickle cell disease is a congenital disorder of the RBCs that can present with pain from vaso-occlusion, but in this case, because the patient is 6 years old and has no past medical issues, sickle cell disease is unlikely. A CBC and a hemoglobin electrophoresis can aid in the diagnosis. In the United States, newborns undergo screening for the presence of sickle cell trait, so this would be known. Enlargement of the spleen might be common in younger patients with sickle cell disease, but the spleen generally atrophies after the first decade. Anemia related to decreased lifespan of the sickled hemoglobin is often chronic in the sickle cell patient.

PEER REVIEW

✓ Leukemia can present with symptoms similar to other more common pediatric viral or bacterial illnesses.

✓ Intracranial hemorrhage is a life-threatening issue in a patient with idiopathic thrombocytopenic purpura but is less likely with a platelet count above 20,000.

✓ Acute lymphoblastic leukemia is the most common type of leukemia.

REFERENCES

Fleisher GR, Ludwig S, et al, eds. *Textbook of Pediatric Emergency Medicine.* 6th ed. Philadelphia, PA: Lippincott, Williams & Wilkins; 2010: 378-379; 875-877; 1033-1038.

Wolfson AB, Hendey GW, Ling LJ, et al, eds. *Harwood-Nuss' Clinical Practice of Emergency Medicine.* 6th ed. Philadelphia, PA: Lippincott, Williams & Wilkins; 2014: 985-990; 1265-1270.

270. The correct answer is D, There is a clear relationship between patient satisfaction and medical liability lawsuits.

Why is this the correct answer?

When patients are unhappy with the care that they receive, they are more likely to look for satisfaction through the medical liability system. This has been shown to be particularly true if they feel their complaints are not being addressed in any other way. Studies indicate that a minimum satisfaction score can identify malpractice risk, and that patient satisfaction survey ratings are associated with complaints and with risk management episodes. This is of particular concern to emergency physicians, who typically have very little time to establish trusting and meaningful relationship with their patients. There are numerous other reasons to place importance on patient satisfaction, including its direct effects on patient census, financial reimbursement, and the increasing focus on patients as consumers of health care services. It is inevitable that every emergency department will receive complaints. Therefore, it is important to have a robust complaint management and service recovery system in place.

Why are the other choices wrong?

When it evaluates hospitals, The Joint Commission looks specifically at the system for addressing complaints. Furthermore, various other regulatory agencies place similar emphasis on complaint management processes in their reviews.

Through various mechanisms, improved patient satisfaction leads to a financial benefit to hospitals, emergency departments, and, in many cases, to individual providers. Health care remains a competitive environment, and dissatisfied patients are more likely to take their business elsewhere, leading to decreased revenue. In recent years, there has been an increased focus on linking patient satisfaction scores with reimbursement. For example, one component of the Affordable Care Act creates a reward system for hospitals based on maintaining high levels of patient satisfaction.

Although increasing emphasis has been placed in recent years on the importance of patient satisfaction, its correlation with quality of medical care and patient outcomes remains controversial. Some studies have linked various measures of quality with satisfaction scores, and others have failed to find a direct relationship or have even found a negative relationship, between the two.

PEER REVIEW

✓ Improved patient satisfaction lessens the likelihood of medical liability suits.
✓ Patient satisfaction has direct implications for hospitals' financial reimbursement.
✓ The link between patient satisfaction and quality of medical care remains controversial.

REFERENCES

Brookes L, Fenton J. Patient Satisfaction and Quality of Care: Are They Linked? Medscape multispecialty, June 11, 2014. http://www.medscape.com/viewarticle/826280. Accessed April 8, 2015.

Fullam F, et al. The use of patient satisfaction surveys and alternative coding procedures to predict malpractice risk. *Medical Care.* 47.5 (2009): 553-559.

Stelfox HT, et al. The relation of patient satisfaction with complaints against physicians and malpractice lawsuits. *Am J Med.* 2005;118.10:1126-1133.

Strauss RW, Mayer TA. Strauss and Mayer's *Emergency Department Management.* New York, NY: McGraw-Hill; 2014:437.

271. The correct answer is C, More than 9%.

Why is this the correct answer?

This case illustrates the signs of severe volume depletion and shock. The patient has likely lost more than 90 mL/kg of his circulating plasma volume, which is more than 9% of his weight. Children who are mildly dehydrated or who fail oral therapy may be treated with intravenous fluids, beginning with a 10 to 20 mL/kg bolus of crystalloid. Inability to establish venous access in a patient such as the one described in the case is an indication for establishing intraosseous access.

Why are the other choices wrong?

Children with less than 3% of their weight lost are unlikely to demonstrate vital sign abnormalities but might have dry mucous membranes. Capillary refill is intact.

Children with 4% to 6% of their weight lost are not likely to be hypotensive or lethargic. But they do manifest other abnormalities on examination such as delayed capillary refill and tachycardia.

This patient has not lost 60% of his weight or all of his water. The total body water content of a human is approximately 60%, which is key to the equation to determine free water deficit/excess in a patient with hypernatremia or hyponatremia, respectively. Free water deficit = $0.6 \times$ weight in kg $\times$ ([current Na/140] − 1).

PEER POINT

Physical examination findings in dehydration in children

	Mild (<3%)	Moderate (6%)	Severe (>9%)
Dry mucous membranes	Yes	Yes	Yes
Delayed capillary refill	No	Sometimes	Yes
Sunken eyes	No	Yes	Yes
Decreased skin turgor	No	Sometimes	Yes
Heart rate	Normal of slightly elevated	Elevated	Elevated
Respiratory rate	Normal	Normal of slightly elevated	Elevated
Blood pressure	Normal	Normal	Decrease
Mental status	Normal	Irritable	Lethargic

PEER REVIEW

✓ In children, blood pressure is not a reliable marker of distress, so treat them for dehydration way before blood pressure becomes unstable.

✓ Most children manifest severe signs and symptoms of dehydration after losing 9% of their plasma volume. Initial replacement should be 10 to 20 mL/kg of crystalloid.

✓ Infants can tolerate a relatively larger percentage of volume loss because they have relatively larger extracellular fluid volume.

REFERENCES

Marx JA, Hockberger RS, Walls RM, eds. *Rosen's Emergency Medicine: Concepts and Clinical Practice*. 8th ed. St. Louis, MO: Elsevier; 2014: 2188-2204.e2.

Tintinalli JE, Stapczynski JS, Ma OJ, et al, eds. *Tintinalli's Emergency Medicine: A Comprehensive Study Guide*. 8th ed. New York, NY: McGraw-Hill; 2012: 843-852.

272. The correct answer is C, Ensures that acutely injured or ill patients receive the most appropriate care.

Why is this the correct answer?

The term regionalization of care refers to a coordinated system of care in which patients with time-critical illness are transported directly to, as the definition reads, "designated facilities in a defined geographic region with the capabilities and resources immediately available to provide appropriate, specialized treatment." Classically this has been considered in the context of trauma centers but more recently has been expanded to include other time-critical diagnoses (TCD) such as STEMI and acute ischemic stroke. The American College of Emergency Physicians has a policy in support of regionalization of care. In addition to providing the most appropriate level of care for patients with TCDs, regionalization also has the benefits of streamlining care, good stewardship of health care resources, and avoidance of duplication of tests. The goal is to concentrate expensive and specialized resources within a geographic region to achieve more coordinated and efficient care, leading to optimal patient outcomes.

Why are the other choices wrong?

Any system of regionalization must incorporate EMS at every level; this is critical. It should include the creation of EMS protocols, the involvement of EMS medical directors, creation of cooperative agreements among EMS agencies across a region, and the incorporation of EMS into funding models. However, because a regionalized system designates specific specialized facilities where patients with time-critical diagnoses should be sent, longer transport times and a greater burden on EMS resources can be the result.

The traditional health care system model relies on transport of patients to the closest facility for "stabilization" before transfer to more definitive care. A regionalized system incorporates EMS protocols such that patients are identified in the field and transported directly from the scene to the regional specialty center, often bypassing a closer facility that lacks the resources to provide the care ultimately needed. One study found that stopping at a local facility for stabilization added an average of 79 minutes to the time to eventual definitive care.

One of the major barriers to the creation of regionalized systems of care is connected to funding and reimbursement. Although it might be in the best interest of a patient with a time-critical diagnosis to be taken directly to a specialty center, the local hospital will experience a direct loss of revenue. If EMS protocols are too broad, a significant amount of overtriage can occur, leading to further diversion of less-critical patients away from the local hospital that might actually be equipped to care for them.

PEER REVIEW

✓ What's the argument for regionalization of care? To ensure that patients with time-critical diagnoses get treated at the facility with the most appropriate resources.

✓ Any system of regionalization must incorporate EMS at all levels.

✓ Regionalization creates economy by concentrating costly resources in designated locations.

REFERENCES

EMS regionalization of care. ACEP Web site. https://www.acep.org/Clinical---Practice-Management/EMSRegionalization-of-Care/. Accessed May 31, 2017.

273. The correct answer is D, Metronidazole 500 mg PO three times daily for 10 days.

Why is this the correct answer?

The patient in this case has symptoms suggestive of *Giardia lamblia* infection. Many patients who harbor *Giardia* are asymptomatic, but acute infection does have good distinguishing features: forceful diarrheal episodes with stool described as foul-smelling and pale. Patients might also report abdominal distention with intermittent abdominal pain and frequent flatulence. Audible borborygmi, or stomach rumbling, might be heard during the physical examination. Treatment includes metronidazole 250 to 750 mg PO three times daily for 5 to 10 days. Alternative treatments include single-dose therapy with tinidazole 2 g PO or furazolidone 100 mg PO once daily for 7 to 10 days. Giardia is the most common cause of diarrhea outbreaks from parasitic origin worldwide. Its mode of transmission is usually the fecal-oral route from water contaminated by animal feces (particularly beavers) infested with trophozoite cysts, and campers are commonly affected. Fecal contamination can also occur through close personal contact.

Why are the other choices wrong?

Azithromycin is used to treat protozoal infection with *Cryptosporidium* or bacterial *Salmonella* species. *Cryptosporidium* is an opportunistic infection seen most commonly in persons with AIDS or in areas without adequate hygiene. Eating exacerbates the watery diarrhea and cramping abdominal pain, and serious infections lead to significant dehydration. Salmonella infection is usually related to improperly cooked food; it causes vomiting and diarrhea.

Ciprofloxacin is used to treat diarrhea from bacterial *Shigella* or *Yersinia* species. *Shigella* can cause severe dysentery (large amounts of watery diarrhea) that can progress to frank bloody diarrhea with a relatively small number of bacterial pathogens. Yersiniosis can also cause bloody diarrhea and is known as an appendicitis mimic due to regionalization in some patients to the ileocecal area.

Iodoquinol is used for treatment of amebic dysentery from *Entamoeba* species, of which abdominal pain from colonic ulceration is a feature, as well as blood-streaked mucous diarrhea. Iodoquinol is used for asymptomatic carriers of the disease, but if symptomatic, metronidazole is added.

PEER REVIEW

- ✓ *Giardia lamblia* is the most common cause of parasite diarrheal outbreaks worldwide.
- ✓ Treatment of *Giardia* infection: metronidazole 250 to 750 mg PO three times a day for 5 to 10 days.
- ✓ Alternatives: single-dose tinidazole 2 g PO or furazolidone 100 mg PO once a day for 7 to 10 days.
- ✓ Audible borborygmi, rumbling from intestinal gas, is a classic physical examination finding in *Giardia* infection.

REFERENCES

Marx JA, Hockberger RS, Walls RM, eds. *Rosen's Emergency Medicine: Concepts and Clinical Practice*. 8th ed. St. Louis, MO: Elsevier; 2014: 1252-1253.

Tintinalli JE, Stapczynski JS, Ma OJ, et al, eds. *Tintinalli's Emergency Medicine: A Comprehensive Study Guide*. 8th ed. New York, NY: McGraw-Hill; 2012: 1081-1083.

274. The correct answer is B, Advanced practice RNs may practice independently in some states.

Why is this the correct answer?

The scope of practice and supervision of advanced practice RNs (APRNs) or nurse practitioners (NPs) varies from state to state. Some states allow APRNs full practice status, allowing them to practice independently, without any physician supervision at all. Others allow for reduced practice status, wherein they may treat and diagnose patients but require physician oversight to prescribe medications. Still other states have restricted practice status, requiring all care by APRNs to be done under the supervision of a physician. The policy of the American College of Emergency Physicians states that "advanced practice registered nurses or physician assistants should not provide unsupervised emergency department care," and that "PAs and APRNs do not replace the medical expertise and patient care provided by emergency physicians."

Why are the other choices wrong?

Advance practice providers may prescribe medications, including controlled substances, in certain states. However, PAs are dependent practitioners who must practice under the supervision of a physician. Advanced practice RNs may prescribe independently in some states but require physician oversight in others.

Physician assistants (PAs) practice medicine under the supervision of a physician. However, the scope of supervision varies widely based on the needs of the employer. Because PAs are considered "dependent practitioners," their scope of practice encompasses whatever the supervising physician delegates. Typically, this scope is determined based on the specific needs and utilization of the emergency department.

Although the required level of physician supervision varies from state to state, advance practice providers in many places might be used to perform all of the same medical care that is performed by emergency physicians. In some locations, state laws and regulations restrict their scope. It is critical that emergency department directors and supervising physicians are aware of their state's specific rules, and that they incorporate this into their supervisory agreements (where supervision is required). That being said, the 2009 Report on PAs in Emergency Medicine found that 70% of surveyed PAs worked in the main emergency department, 20% in fast track, and 10% in urgent care.

PEER REVIEW

✓ Advanced practice RNs may practice independently in some states.

✓ Physician assistants practice under the supervision of a physician.

✓ Advanced practice provider scope of practice and supervision vary by state and by individual emergency department.

REFERENCES

American College of Emergency Physicians. Guidelines Regarding the Role of Physician Assistants and Advanced Practice Registered Nurses in the Emergency Department. ACEP website. Available at: https://www.acep.org/Clinical---Practice-Management/Guidelines-Regarding-the-Role-of-Physician-Assistants-and-Advanced-Practice-Registered-Nurses-in-the-Emergency-Department. Accessed October 11, 2016.

Strauss RW, Mayer TA. Strauss and Mayer's *Emergency Department Management*. New York, NY: McGraw-Hill; 2014:145.

275. The correct answer is A, Erythema multiforme.

Why is this the correct answer?

Erythema multiforme (EM) is a discrete rash known best for its target lesion appearance. There are several culprits; it can be caused by an infection such as herpes simplex virus; by a drug (sulfonamides and other antibiotics, anticonvulsants); by an autoimmune disease; or it can be idiopathic. The classifications of EM are minor and major. A minor presentation is that of a self-limited rash that is affecting mostly the extremities; there are no prodromal symptoms and no mucous membrane involvement. Outpatient treatment with supportive care is appropriate for minor EM. The major form is more severe. It starts with a prodromal viral illness then progresses to a rash that involves palms or soles and mucous membranes. Less than 10% of the body surface is involved. Patients with major EM are typically observed to monitor for further disease progression and treat accordingly.

Why are the other choices wrong?

Kawasaki disease (mucocutaneous lymph node syndrome or infantile polyarteritis) is a childhood vasculitis affecting many organs: skin, mucous membranes, lymph nodes, and vasculature. Diagnostic criteria for Kawasaki disease include fever for more than 5 days, diffuse erythroderma, strawberry tongue, significant cervical lymphadenopathy, bilateral nonexudative conjunctiva injection, edema, and sloughing of extremities. Thrombocytosis might also be present. The most serious complication is vasculitis of the coronary arteries; this can lead to aneurysm, myocarditis, or MI. Treatment consists of hospitalization, high-dose aspirin, intravenous immunoglobulin, and echocardiogram.

Scarlet fever is an exotoxin-mediated illness caused by *Streptococcus pyogenes*. It occurs primarily in young children. It is most often associated with streptococcal tonsillopharyngitis, although it can be seen following other streptococcal infections. Symptoms include fever, headache, malaise, and odynophagia with some occasional vomiting and abdominal pain. This is followed by the appearance of a strawberry tongue and a red exanthem on the soft palate and uvula, called Forchheimer spots. Petechiae might also appear on the flexural surfaces; these are called Pastia lines. The rash, preceded by fever for 1 to 2 days, is a generalized erythroderma with blanching papules. It has a sandpaper-like texture. The exanthem typically resolves in 1 week followed by desquamation of skin (most often on the palms or soles). Penicillin remains the treatment of choice to prevent suppurative complications.

Toxic shock syndrome is a toxin-mediated infection (typically group A streptococcus or *Staphylococcus aureus*) resulting in B-type symptoms (fever, headache, malaise), hypotension, and a rash that looks like a sunburn — diffuse, erythematous, scarlet feverlike with desquamation. It is classically associated with tampons but can also be seen with nasal packing and surgical wounds. Death in these patients is typically related to sepsis and multiorgan system failure. Treatment requires removal of the offending agent, supportive care with fluids, and antibiotics.

PEER REVIEW

✓ The rash of erythema multiforme is best described as discrete target lesions.

✓ The minor form of erythema multiforme is a self-limited rash that doesn't have a prodrome or involve mucous membranes.

✓ The major form of erythema multiforme begins as a prodromal viral illness and progresses to a diffuse rash involving mucous membranes.

REFERENCES

Adams JG, Barton ED, Collings J, et al, eds. *Emergency Medicine: Clinical Essentials*. 2nd ed. Philadelphia, PA: Saunders; 2013: 1598-1618.

Marx JA, Hockberger RS, Walls RM, eds. *Rosen's Emergency Medicine: Concepts and Clinical Practice*. 8th ed. St. Louis, MO: Elsevier; 2014: 1558-1585.

276. The correct answer is B, Postpartum pituitary gland necrosis.

Why is this the correct answer?

Postpartum pituitary gland necrosis (Sheehan syndrome) is a condition that affects women who lose a significant amount of blood and suffer pituitary hypoperfusion and necrosis after childbirth. Presentations range from fairly asymptotic to difficulties with lactation, oligomenorrhea/amenorrhea, and orthostasis. Secondary hypothyroidism and hypoadrenalism can also occur and lead to fatigue, cold intolerance, constipation, weight gain, hair loss, and slowed thinking as well as bradycardia and hypotension. Laboratory abnormalities that can indicate postpartum pituitary gland necrosis include hyponatremia, hypoglycemia, and anemia secondary to resulting adrenal insufficiency. Other mechanisms by which hypopituitarism can result in hyponatremia include decreased free-water clearance by hypothyroidism and direct syndrome of inappropriate antidiuretic hormone (ADH) hypersecretion.

Why are the other choices wrong?

Eclampsia is the development of new-onset seizures between 20 weeks' gestation and 4 weeks postpartum. Pre-eclampsia typically precedes seizures and is hallmarked by hypertension, proteinuria, and/or the development of HELLP (hemolysis, elevated liver enzymes, and low platelets) syndrome. Eclampsia should be suspected in any woman who is between 20 weeks pregnant and 4 weeks postpartum who develops seizures, coma, or encephalopathy.

Subarachnoid hemorrhage (SAH) and vascular dissection should both be considered in the setting of acute headache and hypertension, but it is not specific to pregnancy. Eclampsia, SAH, and dissection can all lead to neurologic abnormalities, including syncope. The patient in this case has had a generalized headache for a week, making the diagnosis of SAH less likely.

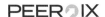

Like SAH, vascular dissection should be considered in this presentation but is not a pregnancy-related condition. They should all be considered in this case; however, the classical laboratory abnormalities seen in adrenal insufficiency (hyponatremia, hypoglycemia, anemia) make Sheehan syndrome a much more likely diagnosis.

PEER REVIEW

✓ Postpartum syncope in addition to polydipsia, hyponatremia, and headache are most suggestive of postpartum pituitary necrosis.

✓ Postpartum eclampsia can occur up to 4 weeks after delivery and the diagnosis should be considered in any patient with headache, visual symptoms, and a blood pressure higher than 140/90.

REFERENCES

Tintinalli JE, Stapczynski JS, Ma OJ, et al, eds. *Tintinalli's Emergency Medicine: A Comprehensive Study Guide*. 8th ed. New York, NY: McGraw-Hill; 2012: 644-652.

Wolfson AB, Hendey GW, Ling LJ, et al, eds. *Harwood-Nuss' Clinical Practice of Emergency Medicine*. 6th ed. Philadelphia, PA: Lippincott, Williams & Wilkins; 2014: 1039.

277. The correct answer is A, Crystallizing of fluid on microscopic examination.

Why is this the correct answer?

The approach to confirming rupture of membranes has three components: pooling of amniotic fluid in the vaginal vault, a positive Nitrazine test result, and ferning revealed on microscopic analysis of amniotic fluid. Of the three findings, ferning is the most specific. It occurs when amniotic fluid dries and sodium chloride crystals precipitate.

Why are the other choices wrong?

When exposed to a flame, vaginal secretions, not amniotic fluid, turn brown. Amniotic fluid turns white and displays the crystallized ferning pattern.

Nitrazine is a pH indicator that is more sensitive than litmus and is often used in the emergency department. Vaginal fluid is mildly acidic with a pH of approximately 4.0 to 5.0 and causes a Nitrazine strip to either remain yellow or turn slightly red (acidic). Amniotic fluid is basic with a pH of 7.0 to 7.5 and turns a Nitrazine strip blue. But for several reasons, a Nitrazine test can have a false-positive result: lubricant use during speculum examination, the presence of semen, blood, or cervical mucus, or concurrent *Trichomonas vaginalis* infection.

When rupture of membranes is suspected, a speculum examination must be performed. Pooling fluid can have various sources: amniotic, vaginal, or urinary, so visualization of pooling is not specific.

PEER REVIEW

✓ The most specific finding for rupture of membranes is ferning — sodium chloride crystal precipitation.

✓ A Nitrazine test can yield a false-positive result for multiple reasons, so it shouldn't be the only test used to confirm rupture of membranes.

✓ Pooling of fluid in the vaginal vault is the least specific sign of rupture of membranes.

REFERENCES

Marx JA, Hockberger RS, Walls RM, eds. *Rosen's Emergency Medicine: Concepts and Clinical Practice*. 8th ed. St. Louis, MO: Elsevier; 2014: 2334, 2340-2341.

Tintinalli JE, Stapczynski JS, Ma OJ, et al, eds. *Tintinalli's Emergency Medicine: A Comprehensive Study Guide*. 8th ed. New York, NY: McGraw-Hill; 2012: Chapter 62 Emergency Delivery; 644-652.

278. The correct answer is B, Panic disorder.

Why is this the correct answer?

Panic disorder is a very common anxious condition characterized by sudden, brief episodes of intense fear that are frequently associated with a variety of somatic complaints, including nausea, vomiting, diaphoresis, tremor, paresthesias, and chest discomfort. Patients may present with tachycardia, hyperventilation, or hypertension. One of every 20 adults can be expected to develop a panic disorder sometime during his or her life. A panic disorder might or might not be associated with agoraphobia, the fear of open places or shopping areas. Patients who experience panic attacks when in public areas are at risk to restrict themselves to their homes. Generalized anxiety disorder, which is also very common, is defined by 6 months of excessive anxiety and worry, but not specifically episodes of panic. It is important to note that a panic disorder is a diagnosis of exclusion, and medical causes for similar symptoms should be excluded first. A panic attack can mimic PE, an MI, asthma, thyrotoxicosis, or even an endocrine-secreting tumor such as a pheochromocytoma. These conditions can likely be excluded on clinical grounds alone, but laboratory testing might be necessary. Most patients with new presentations of anxiety disorders (or any psychiatric symptoms) should have a thyroid-stimulating hormone (TSH) level measured, as hyperthyroidism can mimic schizophrenia, bipolar disorder, and anxiety disorders, and hypothyroidism often leads to depression.

Why are the other choices wrong?

A generalized anxiety disorder is characterized by frequent and prolonged (6 months) periods of worry and anxiousness. This patient describes shorter episodes that are consistent with panic attacks typical of panic disorder.

Pheochromocytoma is a very rare (2 persons per million) condition caused by a catecholamine-secreting tumor. It is characterized by paroxysms of hypertension, tachycardia, tremor, and anxiety. But it is far less likely than the extremely common panic disorder.

Thyrotoxicosis should be considered in any patient with unexplained anxiety and tachycardia. It can be easily excluded by measuring the TSH level. It is typically, but not always, persistent rather than episodic, as described by this patient.

PEER POINT

Anxiety disorders and definitions

- Agoraphobia — Specific fear of open or public places
- Generalized anxiety disorder — At least 6 months of persistent worry and excessive anxiety
- Panic disorder — Episodes of discrete periods of sudden fear, associated with tachycardia, diaphoresis, chest discomfort, and a sense of impending doom
- Specific phobia — Clinically significant anxiety or worry that develops in response to a specific situation or object, leading to avoidance behavior

PEER REVIEW

- ✓ Panic disorder is characterized by episodic, unexpected panic attacks that can be debilitating.
- ✓ Get a thyroid level in new cases of anxiety, depression, and other psychiatric conditions — hyperthyroidism and hypothyroidism can mimic these disorders.
- ✓ Patients with panic disorder might or might not have associated agoraphobia.

REFERENCES

Adams JG, Barton ED, Collings JL, et al, eds. *Emergency Medicine: Clinical Essentials.* 2nd ed. Philadelphia, PA: Elsevier; 2013: 1644-1647.e1.

Tintinalli JE, Stapczynski JS, Ma OJ, et al, eds. *Tintinalli's Emergency Medicine: A Comprehensive Study Guide.* 8th ed. New York, NY: McGraw-Hill; 2012: 1941-1952.

279. The correct answer is B, Copper IUD.

Why is this the correct answer?

Options for emergency contraception include pills such as antiprogestin (ulipristal acetate), progestin only (levonorgestrel), and combined estrogen-progestin oral contraceptive pills and the copper intrauterine device (IUD). There is strong evidence that all four of these forms of emergency contraception are effective at the individual level and that all methods are highly effective within 72 hours of unprotected sex, but the copper IUD does not decrease in efficacy after 120 hours, unlike the others. Findings of a systematic review of 42 studies revealed a failure rate of only 0.14% in more than 7,000 postcoital IUD insertions. Which emergency contraceptive to use depends on a number of factors, including presentation after unprotected sex, patient factors (such as obesity and allergies), cost, and availability.

Why are the other choices wrong?

Antiprogestin (ulipristal acetate) is available by prescription only and has been found to be highly effective and well tolerated. It can be taken up to 5 days after unprotected sex and is believed to be more effective than progestin-only levonorgestrel. However it is not as effective as the copper IUD for the time period specified.

The most commonly used emergency contraceptive is progestin only (levonorgestrel) (Plan B, Plan B One-Step, Fallback Solo, among others). It does not require a prescription and is effective but not as effective as the copper IUD beyond 120 hours.

Both progestin-only and combined pill options have slightly less efficacy when compared to antiprogestin and are associated with a higher incidence of nausea and vomiting. Again, estrogen-progestin pills are not effective for as long a time period as the copper IUD is.

PEER REVIEW

✓ The copper IUD is best for emergency contraception if it has been more than 120 hours since unprotected sexual intercourse.

✓ Antiprogestin is as effective as the more commonly used progestin-only emergency contraceptive option when taken early, more effective when taken later, and has a less caustic side effect profile.

✓ The combined estrogen-progestin emergency contraception pill is more likely to cause nausea and vomiting and is thought to be less effective than other options.

REFERENCES

Cleland K, Zhu H, Goldstuck N, et al. The efficacy of intrauterine devices for emergency contraception: a systematic review of 35 years of experience. *Hum Reprod.* 2012;27(7):1994-2000.

Marx JA, Hockberger RS, Walls RM, eds. *Rosen's Emergency Medicine: Concepts and Clinical Practice.* 8th ed. St. Louis, MO: Elsevier; 2014: 868-869.

Tintinalli JE, Stapczynski JS, Ma OJ, et al, eds. *Tintinalli's Emergency Medicine: A Comprehensive Study Guide.* 8th ed. New York, NY: McGraw-Hill; 2012: 1260-1265.

280. The correct answer is D, Start parenteral antibiotics.

Why is this the correct answer?

Flexor tenosynovitis is an infection of the tendon sheath. This patient is exhibiting the classic Kanavel signs that support a clinical diagnosis. The immediate risk is progression to the deep spaces of the hand and subsequent necrosis and proximal spread, so parenteral antibiotics must be started immediately. Consulting a hand surgeon is the right thing to do in all patients with suspected flexor tenosynovitis, but in this case, it is not the first thing. The initial action must be to start parenteral antibiotics to minimize the risk of deep space infection. Sometimes flexor tenosynovitis can be treated successfully without surgery if it is identified and treated early. Patients with flexor tenosynovitis frequently have a puncture wound as the inciting event; however, many do not have an identifiable cause. The most common bacteria are *Staphylococcus* and *Streptococcus*, but patients who are sexually active and without an identifiable source of infection should also be treated for presumed disseminated gonorrhea. The Kanavel signs are tenderness to palpation over the flexor tendon sheath, symmetric finger swelling, pain with passive extension, and flexed positioning of the digit to minimize pain.

Why are the other choices wrong?

Because of the high risk for deep space infections of the hand, patients with presumed flexor tenosynovitis should not be discharged with oral antibiotics and instructions to see a hand surgeon. Parenteral antibiotics should be started immediately and consultation with a hand surgeon initiated in the emergency department. Sometimes nonsurgical treatment is considered, but this decision must be made in collaboration with the hand surgeon, and the patient would require follow-up within 24 hours.

Immobilizing the finger for comfort is not the priority in a patient with flexor tenosynovitis. This is an infectious emergency of the hand and must be treated preferentially with parenteral antibiotics and consultation with a hand surgeon. A bulky dressing can be placed with elevation of the affected part in early cases, but does not take priority over antibiotics.

Although hand infections involving subcutaneous tissue are routinely managed by emergency physicians with incision and drainage, that is not the right approach to treating flexor tenosynovitis in the emergency department. The flexor sheath where the infection is located is much deeper than the typical abscesses emergency physicians routinely treat with incision and drainage: the sheath is in very close proximity to the tendon, and the treatment is a surgical emergency appropriately managed by a hand surgeon.

PEER POINT

The Kanavel signs — they point to a diagnosis of flexor tenosynovitis

- Tenderness over the flexor tendon sheath
- Symmetric finger swelling
- Pain with passive extension
- Flexed positioning of the digit to minimize pain

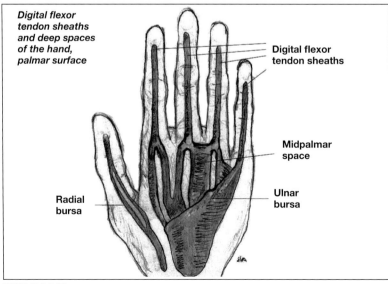

Digital flexor tendon sheaths and deep spaces of the hand, palmar surface

Digital flexor tendon sheaths

Midpalmar space

Radial bursa

Ulnar bursa

PEER Point 25

PEER REVIEW

✓ Most common bacteria in flexor tenosynovitis: *Staphylococcus* and *Streptococcus*. In sexually active patients with no identifiable source of infection, treat for presumed disseminated gonorrhea, too.

✓ Flexor tenosynovitis is diagnosed clinically by recognizing the four Kanavel signs.

✓ Flexor tenosynovitis is a surgical emergency. Start parenteral antibiotics and call a hand surgeon.

REFERENCES

Marx JA, Hockberger RS, Walls RM, eds. *Rosen's Emergency Medicine: Concepts and Clinical Practice*. 8th ed. St. Louis, MO: Elsevier; 2014: 534-569.

Tintinalli JE, Stapczynski JS, Ma OJ, et al, eds. *Tintinalli's Emergency Medicine: A Comprehensive Study Guide*. 8th ed. New York, NY: McGraw-Hill; 2012: 1921-1927.

281. The correct answer is A, Cytomegalovirus.

Why is this the correct answer?

Transplant-related infection is the most likely diagnosis for this patient who is presenting 2 months after renal transplant. Time since the transplant took place is an important factor: in this time period, 1 to 6 months following transplant, viral infections and opportunistic infections are the culprits. Viral infections such as cytomegalovirus (CMV), Epstein-Barr virus, hepatitis, herpes virus, and adenovirus are typically encountered, and the clinical picture depends on the type of virus. The most common causes tend to be UTIs and pneumonia. Infections with CMV typically manifest as pneumonia. An active CMV infection can cause or worsen organ rejection, so in a post-transplant patient, it must be suspected early.

Why are the other choices wrong?

Diverticulitis is the most common GI infection encountered in chronic rejection, that is, more than 6 months after transplant. The incidence of perforation is higher because inflammation is often inhibited by long-term steroid therapy. This patient is only 2 months post-transplant, so diverticulitis is not the most likely cause of his symptoms.

Infection caused by community-acquired organisms — most commonly *S. pneumoniae* — is likely 6 months following transplantation. Community-acquired infections are certainly possible before the 6-month mark, but opportunistic and viral infections should be higher on the differential in this case.

Wound infections, catheter-related infections, other transplant- and procedure-related infections, and colonization of the transplanted organ are prevalent less than 1 month from the time of transplantation. Hospital-acquired infections should be considered as well. Opportunistic infections are much less likely in the first month because the patient is not yet fully immunosuppressed.

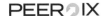

PEER REVIEW

✓ What's causing this transplant-related infection? Good clues are provided by the amount of time that has passed since transplantation. Within the first month, wound infections, abscesses, and catheter-related infections are common.

✓ One to 6 months after transplant, viral infections, commonly cytomegalovirus, and opportunistic infections are likely culprits.

✓ More than 6 months following transplant, consider community-acquired infections, and *S. pneumoniae* in particular.

REFERENCES

Marx JA, Hockberger RS, Walls RM, eds. *Rosen's Emergency Medicine: Concepts and Clinical Practice*. 8th ed. St. Louis, MO: Elsevier; 2014: 2368-2377.e1.

Tintinalli JE, Stapczynski JS, Ma OJ, et al, eds. *Tintinalli's Emergency Medicine: A Comprehensive Study Guide*. 8th ed. New York, NY: McGraw-Hill; 2012: 1039-1047; 2002-2010.

282. The correct answer is A, Gonococcemia.

Why is this the correct answer?

Gonococcemia is a sexually transmitted disease that spreads from a primary site (urethra, cervix, pharynx, prostate), causes bacteremia, and affects other organs. The first stage of disseminated gonococcus infection causes an arthritis or dermatitis syndrome. Arthralgias are very common and are typically migratory, which distinguishes it from the other illnesses in this question. Tenosynovitis can also be seen. The dermatitis consists of varying lesions from maculopapular to pustular, best described as dusky from a hemorrhagic component. Lesions might be seen on the palms or soles or both. During the second stage of dissemination, the rash typically disappears, followed by septic arthritis. In the tertiary stage, several complications can be seen: endocarditis, meningitis, and septic shock. Treatment is intravenous administration of third-generation cephalosporins.

Why are the other choices wrong?

Meningococcemia, most commonly caused by *Neisseria meningitidis* (less commonly *Streptococcus pneumoniae* and very infrequently *Haemophilus influenzae*), can produce a clinical presentation ranging from mild febrile illness to fulminant disease (meningitis, septicemia, and/or meningococcemia) progressing to death within hours. The rash of meningococcemia is erythematous and maculopapular (beginning on the wrists and ankles), spreading centripetally (often sparing the palms and soles), and ultimately forming palpable petechiae and purpura. The sequelae of this condition include disseminated intravascular coagulopathy (DIC), acute respiratory distress syndrome (ARDS), renal failure, multiorgan system failure, and adrenal hemorrhage (Waterhouse-Friderichsen syndrome). A third-generation cephalosporin such as ceftriaxone is often first-line therapy with the addition of vancomycin to cover resistant strains of *S. pneumoniae*. Dexamethasone has been shown to reduce neurologic complications if administered early.

Rocky Mountain spotted fever (RMSF) is a tickborne illness (organism *Rickettsia rickettsii*) that results in fever, headache, muscle aches, abdominal pain, and an erythematous maculopapular rash with centripetal spread (involvement of palms or soles is reported in approximately 50% of cases). The rash eventually becomes petechial; a small proportion of patients has no rash. Shock can ensue within several days of the onset of illness. The diagnosis is clinical, and treatment should begin before confirmatory testing results are available. If unrecognized, the mortality rate associated with RMFS is higher than 30%. However, the mortality rate decreases to 5% with prompt appropriate antibiotic therapy. Doxycycline is the drug of choice.

Syphilis is a sexually transmitted disease caused by a spirochete (*Treponema pallidum*) that initially results in a painless chancre (primary syphilis) that often goes unnoticed and resolves in several weeks. Secondary syphilis occurs after disappearance of the chancre and consists of constitutional symptoms (malaise, headache, sore throat, fever, joint and muscle aches) decreased oral intake, generalized lymphadenopathy, and a mucocutaneous rash. The rash is symmetric, diffuse, and maculopapular (reddish brown) with involvement of hand or soles; it is highly contagious. The lesions rarely appear pustular, which distinguishes it from gonorrhea. Patients might also have other skin findings, including condylomata lata and patchy alopecia. Tertiary syphilis can affect any organ, but cardiovascular and neurologic involvement are most common. Gumma, inflamed necrotic tissue that becomes ulcerative, is also commonly seen in tertiary syphilis. The diagnosis is made clinically, and a high degree of suspicion is required. Treatment of choice is penicillin.

PEER REVIEW

✓ Dissemination of gonorrhea from a primary site — urethra, cervix, pharynx, prostate — via bacteremia results in gonococcemia.

✓ Characteristics of the dermatitis associated with gonococcemia: varying lesions from maculopapular to pustular, dusky pustules.

✓ Rashes that can present with lesions on the palms or soles or both include disseminated gonorrhea, meningococcemia, Rocky Mountain spotted fever, secondary syphilis, hand/foot and mouth disease, Kawasaki disease, erythema multiforme, and toxic shock syndrome.

REFERENCES

Adams JG, Barton ED, Collings J, et al, eds. *Emergency Medicine: Clinical Essentials.* 2nd ed. Philadelphia, PA: Saunders; 2013: 149-158, 1518-1525.

Marx JA, Hockberger RS, Walls RM, eds. *Rosen's Emergency Medicine: Concepts and Clinical Practice.* 8th ed. St. Louis, MO: Elsevier; 2014: 1558-1585; 1785-1808.

283. The correct answer is B, Cardiotocodynamometry.

Why is this the correct answer?

Placental abruption should always be considered in pregnant women who present with acute abdominal or uterine pain with or without bleeding. The most sensitive test for placental abruption is cardiotocodynamometry, which identifies irritability of the uterus, most notably uterine contractions. In addition, the continuous fetal monitoring aspect of this is appropriate to assess fetal wellbeing, with fetal tachycardia or decelerations as a sign of distress. Placental abruption occurs in 1% of pregnancies, and 65% of placental abruptions occur in patients older than 35 years. There is also evidence that black women are at higher risk for placental abruption than are white women. In this case, the first step is to involve an obstetrician because imminent delivery of the baby is needed if the diagnosis is confirmed. The next step is to establish intravenous access and obtain samples for laboratory testing, including a CBC, coagulation panel, fibrinogen level, and fibrin degradation product levels. Fetal monitoring and close monitoring of the mother's vital signs should be continued until the consultant arrives. Both mother and baby might appear stable initially then quickly decompensate if the bleeding gets worse.

Why are the other choices wrong?

Administration of a medication such as terbutaline that acts to stop uterine contractions is not appropriate in this clinical setting when a pregnant patient presents with abdominal pain and vaginal bleeding that is highly suspicious for abruption.

Laboratory testing, including a CBC, coagulation panel, fibrinogen level, and fibrin degradation product levels, is helpful to track, and if abnormal, to guide treatment, especially for patients in disseminated intravascular coagulation from abruption. But in patients with small abruptions or early in the course, these test results can be normal and should not be counted on to make the diagnosis.

Ultrasonography is very specific for diagnosing placental abruption but not sensitive enough to rule it out, especially if there is a retroplacental clot. Magnetic resonance imaging may be used, but only in stable patients.

PEER POINT

Signs and symptoms of placental abruption

Mild abruption

- Pain? Mild uterine tenderness
- Bleeding? None or mild, no coagulopathy
- Vital signs? Maternal, normal; fetal, distress

Severe abruption

- Pain? Uterine, severe or tenderness
- Bleeding? Heavy or none, coagulopathy
- Vital signs? Maternal, hypotension or shock; fetal, distress
- What else? Continuous or repetitive uterine contractions, possibly nausea, vomiting, and back pain

PEER REVIEW

✓ If you're treating a pregnant patient who has painful vaginal bleeding, consider placental abruption.

✓ Don't let diagnostic testing to confirm placental abruption delay definitive treatment in the hands of an obstetrician. Often the ultrasound findings are absent for a retroplacental clot or hematoma that might signify abruption.

✓ In placental abruption, the mother and fetus might be stable at first then decompensate quickly. Monitor vital signs closely and consider obstetrics consultation with emergent delivery with nonreassuring fetal or maternal status.

REFERENCES

Horsager R, Roberts S, Rogers V, et al. Williams Obstetrics. 24th ed. Study Guide. New York, NY: McGraw-Hill; 2015. http://accessmedicine.mhmedical.com.foyer.swmed.edu/content.aspx?bookid=1057&sectionid=59789185. Accessed May 17, 2017.

Shen TT1, DeFranco EA, Stamilio DM, Chang JJ, Muglia LJ A population-based study of race-specific risk for placental abruption. *BMC Pregnancy Childbirth*. 2008;8:43. doi: 10.1186/1471-2393-8-43. http://bmcpregnancychildbirth.biomedcentral.com/articles/10.1

Tintinalli JE, Stapczynski JS, Ma OJ, et al, eds. *Tintinalli's Emergency Medicine: A Comprehensive Study Guide*. 8th ed. New York, NY: McGraw-Hill; 2012: 644-652; 1692-1695.

Wolfson AB, Hendey GW, Ling LJ, et al, eds. *Harwood-Nuss' Clinical Practice of Emergency Medicine*. 6th ed. Philadelphia, PA: Lippincott, Williams & Wilkins; 2014: 689-690.

284. The correct answer is B, Nasal suctioning and supplemental oxygen.

Why is this the correct answer?

Bronchiolitis is an acute infectious illness that causes inflammation of the small airways. Supportive care with supplemental oxygen remains the keystone of therapy, and nasal suctioning can provide benefit. Beyond that, treatment is controversial. Respiratory syncytial virus (RSV) is the most commonly associated virus (70%) with this disease, but parainfluenza, human metapneumovirus, adenovirus, bocavirus, and rhinovirus are frequently implicated as well. Bronchiolitis typically occurs during the winter in children younger than 2 years old. It classically presents initially with common URI symptoms such as rhinorrhea and cough, which then proceed to increased work of breathing, decreased feeding, and wheezing. It is rarely fatal, but it does frequently contribute to hospitalizations. There is increased risk of death in children with low birth weight, with low initial Apgar scores, first-born children, and those born to young mothers. The most common comorbid complication of bronchiolitis is bacterial otitis media (60%). Apnea can occur in younger infants with RSV as well. Routine laboratory evaluations and imaging are not recommended in straightforward presentations of bronchiolitis.

Why are the other choices wrong?

Intravenous fluids and antibiotics are the treatment of choice in a child with severe pneumonia or some other serious bacterial infection. But there is no benefit from this approach in a viral process.

Nebulized L-epinephrine or racemic epinephrine is used in the treatment of upper airway conditions such as croup, which often presents with stridor and a barking cough. No difference has been found between the two isomers of epinephrine in croup. However, there is no supported benefit of this treatment in bronchiolitis.

Continuous albuterol and steroids are most beneficial in children with acute asthma exacerbations, not bronchiolitis. Distinguishing between asthma and bronchiolitis can be challenging because they often present similarly. But in a child younger than 2 years with no asthma risk factors who has concurrent URI symptoms and no improvement after a trial of albuterol, the diagnosis of bronchiolitis is more likely, particularly during peak bronchiolitis months. Studies have not supported the benefit of steroids.

PEER REVIEW

✓ Bacterial otitis media is the most common comorbid condition with bronchiolitis.

✓ If you're treating a wheezing infant, you may consider giving albuterol diagnostically, but keep in mind that the use of albuterol to treat bronchiolitis is controversial.

✓ Bronchiolitis can be associated with apneic events.

REFERENCES

Marx JA, Hockberger RS, Walls RM, eds. *Rosen's Emergency Medicine: Concepts and Clinical Practice*. 8th ed. St. Louis, MO: Elsevier; 2014: 2117-2128.

Tintinalli JE, Stapczynski JS, Ma OJ, et al, eds. *Tintinalli's Emergency Medicine: A Comprehensive Study Guide*. 8th ed. New York, NY: McGraw-Hill; 2012: 793-813.

285. The correct answer is C, Maintain adequate right ventricular filling pressure.

Why is this the correct answer?

Maintaining high right ventricular filling pressures by ensuring adequate intravascular volume status is the mainstay of emergency therapy for pulmonary hypertension; parenteral fluid hydration with normal saline is recommended. Primary, or idiopathic, pulmonary hypertension is rare. It often presents as exercise intolerance, syncope or near syncope, dyspnea on exertion, and shortness of breath, making it difficult to distinguish from a variety of other more common cardiopulmonary disease processes such as asthma, COPD, left ventricular heart failure, and PE. Syncope occurs in up to half of patients with pulmonary hypertension and is typically related to dysrhythmia. There are many secondary causes of pulmonary hypertension, most notably congenital heart disease with unrepaired cardiac shunt.

Why are the other choices wrong?

Decreasing afterload through diuresis is beneficial in left-sided heart failure and, judiciously, in right-sided heart failure, but in this patient without clear evidence of right-sided heart failure and pulmonary hypertension, fluid resuscitation is indicated.

Medications such as prostacyclin analogues and phosphodiesterase inhibitors can decrease pulmonary artery pressure; however, this should be initiated and managed by or in collaboration with a cardiologist. The initial management of pulmonary hypertension should focus on intravascular volume resuscitation to maintain right ventricular filling pressure and ensure adequate cardiac output.

There are no benefits to maintaining pulmonary artery resistance, and the emergency physician should focus on maintaining adequate cardiac output by maintaining preload.

PEER REVIEW

✓ Syncope is a frequent presentation of pulmonary hypertension and is often related to dysrhythmia.
✓ Unrepaired congenital heart disease defects can lead to pulmonary hypertension.

REFERENCES

Marx JA, Hockberger RS, Walls RM, eds. *Rosen's Emergency Medicine: Concepts and Clinical Practice*. 8th ed. St. Louis, MO: Elsevier; 2014: 135-141; 1075-1090.

Tintinalli JE, Stapczynski JS, Ma OJ, et al, eds. *Tintinalli's Emergency Medicine: A Comprehensive Study Guide*. 8th ed. New York, NY: McGraw-Hill; 2012: 409-412.

286. The correct answer is D, Straight blade instead of curved.

Why is this the correct answer?

There are important anatomic variations that must be considered when performing direct laryngoscopy in a pediatric patient. One in particular that applies in this case is that the epiglottis is floppy; it is best lifted with a straight blade rather than a curved one. If the physician is not able to see the vocal cords with a curved blade, switching to a straight one will likely improve visualization of the vocal cords.

Why are the other choices wrong?

Cricoid pressure is optional, but locating the cricoid cartilage in an infant can be difficult. Simple maneuvers accounting for anatomic variations should be attempted first.

Hyperflexion of the neck further misaligns the airway axis, making laryngoscopy increasingly difficult, not easier.

Infants tend to have a larger occiput than adults, which means that the airway anatomy is more forward. This impairs airway visualization. The use of a rolled sheet to align the airway axis is an effective adjustment, but the roll should be placed under the shoulder blade, not the occiput.

PEER POINT

Anatomic variations that make the pediatric airway different from the adult airway

- Large tongue
- Floppy epiglottis
- Large head and occiput
- More anterior and cephalad airway

PEER REVIEW

✓ A straight blade improves visualization of the cords by controlling the floppy epiglottis.

✓ Here's a workaround for the larger occiput in the pediatric airway: put a rolled sheet under the infant's shoulders to help align the airway axis.

REFERENCES

Roberts JR, Custalow CB, Thomsen TW, eds. Roberts and Hedges'; *Clinical Procedures in Emergency Medicine*. 6th ed. Philadelphia, PA: Elsevier; 2014: 72-73.

Tintinalli JE, Stapczynski JS, Ma OJ, et al, eds. *Tintinalli's Emergency Medicine: A Comprehensive Study Guide*. 8th ed. New York, NY: McGraw-Hill; 2012: 716-719.

287. The correct answer is B, Pneumonia.

Why is this the correct answer?

Pneumonia remains the most common cause of death due to complications from *B. pertussis* infection, especially in infants and young children. The complications from *B. pertussis* infection include pneumonia superinfection, CNS complications, subconjunctival hemorrhage, petechiae (particularly above the nipple line), epistaxis, hemoptysis, subcutaneous emphysema, pneumothorax, pneumomediastinum, diaphragmatic rupture, umbilical and inguinal hernias, and rectal prolapse. Many of these complications are secondary to the paroxysms of cough and resulting increased intrathoracic and intra-abdominal pressure. Bradycardia, hypotension, and cardiac arrest can occur in neonates and young infants with pertussis. Severe pulmonary hypertension has also shown increased prevalence in this age group and can lead to systemic hypotension, worsening hypoxia, and increased mortality rates. Antibiotic treatment does not seem to reduce the severity or duration of illness. The primary goal of antibiotic therapy is to reduce infectivity and carriage. Macrolide antibiotics, including erythromycin, azithromycin, or clarithromycin, are primary choices for therapy. Sulfamethoxazole/ trimethoprim is a possible secondary choice for macrolide-allergic patients, but its efficacy has not been proved. Corticosteroids can reduce the severity and course of illness, especially in young, critically ill children. Beta-agonists might have efficacy in patients with reactive airway disease. There is no evidence to support the use of pertussis immunoglobulin. Standard cough suppressants and antihistamines are ineffective. Postexposure prophylaxis is recommended for infants younger than 6 months who are household contacts with confirmed pertussis infection because they have not completed the recommended immunization regimen.

Why are the other choices wrong?

Rupture of the diaphragm is certainly a complication of pertussis, secondary to coughing and increased intrathoracic and intra-abdominal pressure. But it is not the most common cause of death.

Pneumothorax, too, is a complication but not the most common cause of death in patients with pertussis. This diagnosis should be considered if a patient's respiratory effort suddenly increases.

Seizure and encephalopathy are among the CNS complications of pertussis, but neither is the most common cause of death.

PEER REVIEW

✓ Pneumonia is the most common cause of death in pertussis.
✓ Macrolides, not penicillins, are first-line treatment for pertussis infections.
✓ The primary goal of antibiotic therapy in pertussis is to reduce infectivity, not the duration of symptoms.
✓ Infants older than 6 months do not require postexposure prophylaxis.

REFERENCES

Marx JA, Hockberger RS, Walls RM, eds. *Rosen's Emergency Medicine: Concepts and Clinical Practice.* 8th ed. St. Louis, MO: Elsevier; 2014: 1693-1717.

Tintinalli JE, Stapczynski JS, Ma OJ, et al, eds. *Tintinalli's Emergency Medicine: A Comprehensive Study Guide.* 8th ed. New York, NY: McGraw-Hill; 2012: 440-445; 741-747.

288. The correct answer is A, Cranial nerve VII paralysis.

Why is this the correct answer?

Given the patient's presentation, the most likely diagnosis is necrotizing external otitis (formerly known as malignant otitis externa). She has pain on movement of the tragus, along with drainage, which suggests an external process. Symptoms and risk factors that differentiate necrotizing external otitis from the more benign form of otitis externa include high fever (>38.9°C), meningeal signs, and severe otalgia. The patient's history of diabetes also puts her at risk for this type of infection. The most common complication of necrotizing external otitis is paralysis of the seventh cranial nerve. Unlike acute otitis externa, which can be treated with topical antibiotic drops, most infections require parenteral antimicrobial treatment and admission with ENT consultation. Coverage for *Pseudomonas* (ceftazidime 50 mg/kg IV every 8 hours, or methicillin 50 mg/kg IV every 6 hours) is clinically indicated, although a course of oral fluoroquinolones can be attempted if the diagnosis is made early. Magnetic resonance imaging might be indicated to look for osteomyelitis of the skull base.

Why are the other choices wrong?

Given the location of the infection, it is unlikely to spread and develop into an anterior facial cellulitis.

Mastoiditis is an infection of the mastoid bone. It is treated similarly to necrotizing external otitis, with hospitalization for intravenous antibiotic therapy and ENT consultation, but it is not the most common complication.

Perforated tympanic membrane is not common in necrotizing external otitis, and if present, a secondary etiology should be explored.

PEER REVIEW

✓ Patients with acute otitis externa can be treated with topical antibiotic drops as outpatients.

✓ The risk of necrotizing external otitis is higher in immunocompromised patients and presents with systemic symptoms.

✓ Treatment for necrotizing external otitis usually requires hospitalization, intravenous antibiotics, and ENT consultation.

REFERENCES

Brown KD, Banuchi V, Selesnick SH, et al. Diseases of the External Ear. In: Lalwani AK, eds. *CURRENT Diagnosis & Treatment in Otolaryngology—Head & Neck Surgery*. 3rd ed. New York, NY: McGraw-Hill; 2012. http://accessmedicine.mhmedical.com/content.aspx?bookid=386&sectionid=39944089. Accessed May 18, 2017.

Marx JA, Hockberger RS, Walls RM, eds. *Rosen's Emergency Medicine: Concepts and Clinical Practice*. 8th ed. St. Louis, MO: Elsevier; 2014: 931-940.

Tintinalli JE, Stapczynski JS, Ma OJ, et al, eds. *Tintinalli's Emergency Medicine: A Comprehensive Study Guide*. 8th ed. New York, NY: McGraw-Hill; 2012: 757-764.

289. The correct answer is C, Pregnancy.

Why is this the correct answer?

Pregnancy is considered an indication for hyperbaric oxygen (HBO) therapy after carbon monoxide (CO) exposure if the mother has signs of ischemic injury, neurologic deficits, or an elevated carboxyhemoglobin (COHb) level over 15%. High levels of maternal COHb can lead to significant fetal hypoxia and death or permanent neurologic or developmental injury if the CO is not displaced by oxygen. Other indications for considering HBO therapy include COHb levels over 40% (some institutions go as low as levels >25%) and signs of tissue ischemia such as altered mental status, neurologic deficits, myocardial ischemia, cardiac dysrhythmias, and syncope. Carbon monoxide poisoning is known to cause delayed neurologic deficits, and this is the primary reason for considering HBO therapy in these patients and even in asymptomatic patients who have elevated COHb levels.

Why are the other choices wrong?

A low oxygen saturation level can be managed with supplemental oxygen and observation. A chest xray might be warranted to assess for other lung injury from smoke inhalation, but alone, this is not an indicator for HBO therapy. Supplemental oxygen at 100% can reduce the half-life of COHb to 1 hour from the normal 5 hours at room air. Hyperbaric oxygen therapy decreases that half-life even further, to 30 minutes.

Underlying asthma does not increase the likelihood of delayed neurologic sequelae from CO exposure. It might cause the patient to present with some bronchospasm from the inhaled irritant gas and smoke, but it is not an indication for HBO therapy.

Nausea and vomiting are common after smoke and CO exposure and do not indicate a need for HBO therapy or control of the airway if they can be controlled or have resolved.

PEER POINT

Indications for HBO therapy

- Neurologic deficits
- Altered mental status
- Cardiovascular compromise
- Myocardial ischemia
- Syncope
- Dysrhythmia
- COHb level >25%
- Pregnant patient with COHb level >15%

PEER REVIEW

- ✓ Pregnant patient with an elevated COHb? Hyperbaric oxygen therapy is indicated.
- ✓ Neurologic deficits or signs of cardiac ischemia are also indications for HBO.
- ✓ Carbon monoxide poisoning is known to cause delayed neurologic sequelae.

REFERENCES

Marx JA, Hockberger RS, Walls RM, eds. *Rosen's Emergency Medicine: Concepts and Clinical Practice.* 8th ed. St. Louis, MO: Elsevier; 2014: 2036-2043.

Tintinalli JE, Stapczynski JS, Ma OJ, et al, eds. *Tintinalli's Emergency Medicine: A Comprehensive Study Guide.* 8th ed. New York, NY: McGraw-Hill; 2012: 1405-1411.

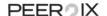

290. The correct answer is C, *Staphylococcus aureus*.

Why is this the correct answer?

S. aureus and *Haemophilus influenzae* are the most common pathogens of childhood pneumonia in patients with cystic fibrosis. Cystic fibrosis is caused by defects in chloride transport in the cellular membranes, which results in reduced ciliary clearance of mucus, thicker mucus, and ultimately, enhanced bacterial adherence to the airway. Patients with cystic fibrosis have pneumonia frequently. An important component of the treatment of pneumonia includes aggressive pulmonary toilet, aerosolized treatments, and mucolytics.

Why are the other choices wrong?

B. cepacia is a common serious pathogen that causes pneumonia in cystic fibrosis patients. Although not the most common cause of pneumonia, infection with this organism is related to increased morbidity and mortality rates.

By age 18, 80% of patients with cystic fibrosis have been colonized with *P. aeruginosa*. Empiric antibiotics generally include a penicillin and aminoglycoside. Typically, an emergency physician should consider expert consultation before treating cystic fibrosis. Investigating the patient's history and evaluation of prior sputum cultures is warranted.

S. pneumoniae is the most common cause of pneumonia overall in both immunocompetent and immunocompromised patients.

PEER REVIEW

✓ *S. aureus* is the predominant cause of pneumonia in cystic fibrosis.
✓ *P. aeruginosa* colonizes 80% of cystic fibrosis patients by the time they are adults.

REFERENCES
Marx JA, Hockberger RS, Walls RM, eds. *Rosen's Emergency Medicine: Concepts and Clinical Practice*. 8th ed. St. Louis, MO: Elsevier; 2014: 2137-2138.
Tintinalli JE, Stapczynski JS, Ma OJ, et al, eds. *Tintinalli's Emergency Medicine: A Comprehensive Study Guide*. 8th ed. New York, NY: McGraw-Hill; 2012: 814-822.

291. The correct answer is C, Magnesium sulfate.

Why is this the correct answer?

The patient's presentation is suggestive of eclampsia, which can occur in the third trimester of pregnancy but can also occur up to 4 weeks postpartum. The initial treatment is magnesium sulfate, 4 to 6 g IV followed by infusion at 1 to 2 g/hr. If the patient has signs of renal insufficiency, the dose should be decreased. Signs of magnesium toxicity include delayed reflexes, flaccid paralysis, hypotension, and respiratory compromise. If the patient continues to have hypertension after magnesium administration, consider a secondary antihypertensive medication such as hydralazine, labetalol, nifedipine, or sodium nitroprusside. All patients require admission to an obstetric care setting with critical care capabilities given the risk for ongoing seizures and complications from magnesium administration.

Why are the other choices wrong?

Hydralazine may be given to control blood pressure in a patient who develops eclampsia with hypertension, but it is considered a secondary agent because magnesium can treat elevated blood pressure when given as the initial therapy for seizure activity.

Although benzodiazepines like lorazepam are an initial first-line agent for seizures, they are not indicated in the treatment of eclampsia. They may be considered if magnesium toxicity is a concern and the patient continues to have seizures.

Phenytoin is also an appropriate antiepileptic agent for typical patients with seizures, but it is not the first-line agent in eclampsia.

PEER REVIEW

✓ Eclampsia can occur up to 4 weeks postpartum.
✓ The side effects of magnesium administration must be monitored closely.
✓ Blood pressure should be controlled with a secondary agent if it is still elevated after magnesium therapy.

REFERENCES

Cunningham F, Leveno KJ, Bloom SL, et al, eds. *Williams Obstetrics*. 24th ed. New York, NY: McGraw-Hill; 2013. http://accessmedicine.mhmedical.com.foyer.swmed.edu/content.aspx?bookid=1057&sectionid=59789184. Accessed May 17, 2017.

Tintinalli JE, Stapczynski JS, Ma OJ, et al, eds. *Tintinalli's Emergency Medicine: A Comprehensive Study Guide*. 8th ed. New York, NY: McGraw-Hill; 2012: 644-652.

292. The correct answer is A, Acute ovarian torsion.

Why is this the correct answer?

What this case illustrates is that, even when there is good Doppler flow on an ultrasound examination, an ovarian torsion cannot be ruled out using ultrasonography alone given concerning clinical symptoms. Ultrasonography can miss the torsion 25% to 50% of the time. Given the high suspicion, an obstetrics consultation for admission and possible surgical exploration is warranted because the ultrasound imaging might have been obtained during a period when the ovary had detorsed. On surgical exploration, an ovarian mass is identified in 50% to 80% of all torsions. Twenty percent to 25% of all ovarian torsions occur during pregnancy. Ovaries larger than 5 cm in diameter are at greater risk for torsion.

Why are the other choices wrong?

Endometrioma is a mass composed of endometrial material that is found within an ovary. A chocolate cyst, as it is called, can rupture with dark viscous fluid (from old blood) found within. It is generally identifiable using ultrasonography for

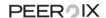

its characteristic thick wall and internal echoes. This condition is often resolved surgically on a nonemergent basis for complaints of recurrent pain or to rule out malignancy.

A corpus luteum cyst is seen in early pregnancy and remains present into the second trimester. It can rupture and cause severe abdominal pain or bleeding, at which point obstetrics consultation is needed. Most commonly, when there is hemorrhage, it occurs within the cyst and does not commonly cause intraperitoneal bleeding or peritoneal signs. This condition is seen only in pregnant patients, and this patient's pregnancy test is negative.

Rupture of an ovarian cyst can also cause severe pain and peritoneal signs. The symptoms tend to be more constant and not intermittently severe. In addition, ruptured ovarian cyst without significant hemorrhage or hemodynamic instability does not need urgent obstetrics consultation. In this case, there is no free fluid described on the ultrasound examination.

PEER REVIEW

- ✓ Suspect an ovarian torsion when a patient presents with intermittent lower quadrant pain even if ultrasound imaging demonstrates good blood flow.
- ✓ If you see an ovary larger than 5 cm on ultrasound, there's a higher likelihood of torsion.
- ✓ An ovarian mass must be ruled out when an ovarian torsion is diagnosed.

REFERENCES

Goh W, Bohrer J, Zalud I. Management of the adnexal mass in pregnancy. *Curr Opin Obstet Gynecol.* 2014;26(2):49-53. doi: 10.1097/GCO.0000000000000048.

Hoffman B, Schorge J, Schaffer J, et al. *Williams Gynecology.* 2nd ed. New York, NY: McGraw-Hill; 2012; Chapter 9: Pelvic Mass. Available at: http://accessmedicine.mhmedical.com/content.aspx?bookid=399§ionid=41722297&jumpsectionID=41724832& Resultclick=2. Accessed May 17, 2017.

Tintinalli JE, Stapczynski JS, Ma OJ, et al, eds. *Tintinalli's Emergency Medicine: A Comprehensive Study Guide.* 8th ed. New York, NY: McGraw-Hill; 2012: 625-628.

293. The correct answer is A, Admission for endoscopy and close monitoring.

Why is this the correct answer?

In the setting of intentional overdose of a large amount of a strongly caustic agent, the appropriate recommendation is admission for close monitoring and serial examinations; endoscopy can be performed to grade the extent of the injury. Serious caustic acid injuries cause coagulation necrosis, a process in which hydrogen ions infiltrate tissues, which leads to killing of cells and formation of an eschar. This eschar protects against deeper injury, and thus caustic acids typically cause less damage than caustic alkalis. Despite this, ingestion of strong acids is associated with a higher mortality rate compared to alkali ingestions because of severe gastric damage. An anion gap acidosis (lactic) might result from tissue injury or impending shock. Of note, some acidic agents (hydrochloric acid) might produce a nongap acidosis, and the acid might be absorbed systemically. Household cleaning agents such as toilet bowl cleaners contain hydrochloric acid. The patient in this question might have some degree of acidosis as indicated by her tachypnea. Psychiatric services are needed, but because she has symptoms of potential gastric injury, she should first be admitted to a medical service for serial abdominal examinations and monitoring for GI bleeding or perforation. Intentional ingestions are associated with higher grades of GI injury.

Why are the other choices wrong?

This patient does not show evidence of chemical burn to the oropharynx or swelling of the upper airway to necessitate airway protection with emergent intubation. She does need endoscopy, which should be obtained in a controlled setting. Endoscopy should be performed within 12 hours of ingestion and not more than 24 hours afterward to avoid GI perforation during the procedure.

Gastric decontamination with activated charcoal is contraindicated in caustic ingestions: charcoal does not bind well to most caustic agents and impairs visualization for endoscopy.

Gastric lavage is not indicated for caustic ingestions. For concern of coingestants, placement of a nasogastric or larger orogastric tube (like the Ewald) is contraindicated until an endoscopy has shown that gastric hemorrhage or perforation is not a risk.

PEER REVIEW

- ✓ Strong caustic acid injuries lead to coagulation necrosis.
- ✓ If you're treating a symptomatic patient who ingested a strong caustic solution intentionally, that patient is at risk for serious injury and should be closely monitored, admitted, and considered for endoscopy.
- ✓ Emetics and neutralizing agents are contraindicated in caustic ingestions.

REFERENCES

Marx JA, Hockberger RS, Walls RM, eds. *Rosen's Emergency Medicine: Concepts and Clinical Practice*. 8th ed. St. Louis, MO: Elsevier; 2014: 1173-1175.

Tintinalli JE, Stapczynski JS, Ma OJ, et al, eds. *Tintinalli's Emergency Medicine: A Comprehensive Study Guide*. 8th ed. New York, NY: McGraw-Hill; 2012: 1314-1318.

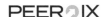

294. The correct answer is D, Stool culture.

Why is this the correct answer?

Yersinia enterocolitica is a gram-negative anaerobic bacterium that can mimic symptoms of appendicitis due to development of ileocecitis. The clinical picture of Yersinia enterocolitis is nonspecific and includes gastroenteritis-type symptoms. One feature that might help differentiate this rarer infection is development of bloody diarrhea. Uncooked pork can be a source. The diagnosis of yersiniosis is difficult to make clinically and requires a positive stool culture or real-time polymer chain reaction (PCR) testing. Standard stool cultures are inadequate; specific techniques are needed. It is not as prevalent as campylobacteriosis or salmonellosis, largely due to modern food processing procedures. *Y. enterocolitica* infection is usually self-limited and resolves without treatment. However, in patients with longstanding illnesses or with significant illness after the return of stool cultures, antibiotic treatment might be considered using trimethoprim-sulfamethoxazole.

Why are the other choices wrong?

Getting an abdominal xray might be helpful if there is suspicion for bowel obstruction, perforation, or volvulus. However, this patient's symptoms are not consistent with these diagnoses.

A CT scan would not be helpful in this case because a normal appendix was visualized on ultrasound examination even with the right lower quadrant pain. In addition, the otherwise benign abdominal examination described with blood-tinged diarrhea should lead to the diagnosis of an infectious disease not diagnosed with imaging.

The patient's appendix appeared normal on the ultrasound examination, so exploratory laparotomy is not warranted.

PEER REVIEW

- ✓ *Yersinia* enterocolitis can look a lot like appendicitis.
- ✓ Yersiniosis is more prevalent in adolescents and young adults.
- ✓ You can't diagnose *Yersinia* enterocolitis clinically; you'll have to get a stool culture or PCR to be sure.

REFERENCES

Marx JA, Hockberger RS, Walls RM, eds. *Rosen's Emergency Medicine: Concepts and Clinical Practice.* 8th ed. St. Louis, MO: Elsevier; 2014: 1238-1239.

Tintinalli JE, Stapczynski JS, Ma OJ, et al, eds. *Tintinalli's Emergency Medicine: A Comprehensive Study Guide.* 8th ed. New York, NY: McGraw-Hill; 2012: 1078-1081.

295. The correct answer is A, Decreased exercise performance is an early symptom.

Why is this the correct answer?

Early symptoms of high-altitude pulmonary edema (HAPE) include decreased exercise performance and dry cough. As HAPE worsens, dyspnea with exertion progresses to dyspnea at rest. Low-grade fever is common, and tachycardia and tachypnea correlate with the degree of illness. The noncardiogenic pulmonary edema in HAPE results from hypoxia-induced pulmonary artery hypertension. This leads to an elevated hydrostatic pressure and capillary leak. Early recognition is critical because HAPE is potentially lethal but initially easily reversible with oxygen administration and descent from altitude.

Why are the other choices wrong?

High-altitude pulmonary edema is noncardiogenic in origin. The noncardiogenic pulmonary edema in HAPE results from hypoxia-induced pulmonary artery hypertension. This leads to an elevated hydrostatic pressure and capillary leak.

High (not low) pulmonary artery pressure due to hypoxia is an essential component in the development of HAPE.

The most important treatments for HAPE are descent and oxygen administration. But phosphodiesterase-5 inhibitors such as sildenafil and tadalafil do blunt hypoxia-induced pulmonary vasoconstriction and have demonstrated some efficacy in prevention and treatment.

PEER REVIEW

✓ Decreased exercise performance is an early symptom of high-altitude pulmonary edema.

✓ Descent and oxygen administration are the cornerstones of high-altitude pulmonary edema treatment.

REFERENCES

Tintinalli JE, Stapczynski JS, Ma OJ, et al, eds. *Tintinalli's Emergency Medicine: A Comprehensive Study Guide.* 8th ed. New York, NY: McGraw-Hill; 2012: 1434-1435.

Wolfson AB, Hendey GW, Ling LJ, et al, eds. *Harwood-Nuss' Clinical Practice of Emergency Medicine.* 6th ed. Philadelphia, PA: Lippincott, Williams & Wilkins; 2014: 1517, 1519.

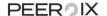

296. The correct answer is C, Discharge with return precautions.

Why is this the correct answer?

Even in the unusual situation described — an actual witnessed bite by a brown recluse spider in an endemic area — discharge with return precautions is appropriate. The majority of actual bites from the brown recluse spider resolve without consequence, and there is currently no known way to predict which patients will develop the rare delayed-onset necrotic wound that might ultimately need skin grafting to repair. There is no treatment proven to prevent the development of necrosis. General wound care and return precautions in case necrosis occurs are appropriate. If necrosis occurs, allowing time for wound edges to demarcate before considering skin grafting is appropriate.

Why are the other choices wrong?

There is currently no commercial antivenom available to treat brown recluse envenomation. Studies in animals do demonstrate efficacy of antivenom but only if administration occurs almost immediately after the envenomation.

Most bites from the brown recluse resolve without consequence. Admission is not needed to monitor for skin necrosis, but return precautions in case it occurs are appropriate.

Prophylactic skin incision is not recommended because, again, the majority of bites resolve without consequence.

PEER REVIEW

✓ Most bites from the brown recluse spider resolve without consequence.

REFERENCES

Hoffman RS, Howland MA, Lewin NA, et al, eds. *Goldfrank's Toxicologic Emergencies.* 10th ed. New York, NY: McGraw-Hill; 2015: 1465-1467.

Tintinalli JE, Stapczynski JS, Ma OJ, et al, eds. *Tintinalli's Emergency Medicine: A Comprehensive Study Guide.* 8th ed. New York, NY: McGraw-Hill; 2012:1373-1374.

297. The correct answer is A, CT angiography.

Why is this the correct answer?

Acute mesenteric ischemia can be difficult to diagnose and is characterized by pain out of proportion to physical examination findings. Patients often have a poor clinical course and rapid deterioration. The primary diagnostic study for acute mesenteric ischemia in the emergency department is CT angiography: it is widely available, highly sensitive and specific (96% and 94% using modern multidetector scanners), and noninvasive. The CT should be obtained with intravenous contrast and, due to the high mortality rate (as high as 90%) of this disease, the need for a prompt diagnosis might override the need for digestion of oral contrast or concerns about elevated creatinine levels. Traditional abdominal angiography is still a gold standard option because it allows simultaneous treatment; however, it might not be as feasible a diagnostic tool due to its invasive nature and requirement for interventional radiology. Mesenteric arterial embolism accounts for 50% of cases of acute ischemia, with the superior mesenteric artery most often affected. Other causes include mesenteric arterial thrombosis, mesenteric venous thrombosis, and nonocclusive mesenteric ischemia.

Why are the other choices wrong?

Magnetic resonance arteriography might be indicated to examine patency of the superior or inferior mesenteric arteries. However, these studies can take a long time to obtain, and MRI is not considered a standard for initial evaluation.

Plain radiographs are nonspecific. In later disease, thumbprinting can be seen with multiple round soft tissue densities appearing in the intestinal lumen from edema and hemorrhage. Very late findings include pneumatosis intestinalis and portal venous gas, which occur with bowel infarction.

Duplex ultrasonography has shown high specificity (92% to 100%) for detection of vascular occlusions, but its sensitivity is limited by difficulty evaluating beyond proximal main vessels. It also might be unable to provide information about complications arising from acute mesenteric ischemia.

PEER REVIEW

✓ What's the classic presentation for acute mesenteric ischemia? Pain out of proportion to physical examination findings.
✓ Occlusions of the superior mesenteric artery are most frequent in acute mesenteric ischemia.
✓ Acting on high clinical suspicion and achieving early diagnosis reduces mortality rates associated with acute mesenteric ischemia.

REFERENCES

Marx JA, Hockberger RS, Walls RM, eds. *Rosen's Emergency Medicine: Concepts and Clinical Practice*. 8th ed. St. Louis, MO: Elsevier; 2014: 1221-1224.

Tintinalli JE, Stapczynski JS, Ma OJ, et al, eds. *Tintinalli's Emergency Medicine: A Comprehensive Study Guide*. 8th ed. New York, NY: McGraw-Hill; 2012: 506.

298. The correct answer is C, Sutures.

Why is this the correct answer?

Of the techniques listed, sutures provide the greatest tensile strength. Horizontal or vertical mattress sutures should be considered in high-tension wounds, especially those located in dynamic areas like extremities. Although suturing can be very time consuming, depending on clinician experience, it has the lowest dehiscence rate.

Why are the other choices wrong?

Adhesive tape has the lowest tensile strength and highest rate of dehiscence. It is also susceptible to moisture.

Staples are quick and easy to apply but can decrease joint movement if they are directly over areas of flexion. Of all the techniques, sutures still provide the greatest tensile strength.

Tissue adhesives like cyanoacrylate should not be used alone in high-tension wounds. Instead, they can be used in addition to deep sutures to provide adequate repair. They also have the lowest infection rates.

PEER POINT

What's good and not so good about different wound closure techniques

Adhesive tape
- ☑ Fast application
- ☑ Least tissue reactivity
- ☑ Lowest infection rate
- ☒ Lower tensile strength than sutures or tissue adhesives
- ☒ Can't get wet
- ☒ Frequently falls off
- ☒ Highest dehiscence rate

Staples
- ☑ Fast application
- ☑ Low tissue reactivity
- ☒ Less precise closure
- ☒ Can interfere with imaging

Sutures
- ☑ Precise closure
- ☑ Greatest tensile strength
- ☑ Lowest dehiscence rate
- ☒ Require anesthesia
- ☒ Time-consuming application
- ☒ Greatest tissue reactivity
- ☒ Require removal (if nonabsorbable)

Tissue Adhesives
- ☑ Fast application
- ☑ Comfortable
- ☑ Resistant to bacteria growth
- ☒ Not useful on hands
- ☒ Lower tensile strength than 5-0 or larger sutures
- ☒ Can't bathe or swim (can shower)
- ☒ Dehiscence over high-tension areas

PEER REVIEW

- ✓ Sutures provide the greatest tensile strength for wound repair.
- ✓ Tissue adhesives have the lowest infection rates of all wound closure techniques.

REFERENCES

Roberts JR, Custalow CB, Thomsen TW, eds. Roberts and Hedges' *Clinical Procedures in Emergency Medicine*. 6th ed. Philadelphia, PA: Elsevier; 2014: 644-655.

Tintinalli JE, Stapczynski JS, Ma OJ, et al, eds. *Tintinalli's Emergency Medicine: A Comprehensive Study Guide*. 8th ed. New York, NY: McGraw-Hill; 2012: 281-288.

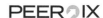

299. The correct answer is C, Discharge her to home with a referral for outpatient endoscopy.

Why is this the correct answer?

In this case, the patient presents with the typical symptoms of esophageal impaction. Because she could initially handle her own secretions, watchful waiting is an appropriate treatment strategy, with endoscopy within 12 to 24 hours. With acute relief, she may be discharged home without further observation. Eosinophilic esophagitis should be considered in patients like this who present with recurrent esophageal food impaction and symptoms of gastroesophageal reflux disease despite the use of antacid medications. Patients typically are nonresponsive to high-dose proton pump inhibitors. Esophageal strictures are commonly seen in these patients, especially if the underlying condition is untreated, and lead to recurrent impactions. Referral for outpatient endoscopy, for both diagnostic and therapeutic purposes, is the correct disposition.

Why are the other choices wrong?

The patient's esophageal food impaction spontaneously passed on its own. It is unnecessary to admit her to the hospital if she remains asymptomatic.

Although the patient does need to see a gastroenterologist for an endoscopy, biopsy, and further workup and management, she can safely do it as an outpatient. Indications for immediate endoscopy include significant distress, impactions that prevent handling of secretions, ingestion of sharp objects or button batteries, and impaction in the esophagus for longer than 24 hours.

Again, the impaction resolved on its own; the patient was able to drink water and had no other symptoms, so observation in the emergency department is not warranted.

PEER REVIEW

- ✓ If you're treating a patient who has recurrent esophageal food bolus impactions and symptoms of gastroesophageal reflux disease despite the use of high-dose proton pump inhibitors, consider eosinophilic esophagitis.
- ✓ Indications for immediate endoscopy in esophageal food impaction: impactions that prevent handling of secretions, ingestion of sharp objects or button batteries, impaction in the esophagus for longer than 12 to 24 hours.

REFERENCES

Marx JA, Hockberger RS, Walls RM, eds. *Rosen's Emergency Medicine: Concepts and Clinical Practice*. 8th ed. St. Louis, MO: Elsevier; 2014: 1173-1175.

Tintinalli JE, Stapczynski JS, Ma OJ, et al, eds. *Tintinalli's Emergency Medicine: A Comprehensive Study Guide*. 8th ed. New York, NY: McGraw-Hill; 2012: 508-514.

300. The correct answer is B, Focal neurologic deficits can occur.

Why is this the correct answer?

The neurologic deficits associated with most toxic and metabolic causes of significant altered levels of consciousness (including hypoglycemia) are typically symmetrical (nonfocal). However, a small but not insignificant number of patients with hypoglycemia presents with focal neurologic deficits, including hemiplegia. The rapid identification and correction of hypoglycemia in all patients, including those with focal neurologic deficits, is critical to avoid severe complications of a rapidly reversible condition and to avoid unnecessary imaging (brain imaging) and potential interventions (thrombolytic therapy).

Why are the other choices wrong?

Although adrenergic symptoms such as diaphoresis and tachycardia are common manifestations of hypoglycemia, bradycardia is less common, and none of these symptoms should be relied on to determine if a patient is hypoglycemic.

Release of the counterregulatory hormone epinephrine in the setting of hypoglycemia can result in a variety of adrenergic symptoms (anxiety, diaphoresis, palpitations, tachycardia, tremors). Hypotension is not expected and is not common.

Syncope is a transient loss of consciousness associated with a loss of postural tone that spontaneously reverses without medical intervention. When a patient becomes comatose from hypoglycemia, the body has exhausted its ability to counteract the hypoglycemia. Spontaneous reversal is very unlikely to occur. Syncope is not a common manifestation of hypoglycemia.

PEER REVIEW

✓ Patients with hypoglycemia — not many, but some — present with focal neurologic deficits, including hemiplegia.

REFERENCES

Tintinalli JE, Stapczynski JS, Ma OJ, et al, eds. *Tintinalli's Emergency Medicine: A Comprehensive Study Guide*. 8th ed. New York, NY: McGraw-Hill; 2012: 360, 1455-1456.

Wolfson AB, Hendey GW, Ling LJ, et al, eds. *Harwood-Nuss' Clinical Practice of Emergency Medicine*. 6th ed. Philadelphia, PA: Lippincott, Williams & Wilkins; 2014: 1014-1015.

301. The correct answer is C, *Mycoplasma pneumoniae*.

Why is this the correct answer?

Patients with sickle cell disease are susceptible to infections from encapsulated organisms because they are functionally asplenic after childhood. Of those infectious conditions, acute chest syndrome is the most common cause of death in this population in the United States. Historically *S. pneumoniae* was the most common cause of acute chest syndrome as a result of this susceptibility. However, current studies show that the most common infections found in sickle cell patients with acute chest syndrome are from atypical bacteria *M. pneumoniae* and *Chlamydia pneumoniae*. Knowledge of the encapsulated organisms is important because coverage of these organisms is an important consideration when selecting adequate broad-spectrum antibiotics. Of the four pathogens listed, only *M. pneumoniae* is not an encapsulated organism, although it remains a common cause of infection in patients with sickle cell disease.

Why are the other choices wrong?

H. influenzae is an encapsulated organism, and it does cause acute chest syndrome in sickle cell patients. However, it is not the most likely pathogen in this case.

Again, according to a national study, *M. pneumoniae* infection is much more common in acute chest syndrome in sickle cell disease than is *K. pneumoniae* infection.

With the broad use of pneumococcal vaccines and penicillin prophylaxis, *S. pneumoniae* now rarely causes acute chest syndrome in patients with sickle cell disease. It is not the most likely culprit in this case.

PEER POINT

Mnemonic for remembering the encapsulated organisms
- **Some** — *Streptococcus pneumoniae*
- **Nasty** — *Neisseria meningitidis*
- **Killers** — *Klebsiella pneumoniae*
- **Have** — *Haemophilus influenzae*
- **Some** — *Salmonella typhi*
- **Capsule** — *Cryptococcus neoformans*
- **Protection** — *Pseudomonas aeruginosa*

PEER REVIEW
- ✓ Patients with sickle cell disease are essentially asplenic after childhood.
- ✓ Patients with asplenia with evidence of infection should be started on broad-spectrum antibiotics that cover encapsulated organisms.
- ✓ Encapsulated organisms: *Streptococcus pneumoniae, Neisseria meningitidis, Klebsiella pneumoniae, Haemophilus influenzae, Salmonella typhi, Cryptococcus neoformans, Pseudomonas aeruginosa.*

REFERENCES

Marx JA, Hockberger RS, Walls RM, eds. *Rosen's Emergency Medicine: Concepts and Clinical Practice*. 8th ed. St. Louis, MO: Elsevier; 2014: 2356-2367.

Tintinalli JE, Stapczynski JS, Ma OJ, et al, eds. *Tintinalli's Emergency Medicine: A Comprehensive Study Guide*. 8th ed. New York, NY: McGraw-Hill; 2012: 1504-1514.

302. The correct answer is C, Dilated bowel with prominent plicae circulares.

Why is this the correct answer?

Knowing that this patient's medical history includes exploratory laparotomy, the entire clinical picture is suggestive of small bowel obstruction (SBO) due to adhesions. Small bowel obstruction is approximately four times more common than large bowel obstruction and accounts for approximately 15% of all emergency admissions for abdominal pain. Classic plain radiographic findings for SBO include distended loops of bowel (>3 cm diameter) and prominent plicae circulares (valvulae conniventes) that go across the entire bowel (the coiled spring sign). These findings are in contrast to haustra of the large intestine, which do not cross the full diameter of the bowel. Generally, the greater the number of distended loops, the more distal the obstruction. Computed tomography has higher sensitivity and specificity in detecting SBO and also provides more information regarding the potential cause of the obstruction.

Why are the other choices wrong?

Bowel wall thickening is generally seen with colonic inflammation in conditions such as diverticulitis. It is generally not seen in SBO.

Haustra are present on the large bowel and do not go all the way across the bowel. Small bowel obstruction is much more common than large bowel obstruction.

A distended U-shaped loop of bowel, often called the coffee bean sign or the bent inner tube sign, is seen in sigmoid volvulus. When the volvulus occurs, the bowel folds back on itself, with the two medial walls touching. Sigmoid volvulus is a cause of large bowel obstruction and occurs when the sigmoid colon twists on the sigmoid mesocolon.

PEER POINT

Severely dilated air-filled small bowel and the coiled spring sign

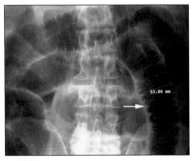

PEER Point 26

PEER REVIEW

✓ Intestinal obstruction accounts for approximately 15% of all emergency admissions for abdominal pain.

✓ Adhesions (postoperative) are the most common cause of small bowel obstruction in the United States, followed by neoplasms and hernias. Gallstone ileus and small bowel volvulus are rarer causes.

✓ Plain radiographs can diagnose small bowel obstruction in 50% to 60% of cases, but CT scanning has increased sensitivity and specificity and can also help determine the etiology of the obstruction.

REFERENCES

Knoop KJ, Stack LB, Storrow AB, et al, eds. *The Atlas of Emergency Medicine.* 4th ed. New York, NY: McGraw-Hill; 2016: 165-199.

Marx JA, Hockberger RS, Walls RM, eds. *Rosen's Emergency Medicine: Concepts and Clinical Practice.* 8th ed. St. Louis, MO: Elsevier; 2014: 1216-1224.e2.

Tintinalli JE, Stapczynski JS, Ma OJ, et al, eds. *Tintinalli's Emergency Medicine: A Comprehensive Study Guide.* 8th ed. New York, NY: McGraw-Hill; 2012: 538-541.

303. The correct answer is B, Ketamine.

Why is this the correct answer?

Ketamine is a dissociative anesthetic and is being used more often for procedural sedation. It has been shown in some cases to cause hypertension and, therefore, might be preferred in patients like this with hypotension. Nausea and vomiting side effects can be abated by presedation antiemetic therapy. Other side effects of ketamine reflect its sympathomimetic properties and include laryngospasm, apnea, angina, and congestive heart failure. Traditionally, ketamine has been contraindicated in patients with increased intracranial pressure and increased intraocular pressure. However, recent evidence questions the relationship of ketamine and increased intracranial and intraocular pressures.

Why are the other choices wrong?

Many different medications and combinations can be used for procedural sedation. But in the setting of hypotension, many of these medications can cause a further drop in blood pressure. Fentanyl provides analgesia, without sedation or is frequently used for pain control because of its brief duration, rapid onset, easy reversibility with naloxone, and lack of histamine release. Certain side effects such as respiratory depression can be easily reversed with an opioid antagonist. A rare side effect of fentanyl is chest wall rigidity. This can be reversed with naloxone, positive pressure ventilation, or a combination.

Benzodiazepines such as midazolam are often used in procedural sedation and provide the additional benefit of amnestic properties. But benzodiazepines does not provide any analgesia and can cause hypotension (not good for this patient), respiratory depression, and paradoxical excitement, in which patients become acutely agitated.

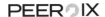

PEER IX

Propofol should not be used in patients with an egg or soy allergy. Common side effects include hypotension and respiratory depression, so this medication might worsen this patient's hypotension.

PEER POINT

Procedural sedation agents, effects, and side effects

Drug	Effects	Side Effects
Etomidate	Sedation, anxiolysis	Respiratory depression, myodonus, nausea, vomiting, adrenocortical suppression
Fentanyl	Analgesia	Respiratory depression, chest wall rigidity
Ketamine	Analgesia, dissociation, amnesia	Laryngospasm, vomiting, agitation, might increase intracranial and intraocular pressures
Midazolam	Sedation, anxiolysis	Can cause paradoxical excitement, oversedation, respiratory depression, hypotension
Propofol	Sedation, anxiolysis	Frequent hypotension and respiratory depression, avoid in egg/soy allergy

Adapted from Roberts and Hedges 6e, Table 33-5

PEER REVIEW

✓ Fentanyl has minimal effect on blood pressure and is optimal for analgesia and procedural sedation in patients with hypotension.

✓ If you use fentanyl and it leads to chest wall rigidity, you can reverse it with an opioid antagonist and positive-pressure ventilation.

✓ Before using ketamine for procedural sedation, be sure to consider the associated complications and contraindications.

REFERENCES

Roberts JR, Custalow CB, Thomsen TW, eds. Roberts and Hedges' *Clinical Procedures in Emergency Medicine*. 6th ed. Philadelphia, PA: Elsevier; 2014: 597-610.

Tintinalli JE, Stapczynski JS, Ma OJ, et al, eds. *Tintinalli's Emergency Medicine: A Comprehensive Study Guide*. 8th ed. New York, NY: McGraw-Hill; 2012: 253-255, 730-733.

304. The correct answer is A, Binds to an H+ K+ ATPase on the gastric parietal cell, blocking H+ secretion.

Why is this the correct answer?

Omeprazole is a proton pump inhibitor (PPI) used in the treatment of conditions caused by excess stomach acid such as gastroesophageal reflux diseases, ulcers, Zollinger-Ellison syndrome, and systemic mastocytosis. It is also used to prevent heartburn and in combination with antibiotics to treat *Helicobacter pylori* infection. Omeprazole acts on the H+ K+ ATPase of the gastric parietal cell, effectively blocking secretion of hydrogen ions. This leads to an increase in the gastric pH, and thus it can inhibit antifungal agents in particular. In addition, it is metabolized through the cytochrome P450 system, which can affect the metabolism of medications with a narrow therapeutic window such as warfarin. Other common PPIs include pantoprazole, lansoprazole, and esomeprazole. Treatment of peptic ulcer disease usually involves initiation of a trial of a PPI or an H2-receptor antagonist.

Why are the other choices wrong?

Histamine-2 receptor antagonists, not PPIs, competitively inhibit the actions of histamine on gastric parietal cells. Common medications in this class include cimetidine, famotidine, and ranitidine.

Sucralfate, not omeprazole, acts by forming a protective barrier that adheres to the ulcer.

The mechanism of action of misoprostol, a prostaglandin analog, increases mucus and bicarbonate production.

PEER REVIEW

✓ Treatment of peptic ulcer disease usually involves trial of a proton pump inhibitor or H2-receptor antagonist.
✓ The mechanism of action of a proton pump inhibitor is blockade of H+ secretion due to binding to an H+ K+ ATPase on the gastric parietal cell.
✓ Histamine-2 receptor antagonists competitively inhibit the actions of histamine on H2 receptors.

REFERENCES

Marx JA, Hockberger RS, Walls RM, eds. *Rosen's Emergency Medicine: Concepts and Clinical Practice*. 8th ed. St. Louis, MO: Elsevier; 2014: 1170-1185.

Tintinalli JE, Stapczynski JS, Ma OJ, et al, eds. *Tintinalli's Emergency Medicine: A Comprehensive Study Guide*. 8th ed. New York, NY: McGraw-Hill; 2012: 514-517.

305. The correct answer is D, It was one of multiple objects ingested.

Why is this the correct answer?

About 80% of the time, foreign body ingestions occur in children 18 to 48 months old. In adults, most cases occur in patients with esophageal disease, prisoners, and psychiatric patients. Indications for urgent endoscopy for swallowed foreign bodies include airway compromise, evidence of perforation, presence of a foreign body for more than 24 hours, ingestion of multiple foreign bodies, ingestion of sharp or elongated objects, and ingestion of button batteries. Physical examination should begin with assessment of the airway. Although the physical examination is often unremarkable, a foreign body can occasionally be visualized in the oropharynx. Often, xrays are obtained to screen for radiopaque objects.

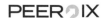

Why are the other choices wrong?

A metallic foreign body does not in itself warrant urgent endoscopy. This does allow the clinician to clearly identify the shape and location of a foreign body and track its movement.

Foreign bodies distal to the pylorus are usually managed expectantly because the vast majority pass through the GI system without complication.

Presence of a foreign body in the esophagus for more than 24 hours, not more than 8 hours, usually warrants endoscopy due to an increased risk of perforation. Watchful waiting for most foreign bodies is safe prior to 24 hours.

PEER POINT

When is urgent endoscopy indicated to remove a foreign body?

If the patient has ingested

- A button battery
- A long or sharp object
- Multiple objects

Or if the patient has

- A foreign body ingested more than 24 hours earlier
- Airway compromise
- Evidence of perforation

PEER REVIEW

- ✓ Who most commonly ingests foreign bodies? Children, patients with esophageal disease, prisoners, and psychiatric patients.
- ✓ If you're treating a patient with a swallowed foreign body, assess the airway — airway compromise or evidence of perforation warrants urgent endoscopy.
- ✓ These objects, if swallowed, warrant urgent endoscopic removal: button batteries, long objects, sharp objects, multiple objects, and objects that have been in there more than 24 hours.

REFERENCES

Marx JA, Hockberger RS, Walls RM, eds. *Rosen's Emergency Medicine: Concepts and Clinical Practice.* 8th ed. St. Louis, MO: Elsevier; 2014: 1170-1171.

Tintinalli JE, Stapczynski JS, Ma OJ, et al, eds. *Tintinalli's Emergency Medicine: A Comprehensive Study Guide.* 8th ed. New York, NY: McGraw-Hill; 2012: 508-514.

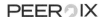
306. The correct answer is B, Malignant hyperthermia.

Why is this the correct answer?

The muscular rigidity present in malignant hyperthermia occurs due to pathology beyond the neuromuscular junction, and therefore a paralytic agent that acts by antagonizing nicotinic receptors on the neuromuscular synapse is ineffective in reversing the rigidity. Malignant hyperthermia is an inherited condition in which there is inappropriate release of calcium from the sarcoplasmic reticulum in skeletal muscle in response to medications such as succinylcholine and certain inhaled anesthetics. Treatment for malignant hyperthermia necessitates immediate administration of dantrolene, an agent that antagonizes the excessive release of calcium from the sarcoplasmic reticulum. Supportive care with cooling and hydration is also critical.

Why are the other choices wrong?

A nondepolarizing agent will resolve the rigidity associated with a dystonic reaction. Dystonic reactions often occur following the administration of a dopamine antagonist and are characterized by sustained involuntary muscular contractions. Anticholinergic agents such as diphenhydramine are effective at reversing dystonic reactions.

A nondepolarizing agent also will resolve the rigidity associated with neuroleptic malignant syndrome and at times is necessary to treat severe cases. Central dopamine depletion is implicated as the cause of neuroleptic malignant syndrome, which manifests classically with lead pipe rigidity, hyperthermia, and depressed level of consciousness.

Finally, a nondepolarizing agent will resolve the rigidity that can occur with serotonin toxicity. Although hyperreflexia and hyperkinesis are more typical of serotonin toxicity, some rigidity can occur, typically more in the lower extremities than the upper extremities.

PEER REVIEW

✓ Malignant hyperthermia manifests with muscle rigidity that won't respond to paralytic agents.
✓ Dantrolene administration is the main treatment for malignant hyperthermia.

REFERENCES

Hoffman RS, Howland MA, Lewin NA, et al. *Goldfrank's Toxicologic Emergencies.* 10th ed. New York, NY: McGraw-Hill; 2010: 386, 945, 949-950, 964-966.

Paden MS, Franjic L, Halcomb SE. Hyperthermia caused by drug interactions and adverse reactions. *Emerg Med Clin North Am.* 2013;31(4):1035-1044.

307. The correct answer is D, Sigmoidoscopy.

Why is this the correct answer?

The radiograph reveals a sigmoid volvulus and is consistent with the patient's signs and symptoms, which include the classic triad of abdominal pain, distention, and constipation. The correct initial management of sigmoid volvulus is usually sigmoidoscopy to attempt endoscopic detorsion. Endoscopic decompression is successful in 50% to 90% of cases. If gangrenous bowel is present or detorsion is not successful, surgery is indicated. The overall mortality rate for sigmoid volvulus approaches 20% and is higher than 50% in patients with gangrenous bowel. Radiographic findings in sigmoid volvulus classically include the "coffee bean sign" or a shape resembling a bent inner tube. The sigmoid is generally displaced from the left iliac fossa and points upward towards the diaphragm. Volvulus can occur at any age but most often affects older adults, mean age 60 to 70 years. Distinguishing sigmoid volvulus from cecal volvulus on abdominal radiographs can be challenging. The "kidney bean sign" is seen in cecal volvulus, and the cecum is generally displaced medially and superiorly, resulting in seeing small bowel in the right iliac fossa rather than large bowel. Cecal volvulus is not amenable to endoscopy due to the proximal nature of the cecum; surgical resection is required.

Why are the other choices wrong?

Initially, if no perforation is present, sigmoidoscopy should be attempted. Surgery is also indicated if the bowel is gangrenous or the reduction attempt is unsuccessful.

Conservative management with a nasogastric tube and bowel rest does not resolve sigmoid volvulus and can allow progression to necrosis.

Reduction barium enema may be attempted for intussusception, but in sigmoid volvulus, especially a case like this one with good radiographic evidence, an enema is not the right choice to resolve the patient's symptoms.

PEER POINT

Common causes of bowel obstruction

Duodenum

- Foreign body (bezoars)
- Stenosis
- Stricture
- Superior mesenteric artery syndrome

Small Bowel

- Adhesions
- Hernia
- Intussusception
- Lymphoma
- Stricture

Colon

- Carcinoma
- Diverticulitis (stricture, abscess)
- Fecal impaction
- Intussusception
- Pseudoobstruction
- Ulcerative colitis
- Volvulus

Adapted from Tintinalli's Emergency Medicine: A Comprehensive Study Guide 8e, © McGraw-Hill Education, Inc.

PEER REVIEW

✓ Volvulus can occur at any age but most often affects adults 60 to 70 years old.

✓ Initial management of sigmoid volvulus is sigmoidoscopy. If that fails or if gangrene is present, surgery is indicated.

✓ What's the mortality rate for sigmoid volvulus? Approaching 20%, and up to 50% if gangrene is present.

REFERENCES

Marx JA, Hockberger RS, Walls RM, eds. *Rosen's Emergency Medicine: Concepts and Clinical Practice.* 8th ed. St. Louis, MO: Elsevier; 2014: 1265-1269.

Tintinalli JE, Stapczynski JS, Ma OJ, et al, eds. *Tintinalli's Emergency Medicine: A Comprehensive Study Guide.* 8th ed. New York, NY: McGraw-Hill; 2012: 538-541.

308. The correct answer is B, Stool antigen.

Why is this the correct answer?

Giardiasis is the most frequently diagnosed parasitic infection in the United States. Stool antigen is the test of choice for confirming the pathogen because it is consistently present in stool, regardless of *Giardia* cyst shedding (which is more variable). The disease is caused by *Giardia lamblia*, which commonly affects hikers and campers who drink contaminated water, adults and children in child care centers, and persons who engage in oral-anal sexual contact. Transmission can be waterborne, foodborne, or fecal-oral. Symptoms vary but generally include diarrhea, excessive flatulence, and abdominal bloating. In severe cases, steatorrhea — excess fat in feces — can develop because saturation of the small bowel with organisms causes malabsorption. A patient experiencing fatty stools might describe them as greasy or sticky, pale, floating, or particularly bad smelling. Metronidazole, tinidazole, and nitazoxanide are among the appropriate therapies for giardiasis.

Why are the other choices wrong?

Serum antibodies against *Giardia lamblia* can be detected; however, this test generally is unhelpful because it cannot differentiate between acute and prior infection.

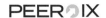

Giardia lamblia is a parasitic infection; therefore, a stool bacterial culture will not be diagnostic.

Giardia cysts are intermittently excreted in stool, leading to false-negative results with microscopy, and organisms quickly break down and become unrecognizable when voided. The sensitivity of the test increases with each repetition; the CDC recommends assessing at least three different samples, but this can be cumbersome and results are dependent on technician expertise. One advantage of stool cultures and ova and parasite studies is their ability to rule out other potential infectious etiologies. If giardiasis is highly suspected, however, stool antigen remains the test of choice.

PEER POINT

The beaver is a common animal reservoir for *Giardia*, hence the common moniker for giardiasis, "beaver fever."

PEER REVIEW

✓ Giardiasis is the most common protozoal infection in the United States.
✓ Suspect giardiasis in any high-risk patient with diarrhea and flatulence. The diagnostic test of choice is stool antigen.
✓ Who is at high risk for giardiasis? Hikers, campers, children who go to daycare, and persons who engage in oral-anal contact.

REFERENCES

Centers for Disease Control and Prevention. Parasites — Giardia. CDC website. Available at: http://www.cdc.gov/parasites/giardia/index.html. Accessed December 2, 2016.

Marx JA, Hockberger RS, Walls RM, eds. *Rosen's Emergency Medicine: Concepts and Clinical Practice*. 8th ed. St. Louis, MO: Elsevier; 2014: 1776.

Tintinalli JE, Stapczynski JS, Ma OJ, et al, eds. *Tintinalli's Emergency Medicine: A Comprehensive Study Guide*. 8th ed. New York, NY: McGraw-Hill; 2012: 1077-1085.

309. The correct answer is D, Urinary retention and fever.

Why is this the correct answer?

Clinical suspicion for an abscess is high in this presentation. The key to correct management lies in determining whether the abscess is perianal or perirectal, which in this case is made challenging by the intensity of the patient's pain. But if the patient also has fever and urinary retention, the deeper and more complicated perirectal abscess is more likely: these findings do not usually accompany perianal abscess. Given the patient's signs, symptoms, and history and the mild leukocytosis, the diagnosis is most likely supralevator abscess, a subtype of perirectal abscess that can lead to urinary retention. The correct disposition for any perirectal abscess is surgical consultation for drainage in the operating room. If the diagnosis were perianal abscesses, drainage could be performed in the emergency department or in an outpatient setting. When draining a perianal abscess, the clinician should make a cruciate incision as close to the anal verge as possible to reduce the risk that a fistulous tract will develop.

Why are the other choices wrong?

Anorectal abscesses, notable for swelling, perianal fluctuant mass, or drainage, may be managed in the emergency department or in an outpatient setting.

Skin changes such as erythema or swelling lateral to the anus are likely signs of developing perianal abscess and not deep infections. Outward signs are not typical in the presentation of supralevator abscess.

Fluctuance above the dentate line anatomically delineates complexity and the need for surgical consultation. An abscess below the dentate line may be treated in the emergency department with incision and drainage.

PEER REVIEW

✓ Uncomplicated perianal abscesses occur below the dentate line and may be drained in the emergent or outpatient setting.
✓ Perirectal abscesses are complicated and require definitive surgical management.

REFERENCES
Breen E, et al. Perianal abscess: Clinical manifestations, diagnosis, treatment. UpToDate Online.
Tintinalli JE, Stapczynski JS, Ma OJ, et al, eds. *Tintinalli's Emergency Medicine. A Comprehensive Study Guide*. 8th ed. New York, NY: McGraw-Hill; 2012: 545-563.

310. The correct answer is D, Tonometry.

Why is this the correct answer?

The acutely painful red eye is a common emergency department presentation. In some cases, patients also report vision changes, as did the patient in this case. The additional clue of a hazy cornea, as shown in the image, makes the complete picture consistent with a diagnosis of acute angle-closure glaucoma. The appearance of the cornea in acute angle-closure glaucoma might also be described as steamy or clouded, with a mid-dilated pupil that is unreactive to light. It can be confirmed with measurement of intraocular pressure (IOP) using a tonometer. Acutely, the IOP can be as high as 60 mm Hg. The normal IOP is between 10 and 20 mm Hg.

Why are the other choices wrong?

Computed tomography should be used to evaluate symptoms concerning for ocular infection, trauma, stroke, or an intracranial lesion causing eye pain or vision changes.

Ocular ultrasound in this patient might reveal narrowing of the anterior chamber. However, tonometry should be performed first to confirm the diagnosis. Ocular ultrasound can also be used in the evaluation of possible retinal detachment, vitreous hemorrhage, and foreign bodies.

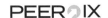

Another cause of eye pain with vision loss is optic neuritis, and ophthalmoscopy is an appropriate test for it because it allows for inspection of the posterior aspect of the eye. In that scenario, ophthalmoscopy might reveal optic disc edema. But in this case, the appearance of the cornea suggests the more likely diagnosis of acute angle-closure glaucoma.

PEER REVIEW

✓ Consider acute angle-closure glaucoma and optic neuritis in patient who present with an acute painful eye and vision loss.

REFERENCES
Roberts JR, Custalow CB, Thomsen TW, eds. Roberts and Hedges' *Clinical Procedures in Emergency Medicine*. 6th ed. Philadelphia, PA: Elsevier; 2014: 1282-1288.
Tintinalli JE, Stapczynski JS, Ma OJ, et al, eds. *Tintinalli's Emergency Medicine: A Comprehensive Study Guide*. 8th ed. New York, NY: McGraw-Hill; 2012: 1572-1575.

311. The correct answer is C, Urinalysis 8 WBC/hpf.

Why is this the correct answer?

The patient in this case has the classic clinical features of mucocutaneous lymph node syndrome, more commonly known as Kawasaki disease (KD). Laboratory test results can be used to determine the presence of KD or incomplete KD. Increased WBCs in the urinalysis likely reflect a sterile pyuria caused by inflammation of the urethra. Since the workup for KD includes evaluating for another etiology, WBCs in the urine without symptoms or bacteria can be seen. Although there is not one definitive test for the diagnosis, Kawasaki disease does have characteristic features that help make the diagnosis, as follows:

• Fever for 5 or more days (and not explained by another disease)

and

• Four of these five other signs and symptoms:
  — Nonpurulent conjunctivitis (often bilateral)
  — Inflammation of the lips or mucous membranes and tongue
  — Nonspecific rash
  — Swelling or redness of hands or feet
  — Cervical adenopathy (often unilateral)

The fever associated with KD is moderate to high and not a low-grade fever. It is important to understand the difference between KD and incomplete KD. Both require prolonged elevated fever, but incomplete KD has only two or three of the additional findings. Kawasaki disease is believed to be due to a diffuse vasculitis, and the most serious sequelae are coronary artery aneurysms. As such, an ECG should be obtained to evaluate for myocarditis and pericarditis. There is an algorithm for laboratory evaluation to aid in the diagnosis of incomplete KD that uses C-reactive protein, erythrocyte sedimentation rate, WBCs with differential, and platelet count. Most patients with KD are admitted for further evaluation and treatment, but this might be dependent on the clinical experience with the disease. There are some sites that see such a high volume of the disease that most of the less acute cases are cared for in an outpatient setting.

Why are the other choices wrong?

An albumin level of 4.2 g/dL is in the normal range. An albumin level below 3 g/dL is one of the criteria that can be used to identify KD.

A platelet count of 80,000 is low. In patients with KD, the platelet count is often elevated after 7 days of the disease, to 450,000 or higher.

The WBC count is often elevated in KD, often 15,000 or higher.

PEER POINT

Classic signs of Kawasaki disease, according to the National Heart, Lung, and Blood Institute

Fever that lasts longer than 5 days even after taking antipyretic medications, as well as:

- Swollen lymph nodes in the neck
- A rash on the midsection of the body and in the genital area
- Red, dry, cracked lips and a red, swollen tongue
- Red, swollen palms of the hands and soles of the feet
- Redness of the eyes

PEER REVIEW

- ✓ Kawasaki disease is a diagnosis of exclusion: there must not be any other diagnosis that can explain the symptoms.
- ✓ In atypical or incomplete Kawasaki disease, there may only be limited clinical findings present with the elevated fever.
- ✓ Get an ECG in the evaluation of Kawasaki disease to look for myocarditis and pericarditis.

REFERENCES
Fleisher GR, Ludwig S, et al, eds. *Textbook of Pediatric Emergency Medicine.* 6th ed. Philadelphia, PA: Lippincott, Williams & Wilkins; 2010: 1157-1164.
Wolfson AB, Hendey GW, Ling LJ, et al, eds. *Harwood-Nuss' Clinical Practice of Emergency Medicine.* 6th ed. Philadelphia, PA: Lippincott, Williams & Wilkins; 2014: 1257-1259.

312. The correct answer is A, Carotid artery.

Why is this the correct answer?

There are two common drainage techniques used in the treatment of peritonsillar abscess: incision and drainage and needle aspiration. During both procedures, the physician must be careful not to cause injury to the carotid artery since it lies posterior and lateral to the tonsil. In needle aspiration in adult patients, the needle should not go more than 1 cm deep to avoid injury to the carotid artery. In children, the distance between the tonsil and the carotid artery is shorter, and involvement by an otolaryngologist might be necessary. If drainage is unsuccessful, a CT scan may be considered. All patients need antibiotic therapy in addition to drainage.

Why are the other choices wrong?

The jugular vein typically lies lateral to the carotid artery and is less likely to be injured.

A peritonsillar abscess should be drained from above and medial to the tonsillar tissue. The actual tonsil should never be incised or aspirated.

The vagus nerve lies in the carotid sheath but is more lateral and seldom injured during drainage of a peritonsillar abscess.

PEER REVIEW

✓ Peritonsillar abscesses can be drained using needle aspiration or incision and drainage.
✓ The carotid artery is the structure most likely to be injured during peritonsillar abscess drainage because it lies posterior and lateral to the tonsil.

REFERENCES

Roberts JR, Custalow CB, Thomsen TW, eds. Roberts and Hedges' *Clinical Procedures in Emergency Medicine*. 6th ed. Philadelphia, PA: Elsevier; 2014: 1303-1308.

Tintinalli JE, Stapczynski JS, Ma OJ, et al, eds. *Tintinalli's Emergency Medicine: A Comprehensive Study Guide*. 8th ed. New York, NY: McGraw-Hill; 2012: 1615.

313. The correct answer is C, Coudé catheter.

Why is this the correct answer?

Urinary retention in a patient this age with this history is most likely caused by a urethral obstruction, which in this case is significant enough to prevent passage of a 14 Fr catheter. The best next step is to try to place a coudé catheter. A coudé catheter has a semirigid curved tip that allows for passage past the urethral obstruction, generally an enlarged prostate gland. A coudé catheter is placed in a similar manner to that used for a Foley catheter, with sterile technique. The shaft of the patient's penis is held vertically and taut with the physician's nondominant hand. After urethral anesthesia with lidocaine is achieved, the tip of the coudé catheter is placed cephalad and advanced until urine is returned. To ensure the tip of the catheter stays cephalad as the catheter is advanced, the physician should reference the position of the balloon port, which faces the same direction. The balloon is then inflated using 5 to 10 mL of sterile water depending on the manufacturer's specifications.

Why are the other choices wrong?

A smaller catheter is not likely to provide enough rigidity to pass by the urethral obstruction. A larger Foley catheter (18 Fr) is sometimes used (because it is stiffer) and can be tried if a coudé catheter is not available.

The use of a catheter over a filiform or hydrophilic guidewire can be considered if the passage of a coudé catheter is not successful. Metal or vascular guidewires should never be used for urethral procedures.

The placement of a suprapubic catheter should be considered if other techniques have failed and urology consultation is not available.

PEER POINT

Steps to troubleshoot urinary retention caused by suspected urethral obstruction

1. Attempt to pass a 14 Fr Foley catheter. *If this fails …*
2. Attempt to pass a coudé catheter. *If that fails …*
3. Consider requesting a urology consultation for possible catheterization using a filiform or flexible cystoscopy. *If consultation is not available or if the clinical situation requires …*
4. Attempt suprapubic tube placement.

PEER REVIEW

✓ When Foley catheterization fails in a patient with urinary retention secondary to urethral obstruction, insertion of a coudé catheter is the preferred next step.
✓ Always use sterile technique when placing a urethral catheter, and fill the balloon with sterile water (not air or saline).
✓ Get a urology consultation if attempts to pass a coudé catheter fail.

REFERENCES

Roberts JR, Custalow CB, Thomsen TW, eds. Roberts and Hedges' *Clinical Procedures in Emergency Medicine*. 6th ed. Philadelphia, PA: Elsevier; 2014: 1132-1139.

Tintinalli JE, Stapczynski JS, Ma OJ, et al, eds. *Tintinalli's Emergency Medicine: A Comprehensive Study Guide*. 8th ed. New York, NY: McGraw-Hill; 2012: 598.

314. The correct answer is C, Apply compression to the anterior nares.

Why is this the correct answer?

Epistaxis is most commonly caused by digital trauma, mucosal irritation from respiratory infection, and chemical irritants such as inhaled medications. Approximately 90% of epistaxis incidents originate from the Kiesselbach plexus, which is located in the anterior nasal septum. So the first step in obtaining hemostasis is to apply direct compression to the cartilaginous portion of the nares by pinching the nose for 10 to 15 minutes. Vasoconstricting agents like cocaine and phenylephrine are also commonly used to stop bleeding. Once there is direct visualization of the bleeding vessel, cauterization should be considered. If bleeding persists, anterior nasal tamponade with ribbons, balloons, or sponges should be performed. If epistaxis continues despite appropriate anterior nasal packing, a posterior nosebleed from the sphenopalatine artery is likely and warrants posterior nasal packing. An otolaryngologist should be consulted if these interventions do not stop the bleeding.

Why are the other choices wrong?

Treatment of elevated blood pressure in a patient with epistaxis is usually not advised in the acute setting because the etiology of the hypertension is most commonly anxiety. Instead, the bleeding should be controlled first and then blood pressure re-evaluated. In severe bleeding, some specialists suggest slow reduction in blood pressure to decrease the hydrostatic pressure and allow for hemostasis.

Blood products and vitamin K should be used as adjuncts to compression and nasal packing, especially if there is concern for coagulopathy. Alone, however, they might not stop the bleeding.

Cauterization is indicated if the bleeding vessel is seen, but it is not the first step in controlling this patient's nosebleed. It can be done chemically with silver nitrate or electrically. An otolaryngologist should perform electrical cauterization due to the risk of perforation.

PEER REVIEW

✓ Anterior epistaxis from the Kiesselbach plexus accounts for most nosebleeds.
✓ If nasal pressure, cautery, and nasal packing don't stop the bleeding, the source is probably posterior.

REFERENCES

Marx JA, Hockberger RS, Walls RM, eds. *Rosen's Emergency Medicine: Concepts and Clinical Practice.* 8th ed. St. Louis, MO: Elsevier; 2014: 938-939.

Roberts JR, Custalow CB, Thomsen TW, eds. Roberts and Hedges' *Clinical Procedures in Emergency Medicine.* 6th ed. Philadelphia, PA: Elsevier; 2014: 1322-1332.

Tintinalli JE, Stapczynski JS, Ma OJ, et al, eds. *Tintinalli's Emergency Medicine: A Comprehensive Study Guide.* 8th ed. New York, NY: McGraw-Hill; 2012: 1688-1692.

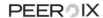

315. The correct answer is C, Methylene blue.

Why is this the correct answer?

This patient is experiencing methemoglobinemia as a result of exposure to chloroquine, the antidote for which is methylene blue. Methylene blue is converted (via a G6PD pathway) to leukomethylene blue, a reducing agent that converts methemoglobin back to hemoglobin. Methemoglobinemia occurs when the ferrous (Fe+2) form of iron in hemoglobin is oxidized to the ferric (Fe+3) form. This form cannot transport oxygen, and there is also a shift in the oxygen dissociation curve that results in an increased affinity of bound oxygen to hemoglobin. Many oxidizing medications have been implicated in methemoglobinemia, including benzocaine, chloroquine, dapsone, phenazopyridine, prilocaine, and primaquine. Symptoms of significant methemoglobinemia reflect those of hypoxia. But the associated cyanosis is due to the color of methemoglobin, not deoxygenated hemoglobin, so oxygen administration does not resolve it. Peripheral pulse oximetry is prone to report a false value of oxygen saturation in patients with significant methemoglobinemia due to inference of light transmission used to detect hemoglobin oxygen saturation. The pulse oximeter reading in patients with methemoglobin concentrations greater than 30% is often near 85%. Diagnosis confirmation is made with co-oximetry to measure the methemoglobin percentage.

Why are the other choices wrong?

Amyl nitrite is an oxidizing agent that induces methemoglobinemia. It can be used by the inhaled route for this purpose as part of the treatment for cyanide poisoning when intravenous access is not available. Methemoglobin has affinity for cyanide, and binding to it forms nontoxic cyanomethemoglobin.

Hydroxocobalamin is a vitamin B12 precursor that is an effective antidote for cyanide poisoning. Hydroxocobalamin binds to cyanide, forming active and nontoxic vitamin B12 (cyanocobalamin). It does not have a role in treating methemoglobinemia.

Sodium thiosulfate is typically administered in conjunction with amyl nitrite or sodium nitrite in the treatment of cyanide poisoning. It helps detoxify cyanide to thiocyanate. It does not have a role in treating methemoglobinemia.

PEER POINT

Methylene blue is the antidote for patients who are blue (cyanotic) from methemoglobinemia.

PEER REVIEW

✓ Methylene blue is the antidotal therapy for significant methemoglobinemia.

✓ Benzocaine, chloroquine, dapsone, phenazopyridine, prilocaine, and primaquine can all cause methemoglobinemia.

✓ Oxygen administration will not improve the cyanosis present in methemoglobinemia.

REFERENCES

Hoffman RS, Howland MA, Lewin NA, et al, eds. *Goldfrank's Toxicologic Emergencies.* 10th ed. New York, NY: McGraw-Hill; 2015: 1615, 1618, 1624.

Tintinalli JE, Stapczynski JS, Ma OJ, et al, eds. *Tintinalli's Emergency Medicine: A Comprehensive Study Guide.* 8th ed. New York, NY: McGraw-Hill; 2012: 1348-1350.

316. The correct answer is C, Administer tetanus toxoid.

Why is this the correct answer?

Current guidelines for a puncture wound like the one described in this case recommend that the patient receive the tetanus toxoid because it has been more than 5 years since her last vaccine. If the patient had a clean minor wound, she would not need a vaccine. Tetanus diphtheria acellular pertussis, Tdap, is the vaccine of choice for persons younger than 65 years who require a Tdap booster given the increased incidence of pertussis. Most reported tetanus cases in the United States have developed following puncture wounds, lacerations, and crush injuries. Therefore, it is important to establish tetanus vaccination status in any patient who presents with a wound.

Why are the other choices wrong?

Tetanus immunoglobulin is not needed in this case and is never given alone. It is typically given in conjunction with the toxoid in a patient who has received fewer than three of the childhood DTaP vaccines or has never received any tetanus vaccines.

Tetanus immunoglobulin is not necessary in this patient given her vaccination history. She needs only the toxoid.

Wound management is completed after the patient has received all of the appropriate treatment. This includes antibiotics for the puncture wound and tetanus toxoid for prophylaxis.

PEER POINT

Tetanus prophylaxis

	Clean Minor Wounds		All Other Wounds	
History of Tetanus Immunization	Administer Tetanus Toxoid?	Administer TIG?	Administer Tetanus Toxoid?	Administer TIG?
Fewer than three doses or unknown	Yes	No	Yes	Yes
Three or more doses				
Last dose within 5 years	No	No	No	No
Last dose within 5 to 10 years	No	No	Yes	No
Last dose more than 10 years ago	Yes	No	Yes	No

Adapted from Tintinalli's 8e, Table 47-2

PEER REVIEW

✓ If you're treating a wound and the patient's tetanus immunization history is incomplete, consider giving both tetanus toxoid and tetanus immunoglobulin.

REFERENCES

Marx JA, Hockberger RS, Walls RM, eds. *Rosen's Emergency Medicine: Concepts and Clinical Practice.* 8th ed. St. Louis, MO: Elsevier; 2014: 765-766.

Tintinalli JE, Stapczynski JS, Ma OJ, et al, eds. *Tintinalli's Emergency Medicine: A Comprehensive Study Guide.* 8th ed. New York, NY: McGraw-Hill; 2012: 321.

317. The correct answer is B, Discharge him with steroid enemas and close follow-up.

Why is this the correct answer?

In this case, the patient's history and clinical presentation are consistent with a diagnosis of acute radiation proctocolitis. Supportive care for mild cases of acute radiation proctocolitis may include steroids (a hydrocortisone enema or foam) to decrease local inflammation and fiber stool softeners to decrease diarrhea. The diagnosis of acute radiation proctocolitis is generally made based on the history, and further evaluation usually is not required. Acute radiation proctocolitis can result in severe disease requiring hospitalization for bowel rest and additional medical therapy; however, treatment is generally supportive. Additionally, bowel perforation can occur and should be considered. Patients with a history of radiation therapy of the pelvis can also present with chronic radiation proctocolitis. This is a diagnosis of exclusion; chronic radiation proctocolitis generally presents within 2 years of therapy but can present at any time. Patients with acute proctitis are at greater risk for chronic disease. As with many cases in emergency medicine, close discussion with the patient's primary care physician or specialist is warranted when making a therapeutic and follow-up plan.

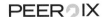

Why are the other choices wrong?

For patients with acute proctocolitis, the diagnosis can generally be made clinically and does not require invasive testing.

The physician should certainly consider complications such as perforation that can be evaluated with CT. But in this case, the patient's history and examination findings do not suggest additional complications; he can be treated with supportive care.

Infectious causes should be considered, and the physician may consider stool testing as appropriate. But again, in this case, the patient does not have symptoms that suggest infection and does not require antibiotics.

PEER REVIEW

✓ Mild cases of acute radiation proctocolitis may be managed with supportive care and outpatient treatment.
✓ If you're treating a patient with acute radiation proctocolitis, consider infection and perforation. Some patients have to be admitted for treatment.
✓ Chronic radiation proctocolitis is a diagnosis of exclusion.

REFERENCES

Marx JA, Hockberger RS, Walls RM, eds. *Rosen's Emergency Medicine: Concepts and Clinical Practice*. 8th ed. St. Louis, MO: Elsevier; 2014: 1273-1274.

Tintinalli JE, Stapczynski JS, Ma OJ, et al, eds. *Tintinalli's Emergency Medicine: A Comprehensive Study Guide*. 8th ed. New York, NY: McGraw-Hill; 2012: 545-563.

318. The correct answer is C, New effusion of unclear etiology.

Why is this the correct answer?

Thoracentesis is not frequently performed in the emergency department. The indications for emergent thoracentesis include possible pleural space infection, relief of dyspnea, and for diagnostic purposes in the evaluation of a new effusion of unclear etiology. The procedure is performed in a manner similar to a paracentesis or central venous access using the Seldinger technique. Lidocaine should be injected to anesthetize the skin and rib space. The finder needle is then walked up and over the rib to minimize the risk of injury to the neurovascular bundle. Air bubbles in the syringe can indicate that the needle has entered the lung parenchyma, so the placement of the needle should be adjusted. A catheter is threaded over the needle, and a stopcock is placed to drain the fluid. Between the eighth and ninth intercostal spaces is the lowest space recommended to minimize complications. Performing a thoracentesis more inferiorly increases the risk of diaphragmatic, splenic, or hepatic injury. The complications associated with thoracentesis include pneumothorax, infection, hemothorax, re-expansion pulmonary edema, air embolism, and intraabdominal hemorrhage.

Why are the other choices wrong?

Bilateral pleural effusions are not an indication for thoracentesis unless they are new effusions causing symptoms or they present with an unclear etiology. Without persistent dyspnea, the thoracentesis does not need to be performed in the emergency department. To minimize complications, thoracentesis can be performed with ultrasound guidance.

Performing a thoracentesis can cause a hemothorax, which is treated with thoracostomy (chest tube placement).

Similarly, pneumothorax can result from the thoracentesis procedure and is treated with placement of a chest tube.

PEER REVIEW

✓ Emergent thoracentesis is rarely indicated in the emergency department, but there are times when it can help in diagnosis and management.
✓ Here are indications for emergent thoracentesis: infection in the pleural space, new effusion with unclear diagnosis, and pronounced dyspnea at rest.
✓ Adding ultrasound guidance to emergent thoracentesis reduces complications.

REFERENCES
Roberts JR, Custalow CB, Thomsen TW, eds. Roberts and Hedges' *Clinical Procedures in Emergency Medicine*. 6th ed. Philadelphia, PA: Elsevier; 2014: 173-188.
Tintinalli JE, Stapczynski JS, Ma OJ, et al, eds. *Tintinalli's Emergency Medicine: A Comprehensive Study Guide*. 8th ed. New York, NY: McGraw-Hill; 2012: 434-436.

319. The correct answer is C, Retained uterine products.

Why is this the correct answer?

Postpartum hemorrhage is defined by more than 500 mL of blood in 24 hours following vaginal delivery. There are two types: early, which occurs 24 hours or less after delivery, and late, which occurs after the first 24 hours and up to 6 weeks after delivery. Retained uterine products of conception are the most common cause of late or delayed postpartum hemorrhage. History of previous curettage, cesarean delivery, multiple births, endometrial infection, and injury are all risk factors that predispose for retention of products. A patient presenting with delayed hemorrhage should undergo a meticulous physical examination; a transvaginal ultrasound examination is the best method to identify retained uterine products of conception.

Why are the other choices wrong?

Coagulation disorders are not often an undiagnosed contributing factor in postpartum hemorrhage. Typically, a type and cross, CBC, and coagulation study are routinely obtained prior to delivery (unless precipitous), and coagulation disorders are diagnosed well prior to delivery. Additionally, primary clotting disorders are fairly uncommon in the general population.

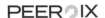

Lacerations to the genital tract (vagina, cervix, uterus) can produce a wide spectrum of bleeding from mild to severe. Lacerations can cause delayed bleeding if they start as a contained hematoma.

Uterine atony occurs when the uterus fails to contract (might feel boggy); this accounts for the majority of early postpartum hemorrhages and should always be treated empirically. Uterine massage stimulates uterine contractions and frequently stops the hemorrhage. If uterine massage is used, care must be taken not to excessively add pressure on the fundus because it can increase the risk of inversion, another cause of early postpartum hemorrhage. Uterine inversion can occur with overly aggressive placental delivery, traction on the cord, or if the placenta fails to separate. This is typically immediately noticed by a mass at the cervical os or introitus and can be repaired by gently pushing the uterus back into position by pressing the tips of fingers together toward the vagina, making contact with the uterine fundus, and using an inward motion along with gentle upward pressure to move the uterus through the cervix.

PEER POINT

The causes of postpartum hemorrhage can be represented by "five T's," listed here by decreasing incidence

- Tone (uterine atony)
- Tissue (retained products of conception)
- Traction (uterine inversion)
- Trauma (lacerations)
- Thrombosis (coagulation disorders)

PEER REVIEW

- ✓ The majority of early postpartum hemorrhage is secondary to uterine atony.
- ✓ Postpartum hemorrhage is defined by hemorrhage of than 500 mL in 24 hours following vaginal delivery and should first be retreated with uterine massage.
- ✓ The majority of delayed postpartum hemorrhage is secondary to retained products of conception.

REFERENCES

Marx JA, Hockberger RS, Walls RM, eds. *Rosen's Emergency Medicine: Concepts and Clinical Practice*. 8th ed. St. Louis, MO: Elsevier; 2014: 2347-2349.

Tintinalli JE, Stapczynski JS, Ma OJ, et al, eds. *Tintinalli's Emergency Medicine: A Comprehensive Study Guide*. 8th ed. New York, NY: McGraw-Hill; 2012: 427-436.

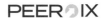

320. The correct answer is C, Obtain a general surgery consultation.

Why is this the correct answer?

Signs and symptoms that suggest a strangulated inguinal hernia include severe pain, skin discoloration, and fever, and this patient has all three. This is a true surgical emergency, and immediate surgical consultation is warranted. Intravenous fluids, analgesia, antibiotics, and preoperative laboratory studies are also indicated. Strangulated hernias typically present with severe, exquisite pain at the hernia site with systemic signs of illness, including a toxic appearance, peritoneal findings, or sepsis. By definition, there is strangulation or vascular compromise of the tissue within the hernia. The history of a recurrent lump in the inguinal area that gets worse with straining or lifting heavy objects is suggestive of an inguinal hernia. Inguinal hernias are the most common type of hernia, occurring in about 75% of all hernias. They tend to be more common in male patients. Hernias can be reducible, incarcerated, or strangulated. A hernia is reducible if it is soft and can be easily pushed back into the peritoneal cavity. An incarcerated hernia is firm, painful, and often nonreducible by direct pressure. Reduction of an incarcerated hernia should be attempted in the emergency department after adequate analgesia is provided; if the attempt is unsuccessful, general surgery should be consulted. After reduction of an incarcerated hernia, observation in the emergency department and serial abdominal examinations are reasonable.

Why are the other choices wrong?

Admitting this patient to the hospital for serial examinations without taking any other action is inappropriate because a strangulated hernia is a surgical emergency.

When a patient exhibits signs of hernia strangulation, which is an acute surgical emergency, reduction should not be attempted in the emergency department. If the bowel is necrotic, there is a risk of sepsis; it should not be pushed back into the peritoneum because there is a likelihood of causing perforation.

Imaging, including plain films of the abdomen, is of limited value in the management of a strangulated hernia. It delays definitive management, which is antibiotics and surgical repair, and it provides no information that will not be revealed during surgery.

PEER POINT

Order of acuity for hernias, from lowest to highest:
Reducible ⇒ Incarcerated ⇒ Strangulated (surgical emergency)

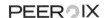

PEER REVIEW

✓ Hernias can be reducible, incarcerated, or strangulated.

✓ A strangulated hernia is an acute surgical emergency — get a surgical consultation and start antibiotics.

✓ Don't try to reduce a strangulated hernia in the emergency department — you might accidentally move necrotic bowel back into the peritoneal cavity.

REFERENCES

Tintinalli JE, Stapczynski JS, Ma OJ, et al, eds. *Tintinalli's Emergency Medicine: A Comprehensive Study Guide*. 8th ed. New York, NY: McGraw-Hill; 2012: 541-545.

Wolfson AB, Hendey GW, Ling LJ, et al, eds. *Harwood-Nuss' Clinical Practice of Emergency Medicine*. 6th ed. Philadelphia, PA: Lippincott, Williams & Wilkins; 2014: 583-587.

321. The correct answer is B, 400 mL.

Why is this the correct answer?

The indications for performing cystourethrography in the setting of pelvic trauma include the inability to void, blood at the meatus, a scrotal hematoma, perineal bruising, an unstable pelvic fracture, and a high-riding prostate. Each of these findings should prompt the physician to perform urethrography before cystography to confirm an intact urethra and assess for possible bladder injuries. An additional indication can be penetrating trauma to the pelvis. Imaging using either xray or fluoroscopy takes place after the infusion of contrast material into the urethra using a Toomey irrigator or a Foley catheter placed at the urethral meatus. After an intact urethra is confirmed, a Foley catheter is then inserted; 400 mL of contrast material is infused by connecting a 60-mL syringe to the catheter with the plunger removed, and then allowing gravity to fill the bladder by lifting the syringe above the plane of the patient. Anteroposterior and lateral images of the pelvis should be evaluated for extravasation in all planes, especially superiorly and posteriorly. If urethral injury is found, placement of a suprapubic catheter might be indicated.

Why are the other choices wrong?

Using only 200 mL of contrast material can lead to a false-negative evaluation of the bladder.

Using 600 mL of contrast material might cause overextension of the bladder.

Similarly, using 800 mL of contrast material is likely to overextend the bladder and can increase the extravasation if there is a bladder injury.

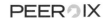

PEER POINT

Intraperitoneal bladder rupture, from LearningRadiology.com

Red arrows indicate extraluminal contrast outside the confines of the normal bladder and spreading into the peritoneal cavity. There is contrast in the left paracolic gutter (yellow arrow), not within the bowel. The intrarenal collecting systems and ureters are visualized because the patient had a contrast-enhanced CT done moments earlier.

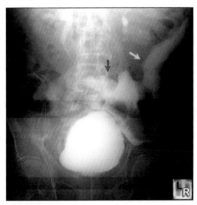

PEER Point 27

PEER REVIEW

✓ Here are the indications for performing cystourethrography in pelvic trauma: penetrating mechanism, inability to void, blood at the meatus, scrotal hematoma, perineal bruising, unstable pelvic fracture, high-riding prostate.

✓ Get a retrograde urethrogram in pelvic trauma before the cystogram because urethral injury prevents safe passage of the Foley catheter and can cause more injury.

✓ Infuse 400 mL of contrast material into the adult bladder to reduce the possibility of a false-negative result for bladder injury.

REFERENCES

American College of Surgeons. *ATLS: Advanced Trauma Life Support, Student Course Manual.* 9th ed. American College of Surgeons; 2012: 132.

Roberts JR, Custalow CB, Thomsen TW, eds. Roberts and Hedges' *Clinical Procedures in Emergency Medicine.* 6th ed. Philadelphia, PA: Elsevier; 2014: 1150-1154.

Tintinalli JE, Stapczynski JS, Ma OJ, et al, eds. *Tintinalli's Emergency Medicine: A Comprehensive Study Guide.* 8th ed. New York, NY: McGraw-Hill; 2012: 1767-1772.

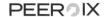

322. The correct answer is C, Schistocytes on peripheral smear.

Why is this the correct answer?

This patient has TTP, or thrombotic thrombocytopenic purpura. The image of the rash shows both purpura (bruises) and petechiae (red and purple dots). It strongly suggests the diagnosis when paired with the clinical findings of anemia, thrombocytopenia, altered mental status, and fever. An additional finding of jaundice might lead the clinician to consider hemolysis. Microangiopathic hemolytic anemia is present in TTP, and a peripheral smear would reveal fragmented RBCs known as schistocytes. Acute renal failure might be present in TTP, along with other renal manifestations such as proteinuria and hematuria, but it is not necessary for confirming the diagnosis. The classic TTP pentad of thrombocytopenic purpura, microangiopathic hemolytic anemia, fluctuating neurologic symptoms, renal disease, and fever is not commonly present. But in the presence of microangiopathic hemolytic anemia with unexplained thrombocytopenia, TTP should always be considered. The cause of TTP is often unknown, but certain medications have been linked to it, including clopidogrel. Hemolytic uremic syndrome (HUS) and TTP are commonly difficult to distinguish from one another, but the absence of diarrhea suggests TTP rather than HUS. Also, HUS is more prevalent in children and has a higher prevalence of renal findings than neurologic findings such as altered mental status, seizures, hemiplegia, paresthesias, vision disturbance, and aphasia; these are more common in TTP. Plasma exchange is the standard of care for patients who present with TTP, and steroid administration frequently accompanies the plasmapheresis. Platelet transfusion is avoided because it can worsen thrombosis in the acute phase. It is done only in instances of life-threatening bleeding, but in conjunction with plasma exchange.

Why are the other choices wrong?

Abnormal coagulation studies are usually seen in patients with disseminated intravascular coagulation. Typically, coagulation study results are normal in TTP because fibrin is not involved in the TTP process.

Colonic inflammation is typically seen in HUS, which is associated with microangiopathic anemia, thrombocytopenia, and renal failure. It usually occurs in children and is caused by a Shiga toxin, *Escherichia coli* 0157:H7, that causes a colonic inflammation and hemorrhagic diarrhea. The patient in this case denies having diarrhea, which means colonic inflammation and a diagnosis of HUS are not likely.

Splenic sequestration occurs when RBCs are trapped in the spleen acutely. It is a finding in other hematologic disorders, including sickle cell disease, but not in TTP.

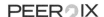

PEER REVIEW

✓ Patients rarely present with all five classic symptoms of TTP, so consider it with any unexplained thrombocytopenia with hemolytic anemia.
✓ Don't do platelet transfusion in TTP. Plasma exchange is the treatment of choice.
✓ Findings that can help you tell HUS and TTP apart: HUS is typically associated with diarrhea and renal manifestations; TTP more commonly has neurologic manifestations.

REFERENCES
Marx JA, Hockberger RS, Walls RM, eds. *Rosen's Emergency Medicine: Concepts and Clinical Practice.* 8th ed. St. Louis, MO: Elsevier; 2014: 1606-1616.
Tintinalli JE, Stapczynski JS, Ma OJ, et al, eds. *Tintinalli's Emergency Medicine: A Comprehensive Study Guide.* 8th ed. New York, NY: McGraw-Hill; 2012: 1513-1518.

323. The correct answer is C, Prepare the patient for escharotomy.

Why is this the correct answer?

In this case, the patient has a circumferential burn causing constriction of the chest wall. It has caused impairment in ventilation necessitating emergent chest decompression with an escharotomy. Failure to recognize the need for decompression can result in respiratory compromise. An escharotomy might also be indicated in circumferential burns of the neck and extremities.

Why are the other choices wrong?

Advising the respiratory therapist to get another ventilator is not the solution. This patient is difficult to ventilate even with a bag-valve-mask device. Getting a new ventilator will not fix the underlying problem.

Needle decompression of the chest is indicated in patients with suspected tension pneumothorax. This patient has a normal xray and equal breath sounds, which excludes the possibility of a tension pneumothorax.

Replacing the endotracheal tube would be indicated if a tube obstruction were suspected or if the tube had become dislodged. This burn patient has gradually become more difficult to ventilate; constriction of the chest due to an eschar must be suspected and appropriate treatment initiated.

PEER POINT

Performing escharotomy, from Life in the Fast Lane

As shown, a full-thickness incision should be made across the top of the chest below the neck, then along both anterior axillary lines down to the bottom of the lung fields at rib 12.

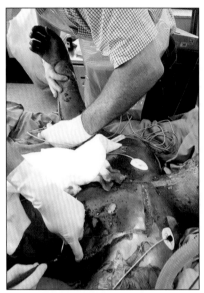

PEER Point 28

PEER REVIEW

✓ Escharotomy is indicated in circumferential burns that result in vascular or ventilatory compromise.

✓ Perform needle decompression in patients with suspected tension pneumothorax.

REFERENCES

Roberts JR, Hedges JR, eds. *Clinical Procedures in Emergency Medicine*. 6th ed. St. Louis, Mo: WB Saunders; 2013: 786-787.

Tintinalli JE, Stapczynski JS, Ma OJ, et al, eds. *Tintinalli's Emergency Medicine: A Comprehensive Study Guide*. 8th ed. New York, NY: McGraw-Hill; 2012: 1404.

324. The correct answer is B, Suspected cellulitis overlying the arthrocentesis site.

Why is this the correct answer?

There is some disagreement among emergency medicine resources related to contraindications for arthrocentesis, with some sources saying that there are no absolute contraindications. But at least one key reference indicates that suspected cellulitis or soft tissue infection overlying the site of arthrocentesis is an absolute contraindication. It is often difficult to distinguish overlying cellulitis or soft tissue infection from a septic joint due to the presence of erythema to the area. Careful

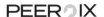

history taking and physical examination must exclude the possibility of overlying infection before arthrocentesis is performed so as not to provide a direct source of bacteria with needle insertion into the joint.

Why are the other choices wrong?

The presence of a heredity clotting factor disorder such as hemophilia is a relative contraindication to arthrocentesis to avoid a complication of hemarthrosis. However, appropriate clotting factors can be given before the procedure to minimize this risk. Atraumatic or traumatic hemarthrosis is a common presentation for patients with hemophilia, and arthrocentesis after clotting factor administration can be therapeutic.

Arthrocentesis is a risk in a patient with bacteremia, but if this diagnosis is occult and the source of the infection is the joint, then obtaining joint fluid is indicated for diagnostic and therapeutic reasons.

The suspicion or presence of fracture in this or other patients is not an absolute contraindication to arthrocentesis. In fact, the discovery of lipohemarthrosis (fat in the bloody joint fluid) confirms an occult fracture.

PEER REVIEW

✓ There is disagreement as to whether aspirating a joint through overlying soft tissue infection is an absolute contraindication; however, it should be avoided.
✓ If you're treating a patient who has an underlying hereditary clotting factor disorder, you can administer clotting factors before performing arthrocentesis.

REFERENCES
Roberts JR, Hedges JR, eds. *Clinical Procedures in Emergency Medicine*. 6th ed. St. Louis, MO: WB Saunders; 2013: 1075-1086.
Sherman S. *Simon's Emergency Orthopedics*. 7th ed. New York, NY: McGraw-Hill; 2015: 45–47.

325. The correct answer is C, Poor feeding.

Why is this the correct answer?

With advances in imaging technology, congenital heart disease (CHD) can be diagnosed in utero or in the newborn nursery. But some disorders are not diagnosed until several weeks of life, when the ductus arteriosus closes, and even then the signs are subtle and easily missed. The most common indicators of CHD are poor feeding with or without sweating, irritability, unexplained hypertension, hepatomegaly, and a pathologic murmur. On presentation to the emergency department, neonates with undiagnosed CHD often have mottled skin, cyanosis, and shock. Shock or cyanosis occurring in the first 2 weeks of life is very alarming, and an undiagnosed CHD should be strongly considered given that the ductus arteriosus is closing. Treatment with prostaglandins can be lifesaving. Other more common diseases such as septic shock must be also be considered and treated as required in the critically ill neonate.

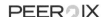

Why are the other choices wrong?

Peripheral edema as a manifestation of heart failure is rare in infants.

Murmurs are common in pediatric patients, present in more than 50% of newborns. Most of these patients have structurally normal hearts and have an "innocent" murmur, for example, grade 1-2 soft with normal split and normal peripheral pulses. Two of the most common murmurs are:

- Peripheral pulmonary stenosis, a midsystolic high-pitched ejection murmur heard best at the left upper sternal border of the pulmonary area, and
- The Still murmur, a low-pitched systolic ejection murmur heard best at the left lower sternal border and often described as musical

Stridor is audible breath sounds that typically originate from the extrathoracic airways. The presence of stridor indicates turbulent flow from a partial obstruction of the upper airways, glottis, or trachea. Congenital stridor presents at birth or within the first few weeks of life and is rarely life threatening. The most common causes include laryngomalacia, subglottic stenosis, bronchogenic cysts, tracheomalacia, gastroesophageal reflux, and foreign body.

PEER REVIEW

- ✓ Here are the subtle indicators of congenital heart disease in neonates: poor feeding with or without sweating, unexplained hypertension, hepatomegaly, and a new pathologic murmur.
- ✓ Signs of heart failure such as edema are uncommon in neonates.
- ✓ Signs of shock in the first weeks of life suggest a congenital heart disease, and treatment with prostaglandins is lifesaving.

REFERENCES

Adams JG, Barton ED, Collings J, et al, eds. *Emergency Medicine: Clinical Essentials*. 2nd ed. Philadelphia, PA: Saunders; 2013: 117-128, 159-166.

Marx JA, Hockberger RS, Walls RM, eds. *Rosen's Emergency Medicine: Concepts and Clinical Practice*. 8th ed. St. Louis, MO: Elsevier; 2014: 151-155, 2139-2167.

326. The correct answer is B, Phrenic nerve.

Why is this the correct answer?

Emergency department thoracotomy is indicated in patients presenting with penetrating chest trauma who have traumatic arrest in the emergency department or shortly before arrival. The procedure involves performing a large chest wall incision, followed by use of the rib spreaders to expose the heart. An incision to the pericardium should be made anterior, or closer to the sternum, to the phrenic nerve, which is a prominent cordlike structure located adherent to the pericardium. Damage to the phrenic nerve can result in unilateral diaphragmatic weakness, which can significantly impair respiratory function. After exposing the heart, the physician must examine it for wounds, which may be repaired with sutures, staples, or the placement of a Foley catheter. It is important to avoid the coronary arteries when placing sutures or staples. Internal cardiac massage may also be performed at this point.

Why are the other choices wrong?

The internal mammary arteries (also referred to as the internal thoracic arteries) are located along the internal aspect of the anteromedial ribcage. When bilateral thoracotomy (clam shell) is performed, these arteries often need to be ligated.

The sympathetic chain ganglia are located along the lateral aspects of the vertebral bodies and are rarely injured during emergency department thoracotomy.

The vagus nerve (also referred to as cranial nerve X) descends from the medulla oblongata along the esophagus to the stomach with multiple branches providing innervation to the heart, lung, and esophagus. The vagus nerve provides the predominant parasympathetic innervation to the body. The vagus nerve courses behind the hilum of the right lung, so it is unlikely to be injured during an emergency department thoracotomy.

PEER POINT

Phrenic nerve in the pericardial sac

This *Gray's Anatomy* illustration is helpful because it is "looking" from the side of the chest you would be if you were performing a thoracotomy. The phrenic nerve is shown in yellow running alongside the pericardiacophrenic artery, in red, on the pericardium.

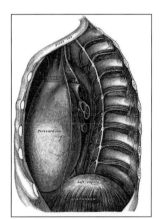

PEER Point 29

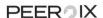
PEER REVIEW

- ✓ Indication for performing thoracotomy in the emergency department: patient presenting with penetrating chest trauma who has a traumatic arrest in the emergency department or shortly before arriving.
- ✓ A left lateral incision is preferred for emergency department thoracotomy because it allows the best exposure of the heart, aorta, and left pulmonary hilum.
- ✓ Avoid the phrenic nerve by cutting more anterior when incising the pericardium.

REFERENCES

Marx JA, Hockberger RS, Walls RM, eds. *Rosen's Emergency Medicine: Concepts and Clinical Practice*. 8th ed. St. Louis, MO: Elsevier; 2014: 294-295.

Roberts JR, Hedges JR, eds. *Clinical Procedures in Emergency Medicine*. 6th ed. St. Louis, Mo: WB Saunders; 2013: 325-339.

Tintinalli JE, Stapczynski JS, Ma OJ, et al, eds. *Tintinalli's Emergency Medicine: A Comprehensive Study Guide*. 8th ed. New York, NY: McGraw-Hill; 2012: 1755-1756.

327. The correct answer is D, WASH regimen.

Why is this the correct answer?

Anal fissures are the most common cause of severely painful acute rectal pain. They are caused by a tear in the anoderm, usually in patients who are constipated, with passage of hard feces. Patients often report seeing bright red blood on the toilet paper or in the stool. Treatment for anal fissures includes the WASH regimen — warm water (sitz bath), analgesic agents, stool softeners, and high-fiber diet. Most fissures are located at the posterior midline where muscle fibers that surround the anus are the weakest. Fissures that are located outside the midline are associated with systemic disease such as HIV, tuberculosis, or Crohn disease. Fissures not treated in a timely manner can become chronic, with a triad of deep ulceration, sentinel pile (edematous and hypertrophic skin), and enlarged anal papillae.

Why are the other choices wrong?

A botulinum toxin injection can, by reducing sphincter pressure, provide some relief from the local spasm and severe pain caused by a fissure. But it is not the initial treatment recommended in the emergency department for an acute rectal fissure. Complications include incontinence of stool that is generally not permanent.

An elliptical incision is used to open and excise the clot from a thrombosed hemorrhoid in the emergency department, but it is not approach to emergency department treatment of anal fissure. If the symptoms of an anal fissure do not improve over 1 to 2 months, a specialist might use an elliptical incision in the surgical excision of the fissure. Sphincterotomy is the most successful treatment for chronic fissures, although not the initial treatment.

Topical nitroglycerin can also be used to decrease the severe pain caused by the anal spasm associated with a fissure. Headaches and flushing are among the side effects of this treatment, so it is not the first-line therapy.

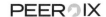

PEER REVIEW

✓ Anal fissures are the most common cause of acute-onset severe rectal pain and can involve rectal bleeding.

✓ Anal fissures are most often found along the posterior midline.

✓ Anal fissures located laterally are associated with systemic disease.

REFERENCES

Marx JA, Hockberger RS, Walls RM, eds. *Rosen's Emergency Medicine: Concepts and Clinical Practice*. 8th ed. St. Louis, MO: Elsevier; 2014: 1276-1281.

Reichman EF. *Emergency Medicine Procedures*. 2nd ed. New York, NY: McGraw-Hill; 2013: 439-443.

Tintinalli JE, Stapczynski JS, Ma OJ, et al, eds. *Tintinalli's Emergency Medicine: A Comprehensive Study Guide*. 8th ed. New York, NY: McGraw-Hill; 2012: 549-550.

328. The correct answer is A, Administer diphenhydramine.

Why is this the correct answer?

The presentation described in this case is an acute dystonic reaction secondary to the administration of the dopamine antagonist metoclopramide, and the patient should receive an antimuscarinic medication such as diphenhydramine. Complications from a single dose of a dopamine antagonist include akathisia (inability to sit still, restlessness), dystonia, and neuroleptic malignant syndrome. Acute dystonic reactions manifest with sustained, involuntary muscular contractions that are often localized to the head and neck. The contractions are often but not always static. Acute dystonic reactions typically occur soon after the offending drug is administered and respond rapidly to appropriate treatment. Characteristic physical findings, temporal association following administration of a dopamine antagonist, and rapid resolution of symptoms with treatment are helpful in distinguishing dystonic reactions from other more serious disorders.

Why are the other choices wrong?

Administering tetanus immunoglobulin would be correct if the patient had tetanus. The involuntary muscular contractions that occur with tetanus often involve the face but are typically recurrent, episodic, and occur in response to trivial stimuli. In contrast, this patient has classic symptoms of an acute dystonic reaction: sustained, involuntary muscular contractions localized to the head and neck soon after being administered a dopamine antagonist (metoclopramide). These findings help distinguish an acute dystonic reaction from other more serious disorders.

Radiographic imaging is not necessary. The patient is experiencing an acute dystonic reaction and should be administered an antimuscarinic agent to reverse it.

An acute dystonic reaction often involves the head and neck and can manifest with signs that provoke concern for the airway. However, response to appropriate treatment with an antimuscarinic agent is rapid, and it should be administered before invasive interventions are considered.

PEER REVIEW

✓ What does an acute dystonic reaction look like? Sustained, involuntary muscular contractions that are often localized to the head and neck.

✓ Antimuscarinic agents such as diphenhydramine and benztropine are first-line treatments for acute dystonic reactions.

REFERENCES

Hoffman RS, Howland MA, Lewin NA, et al. *Goldfrank's Toxicologic Emergencies.* 10th ed. New York, NY: McGraw-Hill; 2010: 964-965.

Wolfson AB, Hendey GW, Ling LJ, et al, eds. *Harwood-Nuss' Clinical Practice of Emergency Medicine.* 6th ed. Philadelphia, PA: Lippincott, Williams & Wilkins; 2014: 1451-1453.

329. The correct answer is C, Hydrofluoric acid.

Why is this the correct answer?

Most acids, when they make contact with skin, cause a coagulative necrosis that limits further penetration. Hydrofluoric acid is a major exception: due to the strong electronegativity of the fluoride ion and corresponding high affinity to its hydrogen ion, deep penetration into tissues can occur. Systemic toxicity results from fluoride binding to calcium and magnesium and can result in life-threatening hypocalcemia and hypomagnesemia. Delayed-onset hyperkalemia from its effect on sodium-potassium ATPase is also possible. Aggressive decontamination of the skin followed by topical application of calcium and/or magnesium preparations can help limit absorption. Initial treatment of systemic toxicity is focused on preventing and treating the hypocalcemia and hypomagnesemia.

Why are the other choices wrong?

Acetic acid, found in some hair-wave neutralizers, is not expected to cause systemic toxicity with topical dermal exposures. Most acids, like acetic acid, can cause coagulative necrosis on skin contact, which limits further acid penetration.

Hydrochloric acid, like most acids, can cause severe dermal burns. Most preparations in products used in homes are so dilute, though, that severe burns are unusual. Hydrochloric acid is not expected to cause systemic toxicity with topical dermal exposures.

Sulfuric acid, the acid often found in car batteries and drain cleaners, is not expected to cause systemic toxicity with dermal exposures.

PEER REVIEW

✓ The primary toxicity seen with topical dermal exposure to most acids is burns, not systemic toxicity.

✓ Hydrofluoric acid, unlike most other acids, can cause systemic toxicity (initially hypocalcemia and hypomagnesemia) after topical dermal exposures.

REFERENCES

Hoffman RS, Howland MA, Lewin NA, et al. *Goldfrank's Toxicologic Emergencies.* 10th ed. New York, NY: McGraw-Hill; 2010: 1315, 1324-1325.

Tintinalli JE, Stapczynski JS, Ma OJ, et al, eds. *Tintinalli's Emergency Medicine: A Comprehensive Study Guide.* 8th ed. New York, NY: McGraw-Hill; 2012: 1405-1408.

330. The correct answer is C, Discharge to home with outpatient follow-up.

Why is this the correct answer?

Household bleach is the most common household alkali. It has a sodium hypochlorite solution of 3% to 6% and a pH of 11; it is fairly dilute and only minimally corrosive to the esophagus. It rarely causes significant injury. Appropriate management of asymptomatic accidental ingestion of a small amount of a low concentration acid or alkali substance includes discharge with outpatient follow-up. Caustic alkali injuries can cause liquefaction necrosis, a process in which the hydroxide ion penetrates deep tissues and causes injury secondary to protein denaturation and lipid saponification.

Why are the other choices wrong?

Certain agents are contraindicated in caustic ingestions: these include the use of a neutralizing agent, which releases heat that can cause additional tissue injury.

Ingestion of industrial-strength bleach or powdered hypochlorite solution is much more likely to result in esophageal injury. Endoscopic evaluation is indicated in patients with these ingestions.

Gastric decontamination with activated charcoal is relatively contraindicated in caustic ingestions because charcoal does not bind well to most caustics and can impair visualization if endoscopy is warranted.

PEER REVIEW

- ✓ Caustic alkali injuries can lead to liquefaction necrosis.
- ✓ Household bleach is the most common household alkali and rarely causes significant injury if ingested in small amounts.
- ✓ Emetics and neutralizing agents are contraindicated in caustic ingestions.

REFERENCES

Hoffman RS, Howland MA, Lewin NA, et al. *Goldfrank's Toxicologic Emergencies*. 10th ed. New York, NY: McGraw-Hill; 2010:1315-1323.

Marx JA, Hockberger RS, Walls RM, eds. *Rosen's Emergency Medicine: Concepts and Clinical Practice*. 8th ed. St. Louis, MO: Elsevier; 2014: 1173-1175.

Tintinalli JE, Stapczynski JS, Ma OJ, et al, eds. *Tintinalli's Emergency Medicine: A Comprehensive Study Guide*. 8th ed. New York, NY: McGraw-Hill; 2012: 1314-1318.

331. The correct answer is A, Bupropion.

Why is this the correct answer?

Flumazenil remains a controversial antidote, but it can be used safely both diagnostically and therapeutically in a very select group of patients. Contraindications to the use of flumazenil include the coingestion of a proconvulsant drug (such as bupropion) and a history of convulsions. Bupropion, both therapeutically and in overdose, can cause convulsions. In the setting of an ingestion of both a benzodiazepine and a proconvulsant drug, flumazenil can reverse the protective effect of the benzodiazepine on seizure prevention and is thus contraindicated. In the setting of an overdose of unknown medications, the presence of findings inconsistent with a pure benzodiazepine overdose or suggestive of a proconvulsant coingestant (such as convulsions, mydriasis, tachycardia, and QRS width prolongation) contraindicates flumazenil administration.

Why are the other choices wrong?

Carisoprodol does not cause convulsions in overdose, and therefore the coingestion of it with a benzodiazepine is not a contraindication for flumazenil administration. Carisoprodol can be associated with myoclonic jerking in overdose that can mimic convulsions, however. There is some evidence that its sedative effects can be reversed with flumazenil.

Gabapentin does not cause convulsions in overdose, so coingestion of it with a benzodiazepine is not a contraindication for flumazenil administration.

Phenobarbital does not cause convulsions in overdose, and, as with the other two agents, coingestion of it with a benzodiazepine is not a contraindication for flumazenil administration. Some patients take phenobarbital for a seizure disorder; the seizure disorder itself is a contraindication to the use of flumazenil, but the medication as a coingestant is not a contraindication.

PEER REVIEW

✓ Here are the contraindications for using flumazenil to reverse benzodiazepine poisoning: the presence of a proconvulsant coingestant and a history of convulsions.

REFERENCES

Hoffman RS, Howland MA, Lewin NA, et al. *Goldfrank's Toxicologic Emergencies*. 10th ed. New York, NY: McGraw-Hill; 2010: 1014-1016.

Tintinalli JE, Stapczynski JS, Ma OJ, et al, eds. *Tintinalli's Emergency Medicine: A Comprehensive Study Guide*. 8th ed. New York, NY: McGraw-Hill; 2012: 1220, 1239, 1240.

332. The correct answer is B, Hypokalemia.

Why is this the correct answer?

This patient's ECG reveals a prolonged QT interval (QTc 541) and flattened T waves inferiorly with U waves seen immediately after the T wave; the amplitude of the U wave greater than the T wave is noted most in the lateral V leads. These findings are consistent with hypokalemia in a patient with hypokalemic periodic paralysis. Hypokalemic periodic paralysis can be an inherited disorder (familial hypokalemic periodic paralysis), or it can occur in the setting of thyrotoxicosis (thyrotoxic periodic paralysis). Both occur from intracellular shifting of potassium. Initial treatment of both types includes oral potassium replacement and close monitoring and rechecking of potassium concentrations to avoid rebound hypokalemia. Thyrotoxic periodic paralysis also requires treatment of the thyrotoxicosis.

Why are the other choices wrong?

Hypernatremia can be associated with muscle weakness, but it would be very unusual for it to be responsible for recurrent episodes of severe weakness. Hypernatremia also does not have characteristic ECG findings. The ECG in this case demonstrates QT interval prolongation, flattened T waves, and U waves, all changes that are characteristic of hypokalemia.

Rhabdomyolysis and various myopathies can present with muscle weakness, and an elevated creatine kinase level can be diagnostic. Due to muscle damage, there is often associated pain. Release of skeletal muscle contents into the blood can lead to acute kidney injury and hyperkalemia. In such a situation, ECG signs of hyperkalemia — peaked T waves and QRS interval prolongation — might manifest, but not the QT interval prolongation, flattened T waves, and U waves typical of hypokalemia.

Both thyrotoxic periodic paralysis and familial hypokalemic periodic paralysis can present with recurrent episodes of severe hypokalemia and associated paralysis. Checking for hyperthyroidism is appropriate in patients who present with such a clinical picture, particularly since other findings of thyrotoxicosis are not always present. In thyrotoxic periodic paralysis, thyroid stimulating hormone is usually so low as to be not measurable (not elevated). Thyrotoxic periodic paralysis occurs most frequently in Asians and typically occurs in the early morning hours after strenuous exercise.

PEER REVIEW

✓ Classic ECG findings in hypokalemia: prolonged QT interval, flattened T waves, and U waves.

✓ Hypokalemic periodic paralysis can be an inherited disorder (familial) or occur in the setting of thyrotoxicosis (thyrotoxic).

✓ If you're treating a patient who presents with hypokalemic periodic paralysis, check for hyperthyroidism.

REFERENCES

Greenberg RD, Daniel KJ. Eye Emergencies. In: Stone C, Humphries RL, eds. *CURRENT Diagnosis & Treatment Emergency Medicine*. 7th ed. New York, NY: McGraw-Hill; 2011. http://accessmedicine.mhmedical.com/content. aspx?bookid=385&sectionid=40357247. Accessed May 18, 2017.

Tintinalli JE, Stapczynski JS, Ma OJ, et al, eds. *Tintinalli's Emergency Medicine: A Comprehensive Study Guide*. 8th ed. New York, NY: McGraw-Hill; 2012: 100, 855.

333. The correct answer is D, Hyponatremia.

Why is this the correct answer?

Hyponatremia is common in hyperglycemic states, including diabetic ketoacidosis (DKA). Hyperglycemia osmotically draws water into the vascular space with a resulting lower serum sodium. Although some refer to this as artificial or pseudohyponatremia, this is not technically correct (the serum sodium is truly low). However, there are correction factors to predict what the serum sodium would be if the glucose were not elevated. Although there has been some suggestion that a larger degree of correction is more accurate, the traditional correction is that, for every 100 mg/dL increase in glucose, there is a corresponding 1.6 mEq/L decrease in sodium. The presence of initial eunatremia or hypernatremia is less common in DKA and signifies an even larger than typical free water deficit. In this situation (in the absence of severe hypovolemia or shock in which normal saline is appropriate), guidelines recommend initiating treatment with 0.45% normal saline.

Why are the other choices wrong?

Hyperglycemic-induced osmotic diuresis typically results in hypocalcemia, not hypercalcemia, in DKA.

Hypophosphatemia (not hyperphosphatemia) is typically present in patients with DKA. Routine repletion of phosphate is not recommended, however. No benefit of routine administration has been demonstrated, and replacement could lead to worsened hypocalcemia.

Presenting hypokalemia is not common in patients with DKA and when present represents a severe total body deficit. In such a situation, potassium administration should begin prior to insulin administration. Insulin administration shifts the potassium intracellularly and can lead to life-threatening hypokalemia. Despite total body depletion, due to the acidosis of DKA causing an extracellular shift of potassium, patients generally present with a serum potassium in the normal or slightly elevated range.

PEER REVIEW

- ✓ Hyponatremia is common in hyperglycemic states, including diabetic ketoacidosis.
- ✓ Hyperglycemia osmotically draws water into the vascular space with a resulting lower serum sodium.
- ✓ If you're treating a patient who has diabetic ketoacidosis presenting with hypokalemia — and this isn't at all common — administer potassium before insulin.

REFERENCES

Tintinalli JE, Stapczynski JS, Ma OJ, et al, eds. *Tintinalli's Emergency Medicine: A Comprehensive Study Guide*. 8th ed. New York, NY: McGraw-Hill; 2012: 1459-1462.

Van Ness-Otunnu R, Hack JB. Hyperglycemic crisis. *J Emerg Med*. 2013;45(5):797-805.

334. The correct answer is C, Epstein-Barr virus.

Why is this the correct answer?

Infectious mononucleosis is a viral syndrome caused by the Epstein-Barr virus. The disease, which commonly affects young, otherwise healthy people, manifests as generalized fatigue, sore throat, and lymphadenopathy. Splenomegaly is present in up to 50% of cases. Blood analysis demonstrates a reactive lymphocytosis and transaminitis. Treatment includes symptom relief; patients should be instructed to abstain from activities like contact sports to avoid the complication of splenic rupture. Pharyngitis associated with mononucleosis occasionally can be misdiagnosed as streptococcal pharyngitis. Antibiotics often trigger a rash in patients with mononucleosis, but the mechanism of this reaction is not well understood. Ampicillin and amoxicillin are the most common culprits; however, rashes also can also be provoked by azithromycin, levofloxacin, and cephalexin.

Why are the other choices wrong?

Coxsackievirus can present with a wide spectrum of clinical diseases, ranging from typical upper respiratory infections to pericarditis or even aseptic meningitis. Rashes related to the coxsackievirus typically manifest as red spots on the palms, soles, and oral mucosa (hand-foot-and-mouth disease) and are unrelated to antibiotic use.

Rashes that develop after antibiotic use in patients with infectious mononucleosis commonly are mistaken for drug-related or allergic reactions, given the timing of onset. However, these rashes are not considered true allergies because patients subsequently can tolerate the same antibiotic without manifesting symptoms.

Pharyngitis associated with mononucleosis commonly is misinterpreted as streptococcal pharyngitis, given its symptom of exudative tonsillitis with cervical lymphadenopathy. Splenomegaly, however, is not seen with streptococcal pharyngitis.

PEER REVIEW

✓ Infectious mononucleosis is caused by the Epstein-Barr virus and commonly affects young, otherwise healthy patients.

✓ Symptoms of infectious mononucleosis: pharyngitis with exudates, posterior cervical lymphadenopathy, and splenomegaly (50%).

✓ When given antibiotics, patients with infectious mononucleosis commonly develop a morbilliform rash.

REFERENCES

Marx JA, Hockberger RS, Walls RM, eds. *Rosen's Emergency Medicine: Concepts and Clinical Practice*. 8th ed. St. Louis, MO: Elsevier; 2014: 1731-1732.

Tintinalli JE, Stapczynski JS, Ma OJ, et al, eds. *Tintinalli's Emergency Medicine: A Comprehensive Study Guide*. 8th ed. New York, NY: McGraw-Hill; 2012: 1044.

335. The correct answer is C, Rectal prolapse.

Why is this the correct answer?

The patient in this question has rectal procidentia or prolapse. Clues from the history include fecal incontinence, constipation, abdominal discomfort, and a prolapsed anal mass. Diagnosis is clinical; visual clues include concentric rings of the rectum protruding through the anus. Concomitant anal sphincter or pelvic floor disorders are not uncommon. Definitive management of rectal prolapse is surgery. Incarceration of the prolapsed tissue is a surgical emergency. Medical management includes adequate dietary fiber and fluid intake.

Why are the other choices wrong?

Although the patient's description of feeling a mass is concerning, physical examination findings show healthy prolapsed tissue.

A prolapsed internal hemorrhoid is generally smaller than the rectum and does not have concentric rings.

A prolapsed uterus is generally seen protruding through the vaginal opening.

PEER REVIEW

✓ What are the clues to rectal prolapse? Fecal incontinence, constipation, abdominal discomfort, and a prolapsed anal mass.

✓ Definitive management of rectal prolapse is surgery, although generally not emergent.

✓ A prolapsed rectum can become incarcerated and strangulated, which is a surgical emergency.

REFERENCES

Marx JA, Hockberger RS, Walls RM, eds. *Rosen's Emergency Medicine: Concepts and Clinical Practice*. 8th ed. St. Louis, MO: Elsevier; 2014: 261-265.

Tou S, Brown SR, Malik AI, Nelson RL. Surgery for complete rectal prolapse in adults. *Cochrane Database Syst Rev*. 2008; :CD001758.

UpToDate. Overview of rectal procidentia (rectal prolapse). Varma et al. 2016.

336. The correct answer is D, Rodent control.

Why is this the correct answer?

The Sin Nombre virus, a strain of Hantavirus that causes hantavirus pulmonary syndrome (HPS), was first discovered in the southwestern United States in 1993. The most common host of this rodent-borne RNA virus is the deer mouse, but other kinds of mice and rats are known to spread disease. Humans typically contract the pathogen by breathing aerosolized particles of rodent urine and feces, often while cleaning. Patients experience nonspecific viral symptoms for 3 to 5 days, followed by pulmonary edema and severe myocardial depression. Treatment is supportive care, usually in an ICU setting. Although the incidence is low, mortality rates are significant (30% to 50%). Rodent control is the primary strategy for disease prevention. In places where carrier rodents are known to live, traps should be placed, holes or gaps should be sealed, and precautions should be taken when cleaning infested areas.

Why are the other choices wrong?

There currently is no vaccination to prevent the Sin Nombre virus.

Ribavirin has been shown to decrease mortality rates in patients with Hantavirus infections that cause hemorrhagic fever with renal syndrome; however, the drug has no proven benefit in the treatment of HPS. No formal recommendation currently exists regarding the use of ribavirin or other antiviral medications for prophylaxis or early cases of HPS; further investigation is required to determine the potential role of these agents.

Although respiratory protection potentially could prevent exposure to airborne urine and feces particles, this approach to prophylaxis is impractical in daily life. Primary rodent control is preferred.

PEER POINT

From the CDC, incidence of hantavirus pulmonary syndrome in the United States

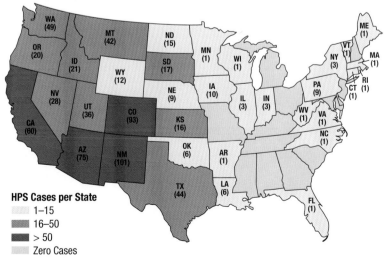

HPS Cases per State
- 1–15
- 16–50
- > 50
- Zero Cases

PEER Point 30

PEER REVIEW

✓ How is Hantavirus spread? Aerosolized particles of rodent urine and feces.

✓ Hantavirus pulmonary syndrome starts out as a mild viral infection but is followed by severe pulmonary edema and myocardial depression.

✓ Rodent control is the best way to prevent the spread of Hantavirus diseases.

REFERENCES

Centers for Disease Control and Prevention. *Hantavirus.* CDC website. Available at: http://www.cdc.gov/hantavirus/. Accessed December 2, 2016.

Marx JA, Hockberger RS, Walls RM, eds. *Rosen's Emergency Medicine: Concepts and Clinical Practice.* 8th ed. St. Louis, MO: Elsevier; 2014: 1720.

337. The correct answer is A, Attempt to remove the object with a moistened cotton applicator.

Why is this the correct answer?

Corneal foreign bodies are most commonly pieces of wood, plastic, or metal. They are typically superficial and tend to be benign most of the time. After the cornea has been appropriately anesthetized, the slit lamp should be used to assess the depth and size of the foreign body. Irrigation of the eye might remove very superficial foreign bodies. If this is not successful, a moistened cotton applicator can be used to dislodge the object. An 18-gauge needle with the bevel up or a burr drill may also be used if other methods are not successful. If a rust ring remains after the foreign body has been removed, a rotating burr can be used to remove superficial rust. Care must be taken to avoid penetrating the cornea. The burr drill should not be used if the rust ring is in the visual axis because this can lead to a vision-impairing scar.

Why are the other choices wrong?

A topical antibiotic such as erythromycin should be prescribed when the patient is discharged; this treatment is similar to that for a corneal abrasion. But the foreign material should be removed first.

It is inappropriate to discharge the patient with ophthalmology follow-up without first attempting to remove the foreign object or at least discussing the plan of care with an ophthalmologist. If the attempt to remove the foreign object is unsuccessful, follow-up with an ophthalmologist within 24 hours is warranted. Patching the eyelid closed has been used in the treatment of corneal abrasions; however, recent evidence suggests no benefit in healing times and a possible increase in infection rates. Thus it is no longer routinely recommended.

Although it is necessary to remove the rust ring, the first step should be to remove the foreign object. Superficial rust can then be removed with the burr drill, or the ophthalmologist can do it at the follow-up appointment. Rust often reaccumulates, so it is not necessary to completely remove the rust if the patient has a follow-up appointment the next day.

PEER POINT

How to remove a corneal foreign body

1. Anesthetize the eye
2. Perform a thorough slit lamp examination to assess the size and depth of the object
3. Remove the object with the use of a slit lamp
4. Attempt to remove the rust ring with a burr drill if the rust is superficial and not in the visual axis
5. Apply topical antibiotic and cycloplegic agents
6. Assess the need for tetanus vaccination
7. Arrange follow-up with an ophthalmologist

PEER REVIEW

✓ Most corneal foreign bodies are wood, plastic, or metal and are usually superficial and benign.

✓ Topical antibiotics should be used after foreign body removal.

REFERENCES
Roberts JR, Hedges JR, eds. *Clinical Procedures in Emergency Medicine.* 6th ed. St. Louis, MO: WB Saunders; 2013: 1273-1277.
Tintinalli JE, Stapczynski JS, Ma OJ, et al, eds. *Tintinalli's Emergency Medicine: A Comprehensive Study Guide.* 8th ed. New York, NY: McGraw-Hill; 2012: 1565.

338. The correct answer is C, Pain control and re-evaluation by primary care physician in 2 to 3 days.

Why is this the correct answer?

According to current guidelines from the American Academy of Pediatrics (AAP), the correct disposition is to provide pain control and instruct the parents to follow up for re-evaluation with their primary care physician in 2 to 3 days. The AAP guidelines, released in February 2013, advise that acute otitis media can be diagnosed in a child presenting with:

- Moderate to severe bulging of the tympanic membrane or new onset of otorrhea not due to acute otitis externa
- Mild bulging of tympanic membrane and recent (less than 48 hours) onset of ear pain (holding, tugging, or rubbing of the ear in a nonverbal child) or intense erythema of the tympanic membrane

The guidelines go on to say that clinicians should not diagnose acute otitis media in children who do not have middle ear effusion. Pain should be actively treated (ibuprofen 10 mg/kg or acetaminophen 15 mg/kg) in those patients who have signs or complaints of discomfort. With regard to antibiotic therapy, the

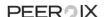
guidelines say treatment is indicated in children 6 months old and older who have severe signs or symptoms; that would be moderate or severe otalgia or otalgia for at least 48 hours or temperature 39°C or higher. For nonsevere acute otitis media in children 24 months old and older, as in the case presented, antibiotic therapy or observation with close follow-up is indicated. Amoxicillin (80 to 90 mg/kg to start) is the drug of choice if the patient has not taken antibiotics in the past 30 days and if he or she has no allergy to penicillin.

Why are the other choices wrong?

Amoxicillin 50 mg/kg is not considered appropriate therapy for acute otitis media. The current standard of care suggests a starting dose of 80 to 90 mg/kg to minimize resistant organisms.

Because amoxicillin is the first-line antibiotic for acute otitis media, azithromycin for a child who does not have a known allergy to amoxicillin is not an appropriate choice. The correct recommended dose for azithromycin is 10 mg/kg for the first dose and 5 mg/kg for the final 4 days.

Follow-up with a primary care physician is an appropriate practice, but this should be done within 48 to 72 hours rather than within 1 week. It is also acceptable to provide the caregiver with a prescription for an antibiotic to be used if the child worsens or fails to improve within the 2- to 3-day timeframe.

PEER REVIEW

- ✓ Don't diagnose acute otitis media unless the patient has an effusion or severe bulging otorrhea without otitis externa, or minimal bulging with intense erythema and acute onset of ear pain.
- ✓ Amoxicillin is the preferred first-line antibiotic and is dosed at 80 to 90 mg/kg. Pain control is an important component of caring for the child with acute otitis media.

REFERENCES

Lieberthal AS, Carroll AE, Chonmaitree T, et al. The diagnosis and management of acute otitis media. *Pediatrics.* 2013;131(3):e964-e999.

Wolfson AB, Hendey GW, Ling LJ, et al, eds. *Harwood-Nuss' Clinical Practice of Emergency Medicine.* 6th ed. Philadelphia, PA: Lippincott, Williams & Wilkins; 2014: 1209.

339. The correct answer is D, Toxin-producing gram-positive causative organism.

Why is this the correct answer?

There are two classically described toxic shock syndromes (TSSs) — one caused by *Staphylococcus aureus* (staph TSS) and one by *Streptococcus pyogenes* (strep TSS). Both causative organisms are gram-positive bacteria that produce toxins that mediate their respective life-threatening syndromes. *S. aureus* (including MRSA) produces toxic shock syndrome toxin-1 (TSST-1) and enterotoxin type B. *S. pyogenes* produces streptococcal pyrogenic exotoxins. These toxins ("super antigens") cause fever, massive systemic inflammatory states, increased vascular permeability, hemodynamic instability, coagulopathy, and multiorgan failure. The hallmark of treatment is supportive care with aggressive antibiotic therapy for gram-positive organisms.

Why are the other choices wrong?

Blood cultures are positive in fewer than 5% of staph TSS cases. However, cultures from retained foreign bodies, mucosal sites, and wounds often are positive and should be collected when possible. In contrast, blood cultures are positive in more than 60% of strep TSS cases.

Strep TSS does not manifest as a rash. On the other hand, staph TSS commonly is associated with erythroderma or exfoliative dermatitis — a diffuse, macular, red/erythematous rash that resembles a painless but severe sunburn. Desquamation occurs between 1 and 3 weeks of symptom onset and most frequently involves the hands and feet. Mucosal involvement is common.

Although staph TSS is associated with retained foreign bodies (classically tampons), strep TSS is unrelated to this etiology. The incidence of staph TSS has decreased since the 1980s when highly absorbent tampons were removed from the market. But tampon use remains a significant risk factor; it is responsible for more than 50% of current cases of staph TSS. Recognition and removal of foreign body nidus is critical to eliminate ongoing toxin production. Risk factors for strep TSS include skin and soft tissue infections, trauma, surgery, childbirth, and viral illnesses. These conditions are also risk factors for non-tampon-mediated staph TSS.

PEER REVIEW

- ✓ Toxic shock syndrome can be caused by two toxin-producing bacteria, *Staphylococcus aureus* and *Streptococcus pyogenes*.
- ✓ Both forms of toxic shock syndrome involve overwhelming systemic inflammation, vascular permeability, hypotension, and multiorgan failure.
- ✓ There are differences between *S. aureus* and *S. pyogenes* toxic shock syndrome that, once recognized, affect diagnosis and treatment decisions.

REFERENCES

Marx JA, Hockberger RS, Walls RM, eds. *Rosen's Emergency Medicine: Concepts and Clinical Practice*. 8th ed. St. Louis, MO: Elsevier; 2014: 1861-1862.

Tintinalli JE, Stapczynski JS, Ma OJ, et al, eds. *Tintinalli's Emergency Medicine: A Comprehensive Study Guide*. 8th ed. New York, NY: McGraw-Hill; 2012: 1017-1021.

340. The correct answer is D, PaO₂ less than 70 mm Hg.

Why is this the correct answer?

Pneumocystis pneumonia (PCP) is one of the most common opportunistic infections in persons who have HIV/AIDS. The disease, which is caused by the fungus *Pneumocystis jirovecii*, can be managed with trimethoprim-sulfamethoxazole for 21 days. Steroids are indicated for the management of severe PCP, as indicated by a PaO_2 less than 70 mm Hg, an A-a gradient of 35 or more, or an oxygen saturation level less than 92% on room air. Common treatment regimens include prednisone (40 mg PO twice daily with a 3-week taper) or methylprednisolone (starting intravenous dose four times a day). Patients who require steroids, whose conditions typically worsen in the days following the initiation of therapy, should be admitted to the hospital. Symptoms of PCP often are insidious and include nonproductive cough, fatigue, malaise, fever, and dyspnea. In the emergency department, the diagnosis is made clinically; confirmatory testing requires direct bronchoscopy and should not be delayed if suspicion is high (for example, patients who have CD4 counts <200 or previous opportunistic infections).

Why are the other choices wrong?

Pneumocystis pneumonia commonly is distinguished on chest xray by diffuse interstitial opacities in a characteristic batwing distribution. These hazy opacities with preserved alveolar and vascular markings often are described as having a ground-glass appearance. However, xray findings are normal in up to 20% of patients with PCP; imaging alone should not be used to rule out the disease. Chest CT can be useful if clinical suspicion remains high despite normal xray findings.

A low CD4 count should prompt consideration for an opportunistic infection; however, this finding should not be used to guide any specific medical therapy. A CD4 count below 500 is considered abnormal; a count below 200 with a concomitant HIV infection is an AIDS-defining finding. Patients with CD4 counts below 200, who are deemed high risk for PCP, should receive antibiotic prophylaxis. Patients with CD4 counts below 100 have an increased susceptibility to toxoplasmosis and *Mycobacterium avium* complex infections, and those with counts below 50 are at increased risk for cytomegalovirus infections.

Serum LDH often is elevated in patients with PCP. Although this finding has a 90% sensitivity for detecting the disease, its specificity is poor. An elevated LDH in the right clinical context should prompt the physician to consider a diagnosis of PCP; however, it should not be used to guide medical management.

PEER POINT

The number needed to treat to see reduced mortality rates with adjunctive steroids for severe pneumocystis pneumonia is nine patients.

PEER REVIEW

✓ Pneumocystis pneumonia is one of the most common opportunistic infections in patients with HIV/AIDS.

✓ Treatment for pneumocystis pneumonia: trimethoprim-sulfamethoxazole for 21 days.

✓ Add steroids to treat severe pneumocystis pneumonia — "severe" meaning Pao_2 less than 70 mm Hg, A-a gradient 35 or more, or oxygen saturation less than 92% on room air.

REFERENCES

Marx JA, Hockberger RS, Walls RM, eds. *Rosen's Emergency Medicine: Concepts and Clinical Practice.* 8th ed. St. Louis, MO: Elsevier; 2014: 1758-1760.

Tintinalli JE, Stapczynski JS, Ma OJ, et al, eds. *Tintinalli's Emergency Medicine: A Comprehensive Study Guide.* 8th ed. New York, NY: McGraw-Hill; 2012: 1052-1053.

341. The correct answer is A, Approximately 20 mg/dL is eliminated per hour in nontolerant individuals.

Why is this the correct answer?

In general, unless the patient has developed a tolerance for ethanol, about 20 mg/dL is eliminated every hour. Alcohol dehydrogenase and the specific cytochrome P450 are the enzymes that metabolize most of the ethanol; both are inducible, and that is why rates of ethanol metabolism are actually higher in chronic drinkers, an estimated 30 mg/dL per hour.

Why are the other choices wrong?

Hepatic alcohol dehydrogenase is the major enzyme responsible for initial ethanol metabolism. A specific cytochrome P450 also metabolizes ethanol but is a minor pathway.

Elimination of ethanol is predominantly by hepatic (not renal) metabolism. Smaller amounts leave the body in sweat and urine.

Zero-order kinetics is the term used to characterize the metabolism of a substance at a fixed amount per hour. This rate of metabolism is rare; with regard to ethanol, it occurs in high concentrations when the enzymes become saturated, which is the case with chronic users and alcoholics. More commonly, among persons with low concentrations of ethanol in the blood and those who are nontolerant, metabolism follows first-order kinetics — a fixed percentage of total ethanol is metabolized per hour.

PEER POINT

Ethanol metabolism kinetics

First-order kinetics

- Ethanol metabolizes at a fixed **percentage** per hour
- Low concentrations of ethanol
- Persons who are not alcohol tolerant
- More common

Zero-order kinetics

- Ethanol metabolizes at a fixed **amount** per hour
- High concentrations of ethanol
- Persons who are alcohol tolerant, chronic, alcoholics
- Less common

PEER REVIEW

- ✓ Approximately 20 mg/dL of ethanol is eliminated from the blood per hour in persons who are not alcohol tolerant.
- ✓ Ethanol metabolism rates are higher in alcoholics and other chronic users because the enzymes that do the work — alcohol dehydrogenase and cytochrome P450 — are inducible.
- ✓ When the enzymes become saturated, metabolism converts to zero-order kinetics — a fixed amount per hour.

REFERENCES

Tintinalli JE, Stapczynski JS, Ma OJ, et al, eds. *Tintinalli's Emergency Medicine: A Comprehensive Study Guide*. 8th ed. New York, NY: McGraw-Hill; 2012: 1244.

Wolfson AB, Hendey GW, Ling LJ, et al, eds. *Harwood-Nuss' Clinical Practice of Emergency Medicine*. 6th ed. Philadelphia, PA: Lippincott, Williams & Wilkins; 2014: 1332.

342. The correct answer is D, Perform a purified protein derivative test now and again in 3 months.

Why is this the correct answer?

It is important to initiate droplet precautions for patients with active tuberculosis (TB) and establish the status of those who have been exposed to the disease. Subcutaneous placement of a purified protein derivative (PPD) skin test is one reliable approach to assessing TB status. The test, which works through a delayed (or type IV) hypersensitivity reaction, is interpreted for positivity within 48 to 72 hours based on the size of the reaction and the patient's underlying risk factors. An interferon-gamma release assay (known commercially as QuantiFERON-TB), which evaluates for cell-mediated immune activity against *Mycobacterium tuberculosis*, can

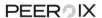

be used as an alternative to the PPD skin test. If the TB test result is negative, the patient should be tested again 3 months after exposure to assess for conversion; the disease can be ruled out if the second test is negative. Up to one-third of patients with a high-risk exposure develop a positive PPD or interferon-gamma release assay result. Any patient with a positive result should undergo clinical examination and chest radiography to assess for active disease and then be treated accordingly.

Why are the other choices wrong?

Isoniazid is appropriate pharmacotherapy for patients with documented latent TB; however, it is inappropriate for the treatment of unconfirmed TB. Although most patients with TB infections (about 95%) never develop active disease, immunocompromised patients (elderly and those with HIV/AIDS) are at greater risk. Latent TB can progress to active disease and should be treated; TB is a public health hazard with high rates of morbidity.

Due to increasing drug resistance with monotherapy, combination or multidrug regimens are preferred for the management of active TB; however, these treatments are not appropriate for unconfirmed cases. In an effort to prevent further drug resistance, direct observed therapy is recommended until the patient is deemed competent to comply with daily medication regimens independently. Therapy typically is required for a minimum of 6 to 9 months based on the patient's underlying health status. These medications should not be administered without consultation with an infectious disease specialist.

Failing to assess a PPD test or interferon-gamma release assay immediately following a high-risk exposure is a mistake. If the initial test results are positive, treatment for latent TB should start immediately; the size of the PPD reaction or interferon-gamma release assay level can help guide management.

PEER REVIEW

- ✓ Infection control for tuberculosis requires testing of high-risk patients and droplet precautions for those with active disease.
- ✓ Individuals who have been exposed to tuberculosis require immediate testing followed by repeat testing at 3 months.
- ✓ Any patient with a positive purified protein derivative test requires a clinical exam and chest xray to rule out active disease.

REFERENCES

Marx JA, Hockberger RS, Walls RM, eds. *Rosen's Emergency Medicine: Concepts and Clinical Practice.* 8th ed. St. Louis, MO: Elsevier; 2014: 1768-1784.

Tintinalli JE, Stapczynski JS, Ma OJ, et al, eds. *Tintinalli's Emergency Medicine: A Comprehensive Study Guide.* 8th ed. New York, NY: McGraw-Hill; 2012: 475-479.

343. The correct answer is B, Foley catheter insertion.

Why is this the correct answer?

When patients present with acute renal failure, the initial action should be to determine the etiology. In this patient's case, the cause is postrenal or obstructive renal failure likely resulting from benign prostatic hyperplasia (BPH). Appropriate initial management consists of placing a Foley catheter. If the patient has recently undergone a urologic procedure, the urologist should place the catheter. Patients who develop renal failure caused by obstruction generally have good recovery of kidney function following relief of the obstruction. The three broad categories within acute renal insufficiency are prerenal (from volume loss or hypotension), renal (intrinsic kidney damage), and postrenal (obstruction within the urinary tract). It is crucial to make this distinction: treatment for each of these is different, and both prerenal and postrenal causes should be ruled out before the diagnosis of intrinsic renal failure can be made. Important clues that indicate obstructive renal failure include history of urinary issues: dribbling, poor urinary stream or frank inability to urinate, lower abdominal discomfort or fullness, and a history of BPH in men. Performing a digital rectal examination might also indicate prostatitis or evidence of an enlarged prostate. In the absence of renal failure, when the patient is discharged from the emergency department, the Foley catheter should remain in place. The patient and family should be provided with clear instructions regarding care for the Foley catheter, signs of infection, and close urologic follow-up.

Why are the other choices wrong?

A fluid bolus would be the correct initial treatment for a patient presenting with prerenal azotemia, a condition suggested by hypotension or tachycardia. The patient in this case does not have those signs. The clues on presentation in this case — decreased urinary stream and suprapubic abdominal discomfort — support the diagnosis of postobstructive renal failure. Additionally, intravenous fluids might help resolve the renal failure, but only after resolution of the obstruction.

A referral to a urologist for follow-up care is appropriate for the patient in this case, but not as the initial management step, and not without placement of the Foley catheter first.

At some point in this patient encounter, insertion of a suprapubic tube might be necessary to drain the bladder. But the first intervention should be to attempt to place the standard 14 to 18 Fr catheter. If that is unsuccessful because of the obstruction, the next step is to try with a coudé acute, or elbowed catheter. If that, too, fails, the suprapubic tube can be considered.

PEER REVIEW

✓ When diagnosing renal failure, consider the cause: prerenal, renal, or postrenal.

✓ Once you've recognized an obstruction, place a Foley catheter — or have the urologist do it if the patient has recently had a urologic procedure.

✓ Generally, patients with obstructive renal failure get kidney function back after appropriate treatment.

REFERENCES

Marx JA, Hockberger RS, Walls RM, eds. *Rosen's Emergency Medicine: Concepts and Clinical Practice*. 8th ed. St. Louis, MO: Elsevier; 2014: 1291-1311.

Tintinalli JE, Stapczynski JS, Ma OJ, et al, eds. *Tintinalli's Emergency Medicine: A Comprehensive Study Guide*. 8th ed. New York, NY: McGraw-Hill; 2012: 597-601.

344. The correct answer is D, Sonographic Murphy sign.

Why is this the correct answer?

Acute cholecystitis is a complication of gallstones and is distinguished from biliary colic by a longer duration of symptoms and a higher intensity of pain. The diagnostic study of choice for acute cholecystitis is abdominal ultrasonography, with a reported sensitivity of 81%. The most sensitive sonographic finding in acute cholecystitis is the sonographic Murphy sign — the ability to reproduce a patient's abdominal pain by compressing the gallbladder with the ultrasound probe when compressing any other surrounding area does not have the same effect. A positive sonographic Murphy sign in addition to the findings of gallstones, has the greatest positive predictive value (.92) for acute cholecystitis. Interestingly, however, the sonographic Murphy sign is very nonspecific, as are the other sonographic signs of cholecystitis — gallbladder wall thickening (>3 mm measured at the anterior gallbladder wall), evidence of cholelithiasis or sludge, and pericholecystic fluid. This patient's sonograms reveal an impacted stone in the neck of the gallbladder. There is marked wall thickening (1.3 cm) and gallbladder distention as measured on the transverse image (width) of 5.27 cm; a Murphy sign is present. Emergency department management of acute cholecystitis includes analgesia, antiemetics, antibiotics, and surgical consultation for cholecystectomy.

Why are the other choices wrong?

Although gallbladder wall thickening is one of the sonographic signs of acute cholecystitis and is evident on this patient's sonograms, it is relatively nonspecific for cholecystitis. It can also be caused by pancreatitis (which often presents with the same symptoms as cholecystitis), ascites, heart failure, or liver disease.

Noncompressibility is a sign of appendicitis, not acute cholecystitis.

As with gallbladder wall thickening, the presence of pericholecystic fluid can be the result of other conditions and is not the most strongly suggestive sign of acute cholecystitis in this presentation.

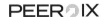

PEER REVIEW

✓ Ultrasonography is the imaging modality of choice to diagnose acute cholecystitis.

✓ Sonographic findings of acute cholecystitis: sonographic Murphy sign, gallbladder wall thickening, evidence of cholelithiasis or sludge, and pericholecystic fluid.

✓ What's the management approach to acute cholecystitis in the emergency department? Symptomatic relief, antibiotics, and surgical consultation.

REFERENCES

Knoop KJ, Stack LB, Storrow AB, et al, eds. *The Atlas of Emergency Medicine*. 4th ed. New York, NY: McGraw-Hill; 2016: 899-902.

Schwartz DT. *Emergency Radiology: Case Studies*. New York, NY: McGraw-Hill; 2008: 210-216.

Tintinalli JE, Stapczynski JS, Ma OJ, et al, eds. *Tintinalli's Emergency Medicine: A Comprehensive Study Guide*. 8th ed. New York, NY: McGraw-Hill; 2012: 517-525.

345. The correct answer is A, *Escherichia coli* 0157:H7.

Why is this answer correct?

In hemolytic uremic syndrome (HUS), kidney function is compromised by blockage of the filtration system with damaged RBCs. According to the National Institute of Diabetes and Digestive and Kidney Diseases, HUS is the most common cause of acute kidney injury in children. And the most common cause of HUS in children is an *Escherichia coli* infection of the digestive system. The bacteria produce a Shiga toxin that leads to the anemia, hemolysis, and low platelet count. In turn, microthrombi are deposited within the kidney glomeruli, leading to kidney damage. The classic presentation of HUS is initial GI symptoms (nausea, vomiting, bloody diarrhea) and a low-grade fever. Within 1 week, symptoms progress to development of microangiopathic hemolytic anemia, kidney failure, and neurologic symptoms such as seizures and encephalopathy. Examination of a peripheral smear shows Burr cells (speculated RBCs). Vital signs might also reveal hypertension. Ingestion of undercooked meat, unpasteurized milk, and contaminated fruits and vegetables is associated with *E. coli* 0157:H7 infection. Treatment for HUS involves intravenous fluids and transfusion as needed. Antibiotics and antimotility agents should be avoided in pediatric patients with diarrheal illness because they might increase the risk for HUS.

Why are the other choices wrong?

Group A *Streptococcus* can be associated with HUS, but it is less common than infection with *E. coli* 0157:H7, and the prodrome is generally pharyngitis, fever, and a rash.

Norovirus is a common cause of nausea, vomiting, and diarrhea in pediatric patients but has not been found to be associated with HUS.

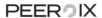

Y. enterocolitica infection is acquired most commonly by eating contaminated food, particularly pork. It causes yersiniosis, an intestinal illness characterized in children by fever, abdominal pain, and (often bloody) diarrhea. It can mimic appendicitis, and patients might present with right lower quadrant abdominal pain. Yersiniosis usually resolves on its own; it does not lead to HUS.

PEER REVIEW

- ✓ Most commonly implicated pathogen in hemolytic uremic syndrome: *E. coli* 0157:H7 and the GI infection it causes, with nausea, vomiting, diarrhea, fever, and abdominal pain.
- ✓ A preceding viral illness could be the cause of hemolytic uremic syndrome in patients who present with renal failure, neurologic symptoms, and microangiopathic hemolytic anemia without GI symptoms.
- ✓ Antibiotics and antimotility agents are generally avoided in pediatric patients with diarrheal illness to prevent hemolytic uremic syndrome.

REFERENCES

Schafermeyer RW, Tenenbein M, Macias CG, et al, eds. *Strange and Schafermeyer's Pediatric Emergency Medicine*. 4th ed. New York, NY: McGraw-Hill; 2015: 486-490.

Tintinalli JE, Stapczynski JS, Ma OJ, et al, eds. *Tintinalli's Emergency Medicine: A Comprehensive Study Guide*. 8th ed. New York, NY: McGraw-Hill; 2012: 1513-1518.

346. The correct answer is D, Strychnine.

Why is this the correct answer?

The clinical manifestations of poisoning with strychnine are very similar to those seen with tetanus. Strychnine antagonizes glycine receptors, one of the major inhibitory neurotransmitters in the spinal cord; tetanus toxin (tetanospasmin) prevents the release of presynaptic glycine. In both situations, because the transmission of glycine is disrupted, recurrent, episodic involuntary muscular contractions occur, often in response to minimal stimuli. Strength differences in regional muscle groups account for why classic findings of opisthotonus (spine and extremities bent forward, body resting on head and heels) and risus sardonicus (sustained facial muscle spasm that appears to produce grinning) can occur. The development of respiratory compromise can be life-threatening, as can hyperthermia, rhabdomyolysis, and severe acidemia that result from excessive muscular contractions. Although the muscular contractions can appear to be convulsions, in strychnine poisoning the sensorium is unaffected. Strychnine poisoning typically has a more rapid onset and shorter duration than tetanus. Supportive care, including benzodiazepines and/or barbiturates to raise the stimulus threshold to initiate muscular contractions, airway control, cooling, and hydration are the mainstays of treatment.

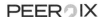

Why are the other choices wrong?

Recurrent, episodic involuntary muscular contractions, often in response to minimal stimuli as seen in strychnine poisoning and tetanus, are not a feature of arsenic poisoning. Acute ingestions of arsenic cause profound vomiting and diarrhea. Hypotension can result from large fluid losses, and cardiac dysfunction can occur from direct toxicity.

Recurrent, episodic involuntary muscular contractions also are not a feature of cyanide poisoning. By inhibition of oxidative phosphorylation in cyanide poisoning, cells are not able to use oxygen. Acute cyanide poisoning is characterized by the rapid onset of coma, apnea, metabolic acidosis, and often hypotension.

Ricin is a toxin derived from the castor bean that disrupts protein synthesis. Ricin poisoning is characterized by initial GI symptoms of vomiting and diarrhea that can be followed by multisystem organ failure, not by recurrent, episodic involuntary muscular contractions.

PEER REVIEW

✓ The clinical manifestations of strychnine poisoning look a lot like those seen with tetanus.
✓ Both strychnine poisoning and tetanus are characterized by recurrent, episodic, involuntary muscular contractions.

REFERENCES
Hoffman RS, Howland MA, Lewin NA, et al, eds. *Goldfrank's Toxicologic Emergencies*. 10th ed. New York, NY: McGraw-Hill; 2015: 1456-1457, 1528.
Wolfson AB, Hendey GW, Ling LJ, et al, eds. *Harwood-Nuss' Clinical Practice of Emergency Medicine*. 6th ed. Philadelphia, PA: Lippincott, Williams & Wilkins; 2014: 320-321e.

347. The correct answer is C, 32-year-old asthmatic who has white plaques in his posterior pharynx and odynophagia and redness.

Why is that the correct answer?

White plaques in the posterior pharynx with associated odynophagia strongly suggest esophageal candidiasis. This pathology typically is found in significantly immunocompromised patients, including those with HIV/AIDS (in whom esophageal candidiasis is an AIDS-defining illness) or cancer with neutropenia. This fungal infection of the esophagus is caused by *Candida albicans*. The presence of thrush or oral candidiasis is not required to confirm the diagnosis. Clinical suspicion should arise in any immunocompromised patient with new odynophagia or oral thrush and concomitant odynophagia. Oral thrush without esophageal involvement should not cause discomfort with swallowing and can occur in immunocompetent patients who regularly use inhaled corticosteroids without rinsing. The diagnosis can be confirmed with upper endoscopy. Esophageal candidiasis is typically treated with fluconazole for 14 to 21 days.

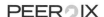

Why are the other choices wrong?

Raised red plaques in the inguinal crease suggest tinea cruris, or jock itch. It can certainly affect immunocompetent persons, but it is so common among healthy persons that its presence alone is not a marker of serious underlying immunocompromise. Tinea cruris is a dermatophyte infection that usually involves the groin but can spread to the buttocks, thighs, and perineum while sparing the genitalia; it is more common in men. The fungus is transmitted by person-to-person contact or autoinoculation from simultaneous tinea pedis or corporis. The lesions, which are similar to those of tinea corporis, classically appear as erythematous, annular plaques with central clearing and sharp demarcated borders that might contain vesicles. The infection should be treated with topical azoles, and the affected areas should be kept clean and dry to prevent recurrences.

Recent travel to the Southwest with associated pulmonary and systemic symptoms should prompt consideration for coccidioidomycosis, or valley fever. The disease can afflict immunocompetent patients who have traveled to endemic areas, including the southwestern United States, regions of Mexico, and South America. Valley fever is usually is self-limited. Symptoms include fever, cough, night sweats, headache, and shortness of breath. Pregnant women and patients with severe disease, known immunosuppression, or underlying cardiopulmonary disorders should be treated with an oral azole antifungal agent such as ketoconazole, fluconazole, or itraconazole.

Tinea versicolor, a common fungal rash caused by *Malassezia furfur*, is not suggestive of an immunocompromised state. The fungus requires oil to grow and, therefore, is more common in teenagers. Although hyperpigmented or hypopigmented, scaly truncal lesions are classic signs of the disease, the rash can be any color, hence the name. First-line treatment is the daily application of topical selenium sulfide shampoo for 1 week. Topical azoles also can be used. Patients should be aware that discoloration can last several months and is not a sign that treatment failed.

PEER REVIEW

✓ Esophageal candidiasis suggests a severe immunocompromised state.

✓ Most fungal skin lesions are not suggestive of an immunocompromised state.

✓ Valley fever can affect immunocompetent hosts and typically is self-limited.

REFERENCES

Marx JA, Hockberger RS, Walls RM, eds. *Rosen's Emergency Medicine: Concepts and Clinical Practice.* 8th ed. St. Louis, MO: Elsevier; 2014: 1558-1585; 1751-1767.

Tintinalli JE, Stapczynski JS, Ma OJ, et al, eds. *Tintinalli's Emergency Medicine: A Comprehensive Study Guide.* 8th ed. New York, NY: McGraw-Hill; 2012: 1652-1666.

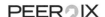

348. The correct answer is B, Lactic acidosis.

Why is this the correct answer?

Cyanide inhibits oxidative phosphorylation and can rapidly lead to apnea, loss of consciousness, convulsions, hemodynamic instability, and death. By inhibiting aerobic metabolism, anaerobic metabolism ensues and a lactic acidosis (not ketoacidosis) develops. Cells are unable to extract oxygen; therefore, a high (not low) venous oxygen saturation is expected. This disruption in oxygen use can lead to "arterialization" of venous blood. Confirmatory cyanide levels are not rapidly available, and antidote administration is required quickly, so a high level of suspicion based on history (smoke exposure, suicide attempt in chemist or jeweler) in combination with clinical manifestations and rapidly available laboratory test results (metabolic acidosis, elevated lactate, elevated venous oxygen saturation) is necessary.

Why are the other choices wrong?

Ketoacids (acetoacetate, beta-hydroxybutyrate) are released in the blood from lipid metabolism. Excess accumulation is responsible for the anion gap acidoses found in diabetic ketoacidosis and alcoholic ketoacidosis. Ketoacids do not accumulate significantly in cyanide poisoning, which is characterized by the accumulation of lactate (lactic acidosis).

By inhibiting oxidative phosphorylation, cyanide prevents cells from using oxygen. In significant cyanide toxicity, venous blood can return "arterialized" with a high (not low) oxygen saturation.

Hydroxocobalamin, an effective antidote for cyanide poisoning, is bright red, and administration causes reddish discoloration of skin, urine, and plasma. Cyanide poisoning itself can cause venous blood to appear arterial but does not cause plasma discoloration.

PEER REVIEW

✓ Laboratory findings that can help you diagnose cyanide poisoning include metabolic (lactic) acidosis and increased venous oxygen saturation.

✓ Hydroxocobalamin is an antidote for cyanide poisoning. It's bright red and can cause reddish discoloration of skin, urine, and plasma.

REFERENCES

Hoffman RS, Howland MA, Lewin NA, et al, eds. *Goldfrank's Toxicologic Emergencies.* 10th ed. New York, NY: McGraw-Hill; 2015: 1602-1606.

Wolfson AB, Hendey GW, Ling LJ, et al, eds. *Harwood-Nuss' Clinical Practice of Emergency Medicine.* 6th ed. Philadelphia, PA: Lippincott, Williams & Wilkins; 2014: 1419-1420.

349. The correct answer is A, Ethylene glycol.

Why is this the correct answer?

Toxicity from ethylene glycol best explains the combination of coma, mild hypothermia, tachypnea, and blood gas that demonstrates a metabolic acidosis with normal respiratory compensation. In an acute metabolic acidosis with normal respiratory compensation, as would be expected in ethylene glycol (and methanol) poisoning, the second two numbers of the pH roughly equate to the P_{CO_2}. Ethylene glycol, typically found in antifreeze, is intoxicating itself and is metabolized, initially by alcohol dehydrogenase, to various toxic metabolites. The result is a progressive anion gap metabolic acidosis. Ethylene glycol, isopropanol, and phenobarbital as sedative-hypnotic agents can cause hypothermia.

Why are the other choices wrong?

Isopropanol (isopropyl alcohol), typically referred to as rubbing alcohol, is converted by alcohol dehydrogenase to acetone, a ketone (not a ketoacid). Isopropanol ingestion can cause coma, but the presentation includes a ketosis, not acidosis.

Phenobarbital can cause coma, but in such a scenario, a respiratory acidosis is expected.

The blood gas analysis in this case demonstrates a metabolic acidosis with normal respiratory compensation, an acid-base scenario that is not typical with salicylate poisoning. Salicylate poisoning in adults characteristically manifests with either with a primary respiratory alkalosis or a combination of a mixed acid-base picture (respiratory alkalosis and metabolic acidosis). Hypothermia also is atypical of salicylate poisoning due to uncoupling of oxidative phosphorylation.

PEER REVIEW

- ✓ In an acute metabolic acidosis with normal respiratory compensation, the second two numbers of the pH should be nearly equal to the P_{CO_2}.
- ✓ The most common acid-base abnormalities in salicylate poisoning are respiratory alkalosis or respiratory alkalosis plus metabolic acidosis.

REFERENCES

Hoffman RS, Howland MA, Lewin NA, et al, eds. *Goldfrank's Toxicologic Emergencies.* 10th ed. New York, NY: McGraw-Hill; 2015: 249-253, 516-527,1346-1357.

Wolfson AB, Hendey GW, Ling LJ, et al, eds. *Harwood-Nuss' Clinical Practice of Emergency Medicine.* 6th ed. Philadelphia, PA: Lippincott, Williams & Wilkins; 2014: 1339-1342, 1346.

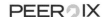

350. The correct answer is B, Causes a metabolic acidosis.

Why is this the correct answer?

Acute mountain sickness (AMS) is a syndrome of high-altitude ascent characterized by headache in combination with one or more symptoms of GI disturbance (anorexia, vomiting), dizziness, fatigue, or sleep disturbance. The etiology of AMS is principally hypoxia. Acetazolamide is a carbonic anhydrase inhibitor that is effective in both preventing and treating AMS. It causes a bicarbonate diuresis resulting in a nonanion gap metabolic acidosis. To maintain serum pH, the body increases ventilation to decrease Pco_2, and as a result serum Po_2 is increased.

Why are the other choices wrong?

Acetazolamide is not an osmotic diuretic. It is a carbonic anhydrase inhibitor.

Acetazolamide causes an increase (not a decrease) in respiratory rate and in doing so increases arterial Po_2.

Acetazolamide decreases hypoxia, which is why it is helpful in both prevention and treatment of AMS.

PEER REVIEW

- ✓ Acetazolamide prevents and treats acute mountain sickness by decreasing hypoxia.
- ✓ Acetazolamide induces a bicarbonate diuresis leading to a nonanion gap acidosis.
- ✓ By inducing a metabolic acidosis, acetazolamide leads to increased ventilation and resulting increased Po_2.

REFERENCES
Tintinalli JE, Stapczynski JS, Ma OJ, et al, eds. *Tintinalli's Emergency Medicine: A Comprehensive Study Guide*. 8th ed. New York, NY: McGraw-Hill; 2012: 1431-1432.
Wolfson AB, Hendey GW, Ling LJ, et al, eds. *Harwood-Nuss' Clinical Practice of Emergency Medicine*. 6th ed. Philadelphia, PA: Lippincott, Williams & Wilkins; 2014: 1517.

351. The correct answer is D, Hyponatremia.

Why is this the correct answer?

Destruction of the adrenal cortex in primary adrenal insufficiency (Addison disease) manifests with signs and symptoms of steroid deficiency (mineralocorticoids, glucocorticoids, gonadocorticoids) and increased adrenocorticotropic hormone (ACTH). The mineralocorticoid aldosterone stimulates the kidneys to reabsorb sodium and to excrete potassium. Aldosterone deficiency contributes to the presence of hyponatremia (seen 90% of the time), and hyperkalemia (seen 60% of the time). Deficiency in the glucocorticoid cortisol can lead to hypoglycemia, a common finding in children and infants. Signs and symptoms of gonadocorticoid deficiency are more common in women and include decreased axillary and pubic hair and decreased libido. Increased ACTH leads to skin hyperpigmentation. Causes of primary adrenal insufficiency include autoimmune disease (most common cause in Western countries), congenital conditions, drugs, hemorrhage, infections (tuberculosis is traditionally a common cause but is uncommon now in Western countries), infiltrative diseases (such as amyloidosis and sarcoidosis), and metastatic cancer.

Why are the other choices wrong?

Cortisol is involved with maintaining euglycemia. Cortisol deficiency in primary adrenal insufficiency leads to hypoglycemia, not hyperglycemia.

Hypercalcemia, not hypocalcemia, is seen in primary adrenal insufficiency. The hypercalcemia is thought to be a result of increased mobilization from bone and diminished renal excretion. It generally corrects quickly with hydration.

Aldosterone causes sodium resorption and potassium excretion. Aldosterone deficiency in primary adrenal insufficiency causes hyperkalemia, not hypokalemia.

PEER POINT

The three types of steroids produced by the adrenal cortex
- Glucocorticoids (cortisol)
- Gonadocorticoids (sex hormones)
- Mineralocorticoids (aldosterone)

PEER REVIEW

✓ Aldosterone deficiency occurs in primary adrenal insufficiency and contributes to the presence of hyponatremia and hyperkalemia.
✓ Cortisol deficiency in primary adrenal insufficiency can lead to hypoglycemia.

REFERENCES
Tintinalli JE, Stapczynski JS, Ma OJ, et al, eds. *Tintinalli's Emergency Medicine: A Comprehensive Study Guide.* 8th ed. New York, NY: McGraw-Hill; 2012: 857, 1479-1481.
Wolfson AB, Hendey GW, Ling LJ, et al, eds. *Harwood-Nuss' Clinical Practice of Emergency Medicine.* 6th ed. Philadelphia, PA: Lippincott, Williams & Wilkins; 2014: 1033-1034, 1053.

352. The correct answer is D, Remove the foreign body endoscopically.

Why is this the correct answer?

The object seen on the radiograph is a button battery. The radiographic clue is a halo or double circle noted on the foreign body. Although coins and other objects are more commonly ingested, they usually require only supportive care. But an ingested button battery or magnet, in contrast, might need to be removed in the emergency department: it can cause an external current that can cause hydrolysis and erosion of the GI tract over time. A button battery that is lodged in the esophagus can cause erosion within a few hours and should be removed as soon

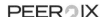

as possible. Management otherwise depends on the age of the patient and the size of the button battery. There is a national button battery hotline that can help in the decision-making process (202-625-3333).

Why are the other choices wrong?

Admission for observation is unlikely to be warranted because the child is in no distress. It is also not an appropriate treatment because the battery simply needs to be removed; it can erode the GI tract over time.

Discharge home with follow-up would be appropriate if the ingested object did not have the potential to damage intestinal tissue. This is often the course of treatment when a child ingests a coin or dull-edged object. There is no advantage in examining the stool in these cases; instead, close follow-up and immediate re-evaluation are indicated for any complaints of abdominal pain or vomiting.

Gastric lavage has fallen out of favor with most toxicologists except in some cases of life-threatening toxic ingestions. It is never used in caustics or hydrocarbon ingestions.

PEER REVIEW

✓ With an ingested foreign body, a halo or double circle indicates a possible button battery.
✓ Endoscopy indications: symptomatic, ingestion of more than 1A magnet, button battery lodged in the esophagus.
✓ Battery ingestion hotline, 202-625-3333

REFERENCES
Fleisher GR, Ludwig S, et al, eds. *Textbook of Pediatric Emergency Medicine.* 6th ed. Philadelphia, PA: Lippincott, Williams & Wilkins; 2010: 279-281.
Wolfson AB, Hendey GW, Ling LJ, et al, eds. *Harwood-Nuss' Clinical Practice of Emergency Medicine.* 6th ed. Philadelphia, PA: Lippincott, Williams & Wilkins; 2014: 1247.

353. The correct answer is B, Calcium gluconate.

Why is this the correct answer?

The cardiac monitor depicts a sinoventricular rhythm (sinusoidal) from severe hyperkalemia, characterized by the absence of P waves, markedly prolonged QRS width, and rates ranging from 30 to 100. Presumably this patient with chronic kidney disease developed worsened renal dysfunction due to volume depletion from vomiting and diarrhea and became hyperkalemic. Recognition and empiric treatment for this life-threatening rhythm are essential. Intravenous calcium is thought to have the most immediate effect and should be administered empirically for such a rhythm. Initial management of severe hyperkalemia includes the following principles:

• Cardiac cell membrane stabilization: intravenous calcium formulations

- Shifting potassium intracellularly: glucose and insulin; nebulized beta agonists; intravenous sodium bicarbonate
- Potassium removal from body: renal excretion with loop diuretics, hemodialysis, and GI binding resins

Recently, several of the classic treatments have fallen into question. The sodium bicarbonate works by causing alkalemia, so it is not effective and might worsen patients with chronic renal failure such as this one. There has been recent recognition that the use of GI binding resins such as sodium polystyrene sulfonate has questionable benefit. In addition, when used in conjunction with sorbitol, patients have an increased risk of colonic necrosis and other GI complications.

Why are the other choices wrong?

The cardiac rhythm depicted is sinoventricular (sinusoidal) from hyperkalemia, so treatment for ventricular tachycardia with an agent such as amiodarone is not indicated. The presence of a markedly prolonged QRS complex (>160 ms) and the absence of tachycardia (rate <100) help distinguish sinoventricular rhythm from ventricular tachycardia.

The correct first step is empiric treatment for hyperkalemia with intravenous calcium; it should be initiated immediately. Magnesium can be administered for ventricular tachycardia, particularly torsades de pointes.

Again, the cardiac rhythm depicted is sinoventricular (sinusoidal) from hyperkalemia, so treatment for ventricular tachycardia with an agent such as procainamide is not indicated. The presence of a markedly prolonged QRS complex (>160 ms) and the absence of tachycardia (rate <100) help distinguish sinoventricular rhythm from ventricular tachycardia.

PEER REVIEW

- ✓ A sinoventricular (sinusoidal) rhythm is a life-threatening manifestation of hyperkalemia.
- ✓ How to recognize a sinoventricular rhythm: absence of P waves, very prolonged QRS widths, and nontachycardic ventricular rates.
- ✓ Intravenous calcium is the first and fastest-acting treatment for life-threatening hyperkalemia.

REFERENCES

Tintinalli JE, Stapczynski JS, Ma OJ, et al, eds. *Tintinalli's Emergency Medicine: A Comprehensive Study Guide*. 8th ed. New York, NY: McGraw-Hill; 2012: 102, 105, 106.

Wolfson AB, Hendey GW, Ling LJ, et al, eds. *Harwood-Nuss' Clinical Practice of Emergency Medicine*. 6th ed. Philadelphia, PA: Lippincott, Williams & Wilkins; 2014: 480, 1048-1050.

354. The correct answer is D, With a normal xray, tenderness and swelling at the physis represent a fracture.

Why is this the correct answer?

The combination of tenderness and soft tissue swelling at the physis commonly describes a pediatric type I Salter-Harris fracture. Because the physis transforms from cartilage into bone and fuses with surrounding bone when growth is complete, a Salter-type fracture cannot occur in grown adults. The Salter-Harris classification scheme for physeal fractures is widely used to categorize pediatric skeletal injuries. In a type I fracture, the fracture extends only through the physis. It might not be visualized on radiographs because of minimal displacement, but it can be identified clinically with tenderness at the physis and adjacent soft tissue swelling. A type II fracture extends from the physis into the metaphysis. In type III, the fracture extends from the physis into the epiphysis and the joint. Type IV fractures cross the epiphysis and the physis, exiting through the metaphysis. The Salter-Harris type V fracture describes a physeal injury that results from a crushing and compressive force. It can be radiologically difficult to diagnose and is more likely to be confirmed after a delay in bone growth.

Why are the other choices wrong?

When evaluating a patient for a suspected fracture, the order for xrays should include at least two views (AP and lateral) taken perpendicular to one another of the injured part. In certain cases, an additional oblique view is also required. Sometimes in pediatric evaluations, an additional view of the contralateral side or comparisons with a radiologic test due to the growing bones are needed. This is not required for diagnosis in most cases.

Adult bones are more dense and less porous than those of children and are therefore less pliable. Pediatric long bones can bow and buckle in response to stress, leading to findings such as torus or greenstick fractures. Adult bones, however, fracture through and through.

A mechanism that would lead to a ligament injury in an adult often leads to a physeal injury in the skeletally immature child. The presence of open physes leaves bones weaker in children compared to adults. Tendons and ligaments attached to the bones can be stronger than the bones themselves. When acute forces are applied to a joint, bony avulsion injuries often result instead of sprains due to this structural imbalance.

PEER REVIEW

✓ Tenderness + soft tissue swelling at the physis + negative radiograph = pediatric type I Salter-Harris fracture.

✓ Pediatric bones are more likely to fracture, although their pliability makes a through-and-though fracture less common.

✓ When you're ordering xrays to evaluate for suspected fracture, get at least two views 90 degrees to each other.

REFERENCES

Chasm RM, Swencki SA. Pediatric orthopedic emergencies. *Emerg Med Clin North Am*. 2010;28:907-926.

Legome E, Shockley LW. *Trauma: A Comprehensive Emergency Medicine Approach*. New York, NY: Cambridge University Press; 2013: 296-298.

Tintinalli JE, Stapczynski JS, Ma OJ, et al, eds. *Tintinalli's Emergency Medicine: A Comprehensive Study Guide*. 8th ed. New York, NY: McGraw-Hill; 2012: 915-934.

355. The correct answer is C, Serial examinations with continuous pulse oximetry monitoring.

Why is this the correct answer?

Because primary blast injury affects air-filled tissue preferentially, lung injury is very common with blast injury. Pulmonary barotrauma is the most common fatal injury to the chest. However, the presentation of pulmonary injury can vary from florid ARDS to mild hypoxia and respiratory difficulty. Mild symptoms can also worsen significantly over several hours, and even the initially asymptomatic patient might decompensate. Although there are no absolute guidelines for observation or admission for low-risk or asymptomatic patients, serial observation of pulmonary status with pulse oximetry checks and examination is generally recommended.

Why are the other choices wrong?

Although patients with severe pulmonary barotrauma should be intubated early in their course, this is not universal for all patients. If the symptomology is mild, observation in a monitored area might also be appropriate. Although considered noninvasive, continuous positive airway pressure can worsen compromised lungs and increase the potential for alveolar rupture and air embolism.

Patients with pulmonary barotrauma have management issues similar to those with pulmonary contusions. Fluids should be administered judiciously to ensure euvolemia and tissue perfusion and avoid fluid overload.

With significant barotrauma, the lung undergoes multiple changes, including hemorrhage, fluid accumulation, and alveolar disruption. High tidal volumes can potentially worsen the already significant lung injury. Patients should be treated in a manner similar to those with ARDS; tidal volume should be kept close to 6 to 7 mL/kg, and peak inspiratory pressures should be limited.

PEER REVIEW

- ✓ Primary blast injuries commonly cause lung injury.
- ✓ Pulmonary injuries can seem mild on presentation and get worse with time, so repeated examinations and SpO_2 monitoring are recommended.
- ✓ In patients with significant lung injury, keep tidal volume at 6 to 7 mL/kg and limit peak inspiratory pressures.

REFERENCES

Bombings: Injury Patterns and Care. ACEP Web site. https://www.acep.org/blastinjury/. Accessed August 30, 2016.

Tintinalli JE, Stapczynski JS, Ma OJ, et al, eds. *Tintinalli's Emergency Medicine: A Comprehensive Study Guide*. 8th ed. New York, NY: McGraw-Hill; 2012: 34-39.

356. The correct answer is C, Perform synchronized cardioversion at 0.5 J/kg.

Why is this the correct answer?

The ECG shows supraventricular tachycardia (SVT). This patient has signs of uncompensated shock with both altered mentation and hypotension. The correct initial approach is synchronized cardioversion at 0.5 to 1 J/kg. Causes of SVT include fever and infections, drug exposure (24%), and congenital heart disease (23%), but most of the time the cause is idiopathic (50%). A child presenting with SVT for the first time should undergo cardiology consultation while in the emergency department, but the prognosis is excellent. Disposition is determined based on the patient's age and whether he or she was treated conservatively (vagal maneuvers or a single dose of adenosine) or warranted further medical interventions (antiarrhythmic medications or synchronized cardioversion).

Why are the other choices wrong?

Adenosine is dosed at 100 mcg/kg and must be delivered intravenously as quickly as possible in a line located as close to the heart as possible (followed with a saline flush for immediate delivery). Because this patient is unstable, cardioversion should be the first treatment, not an antiarrhythmic medication like adenosine.

Defibrillation, using electricity to convert without coordinating or synchronizing with the current rhythm, is not appropriate because the rhythm depicted is SVT. Defibrillation is used for ventricular fibrillation and pulseless ventricular tachycardia.

Vagal maneuvers and adenosine should be used only in patients with stable SVT. They are not appropriate in this child with signs of decompensation. There are many different types of vagal maneuvers, including ice to the face (stimulation of the dive reflex), knee-to-chest position with pushing of the legs, forced exhalation, and even rectal stimulation (used predominantly in neonates and infants).

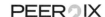

PEER REVIEW

✓ Use synchronized cardioversion at 0.5 to 1 J/kg to convert the rhythm in an unstable patient in supraventricular tachycardia.

✓ Vagal maneuvers may be used in a stable patient in supraventricular tachycardia. For newborns and infants, rectal stimulation is a preferred vagal maneuver.

✓ Infuse adenosine 100 mcg/kg as quickly as possible, and double the dose if the tachyarrhythmia doesn't resolve.

REFERENCES

Fleisher GR, Ludwig S, et al, eds. *Textbook of Pediatric Emergency Medicine*. 6th ed. Philadelphia, PA: Lippincott, Williams & Wilkins; 2010: 492, 596-597.

Wolfson AB, Hendey GW, Ling LJ, et al, eds. *Harwood-Nuss' Clinical Practice of Emergency Medicine*. 6th ed. Philadelphia, PA: Lippincott, Williams & Wilkins; 2014: 474-478.

357. The correct answer is A, Loss of frontalis muscle function.

Why is this the correct answer?

The galea aponeurosis is a fibrous tissue that acts as the fascia of the scalp and inserts into the frontalis muscle, which contributes to facial expression. Loss of function of this muscle, therefore, can have a significant cosmetic impact. Failure to repair a galeal laceration can lead to such a loss of function of the frontalis muscle. Standard of care does not absolutely dictate galeal closure. However, not doing so is associated with increased risk of subgaleal hematoma, poorer cosmetic outcomes, and loss of function of the frontalis muscle.

Why are the other choices wrong?

Galeal closure does not affect the risk of delayed hemorrhage in scalp lacerations. Adequate irrigation and exploration of scalp wounds are essential to evaluate for foreign bodies. Hemorrhage is most likely to occur at the time of injury and repair.

Scalp lacerations can become infected regardless of whether the galea is repaired. There is no clear consensus as to whether galeal repair decreases the risk of subgaleal infection, and it does not decrease the risk of skull osteomyelitis, a rare complication.

There is no increased risk of wound dehiscence if the galea is not repaired as long as the wound is closed appropriately. However, the resulting scar might be wider or more depressed than if the galea had been repaired.

PEER REVIEW

✓ Explore scalp lacerations for galeal injuries.

✓ Here are complications associated with galeal injuries: subgaleal hematoma, poor cosmetic outcome, and loss of function of the frontalis muscle.

REFERENCES

Marx JA, Hockberger RS, Walls RM, eds. *Rosen's Emergency Medicine: Concepts and Clinical Practice*. 8th ed. St. Louis, MO: Elsevier; 2014: 751-766.

Tintinalli JE, Stapczynski JS, Ma OJ, et al, eds. *Tintinalli's Emergency Medicine: A Comprehensive Study Guide*. 8th ed. New York, NY: McGraw-Hill; 2012: 1724-1733.

358. The correct answer is A, Endoscopic retrograde cholangiopancreatography.

Why is this the correct answer?

This patient has acute ascending cholangitis, which is often accompanied by bacteremia and septic shock; it is a surgical emergency. Initial treatment of cholangitis includes stabilization of hemodynamic abnormalities, initiation of broad-spectrum antibiotics, and surgical consultation. Definitive management involves early biliary tract decompression by endoscopic retrograde cholangiopancreatography (ERCP), percutaneous transhepatic cholangiography, or surgery. Ascending cholangitis is most often due to blockage of the common bile duct by a gallstone but can also develop secondary to malignancy or benign stricture. Patients often develop fever, chills, nausea, vomiting, and abdominal pain. The Charcot triad of symptoms includes right upper quadrant pain, fever, and jaundice. When associated with hypotension and altered sensorium due to clinical signs of sepsis, it is described as Reynolds pentad. Common laboratory abnormalities in acute ascending cholangitis include leukocytosis, hyperbilirubinemia, elevated alkaline phosphatase, and increased aminotransferases. Ultrasonography can help detect intrahepatic ductal dilation and also stones in the gallbladder or common bile duct. Studies have shown that the more severe the illness, the more critical the need for urgent biliary decompression using ERCP, which has better results than surgery.

Why are the other choices wrong?

Although intravenous antibiotics are critically important, the definitive management is decompression of the biliary tract. Broad-spectrum choices include piperacillin-tazobactam, imipenem, meropenem, ticarcillin-clavulanate, and ampicillin-sulbactam (with metronidazole).

Although this patient likely requires intravenous fluids and perhaps even vasopressors for hemodynamic stabilization, intravenous fluids alone are not sufficient. If the diagnosis is unclear or there are other competing diagnoses, a CT scan of the abdomen and pelvis might be useful; however, in this case cholangitis is the leading diagnosis.

Oral antibiotics and outpatient follow-up are not appropriate: this patient requires urgent stabilization, intravenous antibiotics, and biliary tract decompression.

PEER POINT

Charcot Triad = Right upper quadrant abdominal pain + fever + jaundice

Reynolds Pentad = Charcot triad + altered mental status + hypotension

PEER REVIEW

✓ Cholangitis is an emergent condition caused by extrahepatic bile duct obstruction and subsequent bacterial infection.

✓ Effective initial management of acute cholangitis requires prompt diagnosis, surgical consultation, initiation of broad-spectrum antibiotics, and early biliary tract decompression.

✓ Biliary tract decompression can be accomplished by endoscopic retrograde cholangiopancreatography, surgically, or transhepatically.

REFERENCES
Marx JA, Hockberger RS, Walls RM, eds. *Rosen's Emergency Medicine: Concepts and Clinical Practice*. 8th ed. St. Louis, MO: Elsevier; 2014: 1203-1204.
Stone CK, Humphries RL. *CURRENT Diagnosis & Treatment Emergency Medicine*. 7th ed. New York, NY: McGraw-Hill; 2011: 227-249.
Wolfson AB, Hendey GW, Ling LJ, et al, eds. *Harwood-Nuss' Clinical Practice of Emergency Medicine*. 6th ed. Philadelphia, PA: Lippincott, Williams & Wilkins; 2014: 900-906; 555-559.

359. The correct answer is D, Restricting intravenous fluids can help prevent the need for positive-pressure ventilation.

Why is this the correct answer?

Patients with traumatic pulmonary contusion might benefit from intravenous fluid resuscitation being restricted to only that which is necessary to support the intravascular volume. Over-resuscitation with intravenous fluids can lead to additional pulmonary edema and hypoxia. When intravenous fluid is necessary, crystalloid solution is theoretically preferred: the concern with colloid solution is sequestration in the alveoli as a sequela of increased permeability and pulmonary capillary leak. However, avoiding colloid solution in these patients is controversial. Both pulmonary toilet and pain control to improve lung expansion and decrease splinting help to improve pulmonary function in patients with severe pulmonary contusion. With regard to the initial evaluation, radiographs obtained early often are not able to show how serious the contusion is. The most severe pulmonary contusions can actually occur without evidence of rib fracture. This is thought to be due to the fact that, in younger patients, the relative elasticity of the chest wall might cause more of the force from blunt trauma to be transmitted to the lungs without fracturing the ribs.

Why are the other choices wrong?

Radiographic findings of pulmonary contusion tend to worsen over the first 72 hours. Computed tomography is better than plain films at defining the initial extent of the contusion, but it, too, can fail to reveal the severity of the contusion initially.

Hemoptysis is a relatively common finding in pulmonary contusion. Auscultation of the chest might reveal rales or decreased breath sounds. Massive hemoptysis is more concerning for pulmonary laceration.

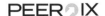

Studies have shown that patients who are intubated and mechanically ventilated have a higher complication rate, including increased length of stay and pneumonia. If the patient is alert, noninvasive positive-pressure ventilation is the preferred treatment for oxygenation.

PEER REVIEW

✓ Remember, initial radiographic findings in pulmonary contusion generally don't reveal the seriousness of the condition.

✓ Pulmonary contusion commonly presents with hemoptysis. And it can occur without rib fracture in younger adults and children.

✓ To improve outcomes in pulmonary contusion, use noninvasive pulmonary support if possible.

✓ And in severe pulmonary contusion, judicious limitation of volume resuscitation can improve outcomes.

REFERENCES

Marx JA, Hockberger RS, Walls RM, eds. *Rosen's Emergency Medicine: Concepts and Clinical Practice*. 8th ed. St. Louis, MO: Elsevier; 2014: 436-437.

Wolfson AB, Hendey GW, Ling LJ, et al, eds. *Harwood-Nuss' Clinical Practice of Emergency Medicine*. 6th ed. Philadelphia, PA: Lippincott, Williams & Wilkins; 2014: 208.

360. The correct answer is C, Roseola infantum.

Why is this the correct answer?

Roseola infantum (also known as exanthema subitum or sixth disease) is caused by human herpesvirus 6 and is a common pediatric infection. It presents as a diffuse maculopapular rash following 3 to 4 days of high fever. The rash often appears as discreet small macules without coalescence that begins centrally and then progresses distally and typically develops after the resolution of the fever. It can be associated with upper respiratory symptoms (lower respiratory symptoms can also be seen), diminished activity, vomiting, and diarrhea, as well as a bulging fontanelle in infants.

Why are the other choices wrong?

Impetigo is caused by either *Staphylococcus aureus* or group A beta-hemolytic *Streptococcus*. The bullous form is almost universally *S. aureus*, as it can produce exfoliative toxins that hydrolyze molecules below the stratum corneum. As opposed to staphylococcal scalded skin syndrome, the blisters are localized and generally start as small vesicles that become flaccid blisters up to 2 cm in diameter. Impetigo also is commonly found in intertriginous regions.

Erythema chronicum migrans is the classic "targetoid" rash associated with Lyme disease. This condition develops 1 to 4 weeks after a tick bite that resulted in transmission of *Borrelia burgdorferi*. Without treatment, the rash clears within 3 to 4 weeks, and only 50% of patients complain of flulike illness with associated fever, headache, chills, and myalgia.

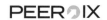

Rubeola, commonly known as measles, has the classic maculopapular rash that starts on the face then spreads down to the trunk and then the extremities. In this case, it is distinguished from roseola because the patient does not have the "three C's" — cough, coryza, and conjunctivitis — rubeola is known for, which generally start a few days before the rash appears.

PEER POINT

Viral illnesses and associated rashes

Disease	Etiology	Characteristic Rash	Presentation	Comments
Erythema infectiosum (fifth disease)	Parvovirus B19	Classic "slapped cheek" erythema on the face initially, then maculopapular rash on the upper extremities that spreads proximally and distally. Fading macular rash appears "lacelike."	Arthralgias and arthritis, circumoral pallor, fever and malaise	Pregnant women exposed are at risk for fetal hydrops. Patients with sickle cell disease are at risk for aplastic anemia.
German measles (rubella)	Togavirus	Pink macules and papules become confluent to form a scarlatiniform rash. Spreads caudally from the face. Forchheimer spots are petechiae on the soft palate.	Malaise, fever, headache, mild conjunctivitis, arthralgia, and prominent adenopathy. Symptoms precede rash by 1–5 days.	In rare cases, thrombocytopenia develops. Strong risk of congenital deformities in the fetus among women who contract rubella in the first trimester.
Hand, foot, and mouth disease	Enteroviruses: Coxsackie virus and echovirus	Oral vesicles that ulcerate, and papules that progress to vesicles on palms and soles	Fever, anorexia, malaise; oral lesions appear 1–2 days after fever, then extremity lesions appear. Decreased oral intake due to pain.	Lesions typically heal in 7–10 days.
Herpangina	Enteroviruses	Vesicular eruptions on posterior pharynx that ulcerate and leave small craters	Fever, headache, sore throat	Lesions heal in 5–10 days.
Measles (rubeola)	Paramyxovirus	Maculopapular, beginning on the face and neck and spreading centrifugally to the trunk and extremities. Koplik spots (white 1-mm lesions) on the buccal mucosa are pathognomonic.	Fever and the "3 C's": cough, coryza, conjunctivitis; symptoms begin 2–4 days before the rash.	Complications include pneumonia and encephalitis.

Table continued on next page

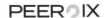

Disease	Etiology	Characteristic Rash	Presentation	Comments
Molluscum contagiosum	Poxvirus	White, waxy papules with central umbilication	Few patients have pruritus.	Lesions can be more extensive in patients with eczema or in immunocompromised patients. Individual lesions resolve in 2 months. Disease can persist for more than 1 year.
Mononucleosis	Epstein-Barr virus	Generalized erythematous rash, petechiae on the soft palate	Fever, malaise, adenopathy	Rash is seen in only 5% of cases primarily. Seen in 100% of patients treated with ampicillin or similar agents.
Mycoplasma	Mycoplasma	Erythematous, maculopapular but seen inconsistently	Frequent cause of exanthems associated with URIs in children	Also associated with erythema multiforme minor and major
Roseola (exanthem subitum)	Human herpesvirus 6	Pink, maculopapular, beginning on the trunk and spreading outward; onset of rash with drop in fever.	High fever (up to 105°C) in a well-appearing infant before the rash; lymphadenopathy; leukopenia on CBC	Associated with intussusception due to lymphoid hyperplasia in GI tract
Varicella	Varicella zoster virus	Pruritic erythematous papules evolving into "dew drop" vesicles then pustules; lesions of various ages; starts on face and scalp.	Fever and malaise; mucosal involvement in many patients; some develop varicella pneumonia.	Lesions resolve after 2 weeks.

PEER REVIEW

✓ Roseola is a common maculopapular rash that often appears after defervescence of a high fever.

✓ Roseola is associated with a bulging fontanelle in infants.

✓ Rubeola is characterized by "3 C's" — cough, coryza, conjunctivitis.

REFERENCES

Fleisher GR, Ludwig S, et al, eds. *Textbook of Pediatric Emergency Medicine*. 6th ed. Philadelphia, PA: Lippincott, Williams & Wilkins; 2010: 514; 937-938.

Wolfson AB, Hendey GW, Ling LJ, et al, eds. *Harwood-Nuss' Clinical Practice of Emergency Medicine*. 6th ed. Philadelphia, PA: Lippincott, Williams & Wilkins; 2014: 258-1e.

361. The correct answer is B, Chest lymphoma.

Why is this the correct answer?

If a PA standing chest xray has been taken with good inspiration and no rotation, any widening of the mediastinum is likely to be genuine. The main pathological causes to consider include masses and widening of vessels. Of the choices listed, chest lymphoma is the most common cause of widened mediastinum, making the diagnosis particularly likely in a patient who reports weight loss and fatigue. The mediastinum is composed of anterior, middle, and posterior compartments. Of the anterior causes of a widened mediastinum, the "four T's" should be considered: (terrible) lymphoma, thymoma, teratoma/germ cell tumor, and thyroid tissue. The middle causes of widened mediastinum, in order by decreasing occurrence, are lymphadenopathy secondary to lymphoma, then sarcoid, then metastatic lung cancer. Of the posterior causes of widened mediastinum, neurogenic tumors are most common.

Why are the other choices wrong?

Pneumomediastinum is a potential complication of Boerhaave syndrome (also associated with tracheobronchial injury) that results in a widened mediastinum in 20% of patients. It can cause a crackling sound known as the Hamman crunch; it is typically heard on chest auscultation coincident with each heartbeat and can be mistaken for a pericardial friction rub. Esophageal rupture in Boerhaave syndrome is likely a result of a sudden rise in intraluminal esophageal pressure produced during vomiting, as a result of neuromuscular incoordination causing failure of the cricopharyngeus muscle to relax. Although these other conditions can be associated with a widened mediastinum, they are particularly uncommon and do not typically present with the same symptoms as lymphoma.

Descending necrotizing mediastinitis is a rare and potentially fatal cause of widened mediastinum. It is caused by the spreading of a head or neck infection to the mediastinum from tonsillitis, dental abscess, or sinusitis. These infections are often polymicrobial and gas producing, which contributes to the widening of the mediastinum.

Although inhalation anthrax can cause a widened mediastinum, it is incredibly rare. Anthrax results in a prodromal viral respiratory illness that lasts about 1 week, but patients generally do not complain of weight loss. This stage is followed by acute hypoxia, dyspnea, or acute respiratory distress with resulting cyanosis. In some patients, mediastinal widening and hilar adenopathy are seen on xray.

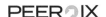

PEER REVIEW

✓ The three compartments of the mediastinum are anterior, middle, and posterior.

✓ Consider the "four T's" of anterior mediastinum widening: (terrible) lymphoma, thymoma, teratoma/germ cell tumor, and thyroid tissue.

✓ The middle causes of widened mediastinum are lymphadenopathy secondary to lymphoma, then sarcoid, then metastatic lung cancer.

REFERENCES

Marx JA, Hockberger RS, Walls RM, eds. *Rosen's Emergency Medicine: Concepts and Clinical Practice*. 8th ed. St. Louis, MO: Elsevier; 2014: 214-222, 2472-2474.

Tintinalli JE, Stapczynski JS, Ma OJ, et al, eds. *Tintinalli's Emergency Medicine: A Comprehensive Study Guide*. 8th ed. New York, NY: McGraw-Hill; 2012: 46-51, 509-510, 967.

362. The correct answer is D, Zygomatic.

Why is this the correct answer?

Because the zygomatic bone does not lie directly over a sinus or the oropharynx, the risk of infection following fracture is lower than it is with the other fractures listed. The zygoma can be fractured as the result of a direct blow, which can lead to an indentation of the cheek and thus cosmetic deformity. An isolated fracture of the zygomatic bone is fairly uncommon. These fractures often require surgical repair due to the resulting deformity of the face. Patients with zygoma fractures can also present with hypesthesia in the distribution of the infraorbital nerve.

Why are the other choices wrong?

Frontal bone fractures often involve the frontal sinus. They are therefore at higher risk for infection. Antibiotic prophylaxis is indicated if the frontal sinus is involved. In general, coverage for sinus infections is similar to that for oral infections: a beta-lactam antibiotic such as penicillin or an extended-spectrum beta-lactam antibiotic such as amoxicillin-clavulanic acid is appropriate, or clindamycin for the penicillin-allergic patient.

Mandibular fractures often involve the teeth and gingiva hidden in the interdental spaces. An open fracture can be difficult to detect without a very careful examination. There is a high risk of infection associated with these fractures for this reason. Antibiotic prophylaxis is indicated if the fracture is open. In general, coverage with a beta-lactam antibiotic such as penicillin or an extended-spectrum beta-lactam antibiotic such as amoxicillin-clavulanic acid is appropriate, or clindamycin for the penicillin-allergic patient.

Orbital fractures often communicate with the frontal, maxillary, or ethmoidal sinuses. They are therefore infection prone, and antibiotic prophylaxis is indicated if the sinuses are involved. Patients should also be instructed regarding nose-blowing precautions.

PEER POINT

Antibiotic prophylaxis for open mandibular fractures or sinus fractures

- Generally, a beta-lactam antibiotic such as penicillin
- Or an extended-spectrum beta-lactam antibiotic such as amoxicillin-clavulanic acid
- Or clindamycin for penicillin-allergic patients

PEER REVIEW

- ✓ Zygomatic arch fractures often require surgery to repair cosmetic deformity.
- ✓ Open fractures of the mandible, orbit, and frontal bone require antibiotic prophylaxis.

REFERENCES

Marx JA, Hockberger RS, Walls RM, eds. *Rosen's Emergency Medicine: Concepts and Clinical Practice*. 8th ed. St. Louis, MO: Elsevier; 2014: 379-380.

Tintinalli JE, Stapczynski JS, Ma OJ, et al, eds. *Tintinalli's Emergency Medicine: A Comprehensive Study Guide*. 8th ed. New York, NY: McGraw-Hill; 2012: 1724-1733.

Wolfson AB, Hendey GW, Ling LJ, et al, eds. *Harwood-Nuss' Clinical Practice of Emergency Medicine*. 6th ed. Philadelphia, PA: Lippincott, Williams & Wilkins; 2014: 160-162.

363. The correct answer is A, Asthma.

Why is this the correct answer?

Pneumomediastinum, as seen on this chest xray, develops when air enters the mediastinum, most commonly from interruption of the tracheobronchial tree or the esophagus. Asthma and COPD can both lead to spontaneous pneumomediastinum or secondary pneumomediastinum due to forceful coughing in the setting of bronchospasm. Chest pain is the most common complaint of patients with this finding. The classic physical findings are subcutaneous emphysema and a sign called the Hamman crunch — a crackling sound caused by the movement of air in the mediastinum heard during systole. Other causes of pneumomediastinum include blunt trauma, mechanical ventilation, marijuana or cocaine inhalation, and forced breathing as in childbirth or severe coughing.

Why are the other choices wrong?

A rapid ascent during diving is a risk factor for pneumomediastinum, as the volume of air within the lungs expands and causes barotrauma. However, a rapid descent decreases the volume of air in the lungs and does not cause barotrauma.

Rheumatic heart disease can lead to valvular disease, including mitral valve stenosis and aortic regurgitation. These lesions cause cardiac murmurs, not the crunching sound heard on chest auscultation in a patient with pneumomediastinum.

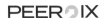

Uremia is a risk factor for pericarditis, and pericarditis produces a pericardial friction rub, but it does not cause a crunching sound. Also, a chest xray might show an enlarged cardiac silhouette but does not produce the radiographic findings seen in this case.

PEER REVIEW

- ✓ Classic chest xray findings in pneumomediastinum: subcutaneous emphysema, pneumopericardium, and air outlining major vessels and bronchi.
- ✓ Physical examination findings in pneumomediastinum include subcutaneous emphysema and a crunching sound during systole.
- ✓ Asthma, environmental factors such as diving or flying, thoracic trauma, and forceful retching are key etiologies of pneumomediastinum.

REFERENCES

Marx JA, Hockberger RS, Walls RM, eds. *Rosen's Emergency Medicine: Concepts and Clinical Practice*. 8th ed. St. Louis, MO: Elsevier; 2014: 431-440, 1113-1123.

Tintinalli JE, Stapczynski JS, Ma OJ, et al, eds. *Tintinalli's Emergency Medicine: A Comprehensive Study Guide*. 8th ed. New York, NY: McGraw-Hill; 2012: 1740-1752.

364. The correct answer is A, Amitriptyline.

Why is this the correct answer?

The ECG in this case demonstrates many of the classic findings seen in poisoning from a tricyclic antidepressant (TCA) such as amitriptyline — tachycardia, widening of the QRS complexes, rightward axis, and tall R wave in lead aVR (lead V1 also demonstrates Brugada syndrome–type morphology). The TCAs have sodium channel-blocking properties that, in overdose, can cause prolonged ventricular depolarization as manifested by QRS prolongation on the ECG. The right bundle branch is more susceptible to the effects of sodium channel blockade, explaining why a terminal rightward axis (large R wave in avR and large S wave in lead I) is often present in the setting of QRS prolongation. The tachycardia typically seen is multifactorial from the antimuscarinic, vasodilatory, and sympathomimetic (from reuptake inhibition of norepinephrine) effects of TCAs. Non-TCAs with sodium channel-blocking effects that can cause similar ECG changes include cocaine, diphenhydramine, lamotrigine, and venlafaxine. Sodium channel blockade leading to QRS prolongation is treated initially with intravenous sodium bicarbonate administration. Intravenous sodium bicarbonate creates systemic alkalinization and an increased concentration of sodium to reverse the process.

Why are the other choices wrong?

The ECG demonstrates QRS prolongation that, although described after the massive overdose of certain selective serotonin reuptake inhibitors (SSRIs) such as fluoxetine, is exceedingly rare.

The ECG demonstrates sinus tachycardia with QRS prolongation. The QRS prolongation is not expected (unless in the setting of ventricular tachycardia) after an overdose of phenelzine, a monoamine oxidase inhibitor (MAOI). Overdoses of MAOIs can cause a biphasic picture in which there is initial hyperadrenergic crisis followed by coma and cardiovascular collapse.

The ECG demonstrates QRS prolongation, a finding not expected after an overdose of trazodone, an atypical antidepressant (not a tricyclic). Sedation and orthostatic hypotension, the latter due to alpha-adrenergic antagonist activity, are typical in significant overdoses.

PEER REVIEW

✓ Here are the typical ECG findings seen after significant overdoses of sodium channel-blocking agents such as tricyclic antidepressants: tachycardia, QRS prolongation, and a prominent R wave in aVR.

✓ Treatment for tricyclic antidepressant overdose is intravenous administration of sodium bicarbonate.

REFERENCES
Hoffman RS, Howland MA, Lewin NA, et al. *Goldfrank's Toxicologic Emergencies*. 10th ed. New York, NY: McGraw-Hill; 2010: 974-975, 997, 1020, 1024.
Mattu A, Tabas JA, Barish RA. *Electrocardiography in Emergency Medicine*. Dallas, TX: American College of Emergency Physicians; 2007: 223-225, 232.
Tintinalli JE, Stapczynski JS, Ma OJ, et al, eds. *Tintinalli's Emergency Medicine: A Comprehensive Study Guide*. 8th ed. New York, NY: McGraw-Hill; 2012: 1215, 1220-1221, 1226.

365. The correct answer is D, Suctioning of the tracheostomy tube.

Why is this the correct answer?

Studies have estimated that 30% of emergency department visits for respiratory distress associated with a tracheostomy are caused by obstruction of the cannula. Obstruction of a tracheostomy tube secondary to a mucus plug, aspiration, blood, or granulation tissue can present as tachypnea, retractions, nasal flaring, hypoxia, cyanosis, reduced oxygen saturation, or increased secretions. Immediate treatment is best performed with preoxygenation, removal of the inner cannula, and suctioning of the stoma. The thick mucus tracheal secretions can cause a ball-valve mechanism, resulting in air trapping and hypoxia. If symptoms do not resolve after two or three attempts at suctioning, then removal of the entire cannula might be required, with repeat suctioning to clear the mucus plug. A red rubber catheter may be used as a guide to exchange the tracheostomy tube. If the appropriately sized tracheostomy tube is not available for reinsertion, then an endotracheal tube can be a temporary substitution. In older children and adults, a double-cannula tracheostomy tube with an inflatable cuff is used to prevent movement of the tube or surrounding air leak. The inner tube can be removed for cleaning and pulmonary toilet.

Why are the other choices wrong?

Common indications for a tracheostomy tube include prolonged mechanical ventilation, anatomical or traumatic obstruction of the upper airway, and difficulty controlling airway secretions. Aside from underlying secretory disorders or myopathy,

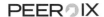

the tracheostomy procedure causes a weakness in the trachea that directly dampens the cough, and patients therefore require pulmonary therapy, chest percussion, and cough assist to routinely clear secretions. This patient, however, has an obstruction of the tracheostomy secondary to mucus plugging, and direct suctioning is required.

Patients with a tracheostomy tube can be prone to pulmonary infections or infection at the stoma; however, this patient is afebrile, making these etiologies less likely. When treating infection of a tracheostomy stoma it is important to use broad-spectrum antibiotics to include coverage for the most common infections: *Staphylococcus aureus*, *Pseudomonas*, and *Candida*.

Patients with a tracheostomy tube in place might present with exacerbation of an underlying cardiopulmonary disease process. However, these patients typically have a progressive course, and this patient had acute onset of symptoms.

PEER POINT

Complications of tracheostomy

Early complications (days to weeks)
- Hemorrhage—postoperative
- Tube dislodgment or obstruction
- Subcutaneous emphysema
- Soft tissue infection
- Pneumothorax, pneumomediastinum

Late complications (>3 weeks)
- Tracheal stenosis or malacia (granulation tissue)
- Tube dislodgment or obstruction
- Equipment failure
- Tracheoinnominate artery fistula
- Tracheoesophageal fistula
- Infection—pneumonia, aspiration

PEER REVIEW

✓ Tracheostomy tubes can get blocked with mucus, aspiration, blood, or granulation tissue.
✓ Obstruction of a tracheostomy tube can present as tachypnea, retractions, nasal flaring, hypoxia, cyanosis, reduced oxygen saturation, or increased secretions.
✓ Pharmacotherapy for an infected tracheostomy stoma: broad-spectrum antibiotics to cover *Staphylococcus aureus*, *Pseudomonas*, and *Candida*.

REFERENCES

Marx JA, Hockberger RS, Walls RM, eds. *Rosen's Emergency Medicine: Concepts and Clinical Practice*. 8th ed. St. Louis, MO: Elsevier; 2014: 2403-2405.

Roberts JR, Hedges JR, eds. *Clinical Procedures in Emergency Medicine*. 6th ed. St. Louis, MO: WB Saunders; 2013: 134-151.

366. The correct answer is D, Slipped capital femoral epiphysis.

Why is this the correct answer?

Slipped capital femoral epiphysis (SCFE) is a displacement of the femoral head. The clinical findings are hip or knee pain with decreased range of motion of the affected hip. To see it on the xray in this case, the diagnostic tool known as the Klein's line can be drawn from the lateral aspect of the femoral neck toward the capitulum. The normal finding is that the line intersects some portion of the epiphysis. If it does not, if there is posterior and inferior displacement of the femoral head, SCFE is the diagnosis. Radiographic findings are often best seen when frog-leg views are taken. Although most cases of SCFE are unilateral, up to 25% can be bilateral, so close inspection of both joints is important. Slipped capital femoral epiphysis is more commonly found in obese children, those weighing above the 95th percentile for their age. It occurs more commonly in males than females (up to 4:1) and in black males most often. The exact cause of SCFE is not known but is believed to be related to an elevated physeal angle leading to increased sheer forces. It is important to distinguish a Salter-Harris type I fracture from SCFE: the Salter-Harris type I fracture disrupts the periosteum, but SCFE does not. The incidence of SCFE is approximately 11 cases per 100,000 children. Treatment requires a surgical pinning of the slip, which, although not emergent, should be performed urgently by an orthopedist. If there is a delay in surgical correction, nonweight bearing is essential to prevent the femoral head from slipping further.

Why are the other choices wrong?

There is no evidence of fracture on the xray. Femoral neck fractures are uncommon in pediatric patients but can be seen in those who are involved in sports with repetitive stressors such as running.

The xray also does not reveal an iliac crest fracture, an injury often related to contraction against resistance such as in hurdling. It can also be seen in athletes participating in sports that involve hard running.

Legg-Calve-Perthes disease is an avascular necrosis disorder affecting the hip. Two factors from the history and presentation help distinguish it from SCFE. First, Legg-Calve-Perthes disease has a slow progression, from discomfort to limp, as opposed to the acute onset seen in SCFE. Second, Legg-Calve-Perthes disease affects children 4 to 9 years old, and children with SCFE are typically older, 8 to 15 years old. Legg-Calve-Perthes disease is associated with shorter children with normal or elevated body mass index (BMI); it is found in 1 of 1,200 children. There is a loss of blood to the femoral head that may lead to bony destruction. In some cases, the disease resolves spontaneously, but in others, it progresses to permanent destruction of the femoral head. Immediate referral to a pediatric orthopedist is warranted and can positively affect prognosis.

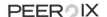

✓ Incidence of SCFE: more common in males than females, more common in obese persons, more common in black males, more likely in a child 8 to 15 years old.

✓ Knee pain can be the presenting symptom in SCFE, so perform a thorough examination and consider getting pelvic/hip xrays.

✓ Once the diagnosis of SCFE is clear, nonweight bearing is essential.

REFERENCES

Fleisher GR, Ludwig S, et al, eds. *Textbook of Pediatric Emergency Medicine.* 6th ed. Philadelphia, PA: Lippincott, Williams & Wilkins; 2010: 1361-1362, 1575-1577.

Wolfson AB, Hendey GW, Ling LJ, et al, eds. *Harwood-Nuss' Clinical Practice of Emergency Medicine.* 6th ed. Philadelphia, PA: Lippincott, Williams & Wilkins; 2014: 288-289, 1168-1172.

367. The correct answer is D, RSI and endotracheal intubation.

Why is this the correct answer?

This patient has experienced a fat embolism to the lungs as a result of his femur fracture. The action to take immediately in this case is to perform RSI with endotracheal intubation to try to correct the hypoxia and provide positive end-expiratory pressure. Bilevel positive airway pressure is contraindicated due to his altered mental status. A fat embolus causes acute rapid hemodynamic compromise with hypoxia from ARDS and systemic signs of DIC. The mortality rate associated with fat embolism is between 5% and 15%. Altered mental status can manifest as agitation or confusion initially. As the disease progresses, patients can develop petechiae, jaundice, and renal failure.

Why are the other choices wrong?

Treatment of a fat embolus includes aggressive supportive care. A fluid bolus to improve this patient's blood pressure is not incorrect, but it is not the most immediate action required.

Pulmonary embolism is high in the differential diagnosis of a patient with hypoxia and recent fracture or immobilization, but the presence of altered mental status and petechiae is more consistent with fat embolism syndrome. A CT pulmonary angiogram can exclude the diagnosis of PE; empiric heparin is not appropriate in this case.

Intralipid infusion is the treatment for lidocaine toxicity. It is not indicated in this case.

PEER REVIEW

✓ Fat embolism syndrome is a rare diagnosis, but consider it in any patient with respiratory distress following a long bone fracture or other significant orthopedic surgery or trauma.

✓ Intubation is the right course of action in a patient with fat embolism syndrome who has hypoxia and altered mental status. Supportive care is the only treatment for fat embolism syndrome.

REFERENCES

Marx JA, Hockberger RS, Walls RM, eds. *Rosen's Emergency Medicine: Concepts and Clinical Practice*. 8th ed. St. Louis, MO: Elsevier; 2014: 511-533.

Tintinalli JE, Stapczynski JS, Ma OJ, et al, eds. *Tintinalli's Emergency Medicine: A Comprehensive Study Guide*. 8th ed. New York, NY: McGraw-Hill; 2012: 1777-1791.

368. The correct answer is B, Identifying disease in infants is difficult because apnea can be the only symptom.

Why is this the correct answer?

Pertussis is the acute and highly contagious respiratory infection caused by *B. pertussis*. Infected infants do not typically develop the characteristic "whooping" cough, and they might present with apneic episodes as the sole symptom, without fever. In fact, even among adults, only one-third of patients develop the characteristic cough. Pertussis arises in three distinct sequential clinical stages: the catarrhal phase, the paroxysmal phase, and the convalescent phase. The catarrhal or prodromal phase begins after an incubation period of approximately 7 to 10 weeks and lasts approximately 1 to 2 weeks. In this early phase, the signs and symptoms include rhinorrhea, low-grade fever, malaise, and conjunctival injection, and in some, apnea. A dry cough usually begins at the end of the catarrhal phase. The paroxysmal phase begins as the fever subsides and the cough increases. Paroxysms of staccato coughing occur 40 to 50 times per day. The patient coughs repeatedly in short exhalations, followed by a single, sudden, forceful inhalation that produces the characteristic "whoop." This phase lasts 1 to 6 weeks or perhaps longer. Recovery from pertussis is gradual; the convalescent stage lasts 2 to 3 weeks. Coughing subsides, but many patients remain susceptible to other respiratory infections.

Why are the other choices wrong?

The *B. pertussis* organism is a small, aerobic, gram-negative coccobacilli that occurs singly or in pairs. It adheres preferentially to ciliated respiratory epithelial cells. The organism elaborates several toxins that act locally and systemically. These toxins include pertussis toxin, dermonecrotic toxin, adenylate cyclase toxin, and tracheal cytotoxin. *B. pertussis* does not invade beyond the submucosal layer in the respiratory tract and is almost never recovered in the bloodstream.

Infectivity is greatest during the catarrhal phase (not the paroxysmal phase). The catarrhal phase begins after a 7- to 10-week incubation period and lasts approximately 1 to 2 weeks. During this time, the disease is clinically indistinguishable from other upper respiratory tract infections.

Vaccination and previous infection do not confer lifelong immunity. Patients require five doses of the DTaP vaccine at ages 2, 4, and 6 months, then again between 15 and 18 months, and between 4 and 6 years. Then every 10 years a booster with Tdap is required to continue immunity. A booster immunization might be required sooner than every 10 years if the patient is exposed to tetanus. Since 1990, the number of *B. pertussis* cases has increased, particularly in the adolescent population, most likely as a result of waning immunity and lack of compliance with episodic booster immunization recommendations.

PEER POINT

From the CDC, the disease progression of pertussis

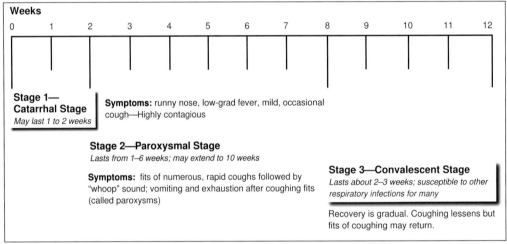

PEER Point 31

PEER REVIEW

✓ Infectivity with *Bordetella pertussis* is greatest during the catarrhal phase of the disease.

✓ Only a third of all adults with pertussis develop the characteristic cough.

✓ Whooping cough can look a lot like any other upper respiratory tract infection in early disease.

✓ Infants with pertussis might have a history of apneic episodes as their only symptom, and they rarely "whoop."

REFERENCES

Marx JA, Hockberger RS, Walls RM, eds. *Rosen's Emergency Medicine: Concepts and Clinical Practice.* 8th ed. St. Louis, MO: Elsevier; 2014: 1693-1717.

Tintinalli JE, Stapczynski JS, Ma OJ, et al, eds. *Tintinalli's Emergency Medicine: A Comprehensive Study Guide.* 8th ed. New York, NY: McGraw-Hill; 2012: 440-445, 741-747.

369. The correct answer is B, Enoxaparin 1 mg/kg subcutaneously.

Why is this the correct answer?

Pulmonary embolism is the likely diagnosis in this case given the patient's history and physical examination. There are also the postpartum and postsurgery risk factors to consider, in addition to tachycardia, tachypnea, and borderline hypoxia. Appropriate emergency department pharmacotherapy is subcutaneous enoxaparin (1 mg/kg) or heparin bolus (80 units/kg) followed by a heparin drip (18 units/kg/hr). Both treatments are considered equally effective in the acute management of PE. Enoxaparin is a reasonable choice for a patient with normal renal function, but heparin should be considered if bleeding is anticipated and rapid reversal becomes necessary.

Why are the other choices wrong?

Alteplase might have a role in the treatment of massive PE, but in this patient who is hemodynamically stable, it is not indicated.

Magnesium sulfate is the treatment of pre-eclampsia, not PE.

Warfarin is indicated for the long-term treatment of PE, but it is not the first-line treatment to start in the emergency department.

PEER REVIEW

✓ Thrombolytic agents might be indicated in massive PE but are not recommended in stable patients.
✓ Either heparin or enoxaparin is first-line treatment for PE in the emergency department.

REFERENCES

Marx JA, Hockberger RS, Walls RM, eds. *Rosen's Emergency Medicine: Concepts and Clinical Practice*. 8th ed. St. Louis, MO: Elsevier; 2014: 1157-1169.

Tintinalli JE, Stapczynski JS, Ma OJ, et al, eds. *Tintinalli's Emergency Medicine: A Comprehensive Study Guide*. 8th ed. New York, NY: McGraw-Hill; 2012: 327, 398.

370. The correct answer is B, Contrast enema.

Why is this the correct answer?

The dermatologic findings in this case are consistent with Henoch-Schönlein purpura (HSP). Because the patient also has, as described by the mother, intermittent abdominal pain and sleepiness, a diagnosis of intussusception should be considered, for which contrast enema is both diagnostic and therapeutic. Henoch-Schönlein purpura can start off as a red and raised rash with an almost urticarial appearance and then progress to the classic purpuric, blue-purple coloration with bruising and tenderness. Associated joint pain or abdominal pain is common. Intussusception is among the complications of HSP, and the symptoms described by the mother provide clues to the abdominal issue: episodic pain associated with increased sleepiness.

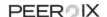

Why are the other choices wrong?

A chest xray is an important consideration in a patient presenting with abdominal pain, but because the patient had no upper respiratory findings, fever, or abnormal pulse oximetry reading, it is unlikely to be helpful.

A Meckel scan should be considered in patients presenting with signs of a Meckel diverticulum, which includes abdominal pain. However, Meckel diverticulitis is usually associated with painless rectal bleeding.

An upper GI series is useful to determine if a patient has a bowel obstruction or volvulus. But the use of an upper GI series is limited by the availability of trained radiologists to perform and interpret the study in pediatric patients. In this case, intussusception is a more likely underlying cause than volvulus given the presence of HSP.

PEER REVIEW

- ✓ The rash of Henoch-Schönlein purpura progresses from erythema to the more classic purpura.
- ✓ Illnesses associated Henoch-Schönlein purpura include intussusception and renal disease.
- ✓ A contrast enema is both diagnostic and therapeutic for intussusception.

REFERENCES

Fleisher GR, Ludwig S, et al, eds. *Textbook of Pediatric Emergency Medicine*. 6th ed. Philadelphia, PA: Lippincott, Williams & Wilkins; 2010: 421-428; 1530.

Wolfson AB, Hendey GW, Ling LJ, et al, eds. *Harwood-Nuss' Clinical Practice of Emergency Medicine*. 6th ed. Philadelphia, PA: Lippincott, Williams & Wilkins; 2014: 842-843; https://www.inkling.com/read/wolfson-harwood-nuss-clinical-practice-emergency-med-6.

371. The correct answer is C, Persistent asystole despite raising core temperature above 32°C (89.6°F).

Why is this the correct answer?

The adage "you're not dead until you're warm and dead" applies to the resuscitation of patients suffering from primary hypothermia (hypothermia directly from a cold environment). It is generally agreed in this situation that if a patient is warmed to a temperature above 32°C (89.6°F) and has persistent asystole, that further resuscitative efforts are futile and can be stopped. But this does not apply to patients suffering cardiac arrest for a different reason who present with secondary hypothermia. Patients with potentially survivable severe hypothermia can appear dead. They can have fixed and dilated pupils, and it can be very difficult to detect a pulse even if one is present. Rigidity mimicking rigor mortis can also be present.

Why are the other choices wrong?

Fixed and dilated pupils can be present in a patient with severe hypothermia in whom successful resuscitation is possible. Patients with severe hypothermia can appear dead, but resuscitative efforts should not stop based on this finding.

Bradycardia is common in patients with severe hypothermia, and even if it is extreme, it does not predict nonsurvivability. Even the presence of initial asystole does not predict nonsurvivability.

An elevated serum potassium level in the setting of primary hypothermia reflects cell death and has prognostic significance. It is not universally agreed on what potassium concentration to use as a cutoff for resuscitation futility; however, it is higher than 6.5 mmol/L. Because the highest recorded serum potassium in a patient successfully resuscitated was 11.8 mmol/L, some recommend using 12 mmol/L as a cutoff to terminate resuscitation.

PEER POINT

"You're not dead until you're warm and dead" applies to the resuscitation of patients suffering from primary hypothermia.

PEER REVIEW

✓ It's appropriate to stop resuscitative efforts in primary hypothermia when there is persistent asystole even after you've raised the core temperature above 32°C (89.6°F).

✓ Patients with potentially survivable severe hypothermia can have fixed and dilated pupils.

REFERENCES

Brown DJ, Brugger H, Boyd J, Paal P. Accidental hypothermia. *N Engl J Med.* 2012;367(20):1930-1938.

Tintinalli JE, Stapczynski JS, Ma OJ, et al, eds. *Tintinalli's Emergency Medicine: A Comprehensive Study Guide.* 8th ed. New York, NY: McGraw-Hill; 2012: 1357-1360.

372. The correct answer is B, Discharge home with precautions to return if he has increased pain.

Why is this the correct answer?

In this case, the patient had an exposure to low voltage. He did not lose consciousness, and he has a normal physical examination and a normal ECG. Appropriate disposition is to provide reassurance and discharge him home with return precautions. The voltage a patient is exposed to and the corresponding current that is transmitted are the major determinants of what complications might ensue. A home electrical outlet, which this patient was exposed to, is low voltage (Australia and Europe 240 volts; United States 120 volts). Low-voltage exposures, depending on the time of exposure and current path, are capable of inducing both immediate (burn injuries, dysrhythmias, respiratory arrest) and delayed (compartment syndrome) injuries. However, if there is no evidence of immediate complications, delayed complications are extremely unlikely. Patients exposed to higher voltages (>600 volts), on the other hand, are at risk for significant complications even in the absence of presenting complications. They should undergo laboratory testing performed (CBC, chemistry, CK, INR), telemetry, and serial examinations, particularly looking for the development of compartment syndrome and rhabdomyolysis.

Why are the other choices wrong?

Admission is not needed. The patient was exposed to low voltage from a home electrical outlet, had no loss of consciousness, and his examination and ECG are normal. It is extremely unlikely that he will develop subsequent complications such as compartment syndrome, dysrhythmias, or rhabdomyolysis. Had the same patient sustained an exposure to more than 600 volts, admission for continuous telemetry and serial arm examinations would be appropriate.

Emergency department observation is not needed either based on the exposure and the lack of worrisome findings. Again, it is extremely unlikely that he will develop compartment syndrome, dysrhythmias, or rhabdomyolysis.

Laboratory testing is not needed given that the voltage the patient was exposed to was 120 volts and he did not lose consciousness and he has a normal ECG and no related abnormalities on physical examination. Under different circumstances such as exposure to more than 600 volts laboratory testing would be indicated.

PEER REVIEW

- ✓ Home electrical outlets are low voltage, and asymptomatic patients who have been shocked by them aren't likely to develop major complications.
- ✓ High-voltage exposures are a different story: exposure to more than 600 volts can lead to delayed complications — compartment syndrome, dysrhythmias, and rhabdomyolysis.

REFERENCES

Tintinalli JE, Stapczynski JS, Ma OJ, et al, eds. *Tintinalli's Emergency Medicine: A Comprehensive Study Guide.* 8th ed. New York, NY: McGraw-Hill; 2012: 1411-1414.

Wolfson AB, Hendey GW, Ling LJ, et al, eds. *Harwood-Nuss' Clinical Practice of Emergency Medicine.* 6th ed. Philadelphia, PA: Lippincott, Williams & Wilkins; 2014: 1527-1529.

373. The correct answer is D, Urine culture.

Why is this the correct answer?

The American Academy of Pediatrics characterizes bronchiolitis as rhinitis, tachypnea, wheezing, cough, crackles, use of accessory muscles, and/or nasal flaring in a child younger than 24 months. This patient presents with a classic history of bronchiolitis but also has fever. Although the risk of bacteremia is low (<1%) in this group of children (younger than 3 months), the continued risk of urinary tract infection warrants consideration. The studies indicate there is an approximately 3% chance of a concomitant urinary tract infection in infants with respiratory syncytial virus bronchiolitis. The evaluation of a patient with bronchiolitis is based on a complete evaluation of past medical history, specifically, any issue with gestational age and/or perinatal complications, immunodeficiency, or history of cardiac or lung disease.

Why are the other choices wrong?

Because the risk for bacteremia is so low, blood culture is not necessary.

Blood work, including CBC count with differential, is not advised in this clinical scenario.

Radiographs are not routinely needed in the evaluation of bronchiolitis, much less in a child with a normal oxygen saturation level who is in no distress. The risk of infiltrates seems to increase in patients with oxygen saturation levels below 92%, but this concern should be weighed against the risks of unnecessary imaging. There is support in the literature that a child with respiratory syncytial virus and an infiltrate on radiograph has no difference in outcome when antibiotics are used.

PEER REVIEW

✓ Fever is common with bronchiolitis, but consider other sources of infection, especially a urinary tract infection.
✓ Radiography is generally not needed in a child if the oxygen saturation level is above 92%.

REFERENCES

Ralston S, Hill V, Waters A. Occult Serious Bacterial Infection in Infants Younger Than 60 to 90 Days With BronchiolitisA Systematic Review. *Arch Pediatr Adolesc Med.* 2011;165(10):951-956. doi:10.1001/archpediatrics.2011.155.

Ralston SL, Lieberthal AS, Meissner HC, et al. Clinical practice guideline: the diagnosis, management, and prevention of bronchiolitis. *Pediatrics.* 2014;134(5):e1474-e1502.

Wolfson AB, Hendey GW, Ling LJ, et al, eds. *Harwood-Nuss' Clinical Practice of Emergency Medicine.* 6th ed. Philadelphia, PA: Lippincott, Williams & Wilkins; 2014: 1230.

374. The correct answer is C, Penicillin.

Why is this the correct answer?

Scarlet fever is an exotoxin-mediated illness caused by infection with *Streptococcus*. It occurs primarily in children. The rash is distinctive — red and rough with a sandpaper-like texture because of the multitude of pinhead-sized lesions. It begins on the face and upper trunk and spreads rapidly within 12 to 48 hours of the start of fever, chills, malaise, and sore throat. Other classic findings of scarlet fever are a red, beefy tongue (strawberry tongue), erythematous lesions or petechiae on the palate (Forchheimer spots), capillary fragility causing petechiae in the flexural surfaces (pastia lines), and facial flushing with circumoral pallor. The rash typically resolves in 1 week followed by desquamation, especially of the palms and soles. Early complications of scarlet fever include infection of lymph nodes, tonsils,

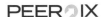

middle ear, and respiratory tract. Late complications include rheumatic fever and acute glomerulonephritis. Treatment is 10 days of oral penicillin VK 50 mg/kg per day (40,000 to 80,000 units) in four divided doses in children or 250 mg four times a day. Intramuscular benzathine penicillin (given as bicillin C-R) is another option; dosing is 300,000 units in patients weighing less than 30 pounds, 600,000 units in patients weighing 31 to 60 pounds, 900,000 units in patients weighing 61 to 90 pounds, and 1.2 million units in patients weighing more than 90 pounds. In patients allergic to penicillin, the treatment is 10 days of erythromycin, 250 mg four times a day in adults or 40 mg/kg per day in children. Other macrolides and certain other cephalosporins may also be used.

Why are the other choices wrong?

Diphenhydramine is an antihistamine, and it would work well for a rash caused by an allergic reaction. But the rash that develops with scarlet fever is exotoxin mediated, not a hypersensitivity reaction: its source, *Streptococcus*, is treated with antibiotics.

The tetracycline family of medications is used to treat several conditions associated with rash, including Rocky Mountain spotted fever and Lyme disease. There is a high resistance of *Streptococcus* to tetracycline, so doxycycline is not a good choice for treatment of scarlet fever. Although many physicians have been reluctant to use tetracyclines in the treatment of children because of concern for dental staining, this outcome has been shown to be less serious than previously thought.

Sulfamethoxazole-trimethoprim is a sulfonamide and is not recommended for treatment of pharyngitis. There is a high level of resistance to sulfonamides for group A beta-hemolytic strep, and it does not seem to eradicate the bacteria in the posterior pharynx even when the culture indicates there might be appropriate sensitivity.

PEER POINT

Skin lesion descriptors and definitions
- Bulla — Fluid-filled circumscribed lesion larger than 0.5 cm in diameter
- Crusts — Dried blood, serum, or purulent exudate on skin surface
- Ecchymosis — Purpura larger than 1 cm
- Erosion — Defect in epidermis only; occurs from physical abrasions, rupture of vesicles and bullae
- Erythema — Red skin appearance due to vasodilation of dermal blood vessels, blanchable
- Induration — Dermal thickening that is palpably thick and firm
- Lichenification — Visible and palpable epidermal thickening with accentuated skin markings
- Macule — Nonpalpable circumscribed area of skin color change
- Nodule — Superficial, elevated, solid lesion larger than 0.5 cm in diameter

- Papule — Superficial, elevated, solid lesion smaller than 0.5 cm in diameter
- Patch — A barely elevated plaque
- Petechiae — Purpura smaller than 3 mm
- Plaque — Plateaulike elevation above the skin surface occupying a large surface area compared with its height
- Purpura — Any skin eruption resulting from extravasated blood; nonblanchable
- Pustule — Vesicle filled with purulent material
- Scales — Flakes of stratum corneum
- Telangiectasia — Small, blanchable superficial capillaries
- Ulcer — Defect that extends into dermis or deeper
- Vesicle — Fluid-filled circumscribed lesion smaller than 0.5 cm in diameter
- Wheal — Papule or plaque of dermal edema

PEER REVIEW

- ✓ The rash associated with scarlet fever is, indeed, red. And it's rough like sandpaper.
- ✓ The scarlet fever rash begins on the face and upper trunk and spreads rapidly, and desquamation occurs after the illness resolves.
- ✓ Treatment of choice for scarlet fever: penicillin.

REFERENCES

Adams JG, Barton ED, Collings J, et al, eds. *Emergency Medicine: Clinical Essentials.* 2nd ed. Philadelphia, PA: Saunders; 2013: 153-154.

Marx JA, Hockberger RS, Walls RM, eds. *Rosen's Emergency Medicine: Concepts and Clinical Practice.* 8th ed. St. Louis, MO: Elsevier; 2014: 1558-1585.

Shulman ST, Bisno AL, Clegg HW, et al. Clinical practice guideline for the diagnosis and management of group A streptococcal pharyngitis: 2012 update by the Infectious Diseases Society of America. *Clin Infect Dis.* 2012;55(10):e86-e102.

Tintinalli JE, Stapczynski JS, Ma OJ, et al, eds. *Tintinalli's Emergency Medicine: A Comprehensive Study Guide.* 8th ed. New York, NY: McGraw-Hill; 2012: 934-953.

375. The correct answer is C, Decreased protein C.

Why is this the correct answer?

Because the liver synthesizes almost all proteins and factors related to coagulation, liver disease causes an impairment of coagulation. Although contradictory, liver disease causes both an increased risk of bleeding because of the decrease in procoagulant proteins and a prothrombotic state because of the decrease in anticoagulant proteins of protein C and antithrombin also synthesized in the liver. This is the reason that patients with advanced liver disease are at increased risk for DVT.

Why are the other choices wrong?

Although many of the proteins and coagulation factors are synthesized in the liver, factor VIII and von Willebrand factor are not. That means that a decrease in factor VIII is not expected with impaired coagulation in patients with advanced liver disease.

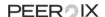

Coagulation factors, including the vitamin K dependent factors, are synthesized in the liver, thus causing an increase in the INR, not a decrease.

Synthesis of coagulation factors in the liver causes an increase in the PT, too, not a decrease. This is typically seen in patients with advanced liver disease, and testing both INR and PT can help determine the severity of disease.

PEER REVIEW

✓ In advanced liver disease, PT and INR increase, while protein C and antithrombin III activity decrease. That's why these patients are at risk for both bleeding and thrombosis.

✓ The vitamin K factors are synthesized by the liver; identifying PT and INR abnormalities can help you assess the severity of liver disease.

✓ Factor VIII and von Willebrand factor are not synthesized in the liver.

REFERENCES

Marx JA, Hockberger RS, Walls RM, eds. *Rosen's Emergency Medicine: Concepts and Clinical Practice*. 8th ed. St. Louis, MO: Elsevier; 2014: 1186-1204.e1.

Tintinalli JE, Stapczynski JS, Ma OJ, et al, eds. *Tintinalli's Emergency Medicine: A Comprehensive Study Guide*. 8th ed. New York, NY: McGraw-Hill; 2012: 1491-1496.

376. The correct answer is C, Normal saline.

Why is this the correct answer?

Acute chest syndrome, defined as a new infiltrate on xray associated with fever, cough, dyspnea, wheezing, or chest pain, is the leading cause of death in sickle cell patients. The approach to treating acute chest syndrome starts with oxygen, hydration, antibiotics, and analgesia. Dehydration should be treated right away because it can further the sickling process. Starting fluid hydration is important to decrease the propensity for cells to sickle. Antibiotics are typically targeted toward atypical pathogens such as *Chlamydia* and *Mycoplasma*. In more severe cases, exchange transfusion can be considered, allowing for a decrease in the number of sickled cells and reticulocytosis. In the same vein, blood transfusions are also frequently used in sickle cell disease and acute chest syndrome and are frequently lifesaving.

Why are the other choices wrong?

Fibrinolysis can be a treatment in sickle cell disease for patients presenting with an acute thrombosis such as PE, but PE is associated with acute chest syndrome less than 5% of the time. The possible increased risk of anticoagulation or fibrinolysis in sickle cell patients with anemia should be considered.

Hydroxyurea is frequently used in sickle cell disease but not as an acute treatment for acute chest syndrome. Rather, it is used in an attempt to prevent a pain crisis and acute chest syndrome by stimulating the production of fetal hemoglobin.

Phlebotomy is the treatment of choice for polycythemia, not sickle cell anemia.

PEER REVIEW

- ✓ What is acute chest syndrome? A new infiltrate on chest xray combined with fever, dyspnea, chest pain, cough, or wheezing.
- ✓ Treatment for acute chest syndrome includes analgesia, hydration, oxygenation, and antibiotics.
- ✓ Sometimes blood transfusion and exchange transfusion are warranted in acute chest syndrome, especially in more severe cases.

REFERENCES

Marx JA, Hockberger RS, Walls RM, eds. *Rosen's Emergency Medicine: Concepts and Clinical Practice*. 8th ed. St. Louis, MO: Elsevier; 2014: 1586-1605.e2.

Tintinalli JE, Stapczynski JS, Ma OJ, et al, eds. *Tintinalli's Emergency Medicine: A Comprehensive Study Guide*. 8th ed. New York, NY: McGraw-Hill; 2012: 1504-1512.

377. The correct answer is B, More aggressive.

Why is this the correct answer?

Africanized bees known colloquially as "killer" bees are hybrids of African honeybees that escaped from laboratories in Brazil and are currently present in most of the southern regions of the United States. The primary distinction between Africanized bees and the more common North American variety is that the Africanized bees are much more aggressive. With a perceived threat, often to the hive, many more bees respond than would those of the North American variety. As a result, a person can sustain a massive number of stings that can lead to rhabdomyolysis and acute kidney injury. Hospital admission is appropriate for patients who have a large numbers of stings.

Why are the other choices wrong?

The venom potencies of Africanized "killer" bees and North American honeybees are thought to be equivalent. The danger lies in the Africanized bees' lower threshold for provocation, heightened response, and resulting increased number of bees that will sting.

Both Africanized bees and North American honeybees are capable of only one sting. When they sting, the barbed stinger apparatus is dislodged from the bee's abdomen, and the bee eviscerates itself. Vespids such as wasps, hornets, and yellow jackets have the ability to withdraw the stinger and sting multiple times. Bumblebees can also sting more than once.

The risk of anaphylaxis is not higher from the sting of an Africanized bee sting than from a North American bee, nor is it related to the number of stings. Although anaphylaxis is the major systemic threat to an individual from most bee stings, in the case of a massive number of stings from an Africanized bee, systemic toxicity results from a direct venom effect.

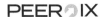

PEER REVIEW

✓ Africanized bees have the same type of venom as other honeybees, but they attack with less provocation and with greater numbers, leading to a larger number of stings.

REFERENCES

Hoffman RS, Howland MA, Lewin NA, et al, eds. *Goldfrank's Toxicologic Emergencies*. 10th ed. New York, NY: McGraw-Hill; 2015: 1472-1473.

Tintinalli JE, Stapczynski JS, Ma OJ, et al, eds. *Tintinalli's Emergency Medicine: A Comprehensive Study Guide*. 8th ed. New York, NY: McGraw-Hill; 2012: 1371-1373.

378. The correct answer is D, Rattlesnake.

Why is this the correct answer?

In this case, the patient has a classic presentation and manifestations of a rattlesnake envenomation, both localized (fang marks, localized progressive swelling and pain) and hematologic (hypofibrinogenemia, thrombocytopenia). Rattlesnake venom is a complex mixture of toxins that can cause local tissue injury, hematologic abnormalities, and neuromuscular effects. A significant number of bites (approximately one-fourth) are considered "dry" in that no local or systemic signs of envenomation occur. Manifestations of envenomation can be quite variable and depend on multiple factors, including the location of the bite, the amount of venom released, and the species of rattlesnake. Localized pain and significant swelling are common. Ecchymosis from bleeding into the skin at the bite site can occur, and hemorrhagic bullae might develop. Myonecrosis can also occur. Hematologic effects can include fibrinolysis and/or thrombocytopenia. Neurologic effects can include local or systemic muscle fasciculations. Initial management of significant or progressive tissue injury and/or severe hypofibrinogenemia or thrombocytopenia is antivenom administration.

Why are the other choices wrong?

Cobras are not native to the United States, and bite victims do not present with coagulopathy in the absence of neurologic effects. The hallmarks of envenomation are immediate pain at the bite site and neurologic dysfunction, including cranial nerve dysfunction, and generalized weakness that can progress to flaccid paralysis. Bronchorrhea, salivation, and vomiting might occur due to parasympathetic stimulation. Edema and skin changes can progress at the site of the bite as well. Coagulopathy is a rare complication from bites of the spitting cobra types.

Coral snakes have small fangs, and bite victims do not present with significant soft tissue damage or coagulopathies. Coral snake venom has primarily neurotoxic effects that can cause respiratory failure. Coral snakes can be identified by black, red, and yellow rings in which the red and yellow rings make contact. "Red on yellow kills a fellow; red on black, venom lacks."

King snakes are nonvenomous, and their bites do not result in venom-induced local tissue damage or coagulopathy. The king snake's physical appearance resembles that of a coral snake except that red rings on the king snake make contact with the black rings. Again, "Red on yellow kills a fellow; red on black, venom lacks."

PEER POINT

Snake rhyme

"Red on yellow kills a fellow" — coral snake

"Red on black, venom lacks" — king snake

PEER REVIEW

✓ Rattlesnake envenomation is characterized by local tissue damage and can be accompanied by hematologic and neurologic effects.

✓ About 25% of rattlesnake bites are dry — no local or systemic signs of envenomation occur.

REFERENCES

Hoffman RS, Howland MA, Lewin NA, et al, eds. *Goldfrank's Toxicologic Emergencies*. 10th ed. New York, NY: McGraw-Hill; 2015: 1537-1546.

Tintinalli JE, Stapczynski JS, Ma OJ, et al, eds. *Tintinalli's Emergency Medicine: A Comprehensive Study Guide*. 8th ed. New York, NY: McGraw-Hill; 2012: 1379-1382.

379. The correct answer is A, Fat emulsion.

Why is this the correct answer?

Administration of intravenous fat emulsion (also referred to as intralipid) should be strongly considered in a patient suffering severe systemic toxicity from a local anesthetic agent such as in this case. Use of fat emulsion as an antidote has been studied most extensively with local anesthetics. Various animal models have demonstrated clear benefit (although not universally so) of fat emulsion administration for systemic toxicity from local anesthetics. Multiple human case reports also suggest benefit with local anesthetics, although there is undoubtedly some reporting bias. Some adverse effects have been reported, but they are not frequent and are typically minor. There are multiple theories as to the mechanism responsible for how lipid emulsion can reverse toxicity. The most prevailing is that lipid emulsion is able to sequester lipid-soluble drugs away from the organ where toxicity is occurring (lipid sink theory). Administration can also be considered in patients suffering toxicity from beta blockers, calcium channel blockers, and tricyclic antidepressants in which standard therapies are not working. Current suggested dosing is a bolus dose of 1.5 mL/kg of 20% lipid emulsion followed by an infusion of 0.25 mL/kg per hour for 30 to 60 minutes.

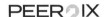

Why are the other choices wrong?

Hydroxocobalamin is a precursor to vitamin B12 that is an effective antidote for cyanide poisoning. It has no known role in the treatment of local anesthetic agent poisoning, which this patient is suffering from.

Pyridoxine (vitamin B6) is used to treat acute toxicity (convulsions and altered level of consciousness) from isoniazid poisoning. Like hydroxocobalamin, it has no known role in the treatment of local anesthetic poisoning.

Sodium nitrite can be used in conjunction with thiosulfate to treat cyanide poisoning. But it has no known role in the treatment of a poisoning such as the one presented in this case.

PEER POINT

Toxic intravenous doses of local anesthetic agents, mg/kg, minimum

- Bupivacaine — 1.6
- Chloroprocaine — 22.8
- Etidocaine — 3.4
- Lidocaine — 6.4
- Mepivacaine — 9.8
- Procaine — 19.2
- Tetracaine — 2.5

Adapted from Goldfrank's Toxicologic Emergencies 10e, Table 67-2

PEER REVIEW

- ✓ If you're treating a patient who has severe systemic toxicity from a local anesthetic agent, strongly consider administering fat emulsion intravenously.
- ✓ You can also consider intravenous fat emulsion in patients suffering toxicity from beta blockers, calcium channel blockers, and tricyclic antidepressants when standard therapies aren't working.

REFERENCES

Hoffman RS, Howland MA, Lewin NA, et al, eds. *Goldfrank's Toxicologic Emergencies.* 10th ed. New York, NY: McGraw-Hill; 2015: 921-930.

Tintinalli JE, Stapczynski JS, Ma OJ, et al, eds. *Tintinalli's Emergency Medicine: A Comprehensive Study Guide.* 8th ed. New York, NY: McGraw-Hill; 2012: 238-240.

380. The correct answer is B, Onset of clinical effects is slower with ingestions than with inhalation.

Why is this the correct answer?

As more states have legalized marijuana in the United States and more edible marijuana-containing products have become available, the number of emergency department visits for marijuana intoxication has increased. One of the dangers of the various edible products is that the clinical effects are slower in onset than they are with inhalation of marijuana. Users, therefore, thinking they have not ingested enough of the product to achieve the desired effects, might consume more prior to symptom onset and unwittingly overdose. Additionally, there has been an increasing number of accidental pediatric exposures. Clinical effects of marijuana intoxication can include conjunctival injection, euphoria, motor incoordination, sedation, slurred speech, and tachycardia. Coma and psychosis are rare, although possible.

Why are the other choices wrong?

Conjunctival injection is common (not rare) with marijuana intoxication.

A positive cannabinoid test on a rapid urine drugs of abuse screen (similar to other potential positives on the test) confirms potential exposure only, not intoxication. False-positive testing is a problem with urine drugs of abuse screens and can occur for the cannabinoid test. Some medications including, NSAIDs and promethazine, can cause inaccurate false-positive testing for cannabinoid. Only comprehensive testing can confirm exposure. Further, true-positive testing confirms exposure to a drug only and not actual intoxication. With chronic use of marijuana, cannabinoids can be detected up to 1 month following use. Urine drugs of abuse testing for cannabinoids is potentially more clinically helpful in children who have consistent manifestations of intoxication.

Transient psychosis is a known but rare (not common) complication that occurs in some individuals after using marijuana.

PEER REVIEW

✓ The clinical effects of marijuana come on more slowly when users ingest it rather than smoke it.

✓ A positive result on a urine drugs of abuse screen for cannabinoids or other drugs does not equate with intoxication from that drug.

REFERENCES

Hoffman RS, Howland MA, Lewin NA, et al, eds. *Goldfrank's Toxicologic Emergencies*. 10th ed. New York, NY: McGraw-Hill; 2015: 1042-1048.

Tintinalli JE, Stapczynski JS, Ma OJ, et al, eds. *Tintinalli's Emergency Medicine: A Comprehensive Study Guide*. 8th ed. New York, NY: McGraw-Hill; 2012: 1263-1264.

381. The correct answer is C, Discharge with instructions to get follow-up care and not return to play.

Why is this the correct answer?

Given the mechanism of injury and the presenting symptoms in this case, concussion is likely. The patient should be kept out of sports until he is evaluated by his primary care physician. If the primary care physician is uncomfortable with concussion monitoring and follow-up, the patient should be referred to a specialist. The CDC has specific guidelines on when a specialist is warranted, as follows: if the symptoms worsen, if they have not resolved in 10 to 14 days, or if the patient has a history of multiple concussions or risk factors for prolonged recovery such as headache syndromes, depression, or mood or developmental disorders.

Why are the other choices wrong?

In general, young athletes with concussion should not leave an emergency department and return to practice or play the same day, nor should a future return to practice or play-date be given at the time of an emergency department visit. There are progressive steps that are taken to return to sports, with monitoring for symptoms and cognitive function along the way by the physician providing follow-up care. Athletes should not progress to the next steps unless they are asymptomatic at the current level.

Because the patient is 16, either the PECARN or the ACEP head injury guideline can be used to help decide if a head CT is warranted. The ACEP guideline applies to persons 16 years old and older, and PECARN to patients younger than 18 years with a GCS score of 14 or 15 and an injury less than 24 hours old. Based on this patient's injury and symptoms, a head CT is not warranted by either guideline.

Although the appropriate length of time to observe a child with a concussion in the emergency department for worsening signs and symptoms has not been definitively established, the PECARN authors recommend a 4- to 6-hour observation period; the likelihood of missing a delayed clinically important traumatic brain injury during this time seems to be rare. Inpatient observation, unless the family is not able to observe the patient at home and follow appropriate instructions, is generally not necessary.

PEER POINT

Is it a concussion?

According to the 2012 Consensus Statement on Concussion in Sport (Zurich conference)

A concussion is:

- A brain injury
- A complex pathophysiologic process that affects the brain
- Induced by biomechanical forces

A concussion is caused by:

- A direct blow to the head, face, or neck or some other part of the body that transmits an impulsive force to the head

A concussion causes:

- Rapid-onset short-lived neurologic function impairment that resolves on its own
- Neuropathologic changes
- Clinical symptoms that reflect functional disturbance rather than structural injury
- Graded clinical symptoms that might or might not include loss of consciousness

Suspect concussion if evaluation of the patient reveals one or more of the following:

- Symptoms, including somatic (headache, nausea, off balance), cognitive (" in a fog," slow), or emotional (rapidly changing)
- Physical signs such as loss of consciousness, amnesia
- Behavior changes such as irritability
- Cognitive impairment such as slowed reaction times
- Sleep disturbance such as insomnia

PEER REVIEW

- ✓ If you're treating a young athlete who has a concussion, resist the temptation — and the parents' pleading — to give a timeframe for safe return to play.
- ✓ When does a patient need a concussion specialist? If symptoms worsen, if they don't resolve in 10 to 14 days, or if the patient has a history of multiple concussions or risk factors for prolonged recovery.

REFERENCES

Centers for Disease Control and Prevention. HEADS UP to Health Care Providers. http://www.cdc.gov/headsup/providers. Accessed January 12, 2017.

Legome EL, Wittels KA, Rogers RL, et al. Imaging in Patients With Mild Traumatic Brain Injury. Dallas, TX: American College of Emergency Physicians; 2015.

Wolfson AB, Hendey GW, Ling LJ, et al, eds. *Harwood-Nuss' Clinical Practice of Emergency Medicine*. 6th ed. Philadelphia, PA: Lippincott, Williams & Wilkins; 2014: 1189-1191.

382. The correct answer is D, Treatment of DVT.

Why is this the correct answer?

Since 2010, the FDA has approved four new anticoagulant drugs, including three factor Xa inhibitors: rivaroxaban, apixaban, and edoxaban. The fourth is a direct thrombin inhibitor, dabigatran. All four of these anticoagulant agents have been approved for the treatment and prevention of venous thromboembolism and nonvalvular atrial fibrillation. The advantage of using one of these new drugs rather than warfarin is not needing blood levels/INR checks and standardized dosing. This ease of use for the patient has prompted an increase in prescribing by physicians in an attempt to increase compliance and get more predictable results. The reversal of these agents is an evolving field of study and an important one for emergency physicians to stay abreast of. At this time, the FDA has approved idarucizumab as a reversal agent for dabigatran, and studies are still being performed on the antidote for the factor Xa inhibitors. Prothrombin complex concentrate is frequently used to reverse the effects of those blockers.

Why are the other choices wrong?

The four newer anticoagulant medications are not indicated to prevent blood clots in patients who have prosthetic heart valves because they do not yet have proven benefit preventing thromboembolic complications from mechanical valves. Several studies are in progress to study the new novel oral anticoagulants, but the only published trial for dabigatran showed an increase in complications when used in prosthetic heart valves.

Nonvalvular atrial fibrillation is a reason to use one of the new oral anticoagulant medications — to prevent potential clot formation. But these newer medications are not indicated for the prevention of atrial fibrillation itself.

The new oral anticoagulant agents do not act as thrombolytic agents: they only inhibit coagulation. Thus they are not useful for treatment in an acute ischemic event such as stroke.

PEER REVIEW

✓ Indications for the newer oral anticoagulant agents: nonvalvular atrial fibrillation and the treatment and prevention of venous thromboembolism.

✓ Advantages of the newer oral anticoagulants: equal efficacy compared to warfarin in the prevention of clot formation, and they don't require frequent INR checks.

REFERENCES

Leung LLK, eds. Direct oral anticoagulants: Dosing and adverse effects. UptoDate. Available at http://www.uptodate.com/contents/direct-oral-anticoagulants-dosing-and-adverse-effects. Accessed January 18, 2017.

Pollack CV Jr., Reilly PA, Eikelboom J, et al. Idarucizumab for dabigatran reversal. N Engl J Med. 2015;373(6):511-520. doi:10.1056/NEJMoa1502000.

Shazly A, Afifi A. RE-ALIGN: First trial of novel oral anticoagulant in patients with mechanical heart valves – The search continues. Glob Cardiol Sci Pract. 2014;2014(1):88-89. doi:10.5339/gcsp.2014.13.

Tintinalli JE, Stapczynski JS, Ma OJ, et al, eds. Tintinalli's Emergency Medicine: A Comprehensive Study Guide. 8th ed. New York, NY: McGraw-Hill; 2012: 1524-1534.

383. The correct answer is D, Piloerection.

Why is this the correct answer?

Opioid withdrawal is characterized by a constellation of clinical manifestations that can include abdominal pain, anxiety, diaphoresis, diarrhea, irritability, myalgias, mydriasis, piloerection (involuntary erection of the skin hairs ["gooseflesh"]), rhinorrhea, vomiting, and yawning. Although very uncomfortable, opioid withdrawal is not life-threatening nor is it characterized by altered level of consciousness.

Why are the other choices wrong?

Constipation is a common manifestation of opioid use, not withdrawal. Diarrhea occurs in withdrawal.

A significant altered level of consciousness, including delirium, is not expected in opioid withdrawal. Delirium should not be attributed to opioid withdrawal.

Miosis is a manifestation of opioid intoxication, not withdrawal. Mydriasis is often present in withdrawal.

PEER REVIEW

✓ Piloerection — goosebumps or gooseflesh — is a classic manifestation of opioid withdrawal.

✓ Do not attribute delirium to opioid withdrawal.

REFERENCES

Hoffman RS, Howland MA, Lewin NA, et al, eds. *Goldfrank's Toxicologic Emergencies*. 10th ed. New York, NY: McGraw-Hill; 2015: 204.

Tintinalli JE, Stapczynski JS, Ma OJ, et al, eds. *Tintinalli's Emergency Medicine: A Comprehensive Study Guide*. 8th ed. New York, NY: McGraw-Hill; 2012: 1255.

384. The correct answer is A, Hypercalcemia.

Why is this the correct answer?

In patients with a history of cancer, hypercalcemia should be considered with the onset of the symptoms described in this case: nausea, lethargy, and an altered mental state. This is especially true in patients with multiple myeloma, leukemia, or breast, lung, or head and neck cancer. In particular, changes of mental status and lethargy should trigger suspicion for possible hypercalcemia. Symptoms of hypercalcemia can be quite varied and nonspecific, but classically lethargy, nausea, anorexia, and confusion ensue. More marked CNS effects such as depression, paranoia, and somnolence can be seen in acute hypercalcemia.

Why are the other choices wrong?

Patients with hyperkalemia are often asymptomatic. They might present with symptoms of generalized weakness, but not depression. Hypokalemia and dehydration (rather than hyperkalemia) are present more typically in patients with neoplasms. In as many as half of patients with hypercalcemia, hypokalemia is also found. Tumor lysis syndrome can cause hyperkalemia, but it develops more commonly in patients being actively treated with chemotherapy.

Hypomagnesemia is not a typical electrolyte abnormality associated with multiple myeloma, and it does not present with the symptoms described in this case. Although hypomagnesemia can cause depression, more typical findings include muscle weakness, ataxia, and paresthesias.

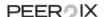

Hyperuricemia (not hypouricemia) is a known complication of multiple myeloma; it can cause acute renal failure.

PEER REVIEW

✓ Electrolyte abnormalities associated with multiple myeloma: hypercalcemia, hyperuricemia, possibly hypokalemia and dehydration.

✓ Consider hypercalcemia in a cancer patient who presents with lethargy, nausea, anorexia, and mental status changes.

REFERENCES

Marx JA, Hockberger RS, Walls RM, eds. *Rosen's Emergency Medicine: Concepts and Clinical Practice*. 8th ed. St. Louis, MO: Elsevier; 2014: 1617-1628.e1.

Tintinalli JE, Stapczynski JS, Ma OJ, et al, eds. *Tintinalli's Emergency Medicine: A Comprehensive Study Guide*. 8th ed. New York, NY: McGraw-Hill; 2012: 1535-1541.

385. The correct answer is A, Administer steroids.

Why is this the correct answer?

Giant cell arteritis (also called temporal arteritis) is a vasculitis affecting the superficial branches of the carotid artery, and more specifically, the superficial temporal artery. Patients with suspected arteritis should be started on steroids immediately in the emergency department; early treatment can prevent the irreversible vision loss that is the major consequence of this disorder. The patient in the case exhibits three of the five American College of Rheumatology criteria for diagnosis, which translates to roughly 93% sensitivity for the diagnosis. The criteria are as follows:

- Age ≥50
- ESR ≥50 mm/h
- New-onset headache
- Tenderness in the temporal area or along the temporal artery or decreased temporal artery pulse
- Abnormal artery biopsy

It is important to recognize that the biopsy can be performed after steroids have been started, and that steroid administration should not be deferred for the biopsy. A delay in treatment can lead to an increase in complications, including vision loss.

Why are the other choices wrong?

The use of color duplex ultrasonography to diagnose giant cell arteritis has been discussed, but it is not the standard of care at this time.

This presentation does not warrant lumbar puncture. Although the patient has a headache with generalized fatigue and body aches, she has no fever, neck pain, or neurologic findings that compel the emergency physician to perform a lumbar puncture for suspected meningitis. Fever can be present in giant cell arteritis;

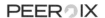

additionally, the temporal tenderness greatly increases the likelihood for giant cell arteritis over meningitis.

An emergent ophthalmology consultation is not needed; the patient should follow up with an ophthalmologist within 1 week for the biopsy. The temporal artery biopsy is the gold standard for diagnosis, but steroids may be started before the biopsy is performed.

PEER REVIEW

✓ If you suspect giant cell arteritis, start treatment with steroids immediately to prevent vision loss.

✓ You can reliably diagnose giant cell arteritis if the patient has three of these five criteria: age ≥50, ESR ≥ 50, temporal tenderness or decreased temporal artery pulse, new-onset headache, abnormal biopsy.

✓ A temporal artery biopsy doesn't have to be done emergently; it can be performed after you start steroids.

REFERENCES

Marx JA, Hockberger RS, Walls RM, eds. *Rosen's Emergency Medicine: Concepts and Clinical Practice*. 8th ed. St. Louis, MO: Elsevier; 2014: 1527-1542.e3.

Tintinalli JE, Stapczynski JS, Ma OJ, et al, eds. *Tintinalli's Emergency Medicine: A Comprehensive Study Guide*. 8th ed. New York, NY: McGraw-Hill; 2012: 1131-1137.

386. The correct answer is B, Discharge with instructions for nasal suctioning and supportive care.

Why is this the correct answer?

The patient in this case appears to have bronchiolitis. The most likely underlying cause is respiratory syncytial virus (RSV), which can be confirmed with point-of-care testing. Appropriate treatment is supportive: he has no fever, and his vital signs are normal for his age given his present illness. Given that he is eating normally, he is likely able to maintain hydration. Children younger than 6 months are obligate nose breathers and have issues with feeding and sleeping when their nasal passages are obstructed. Therefore, the best approach in this case is to teach the father how to perform nasal suctioning and tell him to do it before the baby eats or sleeps to help maintain homeostasis. Supportive care is the key to treatment of the bronchiolitic child. The only other issue to address with the father is apnea. As this child is 4 months old, the likelihood of central apnea is low; this is more common in a neonate 4 weeks old or younger due to the immaturity of the respiratory center. It is important to ask about apnea in any child who appears to have RSV.

Why are the other choices wrong?

Admission is not warranted. The patient has no fever, and his vital signs are normal, and he is able to maintain hydration. Consideration of admitting him is warranted only if he has a history of apnea.

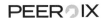

Blood work is not warranted either, and for similar reasons: no fever, otherwise normal vital signs, ability to maintain hydration. There is likely little relevant information to be gleaned from blood testing.

Antibiotics are also not warranted. If the child were febrile, then other infections should be considered, specifically UTI. If he were younger than 1 month, evaluation for significant bacterial infections should be strongly considered.

PEER REVIEW

✓ Children younger than 6 months are obligate nose breathers and can have a hard time breathing while they eat or sleep when their nasal passages are clogged.

✓ Central apnea is an age-dependent risk in children with RSV. Episodes of apnea prior to evaluation or at younger than 1 month warrant admission.

✓ The mainstay of treatment for bronchiolitis is supportive care; these patients often require only frequent nasal suctioning.

REFERENCES
Fleisher GR, Ludwig S, et al, eds. *Textbook of Pediatric Emergency Medicine*. 6th ed. Philadelphia, PA: Lippincott, Williams & Wilkins; 2010: 1004-1006.
Wolfson AB, Hendey GW, Ling LJ, et al, eds. *Harwood-Nuss' Clinical Practice of Emergency Medicine*. 6th ed. Philadelphia, PA: Lippincott, Williams & Wilkins; 2014: 1230-1233.

387. The correct answer is D, Vasoconstriction.

Why is this the correct answer?

This patient likely has Raynaud phenomenon, a vasospasm that occurs when exposure to cold causes a demarcation between ischemic and normal tissue resolving with rewarming. It typically affects the fingers, toes, and possibly the nose and earlobes. It has a predictable pattern: first pallor (white, shown here), representing vasoconstriction, followed by cyanosis (blue) due to ischemia, and then finally a rubor (red) from hyperemia and reperfusion. Raynaud disease can be primary or secondary. Primary is an exaggerated response to the cold without another causal ailment. Secondary Raynaud is the result of another condition and is the most common cutaneous complication of systemic sclerosis.

Why are the other choices wrong?

Hyperemia occurs in the third and last stage of Raynaud phenomenon. It manifests as a rubor following vasoconstriction (pallor) and ischemia (cyanosis).

Ischemia typically manifests as cyanosis and is the second stage following vasoconstriction.

Reperfusion, like hyperemia, occurs in the last stage of a Raynaud phenomenon presentation.

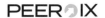

PEER REVIEW

✓ Three stages of a Raynaud vasospasm following cold exposure: pallor (white) from vasoconstriction; cyanosis (blue) from ischemia; rubor (red) from hyperemia and reperfusion.

✓ The symptoms of Raynaud phenomenon resolve with rewarming.

✓ Raynaud disease can be a primary or secondary to various other diseases.

REFERENCES

Kasper DL, Fauci AS, Hauser SL, et al, eds. *Harrison's Principles of Internal Medicine.* 19th ed. New York, NY: McGraw-Hill; 2015: 2163-2165.

Knoop KJ, Stack LB, Storrow AB, et al. *The Atlas of Emergency Medicine.* 4th ed. New York, NY: McGraw-Hill; 2016: 368.

Marx JA, Hockberger RS, Walls RM, eds. *Rosen's Emergency Medicine: Concepts and Clinical Practice.* 8th ed. St. Louis, MO: Elsevier; 2014: 1138-1156.e2.

388. The correct answer is C, NSAIDs.

Why is this the correct answer?

Given the patient's history of sarcoidosis, the most likely diagnosis in this case is erythema nodosum, a vasculitis with many varied causes. Treatment for erythema nodosum is generally supportive with NSAIDs, rest, and elevation of the affected part. The clinical presentation is erythematous or bluish well-circumscribed subcutaneous nodules. They are seen most commonly in the pretibial area but can develop on other extensor surfaces and the torso. Nodules can persist for weeks to months before resolution. Some patients experience a prodrome of malaise, myalgias, and possibly concomitant arthralgias. Although there are many causes for the development of erythema nodosum, including infection and autoimmune disease, the exact cause for a particular case might never be found. If an underlying cause is found, treatment should also be directed toward resolving it. Common causes of erythema nodosum, in addition to sarcoidosis, include viral URI, tuberculosis, ulcerative colitis, and strep infections. Medications, including penicillin, oral contraceptives, sulfonamides, and phenytoin, can also be precipitating factors.

Why are the other choices wrong?

Corticosteroids can be used for erythema nodosum, but they are typically used in cases refractory to NSAIDs.

Intravenous antibiotics are not needed in this case because the underlying cause of the outbreak is most likely an inflammatory disease, not an infectious one.

Similarly, oral antibiotics are not needed because the patient reports a history of sarcoidosis, a likely precipitant of the erythema nodosum.

PEER REVIEW

✓ Erythema nodosum is a vasculitis that can present with tender, erythematous nodules on the pretibial area, torso, or other extensor surface of the body.

✓ Treatment for erythema nodosum is supportive — NSAIDs, rest, and elevation — but if you know the underlying condition, treat it, too.

✓ What causes erythema nodosum? Infections like tuberculosis and strep and URIs. Inflammatory processes like sarcoidosis, and autoimmune disorders. Some medications, like phenytoin, penicillin, oral contraceptives, and sulfonamides. But many times, the cause is never determined.

REFERENCES

Marx JA, Hockberger RS, Walls RM, eds. *Rosen's Emergency Medicine: Concepts and Clinical Practice*. 8th ed. St. Louis, MO: Elsevier; 2014: 1527-1542.e3, 1576.

Tintinalli JE, Stapczynski JS, Ma OJ, et al, eds. *Tintinalli's Emergency Medicine: A Comprehensive Study Guide*. 8th ed. New York, NY: McGraw-Hill; 2012: 1670-1680.

389. The correct answer is D, Soft diet and follow-up with a pediatric dentist in 48 to 72 hours.

Why is this the correct answer?

Most pediatric dental injuries are minor and rarely require significant intervention. In the case presented, there is minimal movement of an intact tooth and some bleeding to the sulcus, which is consistent with a dental concussion. No emergent evaluation is needed; a soft diet with follow-up is the best approach. The periodontal ligament is the soft tissue that maintains the tooth in position, and it can be easily injured with trauma. So it is important for emergency physicians to be familiar with the different traumatic injuries that can occur to the periodontal ligament. Concussion refers to injury without increased mobility or displacement of the tooth but with pain to percussion. Subluxation occurs with injury to the periodontal ligament or other supportive tissues, with increased movement of the tooth but with no displacement. Intrusion indicates dentition that is displaced into the bony socket; there can be associated bony injury to the socket. Lateral luxation occurs with dental displacement from the socket in a lateral direction. Extrusion indicates dentition that is partially displaced out of the bony socket. Avulsion occurs with dentition that is completely displaced out of its socket.

Why are the other choices wrong?

A dental resin bridge is used to anchor a subluxed tooth into position, and its use is reserved for affixing a permanent tooth.

Emergent dental consultation is not required for this case due to the nature of the injury. The tooth is in position and without significant luxation and is a primary tooth. Although an emergent consultation is not needed, urgent dental follow-up is advised.

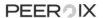

Extraction should be considered only in the setting of dental trauma with a primary tooth that is severely luxated but not avulsed. It might also be performed by a dental specialist if warranted.

PEER POINT

Periodontal ligament injuries and features

- Avulsion — Completely displaced dentition out of its socket
- Concussion — Pain to percussion but no increased mobility or displacement of the tooth
- Extrusion — Partially displaced dentition out of the bony socket
- Intrusion — Displacement of dentition into the bony socket, possible associated bony injury to the socket
- Lateral luxation — Displacement of the tooth from the socket in a lateral direction
- Subluxation — Injury to the ligament or other supportive tissues, increased movement of the tooth but no displacement

PEER REVIEW

- ✓ Pediatric dental concussion warrants dental follow-up but not an emergency consultation.
- ✓ If you're treating a pediatric patient who has a dental concussion, tell the parents to put the child on a soft diet and follow up with a dentist.

REFERENCES
Fleisher GR, Ludwig S, et al, eds. *Textbook of Pediatric Emergency Medicine*. 6th ed. Philadelphia, PA: Lippincott, Williams & Wilkins; 2010: 1289-1297.
Wolfson AB, Hendey GW, Ling LJ, et al, eds. *Harwood-Nuss' Clinical Practice of Emergency Medicine*. 6th ed. Philadelphia, PA: Lippincott, Williams & Wilkins; 2014: 166-173.

390. The correct answer is D, Start intravenous broad-spectrum antibiotics.

Why is this the correct answer?

Descending necrotizing mediastinitis is a life-threatening surgical emergency that often follows an odontogenic infection or thoracic instrumentation. Trauma and esophageal rupture, which can happen with a fish or chicken bone caught in the throat, are common causes. Emergent surgical consultation and intervention are necessary to reduce the risk of death, but of the choices listed, the first priority in emergency department management is to administer broad-spectrum antibiotics intravenously. Airway management should be a priority if needed given the patient's symptoms. Fluid resuscitation and blood pressure support are also critical to the management of these patients. Appropriate antibiotic choices to cover for oral flora

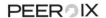

such as anaerobes might include clindamycin plus a third-generation cephalosporin, or vancomycin plus piperacillin-tazobactam. Dental infections can be the preceding event as well, but they have become less common with increased use of antibiotic prophylaxis. Diabetic and immunocompromised patients are at greater risk. Although most patients go to surgery for debridement, some patients are now being treated conservatively and being observed with the antibiotic therapy.

Why are the other choices wrong?

Surgical consultation is critical to the comprehensive treatment of mediastinitis. But the decision-making process of determining when the patient should go to surgery should not delay intravenous administration of antibiotics in these patients.

Endoscopy is not the correct diagnostic study in this case; it is considered a risk factor that precedes the onset of mediastinitis. Computed tomography is the diagnostic imaging test of choice.

Removing a fishbone soon after it becomes lodged in the posterior pharynx is important to prevent soft tissue infections of the throat and neck. But if the patient has already developed mediastinitis, which appears to be the case in this presentation, more aggressive treatment than removing the inciting fishbone is necessary.

PEER REVIEW

- ✓ If you're treating a patient who has descending necrotizing mediastinitis, don't delay intravenous administration of broad-spectrum antibiotics.
- ✓ Descending mediastinitis is an acute surgical emergency that requires immediate surgical consultation and intervention.
- ✓ Imaging modalities of choice in mediastinitis: neck and chest CT with intravenous contrast.

REFERENCES

Marx JA, Hockberger RS, Walls RM, eds. *Rosen's Emergency Medicine: Concepts and Clinical Practice*. 8th ed. St. Louis, MO: Elsevier; 2014: 1170-1185.

Prado-Calleros HM, Jiménez-Fuentes E, Jiménez-Escobar I. Descending necrotizing mediastinitis: systematic review on its treatment in the last 6 years, 75 years after its description. *Head Neck*. 2016;38(Suppl 1):E2275-2283.

Tintinalli JE, Stapczynski JS, Ma OJ, et al, eds. *Tintinalli's Emergency Medicine: A Comprehensive Study Guide*. 8th ed. New York, NY: McGraw-Hill; 2012: 1613-1619.

391. The correct answer is D, Perform immediate RSI.

Why is this the correct answer?

In this case, the patient has been exposed to a pulmonary irritant that is causing bronchospasm and stridor from laryngeal edema. Regardless of what the underlying irritating agent is, he requires immediate rapid sequence induction (RSI) and intubation because of his increasing laryngeal edema and the risk of developing ARDS. In particular, water-soluble irritants can irritate both the upper and lower airways, and if edema is present, early airway control is indicated. Symptoms of

ARDS might not develop for 24 to 36 hours from these pulmonary irritants, but because of the stridor, direct visualization and control of the airway are warranted.

Why are the other choices wrong?

Inhalation injury is the leading cause of death from burns given the significant improvement in fluid management. Bronchospasm is a prominent symptom due to the particles in smoke and the edema from the inflammatory process. Albuterol is indicated as a potential stabilizing measure, but delaying definitive airway management to provide an albuterol treatment is not the right next step for this patient with stridor and impending airway closure.

Corticosteroids have not been shown to be effective at mitigating the symptoms this patient has, and even if they did have an effect, it would take hours.

The contraindications for BiPAP include upper airway obstruction that can be bypassed by endotracheal intubation (as in this case), facial deformity from trauma or other causes that do not allow seal of the mask, decreased respiratory effort from altered level of consciousness, and vomiting or increased secretions There is no role for BiPAP in this patient with upper airway stridor.

PEER REVIEW

✓ Patients who have been exposed to pulmonary irritants might not develop ARDS symptoms for 24 to 36 hours.

✓ Early airway control with intubation is recommended in patients with stridor or hoarseness from an inhaled irritant.

✓ Albuterol can be an effective treatment if bronchospasm dominates the clinical picture

REFERENCES

Marx JA, Hockberger RS, Walls RM, eds. *Rosen's Emergency Medicine: Concepts and Clinical Practice*. 8th ed. St. Louis, MO: Elsevier; 2014: 2036-2043.

Tintinalli JE, Stapczynski JS, Ma OJ, et al, eds. *Tintinalli's Emergency Medicine: A Comprehensive Study Guide*. 8th ed. New York, NY: McGraw-Hill; 2012: 1307-1310.

392. The correct answer is C, Prostaglandin E1 0.05 mcg/kg/min IV.

Why is this the correct answer?

The baby in this case is showing signs of cardiac failure with resultant pulmonary edema. The ECG shows signs of right-sided forces. The clinical signs as well as the ECG suggest tricuspid atresia as a cause of the cyanosis. Prostaglandin E1 (PGE1) is a lifesaving medication in this scenario and must be started as soon as possible. Dosing of the infusion is 0.05 mcg/kg per minute. Side effects of PGE1 include apnea, bradycardia, and hypotension. Beyond initial care, the patient requires ICU admission and a cardiology consultation. Treatment decisions are then made depending on the degree of cardiac defect and patient stability. Definitive repair with cardiothoracic surgery might be delayed until the child grows and matures so that he is better prepared for the surgery.

Why are the other choices wrong?

Atropine is used in pediatric resuscitation for bradycardia related to a vagal cause or as an antisialagogue.

Epinephrine, a staple medication in the resuscitation of a critically ill patient, is not warranted in this patient. He has signs of a cyanotic cardiac defect both clinically and on the ECG, and the addition of epinephrine might cause cardiac instability and prompt worsening shunting of deoxygenated blood.

A fluid bolus using normal saline is contraindicated in this clinical scenario: the child has signs of cardiac dysfunction, and adding fluid could worsen his condition.

PEER POINT

Want to remember congenital heart defects?

Cyanotic — Count to "5"

- 1 Truncus arteriosus (**One** trunk)
- 2 Transposition of the **Two** great vessels
- 3 **Tri**cuspid atresia
- 4 **Tet**ralogy of Fallot
- 5 Total anomalous pulmonary venous return (the **Five**-letter acronym TAPVR)

Acyanotic — Think "left"

- Left-to-right shunting and obstruction of the left ventricular outflow tract, including:
    — Ventricular septal defect
    — Coarctation of the aorta
    — Aortic stenosis
    — Hypoplastic left heart syndrome

PEER REVIEW

✓ Infuse prostaglandin E1 immediately in a neonate with possible congenital cardiac disease.
✓ Side effects of prostaglandin E1: apnea, bradycardia, and hypotension.

REFERENCES

Fleisher GR, Ludwig S, et al, eds. *Textbook of Pediatric Emergency Medicine.* 6th ed. Philadelphia, PA: Lippincott, Williams & Wilkins; 2010: 198-202, 690-699.

Wolfson AB, Hendey GW, Ling LJ, et al, eds. *Harwood-Nuss' Clinical Practice of Emergency Medicine.* 6th ed. Philadelphia, PA: Lippincott, Williams & Wilkins; 2014: 268-269.

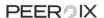

393. The correct answer is D, Perform elective intubation.

Why is this the correct answer?

This patient's signs and symptoms are consistent with laryngotracheal injury secondary to strangulation. The progression of symptoms over the past 30 minutes — worsening hoarseness and the onset of difficulty swallowing — suggests progressive laryngotracheal edema, so the best next step is to get control of the airway. Delaying intubation might be catastrophic if the airway edema progresses to the point where endotracheal intubation is difficult, if not impossible. The essential action the emergency physician must take is to protect the patient's airway.

Why are the other choices wrong?

A swallowing study using diatrizoate meglumine and diatrizoate sodium solution (brand name Gastrografin) certainly might be a good part of this patient's care. However, her presentation is consistent with progressively worsening airway compromise, and stabilization of her airway must be accomplished first before arranging a swallowing study.

Ordering a CT scan of the neck is the right thing to do to determine the extent of the patient's injuries. But stabilization of the airway is crucial and should not be delayed for imaging.

Obtaining AP and lateral neck radiographs might be useful in evaluating injuries to the hyoid bone or cervical spine. But this patient's symptoms are more concerning for soft tissue injury in addition to bony injury, so CT is the most appropriate imaging modality.

PEER POINT

Clues to laryngotracheal injury

- Hoarseness
- Subcutaneous emphysema
- Sore throat
- Stridor
- Painful swallowing

PEER REVIEW

- ✓ If you're caring for a strangulation victim who has signs or symptoms of laryngotracheal injury, be sure to look for airway compromise.
- ✓ Progressive hoarseness, stridor, and difficulty swallowing are consistent with advancing airway compromise and should trigger intubation.

REFERENCES

Tintinalli JE, Stapczynski JS, Ma OJ, et al, eds. *Tintinalli's Emergency Medicine: A Comprehensive Study Guide*. 8th ed. New York, NY: McGraw-Hill; 2012: 1733-1740.

Wolfson AB, Hendey GW, Ling LJ, et al, eds. *Harwood-Nuss' Clinical Practice of Emergency Medicine*. 6th ed. Philadelphia, PA: Lippincott, Williams & Wilkins; 2014: 180-183.

394. The correct answer is C, Meckel scan.

Why is this the correct answer?

Rectal bleeding has many possible causes, and it requires further emergent evaluation, including a rectal examination. In this case, the patient has no signs or history of abdominal pain and has age-appropriate vital signs. Given that history and the large amount of blood, a Meckel diverticulum is a likely cause. A Meckel scan uses a radiolabeled material to determine if there is any ectopic gastric tissue outside of the intestines. If ectopic tissue becomes inflamed, a Meckel diverticulum might present with signs of peritonitis, and surgical intervention is likely required. It is important to note that hypotension is an extremely late sign in pediatric patients with hemorrhage as they can compensate for the loss of up to 25% of their blood volume. As mentioned, the differential diagnosis of rectal bleeding is large, but the appearance of the blood suggests the cause. For example, swallowed foreign body or blood, esophageal varices, and peptic ulcer are suggested by dark blood. The dark, bright blood associated with a Meckel diverticulum is also seen with mesenteric thrombosis, volvulus, intussusception, and systemic disease. Bright blood, suggestive of a point of origin distal to the GI tract, is seen with rectal prolapse, hemorrhoids, fissures, foreign bodies, polyps, and colitis.

Why are the other choices wrong?

Abdominal ultrasonography can be used to determine structural issues or obstructions but does not pick up errant gastric tissue.

A contrast enema is the test of choice when evaluating a patient for intussusception, but it does not show a Meckel diverticulum. Intussusception is more commonly seen in children younger than 12 months, with infants classically indicating abdominal pain with intermittent crying.

As with abdominal ultrasonography, an obstructive abdominal radiographic series can be used to determine structural issues or obstructions but does not identify errant gastric tissue.

PEER POINT

Meckel diverticulum and the commonly quoted "rule of 2s"

- 2% of the population has it
- About 2 inches long (although the average is a bit larger)
- Usually found within 2 feet of the ileocecal valve (varies with age)
- Often found in children younger than 2 years
- Affects males twice as often as females (actually, this is generally true of complications rather than incidence)

Source: http://www.ncbi.nlm.nih.gov/pmc/articles/PMC3207587/

PEER REVIEW

✓ Painless rectal bleeding with or without abdominal pain suggests a Meckel diverticulum.

✓ A Meckel technetium scan is used to look for ectopic gastric tissue.

REFERENCES

Fleisher GR, Ludwig S, et al, eds. *Textbook of Pediatric Emergency Medicine*. 6th ed. Philadelphia, PA: Lippincott, Williams & Wilkins; 2010: 288-289, 1515, 1528.

Wolfson AB, Hendey GW, Ling LJ, et al, eds. *Harwood-Nuss' Clinical Practice of Emergency Medicine*. 6th ed. Philadelphia, PA: Lippincott, Williams & Wilkins; 2014: 1128-1130.

395. The correct answer is C, Physostigmine.

Why is this the correct answer?

The symptoms described in this case are consistent with poisoning from an organophosphorous compound (OP), which is used most commonly in insecticides. Treatment with atropine, diazepam, and pralidoxime are all appropriate. But physostigmine, similar to an OP, is an acetylcholinesterase inhibitor, and its use is contraindicated in the treatment of OP poisoning. Physostigmine can be used both diagnostically and therapeutically in patients with antimuscarinic poisoning. Diagnostically, complete reversal of delirium after administration of physostigmine can potentially prevent further workup. Therapeutically, physostigmine administration can be considered to treat agitation in a patient known to be delirious from an antimuscarinic agent. The presence of convulsions and/or QRS prolongation should preclude use of physostigmine because asystole has occurred with the presence of these in the setting of tricyclic antidepressant poisoning. Acetylcholinesterase breaks down acetylcholine, and its inhibition leads to the accumulation of acetylcholine in synapses. Accumulation at the neuromuscular junction can manifest with fasciculations and muscle weakness, including respiratory paralysis. Accumulation of acetylcholine at preganglionic synapses occurs in both the parasympathetic and sympathetic nervous system, and at postganglionic parasympathetic synapses. The excess cholinergic activity typically manifests more in the parasympathetic side as evidenced clinically by the presence of diaphoresis, diarrhea, hypersalivation, increased respiratory secretions, miosis, and vomiting. Mnemonics that describe these manifestations include SLUDGE and DUMBELS.

Why are the other choices wrong?

Atropine is indicated (not contraindicated), and in addition to aggressive airway management is the cornerstone of initial management of OP poisoning. Atropine is a purely antimuscarinic drug that antagonizes excessive acetylcholine at muscarinic receptors in OP poisoning. Atropine should be given liberally until respiratory secretions, bronchospasm, and cardiovascular instability are reversed. Importantly, atropine does not reverse respiratory paralysis that occurs as a result of excess acetylcholine at nicotinic receptors.

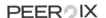

Diazepam should be used to treat OP-related seizures (not those from hypoxia) that can occur with cholinergic crisis. Although it is not currently clear if diazepam should be routinely administered in OP poisoning, some animal studies have demonstrated benefit, and its use is certainly not contraindicated.

The rationale for early pralidoxime administration is to prevent permanent inhibition of acetylcholinesterase by the OP, a process referred to as ageing. Although the routine use of pralidoxime in all OP poisonings has been questioned, its use is not contraindicated.

PEER POINT

SLUDGE mnemonic for cholinergic excess

- <u>S</u>alivation
- <u>L</u>acrimation
- <u>U</u>rinary incontinence
- <u>D</u>iarrhea
- <u>G</u>astrointestinal distress
- <u>E</u>mesis

DUMBELS mnemonic for clinical features of cholinergic toxidrome

- <u>D</u>iarrhea
- <u>U</u>rination
- <u>M</u>iosis/<u>M</u>uscle weakness
- <u>B</u>radycardia/<u>B</u>ronchospasm/<u>B</u>ronchorrhea
- <u>E</u>mesis
- <u>L</u>acrimation
- <u>S</u>alivation/<u>S</u>eizures/<u>S</u>weating

PEER REVIEW

✓ Atropine and aggressive airway management are critical in the initial management of poisonings from organophosphorous compounds.

✓ Physostigmine, like organophosphorous compounds, is an acetylcholinesterase inhibitor. Don't use it in the management of organophosphorous poisoning.

REFERENCES

Hoffman RS, Howland MA, Lewin NA, et al, eds. *Goldfrank's Toxicologic Emergencies*. 10th ed. New York, NY: McGraw-Hill; 2015: 678, 1418-1419.

Tintinalli JE, Stapczynski JS, Ma OJ, et al, eds. *Tintinalli's Emergency Medicine: A Comprehensive Study Guide*. 8th ed. New York, NY: McGraw-Hill; 2012: 1319-1321.

396. The correct answer is C, Get information about the time and amount of ingestion.

Why is this the correct answer?

This patient is in no distress, is able to swallow without difficulty, and her vital signs are normal for her age. The first step in determining what medical care she needs is to get more information about the ingestion — when did it occur, what substance was involved (if known), how much was taken, and what interventions have been performed up to this point. In this age group, the top four ingestions are cosmetics or personal care products, analgesics, cleaning substances (household), and foreign bodies (toys and other miscellaneous items. The top causes of death following ingestion in children are analgesics, fumes or vapors, and cough and cold preparations. The next step is to find out more about the substance and how the ingestion should be managed. The Poison Help Line (1-800-222-1222) is a good resource on toxic ingestions for both clinicians and caretakers. Toxicology specialists can also be helpful. In this specific case, the substance in the glow-stick is actually nontoxic, as are most pediatric ingestions. Although children younger than 6 years account for almost half of all human ingestions, they account for only 1.5% of the fatalities.

Why are the other choices wrong?

Oxygen should be administered to a child who is in respiratory distress or exhibiting signs of hypoxia (clinical or abnormal pulse oximetry/blood gas readings). In those cases, oxygen should be supplied via a nonrebreathing mask to provide the highest oxygen content possible and not via nasal cannula. Because this child has a normal respiratory rate and pulse oximetry reading, this intervention is not warranted.

Activated charcoal is commonly used in the treatment of toxic ingestions because it can bind the toxic agent. But it is important to note that activated charcoal should not be used if the substance ingested is any of the following: caustics, pesticides, hydrocarbons, alcohols, iron, lithium, solvents.

Co-oximetry testing is used to determine the carrying state of hemoglobin to evaluate causes of hypoxia such as for carbon monoxide exposure or in the evaluation of methemoglobin. It has no role in the treatment of the ingestion described in this case.

PEER REVIEW

✓ What you need to find out in all potentially toxic ingestions: when the ingestion occurred and how much of the substance was ingested, always assuming the largest amount possible if not known.

✓ Consider the nature of the ingestion, how the child got the substance, and if a lack of supervision led to it.

✓ Most pediatric ingestions are not toxic, but take advantage of any opportunity to tell a parent or caregiver about The Poison Help Line, 1-800-222-1222.

REFERENCES

Bronstein AC, Spyker DA, Cantilena LR Jr, et al. 2011 Annual Report of the American Association of Poison Control Centers' National Poison Data System (NPDS): 29th Annual Report. *Clin Toxicol (Phila)*. 2012;50(10):911–1164.

Fleisher GR, Ludwig S, et al, eds. *Textbook of Pediatric Emergency Medicine*. 6th ed. Philadelphia, PA: Lippincott, Williams & Wilkins; 2010: 1183.

Wolfson AB, Hendey GW, Ling LJ, et al, eds. *Harwood-Nuss' Clinical Practice of Emergency Medicine*. 6th ed. Philadelphia, PA: Lippincott, Williams & Wilkins; 2014: 1315-1322.

397. The correct answer is D, Chest xray.

Why is the correct answer?

The patient in this case has suffered the most common primary blast injury complication: tympanic membrane perforation. Performing a chest xray is appropriate, looking for evidence of pulmonary barotrauma, as is a period of observation even if the chest xray is normal. Primary blast injuries are those that result from transmitted overpressure on the body, and they occur most frequently at air-tissue interfaces. High air content organ systems are most at risk. In descending order of injury frequency are the tympanic membrane, lung, and bowel. Given the sensitivity of the tympanic membrane to transmitted overpressure, evaluation for perforation should be performed in patients exposed to a blast, and the presence of tympanic membrane rupture should heighten suspicion for other injuries. In an asymptomatic patient with intact tympanic membranes, the development of other primary blast injuries is rare. However, the absence of tympanic membrane rupture alone does not exclude the possibility that other primary blast injuries will develop. Obtaining a chest xray is appropriate in all patients following a blast injury with pulmonary complaints, but also in those who show signs of any primary blast injury, including tympanic membrane rupture even in the absence of pulmonary symptoms (as in this case). An observation period is important because injuries from primary blast injury can manifest in a delayed manner.

Why are the other choices wrong?

Emergency physicians should maintain a low threshold for evaluating patients radiographically following blast injury. However, tympanic membrane rupture alone, which is very common after blast injury, is in itself not an indication to obtain a CT scan of the abdomen. The bowel is the third most common hollow organ to be injured in a blast injury (following the tympanic membrane and lung). However, observation and serial examinations in the asymptomatic patient are appropriate prior to discharge.

Tympanic membrane rupture alone also is not an indication to perform an abdominal ultrasound examination. Ultrasound is not sensitive for the evaluation of bowel injuries, which are the abdominal injuries most common following primary blast injury. A chest xray is much more likely to be of greater yield.

Similarly, tympanic membrane rupture alone is not an indication to perform brain CT following blast injury. Serial examinations in the asymptomatic patient are appropriate prior to discharge.

PEER REVIEW

✓ The most common primary blast injury is tympanic membrane perforation.
✓ The presence of tympanic membrane rupture should raise suspicion for other primary blast injuries.
✓ Should you get a chest xray in a patient who was in close proximity to an explosion? Yes, especially those who have pulmonary complaints, but also for anyone who shows signs of any primary blast injury, like tympanic membrane rupture even without pulmonary symptoms.

REFERENCES
Tintinalli JE, Stapczynski JS, Ma OJ, et al, eds. *Tintinalli's Emergency Medicine: A Comprehensive Study Guide*. 8th ed. New York, NY: McGraw-Hill; 2012: 35-38.
Wolfson AB, Hendey GW, Ling LJ, et al, eds. *Harwood-Nuss' Clinical Practice of Emergency Medicine*. 6th ed. Philadelphia, PA: Lippincott, Williams & Wilkins; 2014: 316-317.

398. The correct answer is D, Fluorescein staining of corneas.

Why is this the correct answer?

In the evaluation of a crying infant, it is important to differentiate between emergent causes of and benign causes. The benign causes of persistent crying are more common. Corneal abrasion is certainly one to consider in this case given that the patient appears well; fluorescein staining of corneas is easily done and should be performed after more serious causes have been eliminated. Normal infant crying is characterized as crying that lasts less than 3 hours per day and is typically present in the afternoon to evening (around 3 pm to 11 pm). There is a long differential that includes life-threatening causes (cardiac arrhythmia, nonaccidental trauma, traumatic brain injury), limb-threatening causes (fracture, hair-tourniquets, wounds), and more benign causes. The crying infant should be evaluated for fractures, skin injury (lacerations, abrasions, hair tourniquets), and nonaccidental trauma. It is important to ensure that the examination rules out the life- and limb-

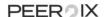

threatening causes, but again, it is more likely that persistent crying has a benign cause. The examination should be conducted with the infant completely undressed, including the diaper, and should focus on conditions that are known culprits in persistent crying.

Why are the other choices wrong?

A CBC count provides no relevant information in the evaluation of a child who has no signs or symptoms of infection or anemia. Murmur is a common finding in younger children and is a normal variant in most.

A chest xray is not warranted in a child with a normal chest examination and no history of illness or trauma.

An echocardiogram is excessive in the evaluation of this clinical finding in an otherwise healthy infant with an innocent murmur.

PEER POINT

Why is this baby still crying? From Pediatric EM Morsels, the mnemonic IT CRIES

- **I** — Infections: meningitis, UTI, sepsis
- **T** — Trauma: intracranial bleed, fracture, nonaccidental trauma
- **C** — Cardiac: arrhythmia
- **R** — Reaction to meds, reflux, rectal or anal fissure
- **I** — Intussusception
- **E** — Eyes: corneal abrasion, foreign body, glaucoma
- **S** — Strangulation, Surgical process: torsion, hernia, tourniquet

PEER REVIEW

- ✓ Baby won't stop crying? Take a systematic approach to checking out possible causes.
- ✓ Be sure to consider fractures, skin injury, and nonaccidental trauma when you're evaluating a crying infant.
- ✓ Corneal abrasions are a common cause of crying in infants and are easily evaluated.

REFERENCES

Fleisher GR, Ludwig S, et al, eds. *Textbook of Pediatric Emergency Medicine*. 6th ed. Philadelphia, PA: Lippincott, Williams & Wilkins; 2010: 203-205.

Wolfson AB, Hendey GW, Ling LJ, et al, eds. *Harwood-Nuss' Clinical Practice of Emergency Medicine*. 6th ed. Philadelphia, PA: Lippincott, Williams & Wilkins; 2014: 1123-1124.

399. The correct answer is D, Reassurance.

Why is this the correct answer?

The clinical scenario presented in this case is classic for a breath-holding spell. Breath-holding spells are first noted in children between 6 and 18 months old and can occur in up to 4.5% of children. There are two classic types: pallid (as in the case presented) and cyanotic (most common). Breath-holding spells are a benign issue and generally do not require further workup in the emergency department. Reassurance of caregivers is the key. This is often achieved by explaining the pathophysiology of what occurred: crying leading to stimulation of the vagal nerve, which then leads to a syncope-type reaction. A good history and physical examination help differentiate benign causes from emergent ones such as seizure and syncope. The exact cause of breath-holding spells is unknown, but there does seem to be a genetic link or familial predilection for them even though they are involuntary.

Why are the other choices wrong?

Chemistry evaluation is not helpful in the examination of a patient following a breath-holding event. Exceptions are evaluations of patients with possible seizure, especially if there is a history of volume loss or dehydration (vomiting, diarrhea, decreased oral intake) and those who continue to be symptomatic.

A neurology consultation is not warranted and is unlikely to yield results in a brief, spontaneously resolving loss of consciousness with a prompt return to baseline. Although these episodes can be mistaken for seizure-like activity, there is no postictal phase, and they often have an emotional trigger.

Noncontrast head CT is likewise not indicated, and for similar reasons. The "Choosing Wisely" campaign encourages minimizing the use of ionizing radiation in children with minor head injury. Because this child has a normal examination, there is no justification for CT.

PEER REVIEW

- ✓ A good history and physical examination are key elements in the evaluation of an apneic child.
- ✓ Consider breathholding in pediatric patients presenting with syncope.
- ✓ Breath-holding spells usually occur for the first time between 6 and 18 months and resolves by or before 6 or 7 years.
- ✓ Avoid head CT in the evaluation of children with minor head injury to prevent unnecessary exposure to ionizing radiation.

REFERENCES

Fleisher GR, Ludwig S, et al, eds. *Textbook of Pediatric Emergency Medicine*. 6th ed. Philadelphia, PA: Lippincott, Williams & Wilkins; 2010: 1650-1651.

Wolfson AB, Hendey GW, Ling LJ, et al, eds. *Harwood-Nuss' Clinical Practice of Emergency Medicine*. 6th ed. Philadelphia, PA: Lippincott, Williams & Wilkins; 2014: 1137-1139, 1146-1147.

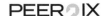

400. The correct answer is C, Hypothermia.

Why is this the correct answer?

Myxedema coma is the most extreme form of hypothyroidism and manifests with signs and symptoms of decreased metabolic rate. Bradycardia, decreased ventilation, hypotension, and severe hypothermia are expected. The buildup of hyaluronic acid in tissues leading to nonpitting facial and pretibial edema is commonly present, although not universal. Treatment involves intravenous thyroxine and corticosteroid administration, passive rewarming, supportive care, and searching for and treating any precipitating stressor such as infection.

Why are the other choices wrong?

Exophthalmos can be seen in Graves disease, the most common cause of hyperthyroidism, not hypothyroidism.

Hypotension (not hypertension) is seen in approximately half of patients presenting in myxedema coma.

In hypothyroidism, hyaluronic acid can build up in tissues and lead to nonpitting edema in the face and pretibial areas.

PEER REVIEW

- ✓ You can expect to see bradycardia, decreased ventilation, hypotension, and severe hypothermia in patients with myxedema coma.
- ✓ Patients with hypothyroidism can have a nonpitting edema on their faces and the fronts of their lower legs.

REFERENCES
Tintinalli JE, Stapczynski JS, Ma OJ, et al, eds. *Tintinalli's Emergency Medicine: A Comprehensive Study Guide*. 8th ed. New York, NY: McGraw-Hill; 2012: 1470-1471, 1474.
Wolfson AB, Hendey GW, Ling LJ, et al, eds. *Harwood-Nuss' Clinical Practice of Emergency Medicine*. 6th ed. Philadelphia, PA: Lippincott, Williams & Wilkins; 2014: 1024.

401. The correct answer is D, Victims who required resuscitation should be taken to an emergency department.

Why is this the correct answer?

Persons who required resuscitative efforts on scene as a result of drowning are at risk for delayed symptomatology, which can include respiratory distress as a result of aspiration and neurologic insult as a result of anoxia. For that reason, transporting these victims to an emergency department for evaluation is warranted.

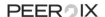

Why are the other choices wrong?

Injuries to the cervical spine occur in less than 0.5% of persons who are drowning, and cervical immobilization in the water is indicated only if head or neck injury is strongly suspected such as can occur in accidents involving diving, waterskiing, surfing, or watercraft.

According to the CDC, accidents (unintentional injuries) are the most common cause of death in persons 5 to 14 years old in the United States, followed by cancer and suicide. Among boys 5 to 14 years old, worldwide, drowning is still a leading cause of death. And in the United States, among children 1 to 4 years old, drowning is the second leading cause of injury-related death. The risk is even higher in countries other than the United States — up to 10 to 20 times. Risk factors for drowning include male and younger than 14 years, as well as low income, rural, poor education, aquatic exposure, alcohol use, and risky behavior, along with lack of supervision. The drowning risk for persons who have epilepsy is 15 to 19 times higher risk than it is for those who do not.

Active efforts to expel water from the airway (using abdominal thrusts or placing the person head down) should be avoided because they delay the initiation of ventilation and greatly increase the risk of vomiting, with a significant increase in mortality rate.

PEER REVIEW

- ✓ Drowning is a leading cause of death in children 1 to 14 years of age worldwide.
- ✓ Factors that increase the likelihood of drowning: male, alcohol use, low income, poor education, rural residency, risky behavior, lack of supervision, history of epilepsy.
- ✓ Cervical spine injuries, although important to consider, are generally rare among drowning victims.

REFERENCES

Kochanek KD, Murphy SL, Xu J, et al.National Vital Statistics Reports. Deaths: Final Data for 2014. Division of Vital Statistics. June 30, 2016. U.S. DEPARTMENT OF HEALTH AND HUMAN SERVICES, Centers for Disease Control and Prevention, National Center for Health Statistics, National Vital Statistics System. Available at https://www.cdc.gov/nchs/data/nvsr/nvsr65/nvsr65_04.pdf. Accessed January 24, 2017.

LLSA Article: Drowning, Current Concepts. *N Engl J Med*. 2012;366:22. nejm.2102. Available at http://www.nejm.org/doi/full/10.1056/NEJMra1013317. Accessed January 24, 2017.

Wolfson AB, Hendey GW, Ling LJ, et al, eds. *Harwood-Nuss' Clinical Practice of Emergency Medicine*. 6th ed. Philadelphia, PA: Lippincott, Williams & Wilkins; 2014: 1524-1526.

402. The correct answer is D, Tracheoinnominate artery fistula.

Why is this the correct answer?

Bleeding after a tracheostomy can be treated by removing the tube and applying silver nitrate or pressure with moist gauze. Erosion into the tracheoinnominate artery can cause life-threatening hemorrhage. This is a rare complication, but when it does occur, it is most common 1 to 3 weeks after the procedure. Immediate treatment should include direct pressure and hyperinflation of the tracheostomy tube cuff with gentle tube traction, which provides direct internal pressure to the bleeding artery. An urgent consultation from ENT or thoracic surgery is necessary to arrange definitive treatment. If bleeding is not controlled with the actions described, then an endotracheal tube should be placed below the bleeding innominate artery with the assistance of a flexible nasopharyngoscope or bronchoscopy and advanced past the tracheostomy tube while withdrawing the tracheostomy tube. An endotracheal tube placed in this manner can be used to ventilate the patient, reduce aspiration of blood, and allow the physician to apply internal digital pressure to the artery while the patient is transferred to the operating room for arterial repair by an ENT or thoracic surgeon.

Why are the other choices wrong?

Portal hypertension resulting in dilation of the esophageal veins can cause life-threatening bleeding if they rupture, but it is not associated with a recent tracheostomy tube placement. Bleeding secondary to esophageal varices can be fatal and requires aggressive airway management, emergent GI consultation, and temporizing measures that might include placement of Sengstaken-Blakemore or Minnesota tubes for balloon tamponade.

The patient's malignancy does increase her risk for PE, and the hypoxia is a worrisome sign. But her recent tracheostomy increases her risk for tracheoinnominate artery fistula formation, which can present with hemoptysis, a seemingly minor sentinel bleed, or severe hemorrhage.

A tracheoesophageal fistula (TEF) is a communication between the trachea and esophagus that can be the result of a congenital malformation. It also can be an acquired condition such as in the case of a tracheostomy-associated TEF. Secondary to a tracheostomy tube placement, TEF can be caused by erosion from an overinflated cuff or direct trauma from the procedure itself. It is best diagnosed with bronchoscopy.

PEER POINT

Steps in assessing a tracheostomy patient with respiratory distress

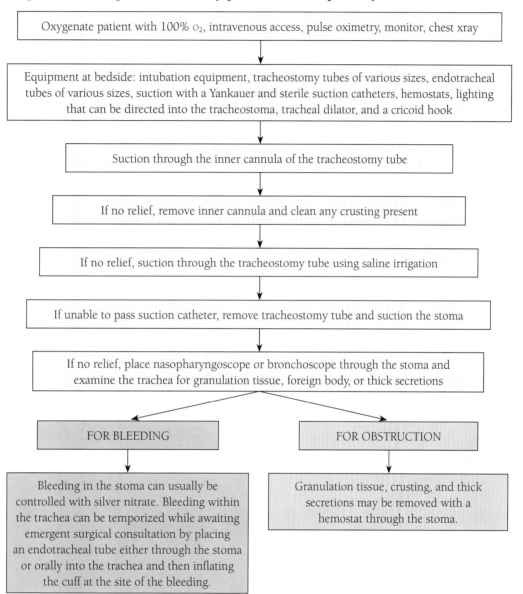

> Oxygenate patient with 100% O₂, intravenous access, pulse oximetry, monitor, chest xray

> Equipment at bedside: intubation equipment, tracheostomy tubes of various sizes, endotracheal tubes of various sizes, suction with a Yankauer and sterile suction catheters, hemostats, lighting that can be directed into the tracheostoma, tracheal dilator, and a cricoid hook

> Suction through the inner cannula of the tracheostomy tube

> If no relief, remove inner cannula and clean any crusting present

> If no relief, suction through the tracheostomy tube using saline irrigation

> If unable to pass suction catheter, remove tracheostomy tube and suction the stoma

> If no relief, place nasopharyngoscope or bronchoscope through the stoma and examine the trachea for granulation tissue, foreign body, or thick secretions

FOR BLEEDING

FOR OBSTRUCTION

Bleeding in the stoma can usually be controlled with silver nitrate. Bleeding within the trachea can be temporized while awaiting emergent surgical consultation by placing an endotracheal tube either through the stoma or orally into the trachea and then inflating the cuff at the site of the bleeding.

Granulation tissue, crusting, and thick secretions may be removed with a hemostat through the stoma.

PEER Point 32

PEER REVIEW

✓ It takes 1 week for a tracheostomy fistula to mature, so don't attempt a blind tube replacement during this time and risk creating a false tract.

✓ You can block a life-threatening esophageal variceal hemorrhage with a temporizing Sengstaken-Blakemore or Minnesota tube.

✓ A tracheoinnominate artery fistula can present as a minor sentinel bleed, hemoptysis, or severe hemorrhage.

REFERENCES

Marx JA, Hockberger RS, Walls RM, eds. *Rosen's Emergency Medicine: Concepts and Clinical Practice*. 8th ed. St. Louis, MO: Elsevier; 2014: 2403-2405.

Tintinalli JE, Stapczynski JS, Ma OJ, et al, eds. *Tintinalli's Emergency Medicine: A Comprehensive Study Guide*. 8th ed. New York, NY: McGraw-Hill; 2012: 1619-1624.

403. The correct answer is A, Congenital adrenal hyperplasia.

Why is this the correct answer?

Congenital adrenal hyperplasia (CAH) is a disorder of steroid synthesis or function. Affected infants typically present between the second and fifth weeks of life; the presentation often is an acute crisis similar to the one described in the case, including hypovolemia and hyponatremia related to the salt wasting. The most common form of the disorder is 21-hydroxylase deficiency, accounting for 90% of cases; it is inherited in a recessive manner. Salt wasting with subsequent clinical manifestations is caused by the altered synthesis of the enzymes involved. Other characteristics due to excess androgen result in virilization that is more obvious in girls and that can lead to a missed diagnosis of a male child at or soon after birth. Although CAH is part of the normal neonatal screening, results might not be available for 3 to 4 weeks. Acute care consists of reversing the shock state as quickly as possible using hydration with isotonic fluids and providing mineralocorticoids using hydrocortisone 50 mg/m^2 per day.

Why are the other choices wrong?

Pavor nocturnus, otherwise known as night terrors, occurs in older children in the early stages of sleep (within the first 2 hours). Affected children are inconsolable but eventually go back to sleep and have no recollection of the event afterward. Pavor nocturnus can affect up to 20% of children, but incidents occur rarely and decrease with age, so treatment is often not required.

Pseudohyponatremia is present in patients with elevated glucose due to a displacement of fluid; it is not present with mild hypoglycemia as seen in this patient. It is often found in a patient in diabetic ketoacidosis. Actual serum sodium can be calculated with the following formula: Sodium + (glucose – 100/100) (for glucose – 100 mg/dL).

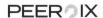
Sepsis must always be considered, regardless of hyperthermia or hypothermia, in the evaluation of a neonate with an alteration from baseline. The abnormal laboratory values in this case are not consistent with this diagnosis, however, making CAH more likely.

PEER REVIEW

✓ Congenital adrenal hyperplasia can present at birth, within 2 to 5 weeks of birth, or during childhood with associated precocious puberty.

✓ Appropriate rehydration and administration of mineralocorticoids are the keys to treatment.

REFERENCES

Fleisher GR, Ludwig S, et al, eds. *Textbook of Pediatric Emergency Medicine*. 6th ed. Philadelphia, PA: Lippincott, Williams & Wilkins; 2010: 768-771.

Wolfson AB, Hendey GW, Ling LJ, et al, eds. *Harwood-Nuss' Clinical Practice of Emergency Medicine*. 6th ed. Philadelphia, PA: Lippincott, Williams & Wilkins; 2014: 257.

404. The correct answer is A, Bupivacaine.

Why is this the correct answer?

Anaphylaxis due to local anesthetic agents is rarely seen. Amides such as bupivacaine that are metabolized in the liver by the cytochrome P450 system very rarely cause allergic reactions. Of all the serious complications related to local anesthetic agents, less than 1% have an IgE-mediated allergic reaction to the ester agents. This occurs because the agents are metabolized by serum pseudocholinesterase into a PABA derivative. If an allergic reaction occurs, the affected area should be infiltrated with 1% diphenhydramine (1 mL of 5% diphenhydramine with 4 mL of normal saline). Anaphylaxis should be treated with epinephrine, antihistamines, steroids, and vasopressors as clinically indicated. If there is concern of prior allergy to an ester agent, patients can receive local anesthesia with diphenhydramine and benzyl alcohol with epinephrine.

Why are the other choices wrong?

Cocaine is an ester agent and can cause an IgE-mediated allergic reaction when used for local anesthesia. A better choice is an amide anesthetic agent such as bupivacaine, levobupivacaine, lidocaine, mepivacaine, prilocaine, or ropivacaine.

Procaine also is an ester, and even though allergic reactions are rare, it is more likely to cause one than is bupivacaine.

Tetracaine also is an ester agent and thus not the best choice in a patient likely to have a history of allergic reactions to local anesthesia.

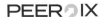

PEER POINT

Worried about allergy to local anesthesia? Remember this mnemonic: Can't Treat Pain with Esters

- **Can't** — Cocaine
- **Treat** — Tetracaine
- **Pain** — Procaine/Chloroprocaine

PEER REVIEW

✓ Allergic reactions to local anesthesia don't happen very often, but when they do, esters are commonly the culprit.

✓ Amide allergies are very rare.

REFERENCES

Roberts JR, Custalow CB, Thomsen TW, eds. Roberts and Hedges' *Clinical Procedures in Emergency Medicine*. 6th ed. Philadelphia, PA: Elsevier; 2014: 538-539.

Tintinalli JE, Stapczynski JS, Ma OJ, et al, eds. *Tintinalli's Emergency Medicine: A Comprehensive Study Guide*. 8th ed. New York, NY: McGraw-Hill; 2012: 239-240.

405. The correct answer is D, Pyridoxine.

Why is this the correct answer?

Neonatal seizures are uncommon events, but they require a different approach to management. As with all seizures, securing the airway and breathing is a priority, as is administration of first-line therapy to stop the seizure. But in a neonate, if seizures do not respond, as they did not in this case, administration of pyridoxine 100 mg IV should be considered. Pyridoxine deficiency is an autosomal recessive issue. It is not common, but it can cause neonatal seizures. Seizures can present in an atypical manner in neonates, with eye deviation alone, episodes of myoclonic jerking, or even facial tics as opposed to the more classic tonic-clonic movements. There is often an underlying abnormality causing the neonatal seizure (altered electrolytes, inborn error of metabolism, hypoxic ischemic injury, sepsis) rather than a seizure disorder, which is more commonly the cause in an older child or adult. Glucose evaluation is critical in the initial evaluation of a seizing child. Children do not have significant glycogen storage and are at risk for hypoglycemia. As in adults, hypoglycemia can masquerade as a myriad of disease process.

Why are the other choices wrong?

Adenosine is used to treat stable supraventricular tachycardia in pediatric patients. This neonate's pulse rate is slightly elevated for his age because of the seizure, but it is not indicative of supraventricular tachycardia.

The same holds true for the low glucose level: it is likely the result of the seizure, not the cause. Rarely is D50 used in pediatric hypoglycemia because it is too hypertonic to be given in a peripheral vein. If there were evidence of hypoglycemia as the cause of the seizure, D10W (5 mL/kg) could be infused.

Although benzodiazepines may be used as a first-line treatment in all other age groups, they must be used cautiously in neonates because of the higher likelihood they will cause respiratory depression. In the neonate, diazepam is a better choice than lorazepam because diazepam has a shorter half-life. In this case, lorazepam is not an appropriate next choice: two doses of benzodiazepines have already been given without effect.

PEER REVIEW

✓ If first-line agents (benzodiazepines) don't resolve a neonatal seizure, consider pyridoxine deficiency as the cause.

✓ Use benzodiazepines carefully in neonates: they're more likely to cause respiratory depression.

✓ Check for low glucose in neonatal seizures — not as a cause, but as an effect.

REFERENCES

Fleisher GR, Ludwig S, et al, eds. *Textbook of Pediatric Emergency Medicine*. 6th ed. Philadelphia, PA: Lippincott, Williams & Wilkins; 2010: 1004-1006.

Surtees R, Wolf N. Treatable neonatal epilepsy. *Arch Dis Child*. 2007;92(8):659-661. doi:10.1136/adc.2007.116913.

Wolfson AB, Hendey GW, Ling LJ, et al, eds. *Harwood-Nuss' Clinical Practice of Emergency Medicine*. 6th ed. Philadelphia, PA: Lippincott, Williams & Wilkins; 2014: 1149-1153.

406. The correct answer is D, Penicillin.

Why is this the correct answer?

The most likely diagnosis in this case is acute rheumatic fever (ARF) with symptoms concerning for arthritis and carditis. Arthritis occurs in 75% of patients with ARF and is classically seen as migratory in large joints with pain out of proportion to findings. Carditis occurs in 30% to 50% of patients with ARF. All patients with ARF should receive antibiotics, and penicillin is the antibiotic of choice (erythromycin in patients allergic to penicillin). In this particular patient, ARF is made evident by migratory polyarthralgia, signs of carditis and pericarditis, and fever with recent streptococcal infection. The diagnosis is confirmed by the Jones criteria. These criteria are as follows:

• A positive strep test

or

• Rising antistreptococcal antibodies

plus

• Two of these major criteria: carditis, new murmur, cardiomegaly/CHF, pericarditis, migratory polyarthritis, chorea, erythema marginatum, subcutaneous nodules

or

• One major criterion

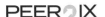

and

- Two of these minor criteria: fever, arthralgia, history of previous rheumatic fever, elevated ESR or CRP, prolonged PR interval

Carditis itself can be indicated by tachycardia, signs of CHF, a new murmur/rub/gallop, while migratory polyarthralgias is the most common symptom. Carditis poses the biggest risk for death and disease in these patients, and recognition is paramount for appropriate diagnosis. Early consultation with cardiology and admission to the hospital are necessary. Traditionally, carditis has often been treated with steroids, although recent data indicate no improvement with their use. Currently, the recommendation is to treat the carditis-associated heart failure with medications typically used for fluid overload and hypoxia as appropriate.

Why are the other choices wrong?

IVIG is not used in ARF; it is commonly used in the treatment of Kawasaki disease.

Methotrexate is typically not indicated in rheumatic fever; it is a medication commonly used to treat rheumatoid arthritis. The arthritis associated with ARF is usually treated with aspirin.

Although NSAIDs are good anti-inflammatory medications, they are not commonly used in ARF. They are used in the treatment of pericarditis, but stronger anti-inflammatory medications are indicated for this patient. The joint manifestations of ARF are generally treated with high-dose aspirin initially, followed by daily aspirin treatment for at least 1 month until symptoms and inflammatory markers are resolved.

PEER POINT

Jones criteria for diagnosing acute rheumatic fever

- A positive strep test or rising strep titers
- Plus two of these major criteria:
    Carditis, new murmur, cardiomegaly/CHF, pericarditis, migratory polyarthritis, chorea, erythema marginatum, subcutaneous nodules
- Or one major criterion from above and two of these minor criteria:
    Fever, arthralgia, history of previous rheumatic fever, elevated ESR or CRP, prolonged PR interval

PEER REVIEW

- ✓ Treat the arthritis associated with acute rheumatic fever with aspirin.
- ✓ All children with acute rheumatic fever should receive penicillin (erythromycin for penicillin-allergic patients) for strep regardless of culture results.

REFERENCES

Marx JA, Hockberger RS, Walls RM, eds. *Rosen's Emergency Medicine: Concepts and Clinical Practice.* 8th ed. St. Louis, MO: Elsevier; 2014: 1106-1112.e1.

Tintinalli JE, Stapczynski JS, Ma OJ, et al, eds. *Tintinalli's Emergency Medicine: A Comprehensive Study Guide.* 8th ed. New York, NY: McGraw-Hill; 2012: 933-934.

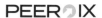

407. The correct answer is B, Perform external rotation of the testis.

Why is this the correct answer?

A genitourinary examination is essential in the evaluation of abdominal pain in any patient. The sudden onset of severe scrotal pain with radiation to the abdomen is a hallmark of testicular torsion. The longer there is diminished blood flow to the testis, the less likely that it can be salvaged. One study indicates that salvage rates drop from around 96% at 4 to 6 hours to 20% after 12 hours. Because this patient's symptoms have already been present for 12 hours, the emergency physician should attempt detorsion of the testis and obtain emergent urologic consultation. The most common direction for testicular torsion is medial (in two-thirds of cases), so the first attempt to correct it is to rotate the testis externally (outward toward the thigh, as if opening a book). Pain relief or return of a normal lie (or both) indicates a successful procedure. If relief is not apparent right away, the emergency physician may attempt detorsion again in the opposite direction. Testicular torsion accounts for 30% of acute scrotal pain presentations and is considered a surgical emergency. Again, timing is crucial. Signs and symptoms of testicular torsion include unilateral pain and swelling with an abnormal lie of the testis (either high riding or horizontal). It is important to note that symptoms alone might not indicate complete obstruction of blood flow but can result from intermittent or diminished blood flow. Further evaluation with ultrasonography and surgical exploration with likely orchiopexy are still warranted even after a successful detorsion.

Why are the other choices wrong?

The longer the testis is starved of blood, the higher the likelihood of permanent injury. Any diagnostic study that delays definitive care should not be obtained. In this case, ordering abdominal and pelvic CT instead of attempting detorsion delays care.

As mentioned above, ultrasonography is part of the evaluation of testicular torsion, but in this case, in which the patient has been in pain for more than 12 hours, the best course of action is to perform the detorsion procedure in an attempt to restore blow flow.

Similarly, consultations are likely needed, but obtaining them is not the best next step in managing this time-sensitive condition.

PEER REVIEW

✓ Hallmark of testicular torsion: severe, sudden-onset scrotal pain with radiation to the abdomen.

✓ Testicular torsion most commonly results from internal rotation, so if you're attempting detorsion, start with external rotation.

✓ Testicular torsion accounts for 30% of acute painful swelling in children, so keep it high in the differential.

REFERENCES

Fleisher GR, Ludwig S, et al, eds. *Textbook of Pediatric Emergency Medicine.* 6th ed. Philadelphia, PA: Lippincott, Williams & Wilkins; 2010: 474-482.

Schafermeyer RW, Tenenbein M, Macias CG, et al, eds. *Strange and Schafermeyer's Pediatric Emergency Medicine.* 4th ed. New York, NY: McGraw-Hill; 2015: 473-474.

Wolfson AB, Hendey GW, Ling LJ, et al, eds. *Harwood-Nuss' Clinical Practice of Emergency Medicine.* 6th ed. Philadelphia, PA: Lippincott, Williams & Wilkins; 2014: 1288-1289.

408. The correct answer is B, Obesity.

Why is this the correct answer?

The B-type natriuretic peptide (BNP) is a counter-regulatory hormone produced by cardiac myocytes in response to increased end-diastolic pressure and volume, as occurs in the setting of heart failure. ProBNP is released into the circulation and cleaved into biologically active BNP and an inactive N-terminal fragment, NT-proBNP, which has a half-life up to six times that of BNP. Patients with a high body mass index tend to have lower levels of BNP and NT-proBNP. Plasma levels of BNP and NT-proBNP correlate with the degree of left ventricular overload, severity of clinical heart failure, and both short-term and long-term cardiovascular mortality rates. Acutely dyspneic patients with BNP lower than 100 pg/mL or NT-proBNP levels lower than 300 pg/mL are very unlikely to have acute decompensated heart failure, whereas those with BNP levels higher than 500 pg/mL or NT-proBNP levels higher than 1,000 pg/mL are very likely to have it. Intermediate levels must be interpreted in the clinical context.

Why are the other choices wrong?

Patients of advanced age tend to have higher levels of BNP and NT-proBNP, not lower.

Patients with pulmonary disease resulting in cor pulmonale and patients with right heart stretch from PE have slightly elevated BNP levels.

As with advanced age, renal insufficiency can falsely elevate BNP slightly; any more significant increases in BNP are the result of heart disease.

REFERENCES

Adams JG, Barton ED, Collings J, et al, eds. *Emergency Medicine: Clinical Essentials*. 2nd ed. Philadelphia, PA: Saunders; 2013: 476-486.

Marx JA, Hockberger RS, Walls RM, eds. *Rosen's Emergency Medicine: Concepts and Clinical Practice*. 8th ed. St. Louis, MO: Elsevier; 2014: 1075-1090.

409. The correct answer is D, Retropharyngeal abscess.

Why is this the correct answer?

Retropharyngeal abscess (RPA) usually occurs in children younger than school age (typically younger than 4 years); it is an infection of the paramedian lymph tissue. In a child of this age, the tissue is still present, but it atrophies as the child develops; this is why RPA is less likely in an older child. Signs and symptoms often include fever and tender cervical lymphadenopathy, usually unilateral. Sore throat and neck pain can also be present; a muffled voice, drooling, and stridor are more ominous signs and indicate increased edema within the airway. The inspiratory lateral xray shown reveals RPA with swelling of the retropharyngeal tissue, classically showing more than 7 mm at C2. Most references recommend CT scanning for making a definitive diagnosis and determining whether the child needs surgery if there is an abscess or if treatment with intravenous antibiotics is appropriate.

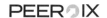

Why are the other choices wrong?

Croup is a viral illness (parainfluenza 1 most commonly, also respiratory syncytial virus, adenovirus, influenza A) that affects the supraglottic airway and typically occurs in children 6 months to 3 years old. Symptoms include an upper respiratory illness, fever, hoarse voice, and the classic barking, seal-like cough, which makes it less likely in this case. Stridor is an indication of airway edema, and it is imperative to ensure that the child has an adequate airway.

Epiglottitis, although markedly less common now with the advent of the *Haemophilus influenzae* type b vaccine, affects patients in a wide age range, from newborn to adult. The average age among pediatric patients ranges from 2 to 7 years. Until development of the Hib vaccine, H. influenzae type b was the most likely causative organism, and it can still cause epiglottitis even in those who are fully immunized. There is now no predominant causative organism, so the infection can be due to *Staphylococcus aureus*, *Streptococcus pneumoniae*, and beta-hemolytic streptococci (groups A and C). Epiglottitis typically presents acutely (within 12 to 24 hours of symptom onset) with several hours of fever and a toxic appearance. There is a history of progressive sore throat, drooling, and dysphagia; severe stridor is usually absent, but the patient might be positioned in the tripod or "sniffing" position, and thus caution should be used when trying to examine the pharynx. Epiglottitis is usually a clinical diagnosis, but an elevated WBC count with a bandemia can be present, and 70% to 90% of blood cultures are positive.

Peritonsillar abscess develops in older children, adolescents, and adults. It is often due to extension of a primary tonsillar infection, typically group A streptococci, but it can be polymicrobial. This can cause the classic findings of an asymmetric pharynx with the affected tonsil deviated medially due to the infection. Although a child might complain of neck pain, there is usually no limitation of movement with peritonsillar abscess, which makes this diagnosis less likely in this case.

PEER POINT

Diseases of the pharynx, larynx, and trachea

Diagnosis	Etiology	Clinical Presentation	Treatment	Comments
Bacterial tracheitis	*S. aureus* (most common)	**Age predominance:** 3 months–13 years but usually <5 years **Symptoms:** Fever, barky cough (unlike epiglottitis and retropharyngeal abscess), sore throat, minimal voice change, no dysphagia **Onset:** 2–7 days of upper respiratory symptoms **Exam:** Toxic appearance, inspiratory and expiratory stridor	Parenteral antibiotics (third-generation cephalosporin plus resistant penicillin) penicillinase or clindamycin, consider vancomycin for MRSA Endotracheal intubation"	Also known as membranous laryngotracheobronchitis Pathophysiology: Bacterial superinfection of the tracheal epithelium with thick mucopurulent secretions Generally more toxic appearing than patients with croup infection Lateral neck radiograph: Normal except for shaggy tracheal air column Complication: Airway obstruction"

Table continued on next page

475

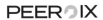

Diagnosis	Etiology	Clinical Presentation	Treatment	Comments
Epiglottitis	*H. influenzae, S. pneumoniae*	**Age predominance:** 3–6 years and adults **Symptoms:** Fever, sore throat, muffled voice, drooling, dysphagia, lack of cough **Onset:** Abrupt, within hours **Exam:** Anxious and toxic appearance, sitting upright in "sniffing" position, drooling, inspiratory stridor	Parenteral antibiotics (second- or third-generation cephalosporin) Nebulized racemic epinephrine (for airway edema) Endotracheal intubation, ideally with fiberoptic laryngoscopy for airway control	**Lateral neck radiograph:** "Thumbprint" sign with swollen epiglottis Avoid manipulation (tongue blade insertion to visualize epiglottis); it can worsen airway occlusion Allow the patient to remain in the most comfortable position (usually upright in the caregiver's lap)
Peritonsillar abscess	Polymicrobial, with the most common bacterial organism being *S. pyogenes*	**Age predominance:** 20–30 years **Symptoms:** Fever, odynophagia, dysphagia, drooling, "hot potato" voice **Exam:** Exudative tonsillitis, unilateral peritonsillar erythema and swelling, trismus, uvular deviation	Aspiration or incision and drainage of abscess Antibiotics (penicillin, cephalosporin, or clindamycin)	Most common deep space infection of the head and neck in adults Suppurative complication of pharyngitis **Complication:** Airway obstruction
Retropharyngeal abscess	Group A beta-hemolytic streptococci (most common) Polymicrobial	**Age predominance:** 6 months–4 years (rare after 4 years because of retropharyngeal lymph node atrophy) **Symptoms:** Fever, sore throat, muffled voice, decreased intake, lack of cough **Onset:** Insidious progression of upper respiratory symptoms for 2–3 days (unlike epiglottitis, which is rapid, within hours) **Exam:** Toxic appearance, dysphagia, hyperextended neck, inspiratory stridor, retropharyngeal mass **Other:** Similar presentation to epiglottitis except for age predominance and symptom onset	Parenteral broad-spectrum antibiotics, including clindamycin Possible endotracheal intubation for airway control	**Children:** Caused by infection of retropharyngeal lymph nodes **Adults:** Caused by local extension of infection (parotitis, otitis media, nasopharyngitis) **Lateral neck radiograph:** Retropharyngeal soft tissue space widening (end-inspiratory, mild neck extension is best quality radiograph to prevent false-positive result) **Definitive imaging:** CT **Complications:** Airway obstruction, mediastinitis, aspiration pneumonia, sepsis

PEER REVIEW

✓ How old is the patient? Retropharyngeal abscess is typical in patients younger than 4 years, and peritonsillar abscess is more likely in older pediatric patients and adults.

✓ Presentation of retropharyngeal abscess: fever and tender lymph nodes unilaterally, and sometimes torticollis.

✓ Be careful when you evaluate the pharynx in a patient who might have upper airway edema — drooling, toxic appearance, tripod or sniffing position, muffled voice.

REFERENCES

Fleisher GR, Ludwig S, et al, eds. *Textbook of Pediatric Emergency Medicine.* 6th ed. Philadelphia, PA: Lippincott, Williams & Wilkins; 2010: 906-907.

Wolfson AB, Hendey GW, Ling LJ, et al, eds. *Harwood-Nuss' Clinical Practice of Emergency Medicine.* 6th ed. Philadelphia, PA: Lippincott, Williams & Wilkins; 2014: 377-381; 1218-1219.

410. The correct answer is A, Emergent orthopedic consultation for surgical management.

Why is this the correct answer?

The patient in this case has sustained a fracture of the proximal third ulna and a dislocation of the radial head, which is known as a Monteggia fracture-dislocation. The definitive repair is open reduction and internal fixation, so the appropriate emergency department intervention is to initiate prompt orthopedic consultation. To make the patient more comfortable in the meantime, the arm may be placed in a temporary splint. Another fracture-dislocation of the forearm is a Galeazzi fracture, which is a distal radius fracture and a dislocation of the distal radioulnar joint. The injury most commonly sustained when a person falls on the outstretched hand (the FOOSH injury) is a distal wrist fracture. When evaluating a possible forearm fracture, it is important to include elbow radiographs, including a lateral view, to examine the position of the radial head. On the lateral film, a horizontal line drawn through the midline of the radial shaft should bisect the capitellum. If this line (the radiocapitellar line) does not bisect the capitellum, the patient has sustained either a facture or a dislocation or was not positioned properly for the radiograph.

Why are the other choices wrong?

Although long arm splinting is appropriate to temporarily immobilize the fracture location of a Monteggia fracture-dislocation, definitive repair is needed emergently to reduce the dislocation and should not be deferred for outpatient management if possible.

The radial head must be surgically reduced in a timely manner, along with internal fixation of the ulna. Again, outpatient management is not appropriate.

A sling does not properly immobilize or manage a Monteggia fracture-dislocation.

PEER POINT

MUGR mnemonic

The two fracture-dislocations can be remembered with the MUGR (or "mugger") mnemonic, indicating which forearm bone is fractured.

<u>M</u>onteggia = <u>U</u>lna / <u>G</u>aleazzi = <u>R</u>adius

PEER REVIEW

✓ A Monteggia fracture is a fracture of the proximal third ulna and a dislocation of the radial head.

✓ Monteggia fractures require surgical management.

✓ If you're evaluating a forearm fracture, get xrays of the elbow to evaluate the radial head: the radiocapitellar line should bisect the capitellum. If it doesn't, suspect a fracture, dislocation, or improper position.

REFERENCES

Sherman S. *Simon's Emergency Orthopedics*. 7th ed. New York, NY: McGraw-Hill; 2015. 112

Tintinalli JE, Stapczynski JS, Ma OJ, et al, eds. *Tintinalli's Emergency Medicine: A Comprehensive Study Guide*. 8th ed. New York, NY: McGraw-Hill; 2012: 1816-1828.

411. The correct answer is A, Acute cerebellar ataxia.

Why is this the correct answer?

The underlying cause of this patient's symptoms is acute cerebellar ataxia, a postinfectious condition that occurs about 2 weeks after a viral illness. It is the most common cause of ataxia in children, found in more than one-third of cases of pediatric ataxia and more common in children younger than 6 years. Infection with coxsackie B virus, echovirus 6, Epstein-Barr virus, influenza, mumps, varicella, and other viruses has been associated with acute cerebellar ataxia. In addition to acute onset, the effects on gait predominate and are worst early on. Effects on the trunk are more pronounced than those on the extremities. The emergency department evaluation of a patient presenting with ataxia must eliminate potential life-threatening causes such as masses, injury, or infection. The examination should evaluate mental status, extraocular movement, gait (if possible), and deep tendon reflexes; cerebellar testing should be performed. In most cases, acute postinfectious cerebellar ataxia resolves on its own in 2 to 3 weeks.

Why are the other choices wrong?

Brain mass is not likely in an acute onset of ataxia, due to its rarity, but an acute intracerebral hemorrhage should be considered. The examination described in the case does not indicate increased intracranial pressure; the patient has a normal mental status and normal vital signs (as opposed to the Cushing triad of hypertension, bradycardia, and an irregular respiratory rate), and there are no signs of papilledema.

Drug ingestion is the second most common cause of ataxia but is more likely to occur in an adolescent or adult. This child is responsive, and there is no history of ingestion, although the emergency physician should always consider this and consider obtaining a drug screen and/or alcohol level as deemed appropriate.

Guillain-Barré syndrome is an ascending demyelinating polyneuropathy associated with decreased or no deep tendon reflexes. It also seems to be a postinfectious process. There is a variant, Miller-Fisher, that causes a descending demyelination and can present with ataxia, areflexia, and ophthalmoplegia. But the patient in this case has intact deep tendon reflexes, so Guillain-Barré syndrome is not the most likely diagnosis.

PEER REVIEW

✓ Most common causes of ataxia in children: acute postinfectious cerebellar ataxia and drug ingestion.

✓ Life-threatening causes of ataxia you have to rule out: hypoglycemia, intracranial infections, intracranial mass, bleed, and stroke.

✓ Getting a thorough history of recent illnesses can help make the diagnosis of both acute postinfectious cerebellar ataxia and Guillain-Barré syndrome.

REFERENCES

Fleisher GR, Ludwig S, et al, eds. *Textbook of Pediatric Emergency Medicine*. 6th ed. Philadelphia, PA: Lippincott, Williams & Wilkins; 2010: 164-167.

Schafermeyer RW, Tenenbein M, Macias CG, et al, eds. *Strange and Schafermeyer's Pediatric Emergency Medicine*. 4th ed. New York, NY: McGraw-Hill; 2015: 323.

Wolfson AB, Hendey GW, Ling LJ, et al, eds. *Harwood-Nuss' Clinical Practice of Emergency Medicine*. 6th ed. Philadelphia, PA: Lippincott, Williams & Wilkins; 2014: 1156-1159.

412. The correct answer is A, 2 cm below the proximal tibial tuberosity.

Why is this the correct answer?

An intraosseous (IO) line provides emergent large-bore access (15 gauge) to an acutely ill patient. Any fluid or medication that would be infused intravenously may be infused through an IO line. The most common location for placement of an IO line is the proximal tibia, approximately 1 to 2 cm below the tibial tuberosity. The needle should be directed perpendicular to and on the flat medial aspect of the bone. If there is any angulation of the IO needle, it should be caudal to avoid any potential injury to the tibial physis. When resuscitation is in progress, vascular access is crucial. In these situations, the likelihood of peripheral intravenous placement is low, especially if the child is in cardiopulmonary arrest or there are signs of shock. Central venous access is possible but costs precious time to establish; therefore, IO placement, which provides a 15-gauge needle, is the best way to access the critically ill child when emergent resuscitation is needed. The limitation of IO infusion is that, due to the narrowed interior of the accessed bone, the fluid might meet increased resistance and cause discomfort. Pressure bags, pumps, and mechanically pushed fluids can be used to overcome the resistance. Premedication with lidocaine (0.5 mg/kg via slow IV push) may be used to diminish discomfort. Contraindications to IO line placement include infection at the site of insertion, bony injury, or prior IO line placement in the site of insertion, as well as a history of bone abnormalities such as osteogenesis imperfecta. Complications of IO lines include infection at the site of insertion, fracture, osteomyelitis, and compartment syndrome, as well as the most common complication: extravasation at the site of insertion.

Why are the other choices wrong?

Again, the most common location for placement of an IO line is the proximal tibia, and not the fibula. The fibula is very small in young children and likely not large enough for IO use in a resuscitation.

The proximal humerus, not the distal humerus, is an acceptable location for an IO line.

Although there are many sites where an IO line may be placed (the proximal tibia, the proximal humeral head, the distal femur, the medial malleolus, and the iliac spine), the sternum, although a possible site, is not a common location for an IO line in either pediatric or adult patients. With this patient in cardiopulmonary arrest, the sternal location of an IO makes it very difficult to provide effective cardiac circulation with CPR.

PEER REVIEW

- ✓ In the care of a critically ill child, when access is needed emergently, intraosseous line placement is an important skill.
- ✓ Insert the intraosseous needle 1 to 3 cm below the anatomic landmark of the proximal tibial tuberosity.
- ✓ Locations for intraosseous line placement: proximal tibia, proximal humeral head, distal femur, medial malleolus, iliac spine.

REFERENCES
Fleisher GR, Ludwig S, et al, eds. *Textbook of Pediatric Emergency Medicine*. 6th ed. Philadelphia, PA: Lippincott, Williams & Wilkins; 2010: 18; 1761.
Wolfson AB, Hendey GW, Ling LJ, et al, eds. *Harwood-Nuss' Clinical Practice of Emergency Medicine*. 6th ed. Philadelphia, PA: Lippincott, Williams & Wilkins; 2014: 1094.

413. The correct answer is B, Infection.

Why is this the correct answer?

Disseminated intravascular coagulation, or DIC, is an acquired disorder characterized by activation of the coagulation system that leads to thrombosis and ultimate consumption of coagulation factors and platelets. Subsequent activation of the fibrinolytic system then causes bleeding. The most common cause of acute DIC is likely infection. In the original historic studies, the etiology of DIC in nearly 40%

of the patients was an infectious process, and 20% of patients with gram-negative sepsis had DIC. This is important to understand because DIC is a consequence of a primary process; thus the management priority is to treat the underlying cause. Chronic DIC, which leads more to clotting than bleeding complications, is caused most commonly by cancer.

Why are the other choices wrong?

In the classic study of clinical and laboratory aspects of DIC, malignancy was the etiology of 6.8% of DIC cases investigated. Among patients with acute leukemia, DIC is most often associated with promyelocytic leukemia. The release of enzymes is increased while the patient is undergoing chemotherapy. Bleeding is the more likely (more than thrombosis) complication.

Transfusion reactions are a less common cause than are infections. In these cases, DIC occurs with severe bleeding, shock, and renal failure.

Trauma was reported as a precipitating factor in DIC in 16.9% of the cases in the original study. The mortality rate for the trauma patients was 30%, lowest of the etiologies; the average mortality rate was 54.7%. Traumatic injuries and complications commonly associated with DIC include brain and crush injuries and burns, as well as hypothermia and hyperthermia, rhabdomyolysis, fat embolism, and hypoxia.

PEER REVIEW

✓ A patient with DIC can have both thrombosis and bleeding because the disorder activates both the coagulation cascade and the fibrinolytic system.

✓ Infection is the most common cause of DIC.

✓ The priority in treating DIC is treating the underlying cause rather than the DIC itself.

REFERENCES

Marx JA, Hockberger RS, Walls RM, eds. *Rosen's Emergency Medicine: Concepts and Clinical Practice*. 8th ed. St. Louis, MO: Elsevier; 2014: 1606-1616.e1.

Siegal T, Seligsohn U, Aghai E, Modan M. Clinical and laboratory aspects of disseminated intravascular coagulation (DIC): a study of 118 cases. *Thromb Haemost*. 1978;39(1):122-134.

Tintinalli JE, Stapczynski JS, Ma OJ, et al, eds. *Tintinalli's Emergency Medicine: A Comprehensive Study Guide*. 8th ed. New York, NY: McGraw-Hill; 2012: 1494.

414. The correct answer is A, Etanercept.

Why is this the correct answer?

Based on the patient's presenting complaints, the most likely diagnosis is tuberculosis. The most likely precipitating factor in the development of infection is her use of etanercept, a biopharmaceutical agent approved for the treatment of the autoimmune diseases ankylosing spondylitis, juvenile rheumatoid arthritis, plaque psoriasis, psoriatic arthritis, and rheumatoid arthritis (RA). In mild or new RA,

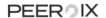

patients typically are treated with NSAIDs or steroids. But if the disease progresses to moderate or severe RA, rheumatologists typically prescribe methotrexate plus an anti-TNF (tumor necrosis factor) medication. Anti-TNF medications such as etanercept are known to cause immunosuppression, which increases the patient's risk of developing severe infections, including sepsis, pneumonia, and tuberculosis. In any patient with RA, it is important to review his or her medication list and look for potential immunosuppressive medications that might be putting the patient at risk for life-threatening infections. Septic arthritis, for example, should be considered in any patient who is taking immunosuppressive drugs who presents with acute arthritis. Etanercept also has been associated with URI and pharyngitis. The overall infection risk is between 50% and 81%.

Why are the other choices wrong?

Fluticasone is sometimes used as an inhaled corticosteroid treatment for asthma. Pulmonary infections can result from the use of fluticasone, but it is not typically associated with tuberculosis.

Metformin is not usually associated with infection or immunosuppressed states, although it is used to treat diabetes. Patients with diabetes are more likely to go from latent to active TB disease, but the medication itself does not cause the immunosuppression.

Methotrexate is a common RA medication and is known to cause flulike illnesses, pulmonary compromise, and renal or hepatic impairment. However, a large longitudinal study has shown that it does not increase the risk of infection in RA patients.

PEER REVIEW

- ✓ In mild rheumatoid arthritis, NSAIDs or steroids are typically the medication of choice.
- ✓ Do other treatments for rheumatoid arthritis have side effects? Anti-TNF medications like etanercept can put patients at risk for sepsis, pneumonia, and even tuberculosis.
- ✓ Side effects of methotrexate: flulike illnesses and hepatic, renal, or pulmonary impairment.

REFERENCES

Doran MF, Crowson CS, Pond GR, et al. Predictors of infection in rheumatoid arthritis. *Arthritis Rheum.* 2002;46(9):2294–2300. doi:10.1002/art.10529.

Marx JA, Hockberger RS, Walls RM, eds. *Rosen's Emergency Medicine: Concepts and Clinical Practice.* 8th ed. St. Louis, MO: Elsevier; 2014: 1501-1517.e2.

Tintinalli JE, Stapczynski JS, Ma OJ, et al, eds. *Tintinalli's Emergency Medicine: A Comprehensive Study Guide.* 8th ed. New York, NY: McGraw-Hill; 2012: 1911-1920; 1934.

415. The correct answer is D, Synchronized cardioversion 100 J.

Why is this the correct answer?

The ECG demonstrates a fast, irregular narrow-complex rhythm consistent with atrial fibrillation with rapid ventricular response. Electrical cardioversion is indicated in an unstable patient with an atrial tachycardia, typically a rate above 150, from a cardiac etiology. Using a biphasic defibrillator with synchronized cardioversion at 100 J, there is a 94% success rate of cardioversion. Synchronized cardioversion synchronizes to the R waves, helping to avoid induction of ventricular fibrillation. Stable patients with atrial fibrillation lasting longer than 48 hours ideally should undergo anticoagulation before cardioversion to minimize risk of thromboembolism. However, an unstable patient or a patient whose risk of developing atrial fibrillation outweighs the risk for thromboembolism should undergo cardioversion. Indications for cardioversion include tachycardia with symptoms of active chest pain, pulmonary edema, lightheadedness, and hypotension. Contraindications include automaticity etiologies of atrial tachycardia such as digitalis toxicity, sinus tachycardia, and multifocal atrial tachycardia. Cardioversion in digitalis toxicity increases the incidence of postshock ventricular tachycardia and ventricular fibrillation.

Why are the other choices wrong?

Adenosine does not convert atrial fibrillation or atrial flutter. It is useful in the treatment of paroxysmal supraventricular tachycardia with Wolff-Parkinson-White syndrome. It has also been used to differentiate narrow-complex tachycardia from monomorphic wide-complex tachycardia. In unstable patients, which includes those with symptoms of altered mental status and hypotension, synchronized cardioversion is the correct treatment.

Pulseless ventricular tachycardia and ventricular fibrillation should be defibrillated with a biphasic defibrillator at 120 J followed by 200 J. Defibrillation is the use of electricity without synchronizing to the R wave.

Diltiazem is commonly used to slow the ventricular rate in patients with atrial fibrillation, but it is contraindicated in patients with hypotension (systolic BP <90). In stable patients with atrial fibrillation with rapid ventricular response, the typical dose of diltiazem is 0.25mg/kg IV bolus, which may be followed with a drip of 5 to 15 mg/hr IV to control the rate.

PEER POINT

Tachyarrhythmias and management

- Atrial fibrillation — Synchronized cardioversion 100-200 J
- Atrial flutter — Synchronized cardioversion 50 J
- Pulseless ventricular tachycardia and ventricular fibrillation — Defibrillation 120 J followed by 200 J
- Stable ventricular tachycardia — Synchronized cardioversion 50 J
- Supraventricular tachycardia — Synchronized cardioversion 50 J

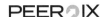

PEER REVIEW

✓ Unstable patients with atrial tachycardia should undergo synchronized cardioversion with 50 J for atrial flutter and 100 to 200 J in atrial fibrillation.

✓ Adenosine is not effective for chemical cardioversion of atrial fibrillation or atrial flutter.

REFERENCES

Page RL, Joglar JA, Caldwell MA, et al. 2015 ACC/AHA/HRS guideline for the management of adult patients with supraventricular tachycardia: a report of the American College of Cardiology/American Heart Association Task Force on Clinical Practice Guidelines and the Heart Rhythm Society. *Circulation*. 2016;133;e506-e574.

Roberts JR, Hedges JR, eds. *Clinical Procedures in Emergency Medicine*. 6th ed. St. Louis, Mo: WB Saunders; 2013: 213-247.

Tintinalli JE, Stapczynski JS, Ma OJ, et al, eds. *Tintinalli's Emergency Medicine: A Comprehensive Study Guide*. 8th ed. New York, NY: McGraw-Hill; 2012: 159.

416. The correct answer is D, Provide reassurance.

Why is this the correct answer?

Febrile seizures are the most common presenting seizure disorder in children. They result from a temperature of 38°C (100.4°F) or more with no evidence of intracranial infection or other defined cause or neurologic disease. There are two major categories: simple and complex. The distinctions are patient age, duration of seizure activity, number of episodes in 24 hours, and generalized as opposed to focal. This patient's seizure activity lasted less than 15 minutes and happened only once; it was generalized, and he is older than 6 months, so it is a simple febrile seizure. Appropriate management is discharge home with reassurance and outpatient follow-up care. Overall, long-term morbidity and mortality rates from febrile seizures are minimal even with prolonged seizure activity.

Why are the other choices wrong?

The risk of significant bacterial infection, including meningitis, in a patient with febrile seizure is the same as it is in a febrile child without seizure. The underlying fever should be evaluated with a thorough history and physical examination; laboratory analysis rarely adds any helpful data and is not needed in the case described. The same is true for imaging studies, and it is important to minimize a child's exposure to ionizing radiation unless it is warranted (focal deficits, alteration of mental status).

Consideration of electrolyte abnormalities is important, and if there is a history to indicate potential loss (vomiting, diarrhea) or impaired intake, then electrolytes should be checked. Glucose level should be determined for any patient presenting for evaluation of seizure to ensure that hypoglycemia, which can be readily treated, is not the underlying cause or is not prolonging the symptoms. But this patient's presentation does not suggest electrolyte abnormality.

Lumbar puncture (LP) should be considered if a child's signs or symptoms are concerning for meningitis or focal neurologic deficit. The American Academy of Pediatrics notes that, in children 6 months to 5 years old, LP should be considered if a child was recently treated with antibiotics, is not up-to-date on vaccinations, or

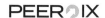

exhibits signs of meningitis or encephalitis. Again, the patient in this case does not meet any of those criteria.

PEER POINT

Febrile seizure: is it simple or complex?

	Simple	Complex
Activity	Generalized	Focal, or focal with a Jacksonian march
Age	6 months to 5 years	Younger than 6 months, older than 5 years
Duration	Less than 15 min	More than 15 min
Episodes in 24 hrs	1	2 or more

PEER REVIEW

✓ When is it OK to reassure and discharge a patient after a febrile seizure? When it's a simple febrile seizure, and when the patient is getting back to baseline and doesn't have signs or symptoms of a more sinister etiology.

✓ Get a baseline glucose if a patient is actively seizing, but otherwise, laboratory and imaging studies aren't all that useful in febrile seizure.

✓ Consider lumbar puncture in a child with febrile seizure if there are focal findings, or a history or physical examination raising concerns of deficit, or the child has been exposed to antibiotics.

REFERENCES

Fleisher GR, Ludwig S, et al, eds. *Textbook of Pediatric Emergency Medicine.* 6th ed. Philadelphia, PA: Lippincott, Williams & Wilkins; 2010: 569-570.

Wolfson AB, Hendey GW, Ling LJ, et al, eds. *Harwood-Nuss' Clinical Practice of Emergency Medicine.* 6th ed. Philadelphia, PA: Lippincott, Williams & Wilkins; 2014: 1149-1153.

417. The correct answer is B, 38-year-old woman with a forehead contusion and a swollen hand.

Why is this the correct answer?

Among victims of blunt trauma, concern for cervical spine injury is common. Fortunately, medical decision support tools such as the NEXUS criteria have been developed and validated to help identify those who are at very low risk for cervical spine injury and in whom cervical spine imaging can be safely avoided. In this case, the crash victim who is the best candidate for transport without immobilization, according to the NEXUS criteria, is the one who does not appear to have been drinking, who does not seem confused, and whose injuries have not likely resulted in neurologic deficit. These are the NEXUS criteria:

- No tenderness at the posterior midline of the cervical spine
- No focal neurologic deficit
- No altered level of alertness
- No evidence of intoxication
- No clinically apparent distracting injury

If the patient meets all of these criteria after blunt trauma, he or she can be cleared from a cervical spine injury without imaging. In this case, the 38-year-old woman meets all the conditions: neither the contusion nor the hand injury is painful enough to distract her from the pain a cervical spine injury would cause. As the authors of the NEXUS study proposed, the benefit of such a validated tool is that it can eliminate a portion of the cervical spine radiographs performed in the United States, and thus substantially reduce health care costs and patients' exposure to ionizing radiation.

Why are the other choices wrong?

Even though he does not complain of injuries on scene, the 22-year-old man must be transported with cervical spine immobilization because he smells of alcohol. This is evidence of possible intoxication, so he does not meet NEXUS criteria and requires cervical spine imaging.

The 45-year-old woman also requires transport with cervical spine immobilization. Although knee pain is not considered a distracting injury, the mild confusion indicates that she does not have a normal level of alertness. That means she does not meet NEXUS criteria and requires cervical spine imaging.

Cervical spine immobilization also is required before transporting the 52-year-old man. The numbness in his hand is concerning for a possible focal neurologic deficit. As a result, this patient does not meet NEXUS criteria and requires cervical spine imaging.

PEER POINT

Features of the cervical spine xray

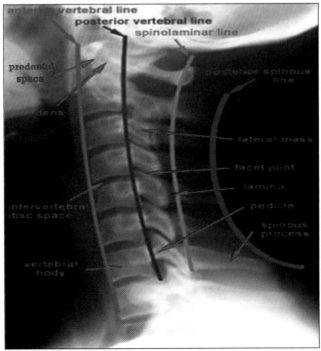

PEER Point 33

PEER REVIEW

✓ You can't clear a cervical spine injury from likely fracture if a blunt trauma victim has any of the five NEXUS criteria findings: focal neurologic deficit, midline spinal tenderness, altered level of consciousness, intoxication, or distracting injury.

REFERENCES

Hoffman JR, Mower WR, Wolfson AB, et al. Validity of a set of clinical criteria to rule out injury to the cervical spine in patients with blunt trauma. *N Engl J Med*. 2000;343:94-99.

Roberts JR, Hedges JR, eds. *Clinical Procedures in Emergency Medicine*. 6th ed. St. Louis, MO: WB Saunders; 2013: 893-903.

Tintinalli JE, Stapczynski JS, Ma OJ, et al, eds. *Tintinalli's Emergency Medicine: A Comprehensive Study Guide*. 8th ed. New York, NY: McGraw-Hill; 2012: 1721-1723.

418. The correct answer is D, Reminder to give aspirin to a patient with a positive troponin.

Why is this the correct answer?

Clinical decision support interventions are tools that are integrated into clinical care workflows to provide information physicians can use to guide clinical decision making. Clinical decision support takes many forms, including documentation templates, order sets, links to reference material, patient status indicators, and rule-based alerts. A reminder to give aspirin to a patient with a positive troponin is an example of a real-time, rule-based alert that uses information on the individual patient's conditions (a positive troponin) combined with medical evidence (patients with acute MI benefit from aspirin) to remind the clinician to perform a specific intervention (administer aspirin). The rule automatically reviews patient information (laboratory test results and medication orders) and displays a reminder to the provider if the patient has a positive troponin and does not have aspirin ordered. If both conditions are not met, no alert is displayed. The alert displays in the provider's workflow and makes it easy to order aspirin or provide an override reason to explain why aspirin is not appropriate for the patient such as allergy to aspirin or active, severe GI bleeding.

Why are the other choices wrong?

Calculation of documentation items needed for a level 5 chart is a rule-based tool for administrative purposes to increase billing charges. It is not a clinical decision support tool and should not influence clinical decision-making.

A list of patient medications is a core feature of the electronic health record. It enables review of the patient's health information but does not provide additional clinical decision-making guidance.

Like the list of medications, links to radiology systems are a core feature and are not intended to influence clinical decision-making.

PEER REVIEW

✓ Clinical decision support interventions are electronic tools that help inform clinical decision-making within the clinician's workflow.

✓ Here are some examples of clinical decision support: documentation templates, order sets, links to reference material, patient status indicators, and rule-based alerts.

✓ Rule-based alerts are a sophisticated type of clinical decision support combining individual patient information and medical evidence to help clinicians at the point of care.

REFERENCES
Strauss RW, Mayer TA, eds. *Emergency Department Management*. New York, NY: McGraw-Hill; 2014:408-413.

419. The correct answer is D, Macro.

Why is this the correct answer?

Documentation is a time-consuming part of the emergency department visit. Many physicians use tools and techniques to help them document faster such as macros, which allow the user to include predetermined text or perform a series of operations with a single keystroke and button click. In this case, the physician likely used a macro to insert a normal examination into the note. When macros are used, the inserted text must be reviewed and edited carefully. In this case, the provider neglected to add the examination of the left arm cellulitis and also failed to indicate the patient had a right-sided below-the-knee amputation (and remove associated right lower extremity normal examination findings). These errors can be difficult to defend in a lawsuit or billing dispute and could lead to Medicare or Medicaid fines under the False Claims Act.

Why are the other choices wrong?

Abbreviations such as RRR for regular, rate, and rhythm are frequently used but might not be universally known and can be misinterpreted by other readers. In this case, the abbreviations are accurate.

Alert fatigue occurs when there are frequent interruptive alerts or reminders and users become desensitized to them and ignore them.

With copy and paste, physicians sometimes find previously recorded notes in the record and copy the content into their own notes. The copied content should be reviewed carefully because it might contain incorrect information or information that no longer applies to the current visit. The examination here is normal, making it more likely that the error resulted from using a macro than from copying and pasting from an earlier note in the patient's record.

PEER REVIEW

✓ Macros, abbreviations, and copy and paste techniques can improve clinical documentation efficiency.

✓ Inaccurate information can be inadvertently added to the documentation when macros and copy and paste are used.

✓ When macros and copy and paste are used, providers should carefully review and edit the documentation.

REFERENCES

Strauss RW, Mayer TA, eds. *Emergency Department Management*. New York, NY: McGraw-Hill; 2014: 401-407.

420. The correct answer is D, Cephalexin.

Why is this the correct answer?

Amoxicillin is a first-generation antibiotic in the penicillin family, which contains medications most commonly associated with allergy. However, close to 90% of patients with reported allergy do not suffer from a true allergy, which occurs in less than 8% of patients who report allergy. Patients who experience anaphylactic symptoms as a result of taking penicillins are four times more likely to experience similar symptoms with cephalosporins, although the risk of anaphylaxis is less than 1%. Specific cephalosporins, primarily first generation, possess a similar R1 side chain that increases the risk of cross reactivity. The risk of anaphylaxis is greater with first-generation cephalosporins such as cephalexin. Third- and fourth-generation cephalosporins possess very low risk of cross reactivity.

Why are the other choices wrong?

Cefepime is a fourth-generation cephalosporin that is very unlikely to induce anaphylaxis in patients with amoxicillin allergy. The risk approaches less than 0.01%.

Cefixime is a third-generation cephalosporin, and its risk profile for anaphylaxis in patients with amoxicillin allergy is similar to that for cefepime, about 0.01%.

Ceftriaxone is another third-generation cephalosporin. Like cefepime and cefixime, it is not likely to cause anaphylaxis in patients with amoxicillin allergy.

PEER REVIEW

✓ Allergic reactions have various causes, but the most commonly implicated medication is penicillin.

✓ First-generation cephalosporins demonstrate the greatest risk of cross reactivity with penicillin, with rates approaching 1% to 8%.

✓ Later-generation cephalosporins demonstrate risk approaching 0.01%.

✓ Parenterally administered medications cause most anaphylactic reactions.

REFERENCES

Marx JA, Hockberger RS, Walls RM, eds. *Rosen's Emergency Medicine: Concepts and Clinical Practice*. 8th ed. St. Louis, MO: Elsevier; 2014: 1543-1557.e2.

Tintinalli JE, Stapczynski JS, Ma OJ, et al, eds. *Tintinalli's Emergency Medicine: A Comprehensive Study Guide*. 8th ed. New York, NY: McGraw-Hill; 2012: 74-79.

421. The correct answer is C, Stevens-Johnson syndrome.

Why is this the correct answer?

Stevens-Johnson syndrome (SJS) is a life-threatening dermatologic condition. It is described as a diffuse rash with target lesions that progresses to blisters and bullae. Hands and soles and mucous membranes are involved, with full-thickness skin necrosis affecting less than 30% of the total body surface area. Stevens-Johnson syndrome is often caused by a drug reaction, although infections and malignancy have also been implicated. It was thought that SJS is part of a continuum of dermatologic conditions starting with erythema multiforme (EM), progressing to SJS, and culminating in toxic epidermal necrolysis (TEN). Currently, there are some who believe that EM is a disease distinct from the other two. Treatment for SJS requires hospitalization in an ICU or burn unit for optimal administration of fluids and electrolytes, control of pain and infection, and cessation of the offending agent.

Why are the other choices wrong?

Erythema multiforme is a discrete rash known best for its target lesion appearance. It is associated with several culprits: infections (HSV), drugs (sulfa and other antibiotics, anticonvulsants), autoimmune diseases, and idiopathic. There are two classifications of EM: minor and major. Minor is a self-limited rash involving mostly the extremities without prodromal symptoms or mucous membrane involvement. Outpatient treatment and supportive care usually are adequate. The major type is more severe, starting with a prodromal viral illness progressing to rash that involves palms and soles and mucous membranes. Treatment typically includes observation to ensure no further disease progression. In both forms, less than 10% of the body surface is involved, so it not the diagnosis for the presentation described.

Staphylococcal scalded skin syndrome (SSSS, or Ritter disease or dermatitis exfoliativa neonatorum) is a diffuse tender scarlatiniform erythematous rash. It causes skin blisters and sloughing (positive Nikolsky sign), but mucous membranes are spared. It is most often seen in infants and has a low mortality rate, less than 5%. Although SSSS is rare in adults, when it does occur it is associated with a much higher mortality rate. An exfoliative toxin in certain strains of *Staphylococcus aureus* causes SSSS. Both SSSS and bullous impetigo are blistering skin diseases caused by the staphylococcal exfoliative toxin. In bullous impetigo, the exfoliative toxins are restricted to the area of infection, and bacteria can be cultured from the blister contents. But in SSSS, the exfoliative toxins spread hematogenously, causing epidermal damage at distant sites; the bullous materials are sterile. Treatment consists of supportive care (fluids and pain control) and eradication of the primary infection.

Toxic epidermal necrolysis (TEN, or Lyell disease) is a life-threatening dermatologic condition characterized by a diffuse erythematous macular rash that coalesces forming bullae; necrosis develops, and the epidermis separates from the dermis. There is both mucosal involvement and Nikolsky sign present. Symptoms first affect the eyes, spread caudal to the thorax and upper extremities, and finally progress to the lower body, involving more than 30% of the body surface area, larger than the condition described in the question. Toxic epidermal necrolysis is most commonly drug induced (sulfa, penicillin, NSAIDs) but has also been associated with infection, malignancy, and vaccines. Persons with AIDS who are taking sulfa prophylaxis have a thousandfold higher risk of developing TEN. Patients are treated in an ICU or burn unit; administration of the offending agent is stopped, and fluids, electrolytes, and pain and infection control are provided. But to date, no specific therapy has proved effective. Despite hospitalization and aggressive resuscitation, the mortality rate for TEN remains high secondary to sepsis and multisystem organ failure.

PEER POINT

Stevens-Johnson syndrome/toxic epidermal necrosis

As noted on DermNet New Zealand, the blisters associated with SJS/TEN come together and form sheets of detaching skin that then expose red, oozing dermis. The second image shows target lesions of the palm seen with erythema multiforme.

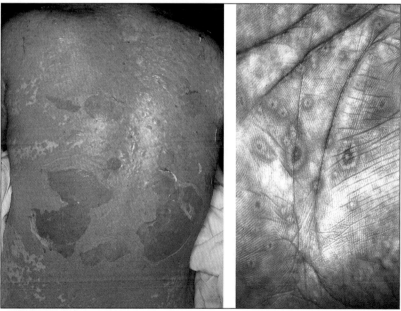

PEER Point 34

PEER REVIEW

✓ Stevens-Johnsons syndrome is a life-threatening condition.

✓ Characteristics of Stevens-Johnson: diffuse rash, target lesion, bullae, involvement of hands or soles and mucous membranes, full-thickness necrosis, less than 30% total body surface area.

REFERENCES

Adams JG, Barton ED, Collings J, et al, eds. *Emergency Medicine: Clinical Essentials.* 2nd ed. Philadelphia, PA: Saunders; 2013: 1598-1610.

Marx JA, Hockberger RS, Walls RM, eds. *Rosen's Emergency Medicine: Concepts and Clinical Practice.* 8th ed. St. Louis, MO: Elsevier; 2014: 1567-1568; 1573.

422. The correct answer is A, Abrupt discontinuation of levodopa-carbidopa.

Why is this the correct answer?

The presentation of the tetrad of altered mental status, autonomic instability, hyperthermia, and muscular rigidity is most consistent with neuroleptic malignant syndrome (NMS). Neuroleptic malignant syndrome is an iatrogenic, idiosyncratic reaction most commonly caused by the administration of drugs that antagonize dopamine receptors, particularly antipsychotic medications. But it occurs much more predictably from the abrupt cessation of dopamine agonists such as those used to treat Parkinson disease, including the combination of levodopa and carbidopa. The muscular rigidity associated with NMS is often described as "lead pipe" in character and is often a distinguishing factor in the diagnosis. Elevated creatinine kinase is a common feature of NMS. Another condition that presents with the NMS tetrad of symptoms (most commonly when a patient reduces or stops taking antiparkinson medications) is an indistinguishable syndrome referred to as Parkinson-hyperpyrexia syndrome. It is a rare but potentially fatal complication associated with Parkinson disease that can lead to acute renal failure, aspiration pneumonia, DVT, PE, and disseminated intravascular coagulation.

Why are the other choices wrong?

Although confusion, hyperthermia, and tachycardia can be features of poisoning from diphenhydramine, the presence of diaphoresis and muscular rigidity are not. Diphenhydramine has both antimuscarinic and sodium-channel blocking properties. Delirium, dry skin, hyperthermia, mydriasis, picking behavior, tachycardia, and urinary retention are all classic features that can occur from the antimuscarinic effects. The sodium channel blocking properties can lead to QRS width prolongation and convulsions. Heat stroke also manifests with altered level of consciousness, hyperthermia, and tachycardia. Patients who are taking antimuscarinic agents such as diphenhydramine might be more predisposed to heat stroke because their ability to sweat is diminished.

Similarly, muscular rigidity and significant hyperthermia (unless in the setting of convulsions) are not expected with poisoning from an organophosphorous (OPs) compound. By inhibiting the enzyme acetylcholinesterase that breaks down acetylcholine, OP poisoning causes excess acetylcholine at various synapses, including the neuromuscular junction (causing fasciculations, respiratory paralysis), and sweat glands (diaphoresis). Excess acetylcholine also occurs at preganglionic sites of both the sympathetic and parasympathetic nervous systems and the postganglionic sites of the parasympathetic nervous system. Although both parasympathetic and sympathetic signs can co-exist, parasympathetic excess typically is most prominent.

Confusion, diaphoresis, hyperthermia, and tachycardia can all occur in the setting of withdrawal from sedative-hypnotic agents such as benzodiazepines and ethanol, but muscular rigidity does not. Hypertension is also expected.

PEER REVIEW

✓ Characteristic finding in neuroleptic malignant syndrome: severe "lead pipe" muscular rigidity.

✓ Neuroleptic malignant syndrome is an idiosyncratic reaction most commonly caused by drugs that antagonize dopamine receptors, particularly antipsychotics.

✓ Neuroleptic malignant syndrome can occur if a patient abruptly stops taking dopamine agonists such as those used to treat Parkinson disease.

REFERENCES
Hoffman RS, Howland MA, Lewin NA, et al, eds. *Goldfrank's Toxicologic Emergencies*. 10th ed. New York, NY: McGraw-Hill; 2015: 668-669, 965, 1108, 1413.
Newman EJ, Grosset DG, Kennedy PG. The parkinsonism-hyperpyrexia syndrome. *Neurocrit Care*. 2009;10(1):136-140. doi: 10.1007/s12028-008-9125-4. Epub 2008 Aug 20.
Wolfson AB, Hendey GW, Ling LJ, et al, eds. *Harwood-Nuss' Clinical Practice of Emergency Medicine*. 6th ed. Philadelphia, PA: Lippincott, Williams & Wilkins; 2014: 797, 1446.

423. The correct answer is C, Poststreptococcal glomerulonephritis.

Why is this the correct answer?

The important clues in this case are the history of pharyngitis, the edema, and what can be assumed to be tea-colored urine. Added to the laboratory findings of hematuria and proteinuria, the clinical presentation is consistent with a diagnosis of poststreptococcal acute glomerulonephritis. It is the most common cause of glomerulonephritis in children 5 to 12 years old and rare in children younger than 3 years. The infection can stem from a streptococcal infection (almost always group A streptococci) from either pharyngitis or a skin infection. The length of time between the pharyngitis and renal symptoms ranges from 1 to 2 weeks; it can take 2 to 3 weeks for renal symptoms to appear following a skin infection. Some patients present with hypertension, which usually resolves in 1 or 2 weeks. Overall, treatment is supportive.

Why are the other choices wrong?

Goodpasture syndrome is an autoimmune disease that attacks collagen in alveoli and glomeruli. The presenting clinical picture in Goodpasture syndrome varies with the tissue affected, but pallor might be present due to bleeding. If the lung is involved, the presentation might include hemoptysis, dyspnea, and cough. If the kidney is involved, the presentation might include hematuria, vomiting, and peripheral edema. But Goodpasture syndrome is very uncommon and more likely in an older child, and it often manifests with symptoms in both pulmonary and renal systems.

Henoch-Schönlein purpura is a diffuse vasculitis without a known cause that can affect many different organ systems. It is associated with arthralgia, diffuse swelling, abdominal pain, and purpura. It typically presents between ages 3 and 15 years; the most common age is between 4 and 7 years. The clinical presentation can include vague lower extremity pain, rash, or signs of nephritis such as hematuria/proteinuria, abdominal pain, vomiting, and/or peripheral edema.

Wegner glomerulonephritis is a triad of sinusitis, pulmonary infiltrates, and glomerulonephritis. Glomerulonephritis and hematuria are rare at presentation.

PEER REVIEW

✓ Poststreptococcal glomerulonephritis is the most common cause of acute glomerulonephritis.

✓ Infection can stem from either pharyngitis or skin infection.Hematuria with oliguria is a concerning sign of kidney disease and warrants further evaluation.

REFERENCES

Fleisher GR, Ludwig S, et al, eds. *Textbook of Pediatric Emergency Medicine*. 6th ed. Philadelphia, PA: Lippincott, Williams & Wilkins; 2010: 1116-1119.

Wolfson AB, Hendey GW, Ling LJ, et al, eds. *Harwood-Nuss' Clinical Practice of Emergency Medicine*. 6th ed. Philadelphia, PA: Lippincott, Williams & Wilkins; 2014: 1280-1282.

424. The correct answer is A, *Amanita* mushroom.

Why is this the correct answer?

Amanita phalloides is a wild growing mushroom, which in addition to a few other *Amanita* species, is responsible for most of the deaths associated with wild mushroom ingestions in the United States. In general, the onset of GI symptoms in fewer than 6 hours is associated with ingestions of less toxic mushroom species. The delayed onset of vomiting and diarrhea is characteristic of poisoning with hepatotoxic *Amanita* species and can portend the development of hepatic failure.

Why are the other choices wrong?

Poisoning from cardiac glycosides, which are found in the oleander plant (*Nerium oleander*), is characterized by the rapid (not delayed) onset of GI symptoms (vomiting). Hepatic failure is not an expected feature. Similar to digoxin (a cardiac glycoside), hyperkalemia occurs due to poisoning of sodium-potassium ATPase and can be used as a predictor of possible dysrhythmias.

Poison hemlock (*Conium maculatum*) contains alkaloids that are similar to nicotine. Poisoning is characterized by the rapid (not delayed) onset of GI symptoms (vomiting). Both parasympathetic and sympathetic symptoms can follow. Convulsions and respiratory failure can ensue, but hepatic failure is not an expected feature.

Poisoning from water hemlock (*Cicuta maculata*) is characterized by rapid (not delayed) onset of GI symptoms and convulsions. Most plant ingestions are accidental and typically occur in children; in contrast, ingestions of water hemlock

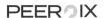

often occur in adults who confuse the plant with similar-appearing edible, nontoxic plants. The toxin present, cicutoxin, is rapidly absorbed, and although not fully characterized, appears to antagonize GABA receptors, explaining why convulsions and status epilepticus are features of poisoning. Hepatic failure is not a feature of this poisoning. Treatment is supportive.

PEER REVIEW

✓ Mushroom toxicity with early vomiting and diarrhea (sooner than 6 hours) generally portends a favorable outcome and less toxic ingestion.

✓ Delayed-onset (after 6 hours) vomiting and diarrhea are characteristic of poisoning from *Amanita* species and are associated with hepatic failure.

REFERENCES

Hoffman RS, Howland MA, Lewin NA, et al, eds. *Goldfrank's Toxicologic Emergencies*. 10th ed. New York, NY: McGraw-Hill; 2015: 1500-1502.

Tintinalli JE, Stapczynski JS, Ma OJ, et al, eds. *Tintinalli's Emergency Medicine: A Comprehensive Study Guide*. 8th ed. New York, NY: McGraw-Hill; 2012: 1419-1420, 1426-1427.

425. The correct answer is B, Hot water immersion.

Why is this the correct answer?

This case describes the classic presentation of a stingray envenomation, the initial treatment for which is hot water immersion. Stingray venom is heat labile, and its effects can be reversed or lessened by immersion in hot (not scalding) water. Stingrays have a whiplike tail that contains a spine surrounded by venom. Envenomation typically occurs when the stingray is threatened, often in the context of being stepped on. When the body of a stingray is stepped on, it reflexively whips its tail and often envenomates the dorsal aspect of the offending foot. Potential complications include anatomic injury from the spine, effects of the venom, and infections. In most cases, the major manifestation of exposure is localized severe pain from the venom itself. Systemic effects are possible but not common. Local skin changes can occur, and occasionally the broken spine or foreign debris can be imbedded in the wound. Further analgesic efforts, including local anesthetic injection, might be required if hot water immersion is insufficient. Antibiotic prophylaxis remains controversial. Other marine envenomations that might benefit from hot water immersion include those from many jellyfish and various fish (catfish, lionfish, stonefish, weeverfish).

Why are the other choices wrong?

Immersing the body part in acetic acid (vinegar) is not beneficial in the treatment of stingray envenomation. Topical application of acetic acid appears to be beneficial in decreasing stinging nematocyst discharge for many (but not all) *Cnidaria* species, commonly referred to as jellyfish. In certain species, acetic acid application can increase nematocyst discharge. Geographic location can help guide whether to use acetic acid. In the United States, where it is more likely to encounter a species

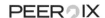

that acetic acid application may cause nematocyst discharge, ocean water can be used instead to aid tentacle removal. In the Indo-Pacific region, where it is more likely to encounter a species that acetic acid application might decrease nematocyst discharge, acetic acid use is appropriate.

The presentation is classic for a stingray envenomation, and hot water (not ice water) is effective because the venom is heat labile.

Currently, there is no antivenom for stingray envenomation. However, there is an antivenom for stonefish envenomation, which typically occurs on the bottom of the foot; significant swelling and erythema at the site of envenomation are typical.

PEER REVIEW

✓ Hot water immersion is an effective treatment for stingray envenomation.

REFERENCES

Hoffman RS, Howland MA, Lewin NA, et al, eds. *Goldfrank's Toxicologic Emergencies*. 10th ed. New York, NY: McGraw-Hill; 2015: 1487-1490, 1494-1496.

Tintinalli JE, Stapczynski JS, Ma OJ, et al, eds. *Tintinalli's Emergency Medicine: A Comprehensive Study Guide*. 8th ed. New York, NY: McGraw-Hill; 2012: 1384-1386.

426. The correct answer is B, Arrange for hyperbaric oxygen treatment.

Why is this the correct answer?

The patient described has a classic presentation of cerebral air embolism, the onset of cerebral symptoms immediately or soon after surfacing after a rapid or uncontrolled ascent. The primary treatment for cerebral air embolism is recompression with hyperbaric oxygen. Administration of 100% oxygen and intravenous fluid is appropriate while arranging the definitive treatment. Cerebral air embolism occurs when air bubbles either transfer from the low pressure venous side via intracardiac (such as via the presence of a patent foramen ovale) or pulmonary arteriovenous shunts to the arterial side or develop spontaneously on the arterial side and embolize to the brain. Typically this occurs in the setting of pulmonary barotrauma from a too-rapid ascent.

Why are the other choices wrong?

Again, administration of 100% oxygen and intravenous fluid with the goal of increasing tissue perfusion is appropriate while arranging for hyperbaric oxygen therapy. But the patient has already manifested classic symptoms of cerebral air embolism and should receive definitive treatment, not monitored for symptom resolution.

Given that the patient has a classic presentation of cerebral air embolism and requires hyperbaric oxygen treatment, initial brain imaging is not necessary, and it should not delay definitive treatment. It would be extremely unlikely that a patient who presents in this classic fashion would have an intracranial hemorrhage, or other etiology that would warrant initial brain imaging.

There is no role for a Valsalva maneuver in the treatment of cerebral air embolus. In fact, performing a Valsalva maneuver while breathing compressed gas during a rapid ascent (as can happen during breath-holding, coughing, or vomiting) can lead to pulmonary barotrauma and cause a cerebral air embolus. Performing a Valsalva maneuver during descent is often done to "clear the ears" (equalize the pressure between the inner ear and outer ear canal). Continuing descent without adequate equalization can lead to barotitis, also known as ear squeeze, characterized by a range of manifestations that can include ear pain, hemotympanum, vertigo, and tympanic membrane perforation.

PEER REVIEW

✓ The definitive treatment for cerebral air embolism is hyperbaric oxygen.
✓ The classic presentation of cerebral air embolism is the presence of cerebral symptoms that occur immediately or soon after surfacing from a rapid or uncontrolled ascent.

REFERENCES

Tintinalli JE, Stapczynski JS, Ma OJ, et al, eds. *Tintinalli's Emergency Medicine: A Comprehensive Study Guide.* 8th ed. New York, NY: McGraw-Hill; 2012: 1392-1394.

Wolfson AB, Hendey GW, Ling LJ, et al, eds. *Harwood-Nuss' Clinical Practice of Emergency Medicine.* 6th ed. Philadelphia, PA: Lippincott, Williams & Wilkins; 2014: 1520-1523.

427. The correct answer is A, Decreasing esophageal balloon pressure by 5 mm Hg every 3 hours.

Why is this the correct answer?

Sengstaken-Blakemore tube insertion can be a lifesaving temporizing procedure for variceal bleeding. But it is not performed frequently because of its associated complications and the development of endoscopic therapies. One significant complication is esophageal or gastric rupture. When bleeding is controlled, the esophageal balloon pressure should be reduced by 5 mm Hg every 3 hours down to a pressure of 25 mm Hg to avoid pressure necrosis. The correct placement of the Sengstaken-Blakemore tube is accomplished with the large balloon advanced completely into the stomach. Appropriate positioning can be confirmed with imaging or by auscultating over the stomach while inserting air in the gastric port. The gastric balloon is initially inflated with about 250 mL of air so that it abuts securely against the gastroesophageal junction. Once fixed, the esophageal balloon is inflated if bleeding persists. The esophageal balloon is inflated to a pressure of no more than 50 mm Hg to control esophageal variceal bleeding. Intragastric balloon pressure should be reassessed frequently after placement; if pressure is increasing, this might signify esophageal placement or migration. Aspiration and airway compromise are concerns during Sengstaken-Blakemore tube placement, so elevation of the head of the bed and endotracheal intubation should be strongly considered.

Why are the other choices wrong?

The gastric balloon should be inflated first, not the esophageal balloon, taking care that it is clearly in the stomach before full inflation. This controls gastric varices, and if bleeding stops after gastric balloon inflation, the esophageal balloon does not have to be inflated.

The esophageal balloon is inflated to a pressure of no more than 50 mm Hg to control esophageal variceal bleeding.

Oral or nasogastric suctioning is necessary after the placement of a Sengstaken-Blakemore tube (not before) to decrease the risk of aspiration because secretions collect above the obstructing tube. Nasogastric tube placement before or after placement does not affect the risk of rupture from Sengstaken-Blakemore tube placement.

PEER REVIEW

✓ Sengstaken-Blakemore tube insertion is an important, lifesaving skill, a temporizing measure when vasoconstrictive medications don't work and endoscopic treatment isn't available.

✓ Be sure to confirm that the gastric balloon is completely in the stomach before inflating it.

✓ Reassess esophageal balloon pressure regularly, and decrease it when possible to avoid pressure ulceration or necrosis.

REFERENCES

Marx JA, Hockberger RS, Walls RM, eds. *Rosen's Emergency Medicine: Concepts and Clinical Practice*. 8th ed. St. Louis, MO: Elsevier; 2014: 251-252.

Reichman EF. Emergency Medicine Procedures. 2nd ed. New York, NY: McGraw-Hill; 2013: 407-414.

Tintinalli JE, Stapczynski JS, Ma OJ, et al, eds. *Tintinalli's Emergency Medicine: A Comprehensive Study Guide*. 8th ed. New York, NY: McGraw-Hill; 2012: 503-506, 563-567.

428. The correct answer is B, Cefotaxime.

Why is this the correct answer?

Hepatorenal syndrome associated with cirrhosis has a significant morbidity rate and a 2-week mortality rate if left untreated. It exists in two types. Type 1 is more critical, marked by oliguria with an increase more than double the serum creatinine within 2 weeks. It can arise spontaneously, but the most common risk factor (up to 25% to 30% of patients) is spontaneous bacterial peritonitis (SBP). A paracentesis should be performed to rule this out, and treatment should be started if there is clinical suspicion. Cefotaxime is the recommended empiric antibiotic because it covers most of the organisms that cause SBP and because of its high ascitic fluid concentrations. Correcting the underlying cause of hepatorenal syndrome might reverse the process, but if there is no etiology found or renal function worsens despite therapies, the definitive treatment is liver transplant. Type 2 hepatorenal syndrome progresses more gradually and might not advance as insidiously.

Why are the other choices wrong?

Use of albumin decreases electrolyte imbalances in patients undergoing paracentesis and helps maintain cardiac output. Large volume paracenteses performed without albumin might actually cause type 1 hepatorenal syndrome as well as hemodynamic compromise. The patient in this case should undergo diagnostic paracentesis for SBP, but albumin by itself does not treat SBP nor reverse hepatorenal syndrome.

N-acetylcysteine is usually used to treat acetaminophen overdose. It has been shown to improve renal function, but the mechanism is unclear. It does not have a role in treatment of liver failure that is not drug related.

Somatostatin analogues like octreotide aid in splanchnic vasoconstriction and are a mainstay for variceal bleeding. There is a potential for benefit in hepatorenal patients due to regulation of splanchnic vasodilation that secondarily causes renal circulatory perfusion problems. This has not yet been validated by clinical trials.

PEER REVIEW

✓ Hepatorenal syndrome is highly associated with spontaneous bacterial peritonitis.
✓ Hepatorenal syndrome is marked by acute serum creatinine elevations and oliguria.
✓ Large volume paracentesis without albumin administration can lead to hepatorenal syndrome due to electrolyte and oncotic shifts.

REFERENCES

Marx JA, Hockberger RS, Walls RM, eds. *Rosen's Emergency Medicine: Concepts and Clinical Practice.* 8th ed. St. Louis, MO: Elsevier; 2014: 1193-1194.

Tintinalli JE, Stapczynski JS, Ma OJ, et al, eds. *Tintinalli's Emergency Medicine: A Comprehensive Study Guide.* 8th ed. New York, NY: McGraw-Hill; 2012: 527-528.

429. The correct answer is B, Colchicine.

Why is this the correct answer?

In about 5% of emergency department presentations for chest pain (not related to MI), the diagnosis is pericarditis. And in the vast majority of these patients, the underlying cause cannot be identified. First-line treatment includes aspirin and other NSAIDs; ibuprofen is effective in most cases and has fewer side effects. Evidence now suggests that the addition of colchicine (1 to 2 mg for the first day and then 0.5 to 1 mg/day for 3 months) to the standard regimen is effective in hastening the resolution of acute symptoms and also preventing recurrence rates, regardless of the cause of the pericarditis. Colchicine is also effective in cases of recurrent pericarditis.

Why are the other choices wrong?

Anti-inflammatory agents are first-line therapy for pericarditis. The pain usually improves significantly within days of ibuprofen therapy. If symptoms persist, an alternative NSAID is indicated. Indomethacin is often used for severe cases because of its stronger anti-inflammatory effect, although it should be avoided in patients with a history of ischemic heart disease because it can decrease coronary blood flow. However, anti-inflammatory medications have not been shown to change the recurrence rate.

Narcotic medications provide pain relief for patients with pericarditis but do not change the course of the disease or reduce the likelihood of recurrence.

The use of corticosteroids is generally reserved for recurrent pericarditis or for the treatment of pericarditis that is unresponsive to aspirin or NSAIDs plus colchicine. Initiation of steroids early in the course of first-time pericarditis might actually be an independent risk factor for recurrence.

PEER REVIEW

- ✓ Ibuprofen is effective in most cases of pericarditis and has fewer side effects than other NSAIDs.
- ✓ Adding colchicine to NSAID treatment can resolve pericarditis symptoms faster and prevent recurrence.
- ✓ Corticosteroids are generally reserved for recurrent pericarditis that doesn't respond to aspirin or NSAID treatment plus colchicine.

REFERENCES

Adams JG, Barton ED, Collings J, et al, eds. *Emergency Medicine: Clinical Essentials*. 2nd ed. Philadelphia, PA: Saunders; 2013: 514-523.

Lilly LS. Treatment of acute and recurrent idiopathic pericarditis. *Circulation*. 2013;127:1723-1726.

Marx JA, Hockberger RS, Walls RM, eds. *Rosen's Emergency Medicine: Concepts and Clinical Practice*. 8th ed. St. Louis, MO: Elsevier; 2014: 1091-1105.

430. The correct answer is A, Consult surgery for laparotomy.

Why is this the correct answer?

The abdominal CT images reveal a "bulls-eye" lesion concerning for intussusception. Definitive treatment is surgical resection of the pathological lesion; otherwise, the intussusception is unlikely to resolve using pneumatic or hydrostatic decompression. With intussusception, the distal segment of bowel is invaginated into an adjacent lumen of the proximal GI tract. This is often called "telescoping," which causes bowel obstruction. Commonly, intussusception is found in children 3 months to 3 years old and can be reduced conservatively with air contrast or barium enema. The classic triad presentation in the pediatric population is cramping abdominal pain, bloody diarrhea ("currant jelly" stool), and a palpable tender mass (sausage shaped). Intussusception is rare in adults and usually secondary to a pathological etiology like malignancy that serves as a lead point for bowel obstruction. Other pathological causes of intussusception include Meckel diverticulum, inflammatory bowel disease, gastric bypass, polyps, adhesions, strictures, and benign neoplasms. Although abdominal CT is the most sensitive diagnostic modality, ultrasonography can be used with classic features such as "pseudokidney" or "doughnut" signs.

Why are the other choices wrong?

Obtaining abdominal CT angiography is unlikely to add helpful information in this patient's case. Ordering this study might be prompted by concern for mesenteric ischemia, which can feature pain out of proportion with the abdominal examination and elevated lactic acid levels.

A barium or air contrast enema is used to treat intussusception in children but is unlikely to resolve bowel obstruction in adults due to other pathological etiologies. In addition, if the lesion causing the intussusception is malignant, there is some concern with release of malignant cells with enema reduction.

Rectal decompression is the initial treatment for sigmoid volvulus. Sigmoid volvulus occurs most commonly in elderly or debilitated patients who suffer from chronic constipation. Despite endoscopic decompression, recurrence is high; surgical intervention is likely necessary.

PEER REVIEW

✓ Adult intussusception is rare and is often due to a pathological lesion such as a carcinoma.

✓ In intussusception, CT imaging shows a lead point with invagination.

✓ Definitive treatment for intussusception in adults is surgical resection.

REFERENCES

Marinis A, Yiallourou A, Samanides L, et al. Intussusception of the bowel in adults: a review. *World J Gastroenterol.* 2009;15(4):407-411.

Marx JA, Hockberger RS, Walls RM, eds. *Rosen's Emergency Medicine: Concepts and Clinical Practice.* 8th ed. St. Louis, MO: Elsevier; 2014: 1216-1218.

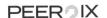

431. The correct answer is A, Esmolol.

Why is this the correct answer?

The primary goal in the medical management of acute aortic dissection is to decrease the blood pressure and heart rate to minimize the aortic shearing force that could worsen the intimal tear and further propagate the dissection. Beta blockers such as esmolol or labetalol should be given first. They effectively reduce blood pressure and shearing force but additionally prevent the reflex tachycardia that occurs with primary administration of vasodilators. The goal systolic blood pressure is 100 to 120 mm Hg, and the goal heart rate is less than 60 beats/min. Note that the blood pressure goal is independent of the patient's baseline blood pressure, unlike the approach to most hypertensive emergencies.

Why are the other choices wrong?

Nicardipine is a vasodilator. It is part of the treatment for acute aortic dissection, but it should be added after the beta blocker. Increased heart rate is a common side effect of vasodilator therapy, so it should not be the first medication given.

Nifedipine is a calcium channel blocker and vasodilator. It can be used as part of the treatment for acute aortic dissection, but it should be added after the beta blocker. As with nicardipine, it can increase heart rate and should not be the first medication given.

Nitroprusside also is a vasodilator and should be administered after a beta blocker.

PEER REVIEW

- ✓ Hemodynamic goals in the treatment of acute aortic dissection: systolic blood pressure 100 to 120, and heart rate less than 60.
- ✓ Give beta blockers first in aortic dissection to reduce blood pressure and shearing forces and prevent reflex tachycardia.
- ✓ Add vasodilators after the heart rate is controlled to further reduce blood pressure as needed.

REFERENCES

Adams JG, Barton ED, Collings J, et al, eds. *Emergency Medicine: Clinical Essentials.* 2nd ed. Philadelphia, PA: Saunders; 2013: 561-570, 592-601.

Marx JA, Hockberger RS, Walls RM, eds. *Rosen's Emergency Medicine: Concepts and Clinical Practice.* 8th ed. St. Louis, MO: Elsevier; 2014: 1124-1128.

432. The correct answer is C, D-dimer.

Why is this the correct answer?

Aortic dissection is deadly and difficult to diagnose. The classic presentation is sudden and severe unrelenting pain in the chest and/or back. There is longitudinal cleavage of the aortic wall by blood, which creates and can propagate a false lumen. When chest pain and acute neurologic or vascular deficits are present, aortic dissection is the most likely diagnosis. Recently D-dimer in several small studies has been increasingly shown to be a sensitive biomarker for ruling out aortic dissection in those with a low pretest probability. Using a risk score to identify those who are low risk such as the aortic detection risk score, with D-dimer has been shown in a large cohort to be accurate and effective. Computed tomographic angiography is the test of choice for diagnosis.

Why are the other choices wrong?

An ABG analysis has no diagnostic utility in suspected acute aortic dissection, although hypotension can lead to acidosis as seen with this testing.

Chest radiography is always obtained in suspected aortic dissection. Assessing for widening of the mediastinum is classically taught; however, this is a poor diagnostic tool with low sensitivity. A tortuous aorta, which is quite common in hypertensive patients, causes a widened mediastinum, in addition to many other etiologies, including tumor, adenopathy, lymphoma, and enlarged thyroid.

Electrocardiography is not diagnostic for aortic dissection, but approximately two-thirds of ECGs are abnormal in patients with dissection. Changes consistent with left ventricular hypertrophy from hypertension can be seen, and ST-segment elevation from dissections involving a coronary artery, or nonspecific changes from generalized coronary artery disease.

PEER REVIEW

✓ D-dimer with low pretest probability (consider use of aortic detection risk score) is sensitive in ruling out an acute aortic dissection.
✓ Chest radiography is not a sensitive screening tool in acute aortic dissection.

REFERENCES

Adams JG, Barton ED, Collings J, et al, eds. *Emergency Medicine: Clinical Essentials.* 2nd ed. Philadelphia, PA: Saunders; 2013: 561-570, 592-601.

Asha SE, Miers JW. A systemic review and meta-analysis of D-dimer as a rule-out test for suspected acute aortic dissection. *Ann Emerg Med.* 2015;66(4):368-378.

Marx JA, Hockberger RS, Walls RM, eds. *Rosen's Emergency Medicine: Concepts and Clinical Practice.* 8th ed. St. Louis, MO: Elsevier; 2014: 1124-1128.

Simony A, Filion KB, Mottillo S, et al. Meta-analysis of usefulness of D-dimer to diagnose acute aortic dissection. *Am J Cardiol.* 2011;107(8):1227-1234.

433. The correct answer is B, Tetralogy of Fallot.

Why is this the correct answer?

Tetralogy of Fallot (TOF) is one of the cyanotic congenital heart diseases that can present during the neonatal period or during infancy and childhood. It is the most common structural congenital heart disease occurring outside the neonatal period. Common physical examination findings in TOF include a right ventricular heave and a harsh systolic ejection murmur with a single second heart sound (without pulmonic valve component). The four features of the TOF defect are:

- A large ventricular septal defect (VSD)
- Right ventricular outflow tract obstruction
- An overriding aorta
- Right ventricular hypertrophy

The murmur of TOF softens as the severity of obstruction worsens because more blood is being shunted across the VSD. In patients with TOF, the severity of the outflow obstruction determines the time of symptom onset and appearance of the disease. Severe obstruction causes cyanosis in the newborn (blue tet), and less severe obstruction (pink tet) can delay diagnosis.

Why are the other choices wrong?

Coarctation of the aorta is a congenital narrowing of the aorta most commonly at the level of the ductus arteriosus. Infants with coarctation are often asymptomatic and have normal oxygen saturation levels as blood bypasses the obstruction when the ductus arteriosus is patent. As the ductus closes, the systemic circulation can be compromised, causing shock. If the narrowing is less severe, the coarctation might not be diagnosed until later in life. Significant physical examination findings are blood pressure and/or perfusion deficits in the upper compared to the lower extremities. A harsh systolic ejection murmur might also be heard radiating from the left axilla to the back.

Tricuspid atresia is characterized by complete absence of the tricuspid valve, a hypoplastic right ventricle, and the presence of a VSD. The size of the VSD determines the amount of pulmonary blood flow. A large VSD can allow for relatively normal pulmonary blood flow and delay detection. Because the left ventricle is the only functional chamber, fluid overload easily occurs, causing heart failure and hepatomegaly in the young. Infants with small VSDs are dependent on the ductus arteriosus for pulmonary blood flow, and tricuspid atresia is often diagnosed during the neonatal period as the ductus arteriosus closes and cyanosis develops. On physical examination, a harsh systolic ejection murmur with a single or split second sound is heard; however, tricuspid atresia is less common in infants and less likely to be the cause of these sounds.

Truncus arteriosus is the presence of a single trunk arising from the heart that functions as both the aorta and the pulmonary artery. A single semilumar valve and

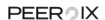

VSD are present, allowing the complete mixing of systemic and pulmonary blood. As the pulmonary resistance falls after birth and blood travels preferentially through the pulmonary circuit, heart failure ensues. The common physical examination findings include a wide pulse pressure with a systolic ejection murmur and a single second heart sound.

PEER POINT

Clinical presentations and causative conditions in congenital heart disease

Clinical Presentation	Conditions in the Neonatal Period	Conditions in Infancy and Childhood
Cyanosis	Tetralogy of Fallot, total anomalous pulmonary venous return, transposition of the great arteries, tricuspid atresia, truncus arteriosus	Eisenmenger complex, tetralogy of Fallot
Arrhythmias		Atrial septal defect, Ebstein anomaly, postsurgical complication after repair of congenital heart defect
Cardiovascular shock	Hypoplastic left heart syndrome, coarctation of the aorta, critical aortic stenosis	Coarctation of the aorta (infants)
Congestive heart failure	Rare: hypoplastic left heart syndrome, patent ductus arteriosus	Atrial septal defect, atrioventricular canal, patent ductus arteriosus, ventricular septal defect
Hypertension		Coarctation of the aorta
Murmur	Patent ductus arteriosus, valvular defects (aortic stenosis, pulmonic stenosis)	Atrial septal defect, outflow obstructions, patent ductus arteriosus, valvular defects (aortic stenosis, pulmonic stenosis), ventricular septal defect
Syncope		Aortic stenosis, Eisenmenger complex, pulmonic stenosis

Adapted from *Tintinalli's Emergency Medicine: A Comprehensive Study Guide,* 8e, Table 126-1

PEER REVIEW

✓ Tetralogy of Fallot is the most common structural congenital heart disease occurring outside the neonatal period.

✓ The tetralogy of Fallot: ventricular septal defect, right ventricular outflow tract obstruction, overriding aorta, right ventricular hypertrophy.

✓ Common physical examination findings in tetralogy of Fallot: right ventricular heave with a harsh systolic murmur and a single second heart sound.

REFERENCES

Adams JG, Barton ED, Collings J, et al, eds. *Emergency Medicine: Clinical Essentials.* 2nd ed. Philadelphia, PA: Saunders; 2013: 117-128, 159-166.

Marx JA, Hockberger RS, Walls RM, eds. *Rosen's Emergency Medicine: Concepts and Clinical Practice.* 8th ed. St. Louis, MO: Elsevier; 2014: 129-134.

434. The correct answer is D, 39-year-old man with layering of cells in the anterior chamber.

Why is this the correct answer?

The disorder shown in this image is a hyphema, a collection of RBCs in the anterior chamber, most often due to trauma. Patients who present with traumatic hyphema may be safely discharged for outpatient management without a consultation from ophthalmology if the hyphema is small and if the patient has no risk factors for complications. If the patient keeps his or her head elevated to at least 30 degrees or sits upright, the RBCs in the anterior chamber layer by gravity. This allows the trabecular meshwork of the superior portion of the eye to remain clear and facilitates drainage of the aqueous humor. The drainage prevents the development of elevated intraocular pressure, which is a complication of hyphema. Patients with a hyphema larger than 25% of the anterior chamber are at higher risk for traumatic glaucoma. They also are at risk for undiagnosed concomitant posterior injury such as retinal detachment or commotio retinae given that ophthalmoscopy is limited in these cases. Ultrasonography can help determine if there is a retinal tear or detachment when the fundus is obscured by blood in the anterior chamber.

Why are the other choices wrong?

A patient with a history of sickle cell disease is at higher risk for obstruction of the trabecular meshwork and elevated intraocular pressure, as well as rebleeding. In the care of such a patient, an ophthalmologist should be consulted when planning disposition. In some centers, these patients might require inpatient management.

The Seidel test is performed by applying fluorescein dye to the injured cornea; the result is positive if a stream of aqueous humor is identified leaking through the cornea. A patient with a positive Seidel test is at risk for having a concomitant corneal perforation or open globe. Such a patient should not undergo ultrasound examination for fear of extruding intraocular contents. Instead, emergent ophthalmologic consultation is required.

An intraocular pressure of 40 is already elevated, and such a patient is high risk. Lowering of the intraocular pressure and ophthalmologic consultation are required prior to discharge. Failure to do so can lead to chronically elevated intraocular pressure and decreased visual acuity, with optic atrophy. Typical glaucoma medications might not successfully lower the elevated intraocular pressure. Generally, these patients are treated surgically to wash the blood out of the anterior chamber.

PEER POINT

High-risk findings in patients with traumatic hyphema

- "Eight-ball" hyphema or involvement of greater than 25% of the anterior chamber
- No light perception or markedly decreased visual acuity
- Sickle cell disease or trait or family history in an untested patient
- History of bleeding diathesis
- Elevated intraocular pressure
- Noncompliance with outpatient instructions due to age or other factors
- Intractable vomiting

PEER REVIEW

✓ Patients with traumatic hyphema should keep their heads elevated to at least 30 degrees.

✓ Measure intraocular pressure in patients with hyphema unless you're concerned about open globe.

✓ You can do an ultrasound examination on a patient with hyphema and decreased visual acuity to look for a torn or detached retina if the fundus is not visible on ophthalmoscopy.

REFERENCES

Nash DL. Hyphema. Medscape website. Available at: http://emedicine.medscape.com/article/1190165-overview. Accessed August 23, 2016.

Tintinalli JE, Stapczynski JS, Ma OJ, et al, eds. *Tintinalli's Emergency Medicine: A Comprehensive Study Guide*. 8th ed. New York, NY: McGraw-Hill; 2012: 1563-1572.

Wolfson AB, Hendey GW, Ling LJ, et al, eds. *Harwood-Nuss' Clinical Practice of Emergency Medicine*. 6th ed. Philadelphia, PA: Lippincott, Williams & Wilkins; 2014: 178.

435. The correct answer is B, Isoproterenol.

Why is this the correct answer?

Infants who have tetralogy of Fallot can become hypoxic during or after feeding or while crying or agitated and then become cyanotic — an event referred to as a tet spell. The underlying pathophysiology is a worsening of the right ventricular outflow obstruction and decreased pulmonary blood flow characteristic of the disorder; the result is worsening cyanosis. Because the goal of treatment is to correct any hypoxia or acidosis that is present, interventions should increase systemic venous return and peripheral vascular resistance. Medications such as isoproterenol, which decrease pulmonary blood flow and increase right-to-left shunt, should be avoided. Supplemental oxygen should be provided; intravenous access should be established to provide fluid boluses, and the patient should be placed on continuous cardiac monitoring. The knee-to-chest position can be used to increase systemic vascular resistance and thus decrease the magnitude of the right-to-left shunt across the VSD.

Why are the other choices wrong?

Bicarbonate (1 mEq/kg) is part of the treatment for a tet spell. It is used to reverse the acidosis that can lead to an increased respiratory rate and cardiac effort.

Morphine (0.1 to 0.2 mg/kg), too, is often used in the management of a cyanotic tet spell because it calms the child and decreases the respiratory rate.

If these measures fail, then a phenylephrine infusion (0.1 mcg/kg/min) may be initiated to increase systemic vascular resistance and drive more blood flow across the right ventricular outflow tract obstruction. Beta blockers such as propranolol are also frequently given to decrease cardiac contractility, therefore decreasing infundibular obstruction at the right ventricular outflow tract.

PEER REVIEW

- ✓ Babies have tet spells when there's worsening of the right ventricular outflow tract obstruction and decreased pulmonary blood flow.
- ✓ Therapeutic options for a tet spell: oxygen, fluids, knee-chest positioning, morphine, bicarbonate, phenylephrine, and propranolol.
- ✓ Anything that decreases pulmonary blood flow or decreases systemic vascular resistance is harmful.

REFERENCES

Adams JG, Barton ED, Collings J, et al, eds. *Emergency Medicine: Clinical Essentials.* 2nd ed. Philadelphia, PA: Saunders; 2013: 117-128, 159-166.

Kato H, Hirose M, Yamaguchi M, et al. Hemodynamic effects of isoproterenol and propranolol in tetralogy of fallot: production and treatment of anoxic spells. *Japanese Circulation Journal.* 1968;31(12):1857-1863. Available at: https://www.jstage.jst.go.jp/a

Marx JA, Hockberger RS, Walls RM, eds. *Rosen's Emergency Medicine: Concepts and Clinical Practice.* 8th ed. St. Louis, MO: Elsevier; 2014: 129-134.

Tintinalli JE, Stapczynski JS, Ma OJ, et al, eds. *Tintinalli's Emergency Medicine: A Comprehensive Study Guide.* 8th ed. New York, NY: McGraw-Hill; 2012: 823-826.

436. The correct answer is D, Request a surgery consultation for an emergent surgical procedure.

Why is this the correct answer?

In the evaluation of a patient who presents with progressive GI bleeding following abdominal aortic aneurysm repair, suspicion should be high for aortoenteric fistula. If the patient is unstable such as the one in this case, consultation for emergent laparotomy for hemorrhage control and bypass surgery is warranted. A stable patient can undergo CT angiography or endoscopy as part of the workup. Aortoenteric fistulas occur most frequently after a surgical aortic graft (secondary fistula) but can occur after endovascular stenting or from unrepaired aneurysms themselves (primary fistula). As an aneurysm enlarges, it can adhere to and erode the bowel wall (most commonly the duodenum), causing a sentinel bleed that then progresses to a massive GI bleed. Erosions can occur by a suture line after endovascular grafting, causing the graft to corrode the surrounding bowel wall. Leakage of bowel contents into the aorta can also lead to abscess formation or infiltration through the aortic wall with subsequent bleeding. The aneurysmal wall might also erode into adjacent venous structures, causing aortovenous fistulae. Aortoenteric fistula has a high mortality rate, and rapid diagnosis is critical.

Why are the other choices wrong?

Proton pump inhibitors like Protonix and somatostatin analogues like octreotide are treatments for variceal bleeding commonly seen in patients with cirrhosis. Hematemesis is a key feature, with melanotic stool a sign of upper GI bleeding.

Transfusion of blood is appropriate in the setting of GI bleed, but an unstable patient should be transfused emergently without waiting for type-specific blood products. This is a temporizing measure until the cause of bleeding is found and stopped.

Endoscopy is a diagnostic tool for workup of aortoenteric fistula, but it is not sensitive or specific. It might help exclude other causes of upper GI bleeding, but visualizing a fistula can be difficult. It might be useful if variceal bleed is discovered, as concomitant endoscopic banding ligation or sclerotherapy can be performed. Computed tomography and angiography are also useful and might be obtained more quickly, but no single test offers high sensitive or specificity.

PEER REVIEW

- ✓ History of abdominal aortic aneurysm or prior surgical repair of an aneurysm + GI bleeding should = suspicion for aortoenteric fistula. The mortality rate is high.
- ✓ Clinical suspicion for aortoenteric fistula must be high: imaging might not reveal a bleed and isn't specific enough to exclude bleeding from fistulae.
- ✓ Surgery is the definitive treatment for aortoenteric fistula. Bypass surgery is the standard, but endovascular options are becoming more popular.

REFERENCES

Marx JA, Hockberger RS, Walls RM, eds. *Rosen's Emergency Medicine: Concepts and Clinical Practice*. 8th ed. St. Louis, MO: Elsevier; 2014: 1131, 1135-1136.

Tintinalli JE, Stapczynski JS, Ma OJ, et al, eds. *Tintinalli's Emergency Medicine: A Comprehensive Study Guide*. 8th ed. New York, NY: McGraw-Hill; 2012: 416-420.

437. The correct answer is C, Oral corticosteroids.

Why is this the correct answer?

Several studies have demonstrated that the prompt use of corticosteroids in asthma patients in the emergency department can improve air flow, thus decreasing both relapse rate and hospital admission rate in both adults and children. The glucocorticoids decrease inflammation of the airways; the type of corticosteroid (short acting or long acting) and the mode (oral, inhaled, IM, IV) all seem to provide the positive response to treatment. Effects of corticosteroids can be seen as rapidly as 2 hours after administration, so administering them early in the emergency department course is important.

Why are the other choices wrong?

Heliox is a combined gas mixture (about 80% helium and 20% oxygen) used to lower effort in patients with critical bronchospasm due to the properties of the inert helium gas. There are no large studies that indicate whether this improves asthma outcomes, such as decreased relapse or intubation rates.

Long-acting beta$_2$-adrenergic receptor agonists are not effective for acute asthma symptoms and have a black box warning against their use for acute symptoms. These medications are intended to be used in conjunction with inhaled corticosteroids for long-term control of symptoms. Short-acting beta$_2$-adrenergic receptor agonists are the key to treatment of acute asthma in the emergency department. Providing repeated treatments by nebulizer or inhaler with a spacer has been shown to provide bronchodilation. Studies have shown that intravenous and subcutaneous short-acting beta$_2$-agonists (epinephrine and terbutaline) do not provide any improvement in outcomes compared to inhaled beta$_2$-adrenergic receptor agonists.

There have been no studies of the use of just oxygen without other treatment modalities to show that oxygen itself can decrease rate of relapse in acute asthma. Use of oxygen via nasal cannula is recommended to keep Sao$_2$ greater than 90% in patients with severe asthma. Hypoxia has been shown to be a factor in death resulting from severe asthma, so oxygenation is important. In addition, the studies show that use of oxygen with nebulized beta$_2$-adrenergic receptor agonists improves outcomes compared to the use of air for nebulization.

PEER REVIEW

✓ Use corticosteroids right away to treat asthma in the emergency department: they can improve air flow and decrease both relapse rates and hospital admission rates.

✓ Short-acting beta$_2$-adrenergic receptor agonists are the key to treatment of acute asthma in the emergency department.

✓ Use oxygen with nebulized beta$_2$-adrenergic receptor agonists instead of air for nebulization.

REFERENCES

Marx JA, Hockberger RS, Walls RM, eds. *Rosen's Emergency Medicine: Concepts and Clinical Practice*. 8th ed. St. Louis, MO: Elsevier; 2014: 941-955.

Tintinalli JE, Stapczynski JS, Ma OJ, et al, eds. *Tintinalli's Emergency Medicine: A Comprehensive Study Guide*. 8th ed. New York, NY: McGraw-Hill; 2012: 468-475.

Wolfson AB, Hendey GW, Ling LJ, et al, eds. *Harwood-Nuss' Clinical Practice of Emergency Medicine*. 6th ed. Philadelphia, PA: Lippincott, Williams & Wilkins; 2014: 423-429.

438. The correct answer is D, Right ventricular diastolic collapse.

Why is this the correct answer?

Tamponade develops when intrapericardial fluid produces pressure sufficient to compress the cardiac chambers, which subsequently impairs ventricular diastolic filling and stroke volume. The pericardium is capable of stretching and can accommodate several liters of fluid when the fluid accumulates very slowly. However, if the fluid accumulates more rapidly, such as in the case of trauma, changing the intrapericardial pressure at once, pericardial tamponade can ensue. Compensatory mechanisms such as tachycardia can temporarily sustain blood pressure, but as the pericardial fluid continues to increase, the compensatory mechanisms begin to fail, resulting in diminished cardiac output, hypotension, and full cardiovascular collapse.

Why are the other choices wrong?

Although beat-to-beat swinging of the heart indicates a large effusion causing electrical alternans, this alone does not suggest impending cardiovascular collapse, especially if the fluid has accumulated gradually.

With pericardial tamponade, pericardial effusion is present on echocardiography with a dilated inferior vena cava without inspiratory collapse. Other findings on echocardiography that are diagnostic of pericardial tamponade include early diastolic right ventricular collapse, late diastolic right atrial collapse, and hemodynamic derangements.

Pulsus paradoxus (drop in systolic blood pressure >10 mm Hg during normal inspiration) can be seen in tamponade, although its presence has limited specificity. Several other conditions that are associated with hypotension or dyspnea can also produce pulsus paradoxus, including massive PE, hemorrhagic shock, and obstructive lung disease.

PEER REVIEW

✓ When pressure from intrapericardial fluid compresses the cardiac chambers, tamponade develops, then ventricular diastolic filling and stroke volume are impaired.

✓ Echocardiographic findings diagnostic of pericardial tamponade: early diastolic right ventricular collapse, late diastolic right atrial collapse, and dilated inferior vena cava.

✓ Findings such as pulsus paradoxus have limited specificity for pericardial tamponade.

REFERENCES

Adams JG, Barton ED, Collings J, et al, eds. *Emergency Medicine: Clinical Essentials.* 2nd ed. Philadelphia, PA: Saunders; 2013: 514-523.

Marx JA, Hockberger RS, Walls RM, eds. *Rosen's Emergency Medicine: Concepts and Clinical Practice.* 8th ed. St. Louis, MO: Elsevier; 2014: 1131, 1135-1136.

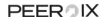

439. The correct answer is A, Administer a third-generation cephalosporin.

Why is this the correct answer?

Spontaneous bacterial peritonitis (SBP) is associated with high mortality rates and should be a consideration in any patient with ascites who presents with fever, chills, malaise, abdominal pain, confusion, hypotension, or general clinical decline. The current treatment of choice is a third-generation cephalosporin (cefotaxime 2 g every 8 hours). Physical examination findings in patients with SBP are often vague. The definitive diagnosis is made by performing diagnostic paracentesis with collection of ascitic fluid for total leukocyte count, PMN count, lymphocyte count, and fluid culture. Positive fluid culture confirms the diagnosis, but antibiotics should be started before results return. The diagnosis is not always clear, as none of these characteristic features is consistently present in all patients, and some patients can even be asymptomatic. The definition of SBP includes a PMN count greater than 250 cells/mm^3; it can be calculated by multiplying the fluid cell count by the percentage of PMNs reported. A total leukocyte count greater than 500 to 1,000 cells/mm^3 strongly correlates with positive fluid cultures. Symptomatic patients with a PMN count less than 250 cells/mm^3 should still be admitted for treatment with antibiotics, with the regimen determined based on culture results.

Why are the other choices wrong?

Combination antibiotic therapy with ampicillin and an aminoglycoside is an alternative to treatment with a cephalosporin. But it has an increased side effect profile with increased risk of nephrotoxicity, so it is not the best course of treatment.

Probiotic therapies have not been shown to increase antibiotic effects or reduce mortality rates, and they have no role in the treatment of SBP. Fluoroquinolone or trimethoprim-sulfamethoxazole prophylaxis for high-risk patients (those who have had SBP before) might prevent future episodes and associated hepatorenal syndrome. However, these are not primary therapies and lead to drug-resistant peritonitis.

Antibiotics should be started based on clinical suspicion and before culture or gram stain results are available. Gram stain is not very sensitive for visualizing bacteria in early SBP, and culture results can be falsely negative; they do not alter management decisions in the inpatient setting.

PEER REVIEW

✓ The presentation of spontaneous bacterial peritonitis is often nondescript, so consider it in any ascitic patient with abdominal pain and fever.

✓ A PMN count greater than 250 cells/mm^3 establishes the diagnosis of spontaneous bacterial peritonitis.

✓ First-line treatment consists of a third-generation cephalosporin.

REFERENCES

Marx JA, Hockberger RS, Walls RM, eds. *Rosen's Emergency Medicine: Concepts and Clinical Practice*. 8th ed. St. Louis, MO: Elsevier; 2014: 1195-1196.

Tintinalli JE, Stapczynski JS, Ma OJ, et al, eds. *Tintinalli's Emergency Medicine: A Comprehensive Study Guide*. 8th ed. New York, NY: McGraw-Hill; 2012: 525-532.

440. The correct answer is C, Paradoxical movement.

Why is this the correct answer?

Flail chest is defined by fractures in three or more adjacent ribs in two or more places, the result of which is that a segment of the chest wall is not connected to the rest of the thoracic cavity. The flail segment moves paradoxically inward during inspiration; this is the classic finding. Flail chest is a cause of death and significant damage because the flail segment is free to indent the lungs and create significant pulmonary contusion at the time of impact. It is, therefore one of the most critical chest wall injuries. Patients who have a flail segment are more likely to have severe pulmonary contusion than those who have rib fractures but no flail segment. Therefore, patients with a flail segment have higher morbidity and mortality rates. Mechanical ventilation is indicated for respiratory failure, hypoxia, or altered mental status of any cause regardless of whether there is a flail segment. The presence of a flail segment should not influence the decision to withhold mechanical ventilation, although it might influence early institution of mechanical ventilation if a patient is not doing well clinically.

Why are the other choices wrong?

Patients with flail chest may demonstrate a wide variation in respiratory insufficiency, but patients typically show tachypnea with decreased tidal volumes and splinting due to pain. Bradypnea, or abnormally slow breathing, is typically not seen in patients with flail chest.

Blunt chest trauma can lead to pneumothorax and hemothorax, resulting in decreased breath sounds, but pulmonary contusion is the most common associated lung pathology in flail chest. Pulmonary contusion does not immediately lead to decreased breath sounds. Due to the limitations of trauma plain films, physical examination is useful in identifying clinically significant flail chest.

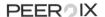

Although flail chest is diagnosed in many patients who exhibit the seatbelt sign, unrestrained passengers in motor vehicle crashes can sustain a flail chest injury and exhibit no seatbelt sign. Flail chest also can occur in a restrained patient who does not present with the seatbelt sign.

PEER REVIEW

✓ Flail chest occurs when three or more adjacent ribs are fractured in two or more places.

✓ Pulmonary contusion is common and often severe with flail chest.

✓ Classic physical finding of flail chest: the flail segment moving paradoxically inward during inspiration.

REFERENCES

Marx JA, Hockberger RS, Walls RM, eds. *Rosen's Emergency Medicine: Concepts and Clinical Practice*. 8th ed. St. Louis, MO: Elsevier; 2014: 433-434.

Wolfson AB, Hendey GW, Ling LJ, et al, eds. *Harwood-Nuss' Clinical Practice of Emergency Medicine*. 6th ed. Philadelphia, PA: Lippincott, Williams & Wilkins; 2014: 205-206.

441. The correct answer is B, Increased use of beta agonists.

Why is this the correct answer?

Numerous factors forecast an increased risk of sudden death due to asthma. One of the most-studied risk factors is increased use of beta agonists via metered-dose inhaler or nebulizer. The increase is likely secondary to delayed formal evaluation of asthma exacerbation in patients using beta agonists. Researchers recently have found that frequent use of short-acting, beta agonists results in tolerance to the medication as well as increased lung reactivity to stimuli. Poor self-perception or physician perception of a patient's asthma and a lack of having or following a formal care plan are also risk factors for asthma-related death. Use of illicit drugs, including heroin and cocaine, has been found to increase the risk for hospitalization, intubation, and fatal asthma. More severe asthma (as indicated by current or recent use of steroids, hospitalization, and intubation within the past year) is also a risk factor for asthma-related death. Finally, recent studies indicate that sensitization to mold is a risk factor for increased asthma severity and death. It is important for emergency physicians to ask patients about these risk factors to educate them and improve treatment plans when needed.

Why are the other choices wrong?

In several studies, smoking was not found to have increased the risk of death in fatal asthma, possibly because the patients were more likely to have the diagnosis of COPD as a cause of death than asthma. One small study in 1996 reported a risk in adult male athletes who were smokers, but this has not been found in more recent studies with larger cohorts.

The use of inhaled corticosteroids has been shown to control patients' asthma symptoms. One study revealed that the use of an average of one or more canisters of inhaled corticosteroids over the prior 3 months decreased the incidence of fatal asthma. Another showed that premature cessation of inhaled corticosteroids increased the risk of fatal asthma.

Patients' reports of the severity of their asthma are highly unreliable. Those who report severe asthma are not more likely to die from asthma, and those who do not accurately perceive the severity of their disease are more likely to die from asthma.

PEER REVIEW

✓ Patients who increase their use of beta-agonists are at higher risk of sudden death from asthma.

✓ Use of inhaled corticosteroids has been shown to control patients' risk of death from asthma.

✓ When patients and physicians fail to realize the severity of asthma, morbidity and mortality rates are higher.

REFERENCES

D'Amato G, Vitale C, Molino A, et al. Asthma-related deaths. *Multidiscip Respir Med.* 2016;11:37.

Marx JA, Hockberger RS, Walls RM, eds. *Rosen's Emergency Medicine: Concepts and Clinical Practice.* 8th ed. St. Louis, MO: Elsevier; 2014: 941-955.

442. The correct answer is D, Wheezing.

Why is this the correct answer?

A foreign body such as a peanut can lodge in any of several anatomic structures in a toddler's pharynx, airway, or esophagus. The presenting symptoms provide a clue to the location of the foreign body and urgency of the need for treatment. A wheezing sound comes from the narrowing of the airways at the level of the bronchus. Most foreign bodies, especially in children, become obstructed at this level because the larynx and trachea are generally larger than the bronchus. A child who is wheezing because of foreign body aspiration but not cyanotic can be watched in the emergency department or admitted for urgent bronchoscopy. Chest xrays generally are not helpful to locate most foreign bodies because most are nonopaque food particles; peanuts are the most frequently identified food culprit. Indirect evidence of a foreign body can be seen on a chest xray with unilateral air trapping or atelectasis on the affected side. Unobserved foreign body aspiration should be considered a possible etiology in any child with unilateral wheezing. If a foreign body is opaque and flat, the location can be determined based on the direction of the item; a flat foreign body appears on edge if in the trachea on an AP image or in the esophagus on a lateral view.

Why are the other choices wrong?

Drooling can occur from a foreign body obstructing the esophagus or the pharynx. Although there might be no airway obstruction, young children drool rather than spit (as adults do) if they cannot swallow their own secretions because of an esophageal obstruction. If a drooling pediatric patient has no respiratory symptoms, including stridor or tachypnea, the foreign body is likely in the esophagus, and a pediatric gastroenterologist should be consulted.

Hoarseness occurs in patients with an obstructing foreign body in the pharynx or larynx generally at the level of the cords or above. An aspirated foreign body can be asymptomatic initially then lead to increasing swelling or granulation tissue resulting in interference with the vocal cords and worsening hoarseness over time. In this situation, an otolaryngologist should be consulted.

Stridor is generally noted with foreign bodies obstructing at the level of the cords or just below in the trachea. This is a much more alarming indication of obstruction, and emergent evaluation, including involvement by a pediatric pulmonologist or otolaryngologist, should be obtained. If the patient is in extremis, the emergency physician can carefully use a laryngoscope to view the larynx and remove a foreign body if it is seen above the cords. If not, intubation can be performed with the attempt to push the tracheal foreign body into one bronchus. Because children generally have larger trachea distally, the foreign body generally does not get stuck again until at the bronchus.

PEER POINT

Chest xray showing a Venezuela 25-cent coin lodged in the upper esophagus of a 9-year-old girl

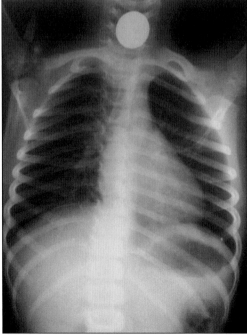

PEER Point 35

PEER REVIEW

✓ Hoarseness and stridor are generally symptoms of a foreign body near the level of the vocal cords or above.

✓ Wheezing is typically heard only with lower respiratory tract or bronchial obstruction from a foreign body.

✓ In a pediatric patient, drooling without airway symptoms can be the clue to an esophageal foreign body.

REFERENCES

Tintinalli JE, Stapczynski JS, Ma OJ, et al, eds. *Tintinalli's Emergency Medicine: A Comprehensive Study Guide.* 8th ed. New York, NY: McGraw-Hill; 2012:427-436.

Wolfson AB, Hendey GW, Ling LJ, et al, eds. *Harwood-Nuss' Clinical Practice of Emergency Medicine.* 6th ed. Philadelphia, PA: Lippincott, Williams & Wilkins; 2014: 1248-1249.

443. The correct answer is A, Disproportionate tachycardia.

Why is this the correct answer?

Myocarditis is an inflammatory condition that causes myocardial damage, usually as a result of infectious, immunologic, or toxin-mediated conditions. It can manifest as mild constitutional symptoms, moderate cardiopulmonary symptoms, or fulminant cardiopulmonary decompensation leading to death. The notable physical examination findings are low-grade fever, tachypnea, and tachycardia. Classically, the tachycardia is out of proportion to the fever. In most adult cases, the myocardial damage is thought to be autoimmune and triggered by a virus (most commonly *Coxsackievirus*) or other infections. In neonates and infants, injury to myocytes is believed to occur more often because of direct injury by the pathogen itself. The clinical manifestations of myocarditis usually begin days to weeks after the acute infection, especially when viruses are implicated as the cause. Only 50% of patients report a recent upper respiratory or GI viral type of infection. The initial symptoms are nonspecific and constitutional: low fever, fatigue, malaise, myalgia, and arthralgia. These mild symptoms are often the reason for initial misdiagnosis or delays in proper diagnosis of this condition. Cardiopulmonary symptoms such as chest pain and dyspnea are also commonly seen. The most common abnormalities on ECG are sinus tachycardia and nonspecific ST-segment or T-wave changes. Chest xrays might reveal signs of congestive heart failure (cardiomegaly, pulmonary vascular redistribution, interstitial edema, frank pulmonary edema). Close attention should be paid to the ABCs of resuscitation because patients with fulminant myocarditis can decompensate rapidly. The mainstay of treatment of myocarditis is primarily supportive with a focus on hemodynamic support and management of complications.

Why are the other choices wrong?

A low-grade fever can be seen in patients who develop myocarditis, but it is not the most suggestive or classic finding of the disease. Fever with night sweats is very characteristic of TB. In fact, only 50% of patients report a recent viral-type upper respiratory or GI infection.

Paroxysmal nocturnal dyspnea is a symptom seen in patients with decompensating heart failure: they wake from sleep to sit upright due to sudden increasing shortness of breath. Although patients with myocarditis can have paroxysmal nocturnal dyspnea with heart failure, it is not the most suggestive symptom of myocarditis.

Pleuritic chest pain is a common symptom of acute pericarditis but is less commonly associated with myocarditis. The progression of myocarditis involves necrosis of the myocardial cells with inflammatory cells leading to fibrosis. This does not lead to the irritation or pleuritic pain associated with pericarditis.

PEER REVIEW

✓ Myocarditis is often misdiagnosed or diagnosed late because the symptoms are nonspecific and constitutional.
✓ Tachycardia out of proportion to fever should raise the suspicion for myocarditis.
✓ *Coxsackievirus* is the most common viral culprit identified in developed countries in myocarditis.

REFERENCES

Adams JG, Barton ED, Collings J, et al, eds. *Emergency Medicine: Clinical Essentials*. 2nd ed. Philadelphia, PA: Saunders; 2013 Chapter 60. Pericarditis, Pericardial Tamponade, and Myocarditis

Marx JA, Hockberger RS, Walls RM, eds. *Rosen's Emergency Medicine: Concepts and Clinical Practice*. 8th ed. St. Louis, MO: Elsevier; 2014:1106-1112.

444. The correct answer is D, Type II diabetes mellitus.

Why is this the correct answer?

Diabetes mellitus (DM) can significantly increase a patient's risk for coronary artery disease, but it is a long-term effect. The young, healthy woman in this case is more likely to have costochondritis; she has typical reproducible pain suggesting a source within the chest wall. Costochondritis is not uncommon in young, healthy patients but should always be a diagnosis of exclusion, taking into account other symptoms and concomitant diseases that can cause chest pain. It is an inflammatory condition of the costochondral junction that can be intermittently sharp followed by dull pain and is reproducible to palpation. Tietze syndrome, as costochondritis is also known, can be worse with inspiration and can be difficult to distinguish from pleurisy, inflammation of the parietal pleura, which is generally not reproducible to palpation. Appropriate management of costochondritis includes pain control with anti-inflammatory medications to treat chest wall pain. Again, with no other associated diseases, other causes for chest pain, such as cardiac disease, pneumothorax, thoracic aortic dissection, and pneumonia, as well as PE, are unlikely given her age and history. Zoster is another consideration if the patient has a rash.

Why are the other choices wrong?

Pregnancy would increase this patient's risk for PE significantly, and symptoms can include the type of sharp pain she reports as ongoing for 3 days. Pain worsening with deep inspiration is a characteristic often noted with PE. It is a leading cause of death in pregnant patients, and classic symptoms are often hard to distinguish from typical findings in pregnancy, including dyspnea.

Rheumatoid arthritis (RA) is another chronic inflammatory autoimmune disease that is associated with increased risk of diseases presenting with chest pain that can cause severe illness or death. These include pericarditis and recurrent venous thrombosis that can lead to PE. The risk of coronary artery disease associated with RA is not as high as that for SLE, but it is still increased, similar to that of type II diabetes. Rheumatoid arthritis can affect any joint, including the costochondral junction, but it is more commonly seen as symmetric disease in the extremity joints and cervical spine.

Patients with systemic lupus erythematosus (SLE) classically have inflammatory symptoms, including of the chest wall, which makes costochondritis a feasible diagnosis for this patient. But what is of more concern is that patients with SLE have a significantly increased risk of coronary artery disease, including young women (20 to 40 years) with findings of fewer traditional cardiac risk factors. Great care should be taken to rule out the possibility of coronary artery disease before diagnosing costochondritis in a patient with SLE.

PEER REVIEW

- ✓ Costochondritis is an inflammatory condition of the costochondral junction that causes sharp pain followed by dull pain.
- ✓ Costochondritis chest pain is typically reproducible on examination.
- ✓ You can treat chest wall pain with anti-inflammatory medications.

REFERENCES

Marx JA, Hockberger RS, Walls RM, eds. *Rosen's Emergency Medicine: Concepts and Clinical Practice.* 8th ed. St. Louis, MO: Elsevier; 2014: 1157-1169, 1527-1542.

Tintinalli JE, Stapczynski JS, Ma OJ, et al, eds. *Tintinalli's Emergency Medicine: A Comprehensive Study Guide.* 8th ed. New York, NY: McGraw-Hill; 2012: 1445-1457, 1911-1921.

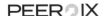

445. The correct answer is D, Toxic megacolon.

Why is this the correct answer?

Toxic megacolon can be the first presentation of inflammatory bowel disease, particularly ulcerative colitis. Plain abdominal radiography shows a long dilated segment of colon, a loss of haustra, and "thumbprinting," which represents submucosal edema and hemorrhage. It might also reveal soft tissue masses in the colonic lumen called "pseudopolyps." Intraabdominal free air indicates perforation. Clinically, symptoms of ulcerative colitis depend on the location affected, but patients generally present with abdominal cramping, diarrhea with blood and mucus, or fecal urgency. Symptoms are intermittent with periods of remission in between. Crohn disease can present similarly but typically has a more insidious and obtuse onset with more extraintestinal manifestations. Its complications include bowel obstruction or abscess formation. Although both entities can lead to toxic megacolon, this progression is thought to be more prominent with ulcerative colitis. Toxic megacolon involves all layers of the colon, resulting in dilation through loss of smooth muscle tone, ileus, and the potential for perforation. Fever, tachycardia, abdominal distention, or hypotension heralds progression of inflammatory bowel disease to toxic megacolon. Treatment consists of reducing colonic decompression with a nasogastric tube and bowel rest, intravenous steroids, intravenous hydration or parenteral nutrition, intravenous antibiotics, and discontinuation of medications that disrupt GI motility. If conservative measures fail, colectomy is warranted.

Why are the other choices wrong?

With colorectal carcinoma, the classic radiographic finding is an apple core lesion. This sign can also be present in Crohn disease and ulcerative colitis. Colorectal carcinoma is not associated with a concerning physical presentation like the one described in this case.

The radiographic finding that signifies volvulus is a dilated coffee bean-shaped colon. Sigmoid volvulus is usually rooted in the left iliac fossa and extends up toward the diaphragm. Cecal volvulus stems from the right iliac fossa and follows an axis extending centrally.

Intussusception is identified, mainly in pediatric patients, by both a target sign and a crescent sign (where the gas from one segment of the intestine is curved into another). Patients generally present with vomiting and crampy abdominal pain. Diarrhea, including bloody stool, is most commonly a late finding.

PEER REVIEW

✓ Inflammatory bowel disease and ulcerative colitis have the same patient demographics, symptoms, and management, but ulcerative colitis has a higher risk for toxic megacolon.

✓ Suspect toxic megacolon when a patient appears unwell and has increasingly frequent abdominal pain or diarrhea, fever, and tachycardia.

✓ An xray won't help in less severe presentations of inflammatory bowel disease, but if you suspect a significant complication like toxic megacolon, get one.

REFERENCES

Marx JA, Hockberger RS, Walls RM, eds. *Rosen's Emergency Medicine: Concepts and Clinical Practice.* 8th ed. St. Louis, MO: Elsevier; 2014: 1269-1272.

Tintinalli JE, Stapczynski JS, Ma OJ, et al, eds. *Tintinalli's Emergency Medicine: A Comprehensive Study Guide.* 8th ed. New York, NY: McGraw-Hill; 2012:492-500.

446. The correct answer is B, Place a large-bore thoracostomy tube.

Why is this the correct answer?

In this patient, clinical suspicion for hemothorax should be high given the penetrating traumatic injury and diminished breath sounds; absent breath sounds and dullness to percussion also fit in the clinical picture. Identification of or strong suspicion for hemothorax in the setting of penetrating trauma should prompt placement of a large-bore thoracostomy tube (at least 32F) in the fifth intercostal space at the anterior axillary line on the affected side. Needle thoracostomy should be performed if there is suspicion for a tension pneumothorax, but tension pneumothorax is less likely in this patient because he does not have hypotension, jugular venous distention, tracheal deviation, or evidence of pneumothorax on chest xray. Bleeding is generally due to injured lung parenchyma, but more significant bleeding can occur with injuries to larger vessels, including intercostal arteries, intermammary arteries, hilar vessels, and the great vessels. Increasingly large hemothoraces can impair venous return and ventilation, resulting in vital sign abnormalities and symptoms and signs of shock. Identification of blood on chest xray is best achieved with upright or lateral decubitus views compared to supine, but these usually cannot be obtained during an acute trauma resuscitation. Hemothorax can be difficult to identify on supine chest radiograph, as the blood layers posteriorly and might not actually obscure the costophrenic angle or cardiac borders, appearing only as a diffuse haziness. This can be true even for large collections greater than 1 L.

Why are the other choices wrong?

Chest CT has the greatest specificity and sensitivity for detecting hemothorax, but transporting this unstable patient to the CT scanner is unwise. His chest xray findings provide enough evidence for significant hemothorax, so chest tube placement should not be delayed.

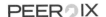

Massive or persistent hemothoraces (>1,500 mL of initial tube output or continued output of >200 mL/hr in the first several hours) should prompt consideration of surgical thoracotomy. Chest tube thoracostomy is still the initial intervention of choice because it can lead to a clinical improvement in the patient's condition.

In a trauma patient with a gunshot wound, transfusion of type-specific packed RBCs is a critical action if there is a likelihood that hemorrhage is causing the concerning vital signs. However, with the classic ABCs of trauma, an emergent airway or breathing problem should be treated first: in this case, placing a chest tube is likely to stabilize the patient's condition. He might still need blood replacement, but if the tachycardia and tachypnea resolve, it might be unnecessary.

PEER POINT

Clinical clues to the diagnosis in chest trauma

- In hemothorax
  - Flat neck veins, slightly decreased breath sounds on affected side
- In both massive (tension) hemothorax and tension pneumothorax
  - Shift of the mediastinum away from the injured hemithorax
  - Breath sounds diminished on the affected side
- In bronchial obstruction, atelectasis, or collapse of the lung
  - Shift of the mediastinum toward the afflicted side

PEER REVIEW

- ✓ Hemothorax can be difficult to identify on a supine chest xray.
- ✓ Standard of care for initial management of hemothorax in penetrating trauma: place a large-bore thoracostomy tube.

REFERENCES

Marx JA, Hockberger RS, Walls RM, eds. *Rosen's Emergency Medicine: Concepts and Clinical Practice*. 8th ed. St. Louis, MO: Elsevier; 2014: 440-442.

Tintinalli JE, Stapczynski JS, Ma OJ, et al, eds. *Tintinalli's Emergency Medicine: A Comprehensive Study Guide*. 8th ed. New York, NY: McGraw-Hill; 2012: 1744-1749.

447. The correct answer is C, Interferon-gamma release assay.

Why is this the correct answer?

The patient in this case has two risk factors that predispose him to TB: he is from Latin America, and he is a farm worker. For efficient and accurate diagnosis of TB, the interferon-gamma release assay (more commonly known by its commercial name, QuantiFERON) is used. This whole blood assay is reportedly 90% to 95% sensitive and has the highest specificity of currently available non–sputum culture testing options available. Results are available within 24 to 48 hours at this time.

Cough is the most common symptom with TB, and it is often the blood-streaked sputum that compels patients to seek care in the emergency department. With active infection, fever occurs during the day, and night sweats occur late in the evening as the fever abates. The chest xray is suggestive of TB with findings that might include hilar or mediastinal lymphadenopathy, but this is most commonly seen in children with TB. Pleural effusions are common, and any lobe can be affected by an infiltrate during active primary infection. A clear chest xray has a high negative predictive value except in HIV-positive patients, in whom it can be falsely negative.

Why are the other choices wrong?

Mycobacterium tuberculosis identification on sputum (or bronchial washing) microscopy with staining for acid-fast bacilli (an AFB smear) can confirm the diagnosis. However, false-negatives on sputum staining occur in more than half of initial studies on patients found to have TB. Sputum culture results are the most accurate method for obtaining the diagnosis but can take weeks to grow. Spontaneous sputum collection, often with early morning sputum, is preferred.

Chest CT with intravenous contrast can help rule out a tumor or an abscess, but it is not the definitive test to diagnose TB. It also has the fastest-available results, but again, is not definitive. Findings on a CT scan include mediastinal lymphadenopathy, cavitary lesions, and miliary nodules. In most algorithms for the diagnostic evaluation of TB, a chest xray suffices for the initial radiographic screening examination.

Mantoux or tuberculin skin testing relies on a patient's hypersensitivity reaction to the *M. tuberculosis* exposure or infection. The result can be falsely positive if a patient has had a BCG (bacille Calmette-Guerin) immunization in the past, and falsely negative if the patient has an immunosuppressive disorder (including HIV), steroid therapy, or chronic illness. The results must be read 72 hours after placing the skin test.

PEER POINT

Who's at risk for TB? Here's what the CDC says

Persons who have been recently infected with TB bacteria, such as:

- Close contacts of a person with infectious TB disease
- Immigrants from areas of the world with high rates of TB
- Children younger than 5 years who have a positive TB test result
- Groups with high rates of TB transmission (homeless persons, injection drug users, persons with HIV infection)
- Those who work or reside in facilities or institutions with people who are at high risk for TB (hospitals, nursing homes, shelters, correctional or residential facilities)

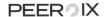

Persons who have weakened immune systems, such as:

- Babies and young children
- People with any of these conditions:
  - Diabetes mellitus
  - HIV infection
  - Low body weight
  - Severe kidney disease
  - Silicosis
  - Substance abuse
  - Head and neck cancer
- People undergoing treatment:
  - With corticosteroids or organ transplant
  - For rheumatoid arthritis or Crohn disease

PEER REVIEW

- ✓ Chest xray findings in primary TB: infiltrate in any lobe and, often, pleural effusion.
- ✓ The confirmatory test to diagnose TB is a sputum collection with culture.
- ✓ The most efficient test to rapidly make a diagnosis is the interferon-gamma release assay (QuantiFERON-Gold Plus).

REFERENCES

Marx JA, Hockberger RS, Walls RM, eds. *Rosen's Emergency Medicine: Concepts and Clinical Practice*. 8th ed. St. Louis, MO: Elsevier; 2014: 1809-1830.

Tintinalli JE, Stapczynski JS, Ma OJ, et al, eds. *Tintinalli's Emergency Medicine: A Comprehensive Study Guide*. 8th ed. New York, NY: McGraw-Hill; 2012: 459-464.

448. The correct answer is B, Perform an ultrasound examination of the testes.

Why is this the correct answer?

When a patient presents with severe scrotal pain following blunt injury, testicular rupture should be suspected. Of such patients who present to the hospital, greater than 40% are found to have testicular rupture. There should be low threshold for imaging, as the degree of internal trauma often does not correlate with what is noted externally. Ultrasonography is the imaging modality of choice. Rupture is characterized sonographically by the identification of the heterogeneous pattern of the testicular parenchyma with the finding of loss of contour definition, indicating disruption of the tunica albuginea. If a rupture, large hematocele, dislocation, or torsion is identified, the patient should undergo urgent surgical intervention within 72 hours, when testicular salvage rates are between 80% and 90%. Surgical intervention after this time has salvage rates of less than 50%. Testicular trauma occurs most commonly while persons are playing sports and usually is the result of a testis being compressed against the symphysis pubis. In addition to exquisite tenderness, signs and symptoms can include nausea, vomiting, urinary retention, and scrotal swelling and ecchymosis. Associated injuries include hematoma or hematocele (identified as a tender, firm scrotal mass that does not transilluminate), testicular dislocation (identified by an empty hemiscrotum), testicular avulsion, testicular torsion, and epididymal injury. These patients can be difficult to examine due to the degree of pain and discomfort.

Why are the other choices wrong?

In some patients with associated abdominal and pelvic injuries, CT is an important imaging study. But the testes are best evaluated by ultrasound, which has a greater than 95% sensitivity for rupture. Ultrasound can show blood flow and velocities for more accurate diagnosis.

Many patients presenting with severe pain after blunt testicular injury can be treated conservatively with analgesics, scrotum support, ice, and urology follow-up. But before making that decision, the clinician should perform an ultrasound examination. Many of these injuries are significant enough to require surgical intervention. If ultrasonography reveals normal-appearing testes and is consistent with simple contusion, the conservative approach is appropriate.

This patient has no obvious external signs of testicular injury requiring immediate urologic consultation and surgical exploration. If the tunica albuginea is not ruptured, conservative, nonsurgical treatment might be appropriate. This patient should first be evaluated using ultrasonography with Doppler studies. Penetrating scrotal trauma, conversely, does require urgent surgical exploration, and initial imaging is not necessary.

PEER REVIEW

✓ Severe scrotal pain following blunt trauma should raise concern for testicular rupture.

✓ Patients with suspected testicular trauma should be evaluated using ultrasonography.

REFERENCES

Marx JA, Hockberger RS, Walls RM, eds. *Rosen's Emergency Medicine: Concepts and Clinical Practice*. 8th ed. St. Louis, MO: Elsevier; 2014: 494-499.

Tintinalli JE, Stapczynski JS, Ma OJ, et al, eds. *Tintinalli's Emergency Medicine: A Comprehensive Study Guide*. 8th ed. New York, NY: McGraw-Hill; 2012: 1771-1772.

449. The correct answer is C, Nitroglycerin.

Why is this the correct answer?

Aortic stenosis (AS) is the third most common form of cardiovascular disease in developed countries after hypertension and coronary artery disease. Significant care should be taken when treating these patients with preload-reducing agents (nitrates) because the sudden decrease in preload can cause severe hypotension, which in turn can lead to decreased coronary flow and worsen ischemia and shock. Diuretics and inotropic agents can also be deleterious and should be used with caution. Management of AS is challenging; judicious use of fluids, maintenance of normal sinus rhythm, and avoidance of nitrates are recommended. The most common causes of AS are calcification of a normal trileaflet aortic valve and a congenital bicuspid aortic valve. Progression of AS is usually quite slow, with symptoms taking decades to manifest in most cases. Auscultation reveals a systolic crescendo-decrescendo murmur associated with diminished and delayed carotid pulses (parvus et tardus), a sustained left ventricular impulse on palpation, and a decreased or absent aortic component of the second heart sound (S_2). An ECG can show left ventricular hypertrophy with a repolarization abnormality, which is seen in 85% of patients with severe AS. Echocardiography is indicated every year for patients with severe AS to assess the severity of the condition, wall thickness, and left ventricle function. Exercise stress testing can lead to complications in patients with symptomatic AS and should not be performed. Once symptoms appear, the average survival time in AS is 2 to 3 years, with a risk for sudden death (<1% per year). Syncope develops in 15% of patients, angina in 35%, and congestive heart failure in 50%.

Why are the other choices wrong?

According to guidelines from the European Society of Cardiology and the European Association for Cardio-Thoracic Surgery, digitalis is recommended for use in patients with AS who are not candidates for surgery. This medication can be used to control the heart rate without the likely complications of hypotension caused by the use of beta blockers and calcium channel blockers.

Lisinopril and other ACE inhibitors can be used to treat hypertension in patients with aortic valve disease, although care should be taken with dosing to avoid hypotension.

No medical treatment has been shown to decrease progression of disease in the aortic valve leaflets, although statins are currently being studied. They have not been shown to worsen symptoms of AS. They are used in patients with AS and atherosclerotic heart disease.

PEER REVIEW

✓ Patients with symptomatic unrepaired aortic stenosis have an expected survival time between 2 and 3 years.

✓ In a patient with aortic stenosis, auscultation reveals a systolic crescendo-decrescendo murmur associated with diminished and delayed carotid pulses (parvus et tardus).

✓ Preload-reducing agents can cause severe hypotension in patients with aortic stenosis, ultimately decreasing coronary blood flow and causing ischemia and shock.

REFERENCES

Adams JG, Barton ED, Collings J, et al, eds. *Emergency Medicine: Clinical Essentials.* 2nd ed. Philadelphia, PA: Saunders; 2013: 524-529.

Marx JA, Hockberger RS, Walls RM, eds. *Rosen's Emergency Medicine: Concepts and Clinical Practice.* 8th ed. St. Louis, MO: Elsevier; 2014: 1106-1112.

Vahanian A, Alfieri O, Andreotti F, et al. Guidelines on the management of valvular heart disease (version 2012): The Joint Task Force on the Management of Valvular Heart Disease of the European Society of Cardiology (ESC) and the European Association for Cardio-Thoracic Surgery (EACTS). *Eur Heart J.* 2012. 33(19):2451-2496.

450. The correct answer is A, Administer oxygen and repeat xray in 4 hours.

Why is this the correct answer?

Traditionally, small pneumothoraces were defined as those occupying less than 20% of one hemithorax. Supplemental oxygen increases the rate of resorption of the pneumothorax by a factor of 4 over 3 to 6 hours, so while patients with small pneumothoraces do not require hospitalization, most physicians choose to observe them until repeat films demonstrate improvement of the pneumothorax. Most pneumothoraces estimated at smaller than 15% are regarded as safe to treat with observation only. In small pneumothoraces, there is less likelihood of persistent air leak and less likelihood of recurrence in those managed with observation alone than in those treated with chest tube insertion. Guidelines for the management of primary spontaneous pneumothorax continue to evolve, and there are many and different systems used to estimate pneumothorax volume, such as the analysis of plain PA chest xrays. Recently, the British Thoracic Society published guidelines regarding the differentiation between large and small pneumothoraces to avoid incorrect estimations of size percentages.

Why are the other choices wrong?

Successful management of a pneumothorax usually requires a therapeutic intervention using thorax drainage. Observation alone is recommended for only those few patients with pneumothorax with minimal clinical symptoms. In the surgical therapy of pneumothorax, VATS (video-assisted thoracic surgery) is the current effective standard treatment. Open posterolateral thoracotomy is the recommend approach in patient with serious illness or complications. The aim is to reduce the recurrence rate of pneumothorax.

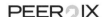

Insertion of a large-bore chest tube is the treatment of choice for hemothorax to encourage drainage; a 28 to 32 Fr chest tube is used in most instances. Smokers have a higher risk of developing pneumothorax.

Studies have shown that needle aspiration has the same outcomes as the placement of a chest tube with less patient discomfort. However, in most patients with a small pneumothorax, no invasive treatment is needed.

REFERENCES

Marx JA, Hockberger RS, Walls RM, eds. *Rosen's Emergency Medicine: Concepts and Clinical Practice*. 8th ed. St. Louis, MO: Elsevier; 2014: 437-440.

Tintinalli JE, Stapczynski JS, Ma OJ, et al, eds. *Tintinalli's Emergency Medicine: A Comprehensive Study Guide*. 8th ed. New York, NY: McGraw-Hill; 2012: 464-468.

451. The correct answer is D, Topical treatment with nifedipine and lidocaine gel.

Why is this the correct answer?

The first line of treatment for anal fissure includes warm sitz baths to reduce anal pressure, laxatives, and a diet with high fiber components to prevent constipation. When first-line therapy is ineffective or chronic anal fissures result, as with the patient in this case, topical agents for analgesia and sphincter pressure reduction are effective. Lidocaine gel applied periodically provides temporary relief of anal pain, and the calcium channel blocker nifedipine in a gel preparation relaxes smooth muscle and decreases anal pressure. Nitroglycerin ointment is also an option but might produce a headache side effect. Anal fissure is characterized by sudden, painful rectal bleeding, and patients typically are constipated and straining to pass hard bowel movements. A superficial tear in the dermis layers of the anus occurs where the anal muscle is weakest, in the posterior midline. Fissures developing in other locations should prompt suspicion for immunocompromised disease states (Crohn disease, HIV, TB). A fissure can become chronic, denoted by a sentinel pile with a skin tag appearance as reactionary hypertrophic skin accumulates at its base. Edematous anal papillae might also be seen or palpated. Spasm of the internal and external anal sphincters often prevents physical examination, exacerbated by severe pain on rectal examination or attempts to perform anoscopy.

Why are the other choices wrong?

Anal dilation to decrease anal pressure or fissurectomy and sphincterectomy might be required for chronic fissure treatment when other therapies are ineffective. It is not an emergent procedure.

Incision and drainage is the correct course of treatment for perianal or ischiorectal abscesses, which can lead to anal fistulae that disrupt sphincter function. Oral antibiotics might be considered if a patient is febrile and the abscess is predominantly superficial.

Intraoperative drainage is recommended for deep ischiorectal, intersphincteric, and supralevator abscesses with or without fistula formation. They can be associated with tender masses that are erythematous, fluctuant, and draining, but generally these abscesses can be difficult to diagnose due to absence of external signs. They are often associated with fever and an elevated WBC count. Surgical management is needed to remove the fistula network and debride the abscess.

PEER REVIEW

✓ Anal fissures are the most common cause of painful rectal bleeding and can be exquisitely painful.

✓ First-line treatment for anal fissure: sitz baths, debulking agents for constipation, and oral analgesics.

✓ Second-line treatment for anal fissure includes topical lidocaine gel and calcium channel blockade.

REFERENCES

Marx JA, Hockberger RS, Walls RM, eds. *Rosen's Emergency Medicine: Concepts and Clinical Practice*. 8th ed. St. Louis, MO: Elsevier; 2014: 1280-1282.

Tintinalli JE, Stapczynski JS, Ma OJ, et al, eds. *Tintinalli's Emergency Medicine: A Comprehensive Study Guide*. 8th ed. New York, NY: McGraw-Hill; 2012: 320-323.

452. The correct answer is B, Dry cough.

Why is this the correct answer?

Atypical pneumonias are generally characterized as those caused by *Legionella pneumophila*, *Chlamydophila pneumoniae*, and *Mycoplasma pneumoniae*, in addition to viruses. The symptoms include fever, dyspnea, and cough. Patients who have an atypical pneumonia tend to describe the cough as "dry"; this nonproductive cough is unlike the cough associated with other bacterial illnesses, which produces sputum. The symptom of dry cough should be considered when selecting an empiric antibiotic, especially if the patient is to be treated as an outpatient. Because *Mycoplasma pneumoniae* is one of the most common etiologies of pneumonia in healthy persons, antibiotic coverage for it should be considered: generally, a macrolide is recommended.

Why are the other choices wrong?

Chest pain, often described as pleuritic pain, is present in up to 50% of patients with pneumonia. This might be caused by inflammation of the parietal pleura by the infiltrate. In addition, 25% of patients with *Streptococcus pneumoniae* infection have a pleural effusion, which can also be symptomatic.

Dyspnea is a more common complaint in patients with pneumonia caused by classic bacterial pathogens, including *Streptococcus pneumoniae* and *Staphylococcus aureus*. It also is common in elderly and immunocompromised patients at high risk for pneumonia caused by *Pseudomonas aeruginosa* and *Haemophilus influenzae*.

Fever, in addition to cough and fatigue, is the one of most common symptoms in patients with all types of pneumonia (75%). It does not help make the distinction between atypical pneumonia and other etiologies. Rigors, the shaking and cold feeling associated with spiking a fever, is a typical symptom found in patients with the most common pneumonia, *Streptococcus pneumoniae*. It can also be common in patients with *Klebsiella pneumoniae*.

PEER REVIEW

✓ Patients who have pneumonia from atypical pathogens complain of a dry, nonproductive cough.

✓ Fever, fatigue, and cough are the most common symptoms of pneumonia.

✓ Here are the atypical pathogens that commonly cause pneumonia: *Legionella pneumophila*, *Chlamydophila pneumoniae*, and *Mycoplasma pneumoniae*.

REFERENCES

Tintinalli JE, Stapczynski JS, Ma OJ, et al, eds. *Tintinalli's Emergency Medicine: A Comprehensive Study Guide*. 8th ed. New York, NY: McGraw-Hill; 2012: 445-456.

Wolfson AB, Hendey GW, Ling LJ, et al, eds. *Harwood-Nuss' Clinical Practice of Emergency Medicine*. 6th ed. Philadelphia, PA: Lippincott, Williams & Wilkins; 2014: 411-418.

453. The correct answer is B, Consult orthopedics emergently for open reduction and repair.

Why is this the correct answer?

This particular injury is called a Galeazzi fracture, a fracture-dislocation of the distal third of the radius associated with dislocation-subluxation of the distal radial ulnar joint, or DRUJ. With Galeazzi fractures, there is a high risk of malunion, loss of function, infection, and chronic pain in adult patients. For this reason, surgical management with internal fixation and possible open reduction is required. The repair should occur promptly, so the emergency physician or another clinician should contact the orthopedic consultant emergently to coordinate care. In children, some Galeazzi fractures are treated conservatively with closed reduction by an orthopedic surgeon. Disruption of the DRUJ can be subtle, so a high suspicion should be maintained when a patient presents with a fracture of the distal third of the radius.

Why are the other choices wrong?

Placing a splint and having the patient follow up later without reducing the patient's fracture increases the likelihood of additional soft tissue injury and malunion. The risk of complication from the fracture drastically increases if closed reduction is not completed. This patient requires orthopedic consultation with open reduction.

Closed reduction can be attempted, but anatomic alignment is rarely held in adults, so open reduction is strongly recommended. Acute operative intervention has been found to provide better outcomes than delayed reconstruction.

Splinting without reduction is not recommended. Orthopedic consultation should take place in the emergency department. Delayed follow-up with orthopedics without reduction of the fracture-dislocation in the emergency department puts the patient at significant risk for a poor outcome from soft tissue injury, conversion to an open fracture, and ultimately possible malunion, loss of function, infection, and chronic pain.

PEER REVIEW

- ✓ Look for fracture-dislocation of the distal radius and ulna after a fall onto an outstretched arm. This injury can't be missed: it requires immediate orthopedic involvement.
- ✓ Skin tenting associated with the Galeazzi fracture-dislocation puts the patient at risk for skin necrosis and conversion to an open fracture.

REFERENCES

Marx JA, Hockberger RS, Walls RM, eds. Rosen's Emergency Medicine: Concepts and Clinical Practice. 8th ed. St. Louis, MO: Elsevier; 2014: 1801-1815, 1826-1828.

Wheeless' Textbook of Orthopedics. Galeazzi's Fracture (Adults). http://www.wheelessonline.com/ortho/galeazzis_fracture_adults_1. Accessed May 21, 2017.

454. The correct answer is C, Nodularity.

Why is this the correct answer?

Fibrocystic changes are the most common cause of breast lesions in women. These noncancerous lesions are described as nodular, mobile, and smooth. As the name describes, the breast tissue develops numerous cystic structures from dilatation of the ducts that are mixed with excessive fibrous tissue. A breast that has undergone these changes can become tender with menstrual cycle changes. Several radiologic imaging techniques have been used to make sure that changes noted on physical examination are not indicative of cancer, including ultrasonography, mammography, and MRI. These changes occur in at least one third of women of child-bearing age. In contrast, cancerous lesions are generally more firm and irregular in shape. Enlarged lymph nodes associated with breast cancer initially are described as rubbery; they become matted and fixed when found in association with breast cancer.

Why are the other choices wrong?

A fluctuant breast mass likely represents an abscess; it can be identified using ultrasonography or mammography. Although the label fibrocystic might imply fluctuance of a mass due to its cystic nature, the small size of the cysts and more prominent dense stromal tissue create the classic bumpy, nonfluctuant feel on palpation of the characteristic fibrocystic changes.

Nipple retraction is a sign found in cancer and not found in fibrocystic changes. The retraction is a result of fibrosis that can pull the nipple toward the breast and chest wall. Bloody, unilateral nipple discharge is another concerning sign that can indicate the presence of a breast carcinoma.

Breast cancer also can cause skin changes, including discoloration, thickening, and dimpling. Classic characteristics of the skin changes in inflammatory breast cancer are skin thickening and an erythema called peau d'orange (orange peel). Some abscesses can cause erythema, but fibrocystic disease does not cause this particular change in the appearance of the skin.

PEER REVIEW

- ✓ Signs of fibrocystic change in a breast include nodularity with a possible tender mass.
- ✓ Concerning signs of possible breast cancer: nipple retraction, discoloration or erythema, and skin thickening.
- ✓ Mammography, ultrasonography, and MRI are all used for diagnosis of breast masses.

REFERENCES

Tintinalli JE, Stapczynski JS, Ma OJ, et al, eds. *Tintinalli's Emergency Medicine: A Comprehensive Study Guide*. 8th ed. New York, NY: McGraw-Hill; 2012: 672-676.

Wolfson AB, Hendey GW, Ling LJ, et al, eds. *Harwood-Nuss' Clinical Practice of Emergency Medicine*. 6th ed. Philadelphia, PA: Lippincott, Williams & Wilkins; 2014: 666-669.

455. The correct answer is B, Low-tidal volume mechanical ventilation.

Why is this the correct answer?

Acute respiratory distress syndrome (ARDS) has been generally defined for decades as Pa_{O_2}/F_{IO_2} less than 300, bilateral pulmonary infiltrates on chest xray, and elevated pulmonary artery pressure greater than18 mm Hg. Although ARDS has been studied extensively, one of the only therapeutic modalities that has been found to reduce mortality rates is careful support of mechanical ventilation, notably, low tidal volume mechanical ventilation (initial tidal volume 6 mL/kg). Over distention of the alveola caused by high tidal volume creates high shear force and injury, worsening the symptoms of ARDS. This is measured as plateau pressures, with the goal of keeping pressures less than 30 mm H_2O. Other strategies for ventilating patients with ARDS include appropriate use of positive end-expiratory pressure, high-frequency oscillatory ventilation, and prone positioning ventilation; these interventions have been shown in studies to decrease mortality rates.

Why are the other choices wrong?

Sepsis is the most common etiology of ARDS. Almost 50% of cases are caused by pulmonary infiltrates, and the mortality rate in these patients is almost 40%. Broad-spectrum antibiotics are the treatment for pneumonia, but they are not the treatment for other conditions that cause the impaired oxygenation and pulmonary infiltrates seen on chest xrays that define ARDS. Other conditions that increase patients' risk for developing ARDS are high-risk surgeries, trauma, pancreatitis, multiple transfusions, and drug overdose.

Historically, packed RBC transfusion was an integral part of early goal-directed therapy for sepsis. More recent recommendations have not included this component of the original protocol. There is no specific support for transfusion for patients with ARDS.

Several studies conducted on prophylactic methylprednisolone to prevent ARDS have demonstrated worse outcomes for the group as a whole, including an increase in infection rates. However, many studies have indicated that early use of steroids in patients with ARDS does improve outcome.

PEER REVIEW

✓ Acute respiratory distress syndrome defined: PaO_2/FIO_2 less than 300, bilateral pulmonary infiltrates on chest xray, and elevated pulmonary artery pressure greater than 18 mm Hg.
✓ Low tidal volume (6 mL/kg initially) mechanical ventilation decreases the risk of ventilator injury to the lungs in patients with ARDS.
✓ Pneumonia is the most common condition in patients who develop ARDS; it also has one of the highest mortality rates.

REFERENCES

Marx JA, Hockberger RS, Walls RM, eds. *Rosen's Emergency Medicine: Concepts and Clinical Practice.* 8th ed. St. Louis, MO: Elsevier; 2014: 1864-1873.

Modrykamien AM, Gupta P. The acute respiratory distress syndrome. *Proc (Bayl Univ Med Cent).* 2015;28(2):163-171.

456. The correct answer is C, Gradual onset dyspnea.

Why is this the correct answer?

Pneumoconiosis is a restrictive lung disease generally resulting from inhaling toxic substances, including coal dust (coal miner's lung, coal workers' pneumoconiosis, black lung disease) and silica. It results in pulmonary fibrosis, which limits total lung volume and decreases oxygen perfusion across the alveoli. Obstructive lung diseases, in distinction, cause symptoms due to increased airway resistance. Patients often have symptoms of dyspnea, but wheezing is heard less often due to the nature of restrictive lung disease. Chest xray reveals numerous nodules larger than 1 cm, generally in the upper part of the lung lobes. Interstitial lung findings (a fine reticular pattern) can appear similar to interstitial pulmonary edema on initial imaging. Treatment is generally based around steroids to prevent further inflammatory response.

Why are the other choices wrong?

Wheezing is not a classic symptom for patients with chronic pneumoconiosis. It can be seen in patients with pneumoconiosis, especially smokers, who generally have worsening disease with a combination of symptoms from COPD and fibrosis.

Chest pain can be caused by numerous pulmonary diseases, but pneumoconiosis is generally not associated with pain. Acute shortness of breath with chest pain in patients with pneumoconiosis might be associated with spontaneous pneumothorax or associated pneumonia.

Productive cough and sputum production can be seen in patients with pneumoconiosis who are smokers and have concomitant chronic bronchitis. Coughing does not distinguish one disease process from another.

PEER REVIEW

✓ Pneumoconiosis is a restrictive lung disease.

✓ Dyspnea worsening over time is the most common symptom of pneumoconiosis.

REFERENCES

Block J, Jordanov MI, Stack LB, et al. *The Atlas of Emergency Radiology*. New York, NY: McGraw-Hill: 2013: 165.

Kasper DL, Fauci AS, Hauser SL, et al, eds. *Harrison's Principles of Internal Medicine*. 19th ed. New York, NY: McGraw-Hill; 2015: Chapter 311. Available at: https://www.cdc.gov/niosh/topics/pneumoconioses/. Accessed May 20, 2017.

Smith DA. Pulmonary Emergencies. In: Stone CK, Humphries RL, eds. *CURRENT Diagnosis & Treatment Emergency Medicine*. 7th ed. New York, NY: McGraw-Hill; 2011.

457. The answer is B, Eyelid eversion.

Why is this the correct answer?

Ocular foreign body is the most likely diagnosis in this case given the patient's history and examination findings. And since the initial examination of the cornea did not reveal imbedded foreign debris, the best next step is to examine the eyelids. The lower lid is inspected by pulling it down with the thumb while the patient looks up. The upper lid is everted by placing the end of a cotton-tipped applicator stick on the crease or base of the upper lid with one hand and pressing gently, then grasping the lashes with the other hand, pulling them down, out, then up and over the cotton tip. Foreign bodies can be so small that they cannot be visualized without magnification, so the use of a loupe or a slit lamp might be necessary. Any debris found can be removed using another cotton-tipped applicator or irrigation. Imbedded corneal foreign bodies may be removed very carefully using a sterile needle; rust rings from imbedded metal can be removed using an ophthalmic burr. Referral to an ophthalmologist is an option if corneal foreign bodies are noted. Fluorescein dye should be used to locate corneal abrasions caused by the debris.

Why are the other choices wrong?

Dilating the patient's pupil to examine the eye is the right course of action to evaluate for possible damage to the retina or the optic nerve; it is indicated when examination of the fundus is necessary but not otherwise possible. Dilation is also indicated to evaluate for traumatic iritis secondary to corneal injury. But in this case, there is no evidence of intraocular injury that warrants dilation before a simple eyelid eversion.

Trauma to the eye in cases like the one presented can result in serious injury, such as perforation of the globe. This is the primary indication for performing the Seidel test as part of a fluorescein examination: the test is positive for globe injury if the diluted fluorescein is seen flowing from a globe rupture site. This patient might eventually undergo a fluorescein examination and evaluation for the Seidel sign, but not as the next step in his care.

Slit lamp examination is valuable in the evaluation of many ophthalmologic conditions, including traumatic corneal injuries caused by foreign bodies. It is crucial in the diagnosis of anterior chamber injury or posterior chamber disease, and it is part of a normal ophthalmologic examination. But in this case, as with the Seidel test, even though it might be needed eventually to complete a thorough examination of the patient's eye, it is not the next step in this evaluation.

PEER REVIEW

✓ When you suspect foreign body secondary to a traumatic eye injury, evert the upper eyelid to look for hidden debris.
✓ To evert the upper eyelid, place the applicator stick at the base of the lid, then pull the lashes down and out and flip the lid over the applicator tip.

REFERENCES
Reichman EF. *Emergency Medicine Procedures*. 2nd ed. New York, NY: McGraw-Hill; 2013: 1016-1019.
Roberts JR, Hedges JR, eds. *Clinical Procedures in Emergency Medicine*. 6th ed. St. Louis, MO: WB Saunders; 2014: 1261-1277.

458. The answer is C, Temporal.

Why is this the correct answer?

The annual incidence of skull fractures is 2 per 1,000 infants and 0.5 to 1 per 1,000 children and adolescents. Most fractures in infants are linear skull fractures; these are more concerning when they traverse underlying vascular regions, including the middle meningeal groove. Temporal bone fractures are not the most common among skull fractures, but they have been associated with a higher risk of intracranial bleeding due to their proximity to underlying cerebral vasculature (middle meningeal artery). Infants are at higher risk of fracture than are older pediatric patients because of the immaturity of the bony skull; this risk decreases after the first year of life. Falls from only 4 to 5 feet can cause significant injury: 50% of infants found to have a skull fracture fell from less than this height. The classic basilar skull fracture is a linear fracture generally through the temporal bone with signs of hemotympanum or Battle sign (ecchymosis behind the ear) or raccoon eyes (ecchymosis around the eyes). A linear skull fracture is the most common manifestation, and plain radiographs of the skull might miss 25% or more of these injuries. Intracranial injury is possible in infants with a skull fracture, so CT is recommended for patients in whom imaging is indicated. There are several validated guidelines that help determine which infants and children should have CT imaging, including the PECARN, CATCH, and CHALICE decision rules. Clinical findings often include overlying swelling, but palpable bony abnormalities are rare in the linear or minimally depressed skull fracture. The patient also should be evaluated for clinical findings of head injury, including level of consciousness, vomiting, and seizures. Few infants require any specific treatment with just a simple skull fracture. The causes of skull fractures in infants include fall, motor vehicle crash or other blunt trauma event, and nonaccidental injury. Abuse must be a consideration: skull fractures are the second most common injury seen in these cases. In children and adolescents, skull fractures are most likely the result of motor vehicle trauma or sports-related injury.

Why are the other choices wrong?

The least likely bone to be injured in skull fracture is the frontal bone. The thickness of the frontal skull protects it from injury, so it indicates great force if fractured and a high likelihood of associated traumatic brain injury, which might or might not be associated with intracranial bleeding. Given the child's proportionately heavier head and uncoordinated gait, forehead injuries are more common in infants and young children.

In infants, the parietal bone is the most likely to be fractured (up to 70% of all skull fractures), but the injury is less likely to cause intracranial bleeding. A large parietal scalp hematoma can indicate a skull fracture or traumatic brain injury, or both.

Facial fractures overall and zygomatic fractures in particular are not common in children. The zygoma structures are part of the midface, positioned between the mandible and cranium. Most of the force of a traumatic impact to this area is absorbed by the mandible and cranium. Likely findings in zygomatic fractures are enophthalmos, exophthalmos, diplopia, and difficulty opening the mouth, along with bony stepoffs at the orbital rim and a loss of malar projection.

PEER REVIEW

- ✓ Of all skull fractures, a fracture of the temporal bone is the most likely to be associated with intracranial bleeding in infants and young children.
- ✓ Most frequently fractured bone of the skull in infants and children: parietal.
- ✓ Use validated clinical decision rules to determine whether an infant or young child with a scalp or head injury should undergo CT.

REFERENCES

Marx JA, Hockberger RS, Walls RM. *Rosen's Emergency Medicine: Concepts and Clinical Practice.* 8th ed. St. Louis, MO: Elsevier; 2014: 339-367.

Shah BR, Lucchesi M, Amodio J, et al, eds. *Atlas of Pediatric Emergency Medicine.* 2nd ed. New York, NY: McGraw-Hill; 2013: Fractures of the Zygomatic Complex and Zygomatic Arch.

Tintinalli JE, Stapczynski JS, Ma OJ, et al, eds. *Tintinalli's Emergency Medicine: A Comprehensive Study Guide.* 8th ed. New York, NY: McGraw-Hill; 2012: 1724-1733.

459. The answer is B, Mannitol.

Why is this the correct answer?

The treatment and amelioration of increased intracranial pressure (ICP) is one of the most important steps in the management of the multiple trauma patient. Mannitol is very effective, with a slightly delayed effect on the oncotic forces at work within the cranial cavity. Indicated in patients with impending herniation or evidence of increased ICP from trauma, mannitol is given as a bolus to lower ICP via osmotic diuresis and increase plasma expansion. A continuous mannitol drip can increase the chance of hypovolemia and is thus not recommended.

Why are the other choices wrong?

Hyperventilation after intubation has been used as a rapid intervention to lower ICP. It can be used for impending herniation or as a lifesaving therapeutic measure. But more recent studies indicate that patients with traumatic brain injury have a worse prognosis if hyperventilation is used in any prolonged manner, and that it should be avoided especially in the first 24 hours.

Neuromuscular paralysis is part of the process of rapid sequence intubation, but it does not in itself contribute to reduction of ICP. Successful intubation to manually control the patient's respiratory rate and ventilation volume is made more successful with the use of neuromuscular blockers. Complete paralysis allows mechanical hyperventilation while the patient is on the ventilator.

The value of steroids in the care of patients with increased ICP from other processes, including cancer, is debatable. Several large studies have shown that steroids are not effective in treating patients with traumatic brain injury.

PEER REVIEW

- ✓ Mannitol is recommended to control increased ICP in patients with acute traumatic brain injury.
- ✓ The use of hyperventilation worsens the prognosis of patients with acute traumatic brain injury.

REFERENCES

Marx JA, Hockberger RS, Walls RM. *Rosen's Emergency Medicine: Concepts and Clinical Practice*. 8th ed. St. Louis, MO: Elsevier; 2014: 347-351.

Wolfson AB, Hendey GW, Ling LJ, et al, eds. *Harwood-Nuss' Clinical Practice of Emergency Medicine*. 6th ed. Philadelphia, PA: Lippincott, Williams & Wilkins; 2014: 156-157.

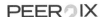

460. The answer is D, Traumatic iritis.

Why is this the correct answer?

In the case described, the patient has sustained blunt trauma to the globe resulting in contusion and spasm of the ciliary body and iris, a condition called traumatic iritis or iridocyclitis. These findings are classic for this disorder. Traumatic iritis is characterized by a deep, aching eye pain, decreased visual acuity, injection of the limbus of the affected eye, both direct and consensual photophobia, and cells and flare in the anterior chamber. The patient can have a low intraocular pressure, generally only seen with uveitis (including iritis and iridocyclitis), which is thought to be the result of decreased production of aqueous fluid and increased outflow associated with the inflammatory state. The presence of a sluggish pupil on the affected side is attributed to the ciliary spasm. In severe traumatic iritis, a hypopyon (layering of white blood cells in the anterior chamber) can be visualized. Treatment for traumatic iritis consists of topical cycloplegic agents and oral pain medications.

Why are the other choices wrong?

Endophthalmitis is a severe infection of the deep structures of the eye that usually follows cataract or other eye surgery or penetrating trauma. The patient presents with fever, diffuse redness, and white blood cells in the anterior chamber. The cornea is described as hazy in patients with endophthalmitis, another finding that distinguishes it from acute iritis.

Hyphema is a pooling or layering of red blood cells in the anterior chamber of the eye resulting most commonly from trauma, such as tears or lacerations of the deep structures. These findings are best visualized with the patient sitting up; treatment recommendations include keeping the patient upright at least 45 degrees to allow the cells to sink with gravity in the anterior chamber to avoid obstructing the outflow track, which would cause increased intraocular pressure. There is no such finding in traumatic iritis.

Scleritis is an inflammatory disorder of the sclera associated with photophobia and severe boring pain. It presents with reddish or bluish discoloration from the inflamed scleral vessels within the edematous white outer coating of the eye. Scleritis is treated with NSAIDs and possibly steroids.

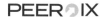

PEER REVIEW

✓ Characteristics of iritis: eye pain, decreased visual acuity, injection of the limbus, cells and flare in the anterior chamber, and direct and consensual photophobia.

✓ A hypopyon, layering of white blood cells in the anterior chamber, can be visualized in patients with severe iritis or endophthalmitis.

✓ Low intraocular pressure can be seen in patients with uveitis, including iritis or iridocyclitis.

REFERENCES

Marx JA, Hockberger RS, Walls RM. *Rosen's Emergency Medicine: Concepts and Clinical Practice*. 8th ed. St. Louis, MO: Elsevier; 2014: 184-197.

Tintinalli JE, Stapczynski JS, Ma OJ, et al, eds. *Tintinalli's Emergency Medicine: A Comprehensive Study Guide*. 8th ed. New York, NY: McGraw-Hill; 2012: 1543-1579.

Bibliography

ACEP Excited Delirium Task Force. White paper report on excited delirium syndrome. ACEP Web site. http://www.fmhac.net/assets/documents/2012/presentations/krelsteinexciteddelirium.pdf. Accessed May 31, 2017.

EMS regionalization of care. ACEP Web site. https://www.acep.org/Clinical---Practice-Management/EMS-Regionalization-of-Care/. Accessed May 31, 2017.

Adams JG, Barton ED, Collings J, et al, eds. *Emergency Medicine: Clinical Essentials.* 2nd ed. Philadelphia, PA: Saunders; 2013.

Adour KK. Otological complications of herpes zoster. *Ann Neurol.* 1994;35 Suppl:S62.

American Medical Association. *Current Procedural Terminology, 2016 Professional Edition.* Chicago, IL: AMA; 2017: 608, 771, 772.

Bombings: Injury Patterns and Care. ACEP Web site. https://www.acep.org/blastinjury/. Accessed August 30, 2016.

American College of Emergency Physicians. Guidelines Regarding the Role of Physician Assistants and Advanced Practice Registered Nurses in the Emergency Department. ACEP website. Available at: https://www.acep.org/Clinical---Practice-Management/Guidelines-Regarding-the-Role-of-Physician-Assistants-and-Advanced-Practice-Registered-Nurses-in-the-Emergency-Department/. Accessed October 11, 2016.

American College of Surgeons. *ATLS: Advanced Trauma Life Support, Student Course Manual.* 9th ed. Chicago, IL: American College of Surgeons; 2012: 132.

American Psychiatric Association. *Diagnostic and Statistical Manual of Mental Disorders.* 5th ed. Washington, DC: American Psychiatric Association; 2013.

Asha SE, Miers JW. A systematic review and meta-analysis of D-dimer as a rule-out test for suspected acute aortic dissection. *Ann Emerg Med.* 2015;66(4):368-378.

Barkun AN, Bardou M, Kuipers EJ, et al. International consensus recommendations on the management of patients with nonvariceal upper gastrointestinal bleeding. *Ann Intern Med.* 2010;152(2):101-13. doi: 10.7326/0003-4819-152-2-201001190-00009.

Birks EJ, Tansley PD, Hardy J, et al. Left ventricular assist device and drug therapy for the reversal of heart failure. *N Engl J Med.* 2006;355:1873-1884.

Bitterman RA. *EMTALA: Providing Emergency Care Under Federal Law.* Irving, TX: American College of Emergency Physicians; 2001: 103-117.

Block J, Jordanov MI, Stack LB, et al. *The Atlas of Emergency Radiology.* New York, NY: McGraw-Hill: 2013: 165.

Botma M, Bader R, Kubba H. 'A parent's kiss': evaluating an unusual method for removing nasal foreign bodies in children. *J Laryngol Otol.* 2000;114(08):598-600.

Brady WJ, Truwit JD. *Critical Decisions in Emergency and Acute Care Electrocardiography.* Hoboken, NJ: Blackwell Publishing, Ltd.; 2009: 43-44.

Brady WJ, Ferguson J, Perron A. Myocarditis. *Emerg Med Clin NA.* 2004;22:865-885.2.

Breen E, Bleday R, Weiser M, et al, eds. Perianal abscess: Clinical manifestations, diagnosis, treatment. UpToDate online. http://www.uptodate.com/contents/perianal-and-perirectal-abscess. Accessed May 31, 2017.

Broder J. *Diagnostic Imaging for the Emergency Physician.* Philadelphia, PA: Saunders; 2011.

Bronstein AC, Spyker DA, Cantilena LR Jr, et al. 2011 Annual Report of the American Association of Poison Control Centers' National Poison Data System (NPDS): 29th Annual Report. *Clin Toxicol (Phila).* 2012;50(10):911-1164.

Brookes L, Fenton J. Patient Satisfaction and Quality of Care: Are They Linked? Medscape multispecialty. June 11, 2014. http://www.medscape.com/viewarticle/826280. Accessed April 8, 2015.

Brown DJ, Brugger H, Boyd J, Paal P. Accidental hypothermia. *N Engl J Med.* 2012;367(20):1930-1938.

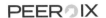

Brown KD, Banuchi V, Selesnick SH, et al. Diseases of the External Ear. In: Lalwani AK, eds. *CURRENT Diagnosis & Treatment in Otolaryngology—Head & Neck Surgery*. 3rd ed. New York, NY: McGraw-Hill; 2012. http://accessmedicine.mhmedical.com/content.aspx?bookid=386&sectionid=39944089. Accessed May 18, 2017.

Brunicardi FC, Andersen DK, Billiar TR, et al. *Schwartz's Principles of Surgery*. 10th ed. New York, NY: McGraw-Hill; 2015.

Butt F, Yuan-Shin F. Benign Diseases of the Salivary Glands. In: Lalwani AK, eds. *CURRENT Diagnosis & Treatment in Otolaryngology—Head & Neck Surgery*. 3rd ed. New York, NY: McGraw-Hill; 2012. Accessed May 18, 2017.

Buttaravoli P, Leffler SM. *Minor Emergencies*. 3rd ed. Philadelphia, PA: Elsevier; 2012:183-184.

Callaway CW, Donnino MW, Fink EL, et al. Part 8: post–cardiac arrest care: 2015 American Heart Association Guidelines Update for Cardiopulmonary Resuscitation and Emergency Cardiovascular Care. *Circulation*. 2015;132(18 Suppl 2):S465–S482.

Centers for Disease Control and Prevention. About shingles (herpes zoster). CDC website. http://www.cdc.gov/shingles/about/index.html. Accessed August 16, 2016.

Centers for Disease Control and Prevention. About SUID and SIDS. CDC website. http://www.cdc.gov/sids/aboutsuidandsids.htm. Accessed August 14, 2016.

Centers for Disease Control and Prevention. Adenoviruses. CDC website. https://www.cdc.gov/adenovirus/index.html. Accessed September 15, 2016.

Centers for Disease Control and Prevention. Hantavirus. CDC website. http://www.cdc.gov/hantavirus/. Accessed December 2, 2016.

Centers for Disease Control and Prevention. HEADS UP to Health Care Providers. http://www.cdc.gov/headsup/providers. Accessed January 12, 2017.

Centers for Disease Control and Prevention. Parasites - Giardia. CDC website. http://www.cdc.gov/parasites/giardia/index.html. Accessed December 2, 2016.

Centers for Disease Control and Prevention. Pneumococcal disease. CDC website.

https://www.cdc.gov/pneumococcal/clinicians/clinical-features.html. Accessed May 23, 2017.

Centers for Disease Control and Prevention. Rabies vaccine. CDC website.

https://www.cdc.gov/rabies/medical_care/vaccine.html. Accessed May 23, 2017.

Centers for Disease Control and Prevention. Rocky Mountain spotted fever (RMSF). CDC website. http://www.cdc.gov/rmsf/index.html. Accessed August 17, 2016.

Chasm RM, Swencki SA. Pediatric orthopedic emergencies. *Emerg Med Clin North Am*. 2010;28(4):907-26.

Cleland K, Zhu H, Goldstuck N, et al. The efficacy of intrauterine devices for emergency contraception: a systematic review of 35 years of experience. *Hum Reprod*. 2012;27(7):1994-2000.

Crawford MH. *CURRENT Diagnosis & Treatment: Cardiology*. 3rd ed. Philadelphia, PA: Elsevier; 2010:847-859.

Cunningham F, Leveno KJ, Bloom SL, et al, eds. *Williams Obstetrics*. 24th ed. New York, NY: McGraw-Hill; 2013. http://accessmedicine.mhmedical.com.foyer.swmed.edu/content.aspx?bookid=1057&sectionid=5978918. Accessed May 17, 2017.

D'Amato G, Vitale C, Molino A, et al. Asthma-related deaths. *Multidiscip Respir Med*. 2016;11:37.

de Caen AR, Berg MD, Chameides L, et al. Part 12: pediatric advanced life support: 2015 American Heart Association Guidelines Update for Cardiopulmonary Resuscitation and Emergency Cardiovascular Care. *Circulation*. 2015;132(suppl 2):S526–S542. http://circ.ahajournals.org/content/132/18_suppl_2/S543. Accessed October 12, 2016.

Diagnostic and Statistical Manual of Mental Disorders: DSM-5. 5th ed. Washington, D.C.: American Psychiatric Association; 2013. http://dx.doi.org.foyer.swmed.edu/10.1176/appi.books.9780890425596.dsm17. Accessed May 26, 2017.

Doran MF, Crowson CS, Pond GR, et al. Predictors of infection in rheumatoid arthritis. *Arthritis Rheum.* 2002;46(9):2294-2300.

Edlow JA, Caplan LR. Avoiding pitfalls in the diagnosis of subarachnoid hemorrhage. *N Engl J Med.* 2000;342:29.

Edlow JA, Panagos PD, Godwin SA, et al. Clinical policy: Critical issues in the evaluation and management of adult patients presenting to the emergency department with acute headache. *Ann Emerg Med.* 2008;52(4):407-436.

Eifling M, Razavi M, Massumi A. The evaluation and management of electrical storm. *Tex Heart Inst J.* 2011;38(2):111-121.

Einav S, Kaufman N, Sela HY. Maternal cardiac arrest and perimortem caesarean delivery: evidence or expert-based? *Resuscitation.* 83:10 (2012): 1191-1200.

Fleisher GR, Ludwig S, et al, eds. *Textbook of Pediatric Emergency Medicine.* 6th ed. Philadelphia, PA: Lippincott, Williams & Wilkins; 2010.

Forthofer RN, Lee ES, Hernandez M. *Biostatistics: a guide to design, analysis, and discovery.* 2nd ed. Philadelphia, PA: Academic Press; 2007.

Friedman NR, Scholes MA, Yoon PJ. *CURRENT Diagnosis & Treatment: Pediatrics.* 22nd ed. Available in part for free and in full with a subscription. http://accessmedicine.mhmedical.com/content. aspx?bookid=1016&sectionid=61597764&jumpsectionID=61597883&Resultclick=2. Accessed May 31, 2017.

Fullam F, Garman AN, Johnson TJ, Hedberg EC. The use of patient satisfaction surveys and alternative coding procedures to predict malpractice risk. *Med Care.* 2009; 47(5):553-559.

Gilbert DN, Chambers HF, Eliopoulous GM, et al, eds. *The Sanford Guide to Antimicrobial Therapy* 2015. 2015: 72-76.

Goh W, Bohrer J, Zalud I. Management of the adnexal mass in pregnancy. *Curr Opin Obstet Gynecol.* 2014;26(2):49-53.

Gower LEJ, O'Keefe Gatewood M, Kang CE. Emergency department management of delirium in the elderly. *West J Emerg Med.* 2012;13(2): 194-201.

Greenberg RD, Daniel KJ. Eye emergencies. In: Stone C, Humphries RL, eds. *CURRENT Diagnosis & Treatment Emergency Medicine.* 7th ed. New York, NY: McGraw-Hill; 2011.

Grover CA, Close RJH, Wiele ED, Villarreal K, Goldman LM. Quantifying drug-seeking behavior: a case control study. *J Emerg Med.* 2012;42(1):15-21.

Hall JB, Schmidt GA, Wood LDH. *Principles of Critical Care.* 3rd ed. New York, NY: McGraw-Hill; 2005: 801-814.

Hamilton C, Stany M, Gregory W, et al. Gynecology. In: Brunicardi F, Andersen DK, Billiar TR, et al, eds. *Schwartz's Principles of Surgery.* 10th ed. New York, NY: McGraw-Hill; 2015. http://accessmedicine.mhmedical. com/content.aspx?bookid=980&sectionid=59610883. Accessed May 18, 2017.

Han JH, Zimmerman EE, Cutler N, et al. Delirium in older emergency department patients: recognition, risk factors, and psychomotor subtypes. *Acad Emerg Med.* 2009;16(3):193-200.

Hay WW Jr., Levin MJ. *Current Diagnosis & Treatment: Pediatrics.* 23rd ed. New York, NY: McGraw-Hill; 2016. http://accessmedicine.mhmedical.com/content.aspx?bookid=1795&sectionid=125740558. Accessed May 18, 2017.

Hobgood C, Harward D, Newton K, et al. The educational intervention "GRIEV_ING" improves the death notification skills of residents. *Acad Emerg Med.* 2005;12(4):296-301. http://onlinelibrary.wiley.com/ doi/10.1197/j.aem.2004.12.008/epdf. Accessed October 20, 2016.

Hockberger RS, Rothstein RJ. Assessment of suicide potential by nonpsychiatrists using the SAD PERSONS scale. *J Emerg Med.* 1988;6:99-107.

Hollands H, Johnson D, Brox AC, et al. Acute-onset floaters and flashes: is this patient at risk for retinal detachment? *JAMA.* 2009;302(20):2243-2249.

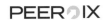

Hoffman B, Schorge J, Schaffer J, et al. *Williams Gynecology*. 2nd ed. New York, NY: McGraw-Hill; 2012; Chapter 9: Pelvic Mass. http://accessmedicine.mhmedical.com/content.aspx?bookid=399&sectionid=41722297&jumpsectionID=41724832&Resultclick=2. Accessed online on March 6, 2015.

Hoffman JR, Mower WR, Wolfson AB, et al. Validity of a set of clinical criteria to rule out injury to the cervical spine in patients with blunt trauma. *N Engl J Med*. 2000;343:94-99.

Hoffman RS, Howland MA, Lewin NA, et al. *Goldfrank's Toxicologic Emergencies*. 10th ed. New York, NY: McGraw-Hill; 2015.

Horsager R, Roberts S, Rogers V, et al. *Williams Obstetrics*. 24th ed. Study Guide. New York, NY: McGraw-Hill; 2015. http://accessmedicine.mhmedical.com.foyer.swmed.edu/content.aspx?bookid=1057&sectionid=5978918. Accessed May 17, 2017.

Infective Endocarditis in Adults: Diagnosis, Antimicrobial Therapy, and Management of Complications (AHA) (Endorsed by IDSA). *Circulation*. 2015;132:1-53.

January CT, Wann LS, Alpert JS, et al. 2014 AHA/ACC/HRS guideline for the management of patients with atrial fibrillation: a report of the American College of Cardiology/American Heart Association Task Force on Practice Guidelines and the Heart Rhythm Society. *J Am Coll Cardiol*. 2014;64(21):2305-2307.

Kasper DL, Fauci AS, Hauser SL, et al, eds. *Harrison's Principles of Internal Medicine*. 19th ed. New York, NY: McGraw-Hill; 2015: 2163-2165.

Kato H, Hirose M, Yamaguchi M, et al. Hemodynamic effects of isoproterenol and propranolol in tetralogy of fallot: production and treatment of anoxic spells. *Japanese Circulation Journal*. 1968;31(12):1857-1863. https://www.jstage.jst.go.jp/a. Accessed May 31, 2017.

Kishiyama JL. Disorders of the immune system. In: Hammer GD, McPhee SJ, eds. *Pathophysiology of Disease: An Introduction to Clinical Medicine*. 7th ed. New York, NY: McGraw-Hill; 2013. http://accessmedicine.mhmedical.com/content.aspx?bookid=961&sectionid+=53555684. Accessed May 18, 2017.

Kline JA, Mitchell AM, Kabrhel C, Richman PB, Courtney DM. Clinical criteria to prevent unnecessary diagnostic testing in emergency department patients with suspected pulmonary embolism. *J Thromb Haemost*. 2004;2(8):1247-1255.

Knoop KJ, Stack LB, Storrow AB, et al. *The Atlas of Emergency Medicine*. 4th ed. New York, NY: McGraw-Hill; 2016.

Kochanek KD, Murphy SL, Xu J, et al. National Vital Statistics Reports. Deaths: Final Data for 2014. Division of Vital Statistics. June 30, 2016. U.S. DEPARTMENT OF HEALTH AND HUMAN SERVICES, Centers for Disease Control and Prevention,

National Center for Health Statistics, National Vital Statistics System. https://www.cdc.gov/nchs/data/nvsr/nvsr65/nvsr65_04.pdf. Accessed January 24, 2017.

Kovala CE, Rakitab R; AST Infectious Diseases Community of Practice. Ventricular assist device related infections and solid organ transplantation. *Am J Transplant*. 2013;13: 348–354.

Kuo CY, Parikh SR. Bacterial tracheitis. *Pediatr Rev*. 2014;35(11):497-499.

Lalwani AK. *Current Diagnosis & Treatment: Otolaryngology - Head and Neck Surgery*. 3rd ed. New York, NY: McGraw-Hill; 2012.

Laudenbach JM, Simon Z. Common dental and periodontal diseases: evaluation and management. *Med Clin N Am*. 2014;98:1239-1260.

Lavonas EJ, Drennan IR, Gabrielli A, et al. Part 10: Special circumstances of resuscitation: 2015 American Heart Association Guidelines Update for Cardiopulmonary Resuscitation and Emergency Cardiovascular Care. *Circulation*. 2015;132(Suppl 2):S501-S518.

Legome E, Shockley LW. *Trauma: A Comprehensive Emergency Medicine Approach*. New York, NY: Cambridge University Press; 2011:129-143.

Leung LLK, eds. Direct oral anticoagulants: Dosing and adverse effects. UptoDate. http://www.uptodate.com/contents/direct-oral-anticoagulants-dosing-and-adverse-effects. Accessed January 18, 2017.

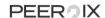

Lieberthal AS, Carroll AE, Chonmaitree T, et al. The diagnosis and management of acute otitis media. *Pediatrics*. 2013;131(3):e964-e999.

Lilly LS. Treatment of acute and recurrent idiopathic pericarditis. *Circulation*. 2013;127:1723-1726.

Link MS, Berkow LC, Kudenchuk PJ, et al. Part 7: Adult Advanced Cardiovascular Life Support: 2015 American Heart Association Guidelines Update for Cardiopulmonary Resuscitation and Emergency Cardiovascular Care. *Circulation*. 2015;132(18 Suppl 2):S444-S464.

LLSA Article: Drowning, Current Concepts. *N Engl J Med*. 2012;366:22. nejm.2102. http://www.nejm.org/doi/full/10.1056/NEJMra1013317. Accessed January 24, 2017.

Macfadyen CA1, Acuin JM, Gamble C. Systemic antibiotics versus topical treatments for chronically discharging ears with underlying eardrum perforations. *Cochrane Database Syst Rev*. 2006;(1):CD005608.

Mahmood AR, Narang AT. Diagnosis and management of the acute red eye. *Emerg Med Clin North Am*. 2008;26:35-55.

Manning L, Robinson TG, Anderson CS. Control of blood pressure in hypertensive neurological emergencies. *Curr Hypertens Rep*. 2014;16:436.

Marinis A, Yiallourou A, Samanides L, et al. Intussusception of the bowel in adults: a review. *World J Gastroenterol*. 2009;15(4):407-411.

Marx JA, Hockberger RS, Walls RM. *Rosen's Emergency Medicine: Concepts and Clinical Practice*. 8th ed. St. Louis, MO: Elsevier; 2014.

Mattu A, Brady WJ, et al (eds). *Cardiovascular Emergencies*. Dallas, TX: American College of Emergency Physicians Publishing; 2014.

Mattu A, Tabas JA, Barish RA. *Electrocardiography in Emergency Medicine*. Dallas, TX: American College of Emergency Physicians; 2007: 223-225, 232.

McCormack RF, Hutson A. Can computed tomography angiography of the brain replace lumbar puncture in the evaluation of acute-onset headache after a negative noncontrast cranial computed tomography scan? *Acad Emerg Med*. 2010;17(4):444-451.

McGuire LC, Cruickshank AM, Munro PT. Alcoholic ketoacidosis. *Emerg Med J*. 2006;23(6):417-420.

Modrykamien AM, Gupta P. The acute respiratory distress syndrome. *Proc (Bayl Univ Med Cent)*. 2015;28(2):163-171.

National Institute on Drug Abuse. Are there effective treatments for tobacco addiction? NIDA website. https://www.drugabuse.gov/publications/research-reports/tobacco/are-there-effective-treatments-tobacco-addiction. Accessed October 9, 2016.

NAEMSP EMS Text, Prehospital Triage for Mass Casualties, Volume 4, Chapter 2.

Nash DL. Hyphema. Medscape Web site. http://emedicine.medscape.com/article/1190165-overview. Accessed August 23, 2016.

Neurocognitive Disorders Diagnostic and Statistical Manual of Mental Disorders. 5th ed. American Psychiatric Association; 2013. http://dx.doi.org.foyer.swmed.edu/10.1176/appi.books.9780890425596.dsm17. Accessed May 19, 2017.

Newman EJ, Grosset DG, Kennedy PG. The parkinsonism-hyperpyrexia syndrome. *Neurocrit Care*. 2009;10(1):136-140. doi:10.1007/s12028-008-9125-4. Epub 2008 Aug 20.

Nolan TW. System changes to improve patient safety. *BMJ*. 2000;320(7237):771-773.

O'Connor RE, Al Ali AS, Brady WJ, et al. Part 9: Acute Coronary Syndromes - 2015 American Heart Association Guidelines Update for Cardiopulmonary Resuscitation and Emergency Cardiovascular Care. *Circulation*. 2015;132(18 Suppl 2):S483-500.

Olson KR. *Poisoning & Drug Overdose*. 6th ed. New York, NY: McGraw-Hill; 2012. http://accessmedicine.mhmedical.com.foyer.swmed.edu/content.aspx?bookid=391&sectionid=42069956. Accessed May 17, 2017.

Paden MS, Franjic L, Halcomb SE. Hyperthermia caused by drug interactions and adverse reactions. *Emerg Med Clin North Am*. 2013;31(4):1035-1044.

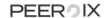

Page RL, Joglar JA, Caldwell MA, et al. 2015 ACC/AHA/HRS guideline for the management of adult patients with supraventricular tachycardia: a report of the American College of Cardiology/American Heart Association Task Force on Clinical Practice Guidelines and the Heart Rhythm Society. *Circulation.* 2016;133;e506-e574.

Pai S, Parikh SR. Otitis Media. In: Lalwani AK, eds. *CURRENT Diagnosis & Treatment in Otolaryngology—Head & Neck Surgery.* 3rd ed. New York, NY: McGraw-Hill; 2012. http//accessmedicine.mhmedical.com/content.aspx?bookid=386&sectionid=39944091. Accessed May 18, 2017.

Pavan-Langston D. Herpes zoster ophthalmicus. *Neurology.* 1995;45(12 Suppl 8):S50.

Petersen AS, Barloese MC, Jensen RH. Oxygen treatment of cluster headache: a review. *Cephalalgia.* 2014;34(13):1079-1087.

Pollack CV Jr., Reilly PA, Eikelboom J, et al. Idarucizumab for dabigatran reversal. *N Engl J Med.* 2015;373(6):511-520. doi:10.1056/NEJMoa1502000.

Prado-Calleros HM, Jiménez-Fuentes E, Jiménez-Escobar I. Descending necrotizing mediastinitis: systematic review on its treatment in the last 6 years, 75 years after its description. *Head Neck.* 2016;38(Suppl 1):E2275-2283.

Ralston S, Hill V, Waters A. Occult serious bacterial infection in infants younger than 60 to 90 days with bronchiolitis: a systematic review. *Arch Pediatr Adolesc Med.* 2011;165(10):951-956. doi:10.1001/archpediatrics.2011.155.

Ralston SL, Lieberthal AS, Meissner HC, et al. Clinical Practice Guideline: The Diagnosis, Management, and Prevention of Bronchiolitis. *Pediatrics.* 2014;134:e1474–e1502.

Reichman EF. *Emergency Medicine Procedures.* 2nd ed. New York, NY: McGraw-Hill; 2013: 439-443.

Revel MP, Sanchez O, Couchon S, et al. Diagnostic accuracy of magnetic resonance imaging for an acute pulmonary embolism: results of the 'IRM-EP' study. *J Thromb Haemost.* 2012;10(5):743-750.

Richmond JS, Berlin JS, Fishkind AB, et al. Verbal de-escalation of the agitated patient: consensus statement of the American Association for Emergency Psychiatry Project BETA De-escalation Workgroup. *West J Emerg Med.* 2012;13(1):17-25.

Riordan-Eva P, Cunningham E. *Vaughan & Asbury's General Ophthalmology.* 18th ed. New York, NY: McGraw-Hill; 2011. http://accessmedicine.mhmedical.com/content.aspx?bookid=387&sectionid=40229328. Accessed May 16, 2017.

Roberts JR, Hedges JR, eds. *Clinical Procedures in Emergency Medicine.* 6th ed. St. Louis, MO: WB Saunders; 2014.

Roberts-Thomson KC, Lau DH, Sanders P. The diagnosis and management of ventricular arrhythmias. *Nat Rev Cardiol.* 2011;8(6):311-321.

Rose EA, Gelijns AC, Moskowitz AJ et al: Long-term use of a left ventricular assist device for end-stage heart failure. *N Engl J Med.* 2001; 345:1435-1443.

Rowe BH, Spooner CH, Ducharme FM, et al. Corticosteroids for preventing relapse following acute exacerbations of asthma. *Cochrane Database Syst Rev.* 2007; (3): CD000195.

Schafermeyer RW, Tenenbein M, Macias CG, et al, eds. *Strange and Schafermeyer's Pediatric Emergency Medicine.* 4th ed. New York, NY: McGraw-Hill; 2015.

Shah BR, Lucchesi M, Amodio J, et al, eds. *Atlas of Pediatric Emergency Medicine.* 2nd ed. New York, NY: McGraw-Hill; 2013: Fractures of the Zygomatic Complex and Zygomatic Arch.

Shazly A, Afifi A. RE-ALIGN: First trial of novel oral anticoagulant in patients with mechanical heart valves—The search continues. *Glob Cardiol Sci Pract.* 2014;2014(1):88-89. doi:10.5339/gcsp.2014.13.

Shen TT1, DeFranco EA, Stamilio DM, et al. A population-based study of race-specific risk for placental abruption. BMC Pregnancy Childbirth. 2008;8:43. doi: 10.1186/1471-2393-8-43. http://bmcpregnancychildbirth.biomedcentral.com/articles/10.1186/1471-2393-8-43.

Sherman S. *Simon's Emergency Orthopedics.* 7th ed. New York, NY: McGraw-Hill; 2015.

Shulman ST, Bisno AL, Clegg HW, et al. Clinical practice guideline for the diagnosis and management of group A streptococcal pharyngitis: 2012 update by the Infectious Diseases Society of America. *Clin Infect Dis*. 2012;55(10):e86-e102.

Sidberry GK, Iannone R, eds. *The Harriet Lane Handbook: A Manual for Pediatric House Officers*. 15th ed. St. Louis, MO: Mosby; 2000: 257-258.

Siegal T, Seligsohn U, Aghai E, Modan M. Clinical and laboratory aspects of disseminated intravascular coagulation (DIC): a study of 118 cases. *Thromb Haemost*. 1978;39(1):122-134.

Silvers SM, White RD, Yannopoulos D, Donnino MW. Part 7: adult advanced cardiovascular life support: 2015 American Heart Association Guidelines Update for Cardiopulmonary Resuscitation and Emergency Cardiovascular Care. *Circulation*. 2015; 132(suppl 2):S444–S464.

Simony A, Filion KB, Mottillo S, et al. Meta-analysis of usefulness of D-dimer to diagnose acute aortic dissection. *Am J Cardiol*. 2011;107(8):1227-1234.

Singer M, Deutschman CS, Seymour C, et al. The Third International Consensus Definitions for Sepsis and Septic Shock (Sepsis-3). *JAMA*. 2016;315(8):801-810. doi:10.1001/jama.2016.0287.

Smith DA. Pulmonary Emergencies. In: Stone CK, Humphries RL, eds. *CURRENT Diagnosis & Treatment Emergency Medicine*. 7th ed. New York, NY: McGraw-Hill; 2011.

Stelfox HT, Gandhi TK, Orav EJ, Gustafson ML. The relation of patient satisfaction with complaints against physicians and malpractice lawsuits. *Am J Med*. 2005;118(10):1126-1133.

Stephan M, Carter C, Ashfaq S, et al. Pediatric Emergencies. In: Stone C, Humphries RL, eds. *CURRENT Diagnosis & Treatment Emergency Medicine*. 7th ed. New York, NY: McGraw-Hill; 2011. http://accessmedicine.mhmedical.com/content. aspx?bookid=385&sectionid=40357266. Accessed May 18, 2017.

Sterns RH. Disorders of plasma sodium—causes, consequences, and correction. *N Engl J Med*. 2015;372(1):55-64.

Stone CK, Humphries RL, eds. *CURRENT Diagnosis & Treatment Emergency Medicine*. 7th ed. New York, NY: McGraw-Hill; 2011.

Strauss RW, Mayer TA, eds. *Emergency Department Management*. New York, NY: McGraw-Hill; 2014.

Sullivan JH. Orbit. In: Riordan-Eva P, Cunningham ET, Jr, eds. *Vaughan & Asbury's General Ophthalmology*. 18th ed. New York, NY: McGraw-Hill; 2011. http://accessmedicine.mhmedical.com/content. aspx?bookid=387&sectionid=40229330. Accessed May 16, 2017.

Surtees R, Wolf N. Treatable neonatal epilepsy. *Arch Dis Child*. 2007;92(8):659-661. doi:10.1136/adc.2007.116913.

Szpilman D, Bierens JJ, Handley AJ, et al. Drowning. *N Engl J Med*. 2012;366(22):2102-2110.

Tintinalli JE, Stapczynski JS, Ma OJ, et al, eds. *Tintinalli's Emergency Medicine: A Comprehensive Study Guide*. 8th ed. New York, NY: McGraw-Hill; 2012.

Tintinalli J, Benegal V. Psychosis among substance users. *Curr Opin Psychiatry*. 2006;19(3):239-245. http://www.medscape.com/viewarticle/528487_5. Accessed October 8, 2016.

Todd SR, Dahlgren FS, Traeger MS, et al. No visible dental staining in children treated with doxycycline for suspected Rocky Mountain Spotted Fever. *J Pediatr*. 2015;166(5):1246-1251.

Tou S, Brown SR, Malik AI, Nelson RL. Surgery for complete rectal prolapse in adults. *Cochrane Database Syst Rev*. 2008; CD001758.

Trobe JD. *The Physician's Guide to Eye Care*. 4th ed. San Francisco, CA: American Academy of Ophthalmology; 2012.

UptoDate. http://www.uptodate.com/contents/approach-to-acute-upper-gastrointestinal-bleeding-in-adults#H9942856, paragraph on Somatostatin and its Analogues. Accessed May 31, 2017.

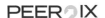

Vahanian A, Alfieri O, Andreotti F, et al. Guidelines on the management of valvular heart disease (version 2012): The Joint Task Force on the Management of Valvular Heart Disease of the European Society of Cardiology (ESC) and the European Association for Cardio-Thoracic Surgery (EACTS). *Eur Heart J.* 2012. 33(19):2451-2496.

Valeri MR, Sullivan JH, Correa ZM, et al. *Vaughn & Asbury's General Ophthalmology.* 18th ed. New York, NY: McGraw-Hill; 2011. http://accessmedicine.mhmedical.com/content.aspx?bookid=387&sectionid=40229321. Accessed May 16, 2017.

Van Ness-Otunnu R, Hack JB. Hyperglycemic crisis. *J Emerg Med.* 2013;45(5):797-805.

Varma MG, Steele SC, Weiser M, et al, eds. Overview of rectal procidentia (rectal prolapse). UpToDate. http://www.uptodate.com/contents/overview-of-rectal-procidentia-rectal-prolapse?source=search_result&search=Overview+of+rectal+procidentia+%28rectal+prolapse%29&selectedTitle=1%7E150. Accessed May 31, 2017.

Wheeless' Textbook of Orthopedics. Galeazzi's Fracture (Adults). http://www.wheelessonline.com/ortho/galeazzis_fracture_adults_1. Accessed May 21, 2017.

Winters ME, Bond MC, DeBlieux P, et al (eds). *Emergency Department Resuscitation of the Critically Ill.* Dallas, TX: American College of Emergency Physician Publishing; 2011.

Wipperman JL, Dorsch JN. Evaluation and management of corneal abrasion. *Am Fam Physician.* 2013;87(2):114-120.

Wolf SJ, Lo B, Shih, Rd, et al. Clinical policy: critical issues in the evaluation and management of adult patients in the emergency department with asymptomatic elevated blood pressure. *Ann Emerg Med.* 2013;62:59-68.

Wolfson AB, Hendey GW, Ling LJ, et al. eds. *Harwood-Nuss' Clinical Practice of Emergency Medicine.* 6th ed. Philadelphia, PA: Lippincott, Williams & Wilkins; 2014.

Zun L, Chepenik LG, Mallory MNS. *Behavioral Emergencies for the Emergency Physician.* Cambridge, NY: Cambridge; 2013.

Index

B

back pain, spinal epidural abscess and, 210–211. *see also* low back pain

bacteremia, contraindication to arthrocentesis, 377

bacteria, encapsulated organisms, 349. *see also specific* bacteria

bacterial meningitis, causative organisms, 151–152

bacterial tracheitis, 164-165, 182-183, 475

bad news, communication of, 245–246

bag-valve-mask (BVM) positive pressure technique, 69

balanoposthitis, 139, 187

"bamboo spine," 117

barium enemas, 356, 501

bark scorpion, 16–18, 17f

barotitis, 497

barotrauma, pulmonary, 411–412

basilar artery aneurysms, 292

bath salts, sympathomimetic toxidrome and, 24–25

bats, rabies and, 299–300

BCG (bacille Calmette-Geurin) immunization, 523

bee stings, 437–438

bees, Africanized *versus* honeybees, 437–438

Bell palsy, 66–67, 309. *see also* idiopathic facial paralysis

benign intracranial hypertension. *see* idiopathic intracranial hypertension (IIH)

benign paroxysmal positional vertigo (BPPV), 3–4

benign prostate hypertrophy, hematuria and, 149

benign prostatic hyperplasia (BP), 398

bent inner tube sign, 350

benzodiazepines
    for cocaine intoxication, 291
    in cocaine toxic patients, 237
    in LSD intoxication, 252
    overdose, 128, 182
    pharmacologic restraint using, 247
    for postpartum seizures, 339
    for seizures, 79–80

benztropine, 128, 154–155, 514–515

beta blockers
    in aortic dissection, 199, 502
    contraindication, 186
    in hypertrophic cardiomyopathy, 222
    in STEMI, 88
    in tetralogy of Fallot spells, 508
    in thyroid storm, 15
    topical, 131
    toxicity, 439–440

beta$_2$-adrenergic receptor agonists, 510

beverages, effervescent, 153

bicarbonate, 252, 276, 508

bile duct obstruction, extrahepatic, 414–415

bilevel positive-pressure ventilation (BiPAP), 54–55, 453

billing, 51, 238–239

bipolar disorders, 12, 20–21, 155

black widow spider envenomation, 17

bladder
    identification of injuries to, 71–72
    incomplete emptying, 149
    intraperitoneal rupture, 373f
    rupture presentation, 93–94

bladder cancer, 148–149

blast injuries, 411-412, 460–461

bleach, ingestion of, 383

blood glucose, fingerstick, 187

blood types, 63–64

bloody stools in infants, 224

blunt trauma
    chest, 513
    diaphragmatic rupture with herniation, 105–106
    patient transport after, 485
    testicular rupture and, 524–525

body language, de-escalation and, 247–248

body volume loss, calculation of, 315–316

Boerhaave syndrome, 303–304, 419

borborygmi, audible, 317

Bordetella pertussis, 334–335, 427–428

Borrelia burgdorferi, Lyme disease and, 416

botulinum toxin, 380

botulism, infant, 27–28

botulism immune globulin, 27–28

Bouchard nodes, osteoarthritis and, 116–118

Boutonnière deformity, 117, 117f

bovine spongiform encephalopathy, 37

bowel dilation, 350

bowel obstruction, 356–357, 500

bowel wall erosion, 508

bowel wall thickening, 350

brachial cleft cysts, 270–271

brachial plexus injury, fetal, 32–33

bradypnea, definition of, 513

bradyarrhythmias, 82

bradycardias, 282–283, 431

bradykinin, metabolism of, 102–103

brain masses, ataxia and, 478

brainstem, infarction of, 127

breast, 531–532

breast cancer, 532

breast milk jaundice, 255

breath-holding spells, 463

bronchial obstruction, 522

bronchiolitis
    characteristics of, 432–433
    presentation, 183, 331–332, 447–448

bronchospasm, 337, 452–453

brown recluse spider envenomation, 17, 344

Brugada syndrome, 192, 263–264

B-type natriuretic peptide (BNP), levels of, 474

bulimia nervosa, electrolyte abnormalities in, 283–284

bulla, description of, 434

bullous pemphigoid, 11–12

"bulls-eye" lesion, 500

bupivacaine, 439–440, 469–470

bupropion, contraindications, 283, 384

Burkholderia cepacia pneumonia, 338

burn patients, Parkland formula for, 81

burns
    circumferential, 375–376
    escharotomy in, 375–376
    first-degree, 81–82
    inhalation injury, 453
    oropharynx, 178–179
    partial thickness, 81